Practical Paediatric Problems in Primary Care

Edited by

Michael Bannon

Postgraduate Dean and Honorary
Consultant Paediatrician,
Oxford.

Yvonne Carter

Dean and Professor of General Practice and Primary Care,
Warwick Medical School,
University of Warwick.

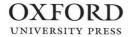
OXFORD
UNIVERSITY PRESS

OXFORD

UNIVERSITY PRESS

Great Clarendon Street, Oxford OX2 6DP

Oxford University Press is a department of the University of Oxford.
It furthers the University's objective of excellence in research, scholarship,
and education by publishing worldwide in

Oxford New York

Auckland Cape Town Dar es Salaam Hong Kong Karachi
Kuala Lumpur Madrid Melbourne Mexico City Nairobi
New Delhi Shanghai Taipei Toronto

With offices in

Argentina Austria Brazil Chile Czech Republic France Greece
Guatemala Hungary Italy Japan Poland Portugal Singapore
South Korea Switzerland Thailand Turkey Ukraine Vietnam

Oxford is a registered trade mark of Oxford University Press
in the UK and in certain other countries

Published in the United States
by Oxford University Press Inc., New York

A catalogue record for this title is available from the British Library

Library of Congress Cataloging in Publication Data
(Data available)

Library of Congress Cataloging-in-Publication Data

Practical paediatric problems in primary care / [edited by] Michael J. Bannon and
Yvonne Carter.
    p. ; cm.
  Includes bibliographic references and index.

  ISBN-13: 978–0–19–852922–4 (alk. paper)

1. Pediatrics--Handbooks, Manuals, etc. 2. Primary care (Medicine)--Handbooks,
manuals, etc. I. Bannon, Michael J., Dr. II. Carter, Yvonne, 1959-
  [DNLM: 1. Pediatrics. 2. Primary Health Care. WS 200 P8947 2007]
  RJ48.P73 2007
  618.92--dc22

                                                                2006100012

Typeset in Minion
by Cepha Imaging Pvt. Ltd., Bangalore, India
Printed in Great Britain
on acid-free paper by
Ashford Colour Press Ltd., Gosport, Hampshire

ISBN 978–0–19–852922–4 (pbk: alk. paper)

10 9 8 7 6 5 4 3 2 1

Foreword

As a practising GP, I know just how important the care of children is in primary care. In the recent past I have to deal with a newborn baby with feeding problems, a child with suspected non-accidental injury, a child with special needs, chest pain in an adolescent, and a new diagnosis of childhood cancer. In addition our practice is planning the implementation of changes to the national immunization programme. These authentic examples show that the care of children impinges on many aspects of primary care on a daily basis and involves the majority of practice team members. It is therefore essential that services for children and clinical care is of a high standard. I know that practices need support in delivering this quality care, and for parents, early diagnosis of a sick child is essential.

So I welcome this book, from two respected doctors—a husband and wife team—with special expertise and interest in paediatrics. Mike Bannon is a Consultant Community Paediatrician and Postgraduate Dean while Yvonne Carter is a senior academic GP and Dean of a new Medical School. They met at Alder Hey Children's Hospital nearly 20 years ago! Their passion and commitment to improving the care of children is therefore clear with a long track record of publishing in the area. The book is one of the most effective texts that I have read on paediatrics in primary care. It is a thoughtful book, well researched, up to date and follows a comprehensive and practical approach for multidisciplinary teams, including vital chapters on safeguarding children.

The Royal College of General Practitioners (RCGP) is the largest medical royal college in the UK. The RCGP has led the way in driving up standards in general practice over the last 50 years by setting standards and promoting the education and training of GPs. Healthcare professionals are now clearly expected to demonstrate accountability for the standard of their work to patients, their peers, the health service and regulators. Integral to this is a sound system of continuing professional development that this book will support. As a GP appraiser, I know that aspects of child health such as safeguarding children feature frequently as identified learning needs in personal development plans. As Chairman of the RCGP, I want to state clearly how important the care of children is in primary care. I want general practice to play a stronger role in driving up standards in paediatrics through improved training. I have no doubt that this book will be a valuable contribution to improving healthcare for children.

Dr Mayur Lakhani FRCP FRCGP
Chairman of Council
Royal College of General Practitioners
London SW1 7PU

Contents

List of Contributors

Gill Adams
Consultant Ophthalmic Surgeon
Moorfields Eye Hospital
London

Shubha Allard
Consultant Haematologist
Barts and the London Hospital

Michael Bannon
Postgraduate Dean and Honorary
Consultant Paediatrician
Oxford

Jane Barlow
Reader in Public Health
Warwick Medical School
The University of Warwick

Ruth Bastable
General Practitioner
Cambridge

Helen Bedford
Senior Lecturer
Institute of Child Health
London

Mark Bloch
Consultant Anaesthetist
Chelsea and Westminster Hospital
London

Jackie Bucknall
Consultant Paediatrician
Homerton University Hospital
London

Yvonne Carter
Dean and Professor of General Practice
and Primary Care
Warwick Medical School
The University of Warwick

Andrew Clark
Consultant Immunologist
Addenbrooke's Hospital
Cambridge

Tim Cole
Professor of Medical Statistics
Institute of Child Health
London

Dee Dawson
Medical Director
Rhodes Farm Clinic
The Ridgeway
London

Justine Dempsey
Head of Nutrition and Dietetic Services
Northwick Park and St Mark's Hospitals
Harrow

Barbara Dulley
Orthoptist
Moorfields Eye Hospital
London

Deborah Eastwood
Consultant Orthopaedic Surgeon
Royal National Orthopaedic Hospital
Stanmore

Daryl Efron
Consultant Paediatrician
Royal Children's Hospital
Melbourne

David Elliman
Consultant in Community Child Health
Great Ormond Street Hospital
for Children
London

David Foreman
Consultant and Honorary Senior Lecturer
in Child and Adolescent Psychiatry
Child and Adolescent Mental
Health Services
Nobles Hospital
Isle of Man

Rodney Franklin
Consultant Paediatric Cardiologist
Royal Brompton and Harefield
NHS Trust

Helen Goodyear
Consultant Paediatrician
Heart of England NHS Foundation Trust

Paul Gringras
Paediatric Neurodisability Consultant
Evelina Children's Hospital Guys and
St Thomas' NHS Foundation Trust
London

Parvis Habibi
Reader and Consultant
Paediatric Intensive Care and Respiratory
Medicine Department of Paediatrics
Imperial College London

Pandora Hadfield
ENT Consultant
The Royal Surrey County Hospital
Guildford and St Peter's Hospital
Chertsey

Mainga Hamaluba
Paediatric Specialist Registrar
Oxford Deanery

Celia Harding
Lecturer in Learning Disabilities
City University
London

Peter Hill
Consultant in Child and Adolescent
Psychiatry
Department of Psychological Medicine
Great Ormond Street Hospital for Children
London

Jeremy Hull
Consultant Paediatrician
Department of Paediatrics
John Radcliffe Hospital
Oxford

Warren Hyer
Consultant Paediatrician and Paediatric
Gastroenterologist
Northwick Park and St Mark's Hospitals
Harrow

Fernando Isaza
Consultant Paediatrician
Northwick Park and St Mark's Hospitals
Harrow

Benjamin Jacobs
Consultant Paediatrician
Northwick Park and St Mark's Hospitals
Harrow

Lionel Jacobson
Honorary Lecturer
Department of General Practice
University of Wales College of Medicine
Cardiff

Sandeep Jayawant
Consultant Paediatric Neurologist
John Radcliffe Hospital
Oxford

Daniel Kelly
Reader in Cancer and Palliative Care
Faculty of Health and Social Science
Middlesex University
London

Fauzia Khan
Community Paediatrician
St George's Centre
Leeds

Peter Lachman
Consultant Paediatrician
Royal Free Hospital
London

Mayur Lakhani
Chairman of Council
Royal College of General Practitioners
London

Daniel Leff
Clinical Research Fellow
Division of Surgery, Oncology,
Reproductive Biology and Anaesthetics
Imperial College
London

Maria Luscombe
Speech and Language Therapist
Northwick Park and St Mark's Hospitals
Harrow

Stephen Marks
Consultant Paediatric Nephrologist
Great Ormond Street Hospital for
Children
London

Peter McDonald
Consultant General Surgeon
Northwick Park and St Mark's Hospitals
Harrow

Richard Nicholl
Consultant Neonatologist
Northwick Park and St Mark's Hospitals
Harrow

Frank Oberklaid
Professor and Director
Centre for Community Child Health
University of Melbourne

Diane Owen
Academic Fellow
Department of General Practice
University of Wales College of Medicine,
Cardiff

Andrew Pollard
Reader in Paediatric Infection/Immunity
Department of Paediatrics
University of Oxford

Michael Preece
Professor of Child Health and Growth
Institute of Child Health
London

Cecil Reid
Consultant Haematologist
Northwick Park and St Mark's Hospitals
Harrow

John Reilly
Professor of Paediatric Energy
Metabolism University of Glasgow

Mary Rudolf
Professor of Child Health
University of Leeds

Aziz Sheikh
Professor of Primary Care Research and
Development
University of Edinburgh

Doug Simkiss
Senior Lecturer in Child Health
Warwick Medical School
The University of Warwick

Zdenek Slavik
Consultant Paediatric Cardiologist
Royal Brompton and Harefield NHS Trust
London

Laura Stewart
Community Paediatric Dietitian
Royal Hospital for Sick Children
Edinburgh

Richard Trompeter
Consultant Paediatric Nephrologist
Great Ormond Street Hospital for
Children
London

Angela Underdown
Associate Professor
Institute of Education
The University of Warwick

David Vickers
Consultant Community Paediatrician
Cambridge

Jonathan Williams
Visiting Research Associate
Institute of Psychiatry
De Crespigny Part
London

David Wilson
Senior Lecturer in Paediatric
Gastroenterology and Nutrition
Royal Hospital for Sick Children
Edinburgh

Introduction

Michael Bannon and Yvonne Carter

In the UK, general practitioners (GPs) and other members of the Primary Health Care Team (PHCT) undertake an enhanced role in the provision of healthcare for children. In the first instance, they see a number of children who present with an acute illness that requires a professional opinion. In addition, they are now responsible for the majority of child health promotional and surveillance activities including developmental checks and immunization. They increasingly undertake a shared role with secondary care for children who have chronic illness such as asthma. GPs, because of their unique and sustained relationships with families, provide continuing support for needy and vulnerable children, including families, where there are concerns regarding child protection and/or domestic violence. The last 3 years in the UK have seen great changes in our thinking about children and, in particular, how we respond to children in need of child protection. Following publication of the Laming Inquiry (2003) there have been a considerable number of publications focusing on the need to prioritize services for children.

Following the emergence of Primary Care Organizations, GPs have further important roles in child health. They can now influence configuration and commissioning of services at a local level and also fulfil an important role in public health. At least 25% of GP consultations are with children. It is therefore important that GPs continue to update their knowledge and skills necessary to address the healthcare needs of this population group. In the past most (but not all GPs) have completed 6 months of training in child health at Senior House Officer (SHO) level during vocational training. However, child health is a complex and varied subject and few GPs will have had exposure to all relevant aspects of paediatrics during such a short period. Children do not represent a homogeneous population and several ages of childhood are recognized, each with its unique set of illnesses and problems: the neonate, infant, pre-school child, school age child, and the adolescent. Whereas many paediatricians subspecialize to a degree and may preferentially treat children of a defined age, e.g. neonates, GPs provide care for the entire age range of childhood. Furthermore, both the childhood population and their illnesses change with time. New illnesses, such as HIV have appeared and others, not seen for many years (such as rickets, tuberculosis, congenital rubella syndrome) have returned. It is important that GPs keep abreast of these developments. A comprehensive knowledge of varied aspects of child health is needed: recognition and initial management of the acutely ill child, developmental surveillance, immunization, collaborative treatment of chronic illness and psycho-social issues. A new curriculum for general practice has been defined by the

Royal College of General Practitioners (http://gpcurriculum.co.uk/curriculum/curriculum_link.htm). This document, which will be implemented during 2007, represents an innovative and evidence-based approach with respect to education and training of future GPs. It anticipates the challenges that will arise as a result of Modernising Medical Careers and the standards set by the new Postgraduate Medical Education and Training Board (PMETB). Care of young people and children is comprehensively covered in the curriculum statement.

The overall aim of this book is provide GPs and other PHCT members with a practical textbook that will be highly relevant to child health in the twenty-first century. It is not the intention to provide a comprehensive text that covers all aspects of childhood illness in terms of epidemiology and pathology. There are in existence other books that achieve this objective and in any case much is already available via the World Wide Web for primary care doctors. Rather, the book will undertake a focused, problem-orientated approach based upon the more common childhood problems currently encountered by GPs. A practical approach is envisaged whereby solutions to clinical scenarios are provided, based upon current, best available evidence. In each case, contributing authors were asked to ensure that their approach is relevant and sensitive to primary care.

The authors have tried to ensure a primary care orientated approach in each chapter. Hence the more common presentations of childhood illness and disorders as they present to GPs are dealt with along with sufficient but not exhaustive background theoretical information.

References

Lord Laming: Inquirm into the death of Victoria Climbié. London: Stationery Office, 2003.

Chapter 2

Recognition and initial management of the sick child

Mark Bloch and Parvis Habibi

Goals of the chapter

All clinicians need to be able to recognize the symptoms and signs of the sick child as early as possible. This chapter attempts to give an understanding of the 'first principles' with regards to both the well child as well as some insight into the aetiology, symptoms, and signs of the child who has the potential to or is becoming seriously ill. It describes a systematic approach to the initial and ongoing assessment of these children. Management options will be described, including a mention of the non-technical skills required for good clinical practice in an attempt to improve patient outcome and practitioner confidence.

Spectrum of paediatrics

When describing pathophysiology in paediatrics, it is important to understand the age-related differences and developments in the normal physiology of our patients. Understanding the spectrum of paediatrics (Table 2.1) enables one to have a baseline from which to describe the normal and therefore the abnormal. By using neonatal and infant physiology as a starting point, one may then extrapolate remembering that there are no absolutes, rather a spectrum of degrees with marked intra- and interpatient variations exists. Pharmacological agents and ongoing pathophysiology further influence this.

First principles

By understanding normal anatomy and physiology, one can then decide if variations have the potential to lead to patient harm. Although all organ systems are important with regards to the overall well-being of the child, with regards to early recognition of deterioration in the patient's clinical condition, several of the systems appear more relevant then others. Please see Table 2.2 for some normal neonatal values.

The unique anatomic features of the airways in children under a year of age leave little reserve or margin of safety. A large occiput may require manipulation to achieve the

Table 2.1 Spectrum of the paediatric patient

Terminology	Age
Premature	<37 weeks
Neonate	4 weeks post-term delivery
Infant	1 year post term delivery
Toddler	2 years
Child	Up to teenage years
Adolescence	Teenage years
Adult	3rd decade onwards

neutral position. There is an increased likelihood for airways obstruction due to several factors including:

◆ relatively large tongue and more submental soft tissue

◆ a 'large floppy' epiglottis and possibly other supraglottic structures

◆ a high and anterior larynx with the narrowest portion being situated at the level of the cricoid cartilage.

Table 2.2 Age-related normal values

Parameter	Neonate (3 kg)	1 month (4 kg)	1 year (10 kg)	Adult
Respiratory rate/min	35–55	30–55	25–35	12–20
PaO$_2$ in room air	65–85 mmHg 8.6–11.3 kPa			85–95 mmHg 11.3–12.6 kPa
PaCO$_2$	30–38 mmHg 4–5 kPa			36–44 mmHg 4.8–5.8 kPa
pH	7.3–7.4			7.36–7.44
SBP (mmHg)*	50–70	60–90	80–110	95–140
DBP (mmHg)	30–50	45–60	50–80	60–85
Heart rate/min	120–160	120–160	90–120	60–90
Haemoglobin (g/dl)/ haematocrit (%)	19 / 60	14.2 / 43 (10.7@8 weeks)	11.6 / 35	13–15 / 39–45
Intravascular volume	90 ml/kg	80–85 ml/kg	75–80 ml/kg	70–75 ml/kg
Glomerular filtration rate (ml/min/1.7 m^2)	20	60	80	120

SBP, systolic blood pressure; DBP, diastolic blood pressure.

*1–10 years 5th centile for SBP = 70 + (age × 2)

Mean arterial pressure (MAP) = DBP + 1/3 × (SBP − DBP)

weight = 2 × (age + 4)

When air flows through a tube there is a pressure difference between the ends. This pressure difference differs for laminar versus turbulent flow. The pressure-flow characteristics for laminar flow are described by Poiseuille's equation (West 2000):

$$\acute{\upsilon} = \frac{P\pi r^4}{8nl}$$

Where $\acute{\upsilon}$ is the volume flow rate, P the driving pressure, r radius, n viscosity and l length this leads to:

$$R = \frac{8nl}{\pi r^4}$$

When airflow is turbulent, as may be seen during crying or with increased work of breathing, the resistance to airflow may be even greater (Davis 2002). The increased work of breathing may directly be due to the airways problem or may be due to altered pulmonary compliance resulting from pathology related to the lungs (alveoli and/or lung parenchyma) or to the chest wall. This illustrates the critical importance of airways radius, which in these young children is relatively more important. For example, if an infant develops 1 mm of circumferential oedema this will increase the resistance by a factor of 16 times. If there were turbulent flow, as described above, then this would increase the work of breathing 32-fold. This is compounded by the lack of reserve and other organ systems' response to hypoxaemia, hypoxia, and hypercapnoea. All the above is also relevant when looking at children who are intubated but breathing spontaneously.

Within the respiratory system the most important factor that distinguishes the neonate from the older patient is oxygen consumption. In the neonate this approaches 6 ml/kg compared with approximately 3 ml/kg in the adult (Stoelting and Dierdorf 2002). To accomplish this, the alveolar ventilation is doubled in the neonate by increasing the breathing rate (tidal volumes on a weight basis in the child and in the adult are similar). The neonate's lungs are immature with a 10-fold increase in number of small airways up to adulthood. The vital capacity in the newborn is approximately half that seen in adults on a weight basis and the baby's lung at functional residual capacity is near to the closing volume. There is increased diaphragmatic breathing in the newborn; however, the diaphragm is easily fatigued.

Adapting to survival in an extra-uterine environment has certain implications in relation to the cardiovascular system in the paediatric patient. *In utero* there is a high pulmonary vascular resistance and low systemic vascular resistance with right to left shunting of blood through the foramen ovale and ductus arteriosus. There is a right ventricular dominance at birth that evolves to left ventricular dominance by about 5 months of age. The increased pulmonary blood flow with the onset of spontaneous ventilation, accompanied by an increase in systemic vascular resistance with clamping of the umbilical cord, is usually well tolerated. The anatomic closure of the foramen ovale occurs between 3 months and a year of age (although a percentage of adult patients will have 'probe patent' foramen ovale). Functional and anatomical closure of the ductus arteriosus occurs from 10 to 15 hours after birth up to 6 weeks (Stoelting and Dierdorf 2002).

During the above transitional periods, the baby may revert to a fetal circulation if exposed to certain stresses, for example: arterial hypoxaemia, acidosis, and conditions associated with a high pulmonary vascular resistance. On a weight basis, the newborn has a large circulating blood volume (approximately 80 ml/kg); however, there is a small actual volume, which becomes relevant with certain pathologies.

Oxygen flux is the delivery of oxygen to the tissues and is equal to: 'cardiac output $\times$ oxygen carrying capacity of the blood (comprising that carried by the haemoglobin and the small dissolved component in the blood)' (West 2000).

this is equal to:

$$(HR \times SV) \times (1.39 \times Hb \times SaO_2/100) + 0.003 \text{ (per 100 ml blood/mmHg } PO_2)$$

where HR is heart rate, SV is stroke volume, Hb is haemoglobin and 1 gram of pure Hb can combine with 1.39 ml of O_2.

There are several important differences with regards to normal infant physiology and maintaining oxygen flux, these include:

1. Neonates are dependent on heart rate to maintain cardiac output and blood pressure as they have less ability to increase myocardial contractility and implement vasoconstrictive responses. They therefore do not tolerate a decrease in intravascular fluid volume as well as may be seen in an older patient.

2. Haemoglobin F (fetal) makes up part of the haemoglobin of the newborn and is gradually replaced over the first year or so of postnatal life. This becomes relevant in the context of the oxygen dissociation curve whose shape provides several physiological advantages both in the alveoli and in the peripheral tissues. Here it is important to understand the relationships between PaO_2, SaO_2, and most importantly O_2 concentration, which represents the actual amount of oxygen that can be delivered to the cells. The curve may be shifted to the right by factors including an increase in $[H^+]$, PCO_2, temperature and 2,3-diphosphoglycerate and this leads to improved O_2 unloading in the tissues. The curve may be shifted left due to factors opposite to the above and due to the presence of increased concentrations of fetal haemoglobin, being one of the reasons for the higher haemoglobin concentration in the newborn.

3. Ventilation to perfusion (V-Q) mismatch or, at the end of the spectrum, a shunt will lead to a reduction in oxygen concentration in the blood and an increase in carbon dioxide. There may then be an increase in the tissue extraction ratio in an attempt to maintain oxygen delivery and this may lead to worsening hypoxaemia particularly if the child is unable to compensate by increasing cardiac output.

Human physiology is designed with several feedback systems. The autonomic nervous system plays a vital role with regards to maintaining normal homeostasis within all organ systems and enabling increased capacity of various organs to attempt survival strategies should the organism require this. Most organs have dual autonomic innervations with input from sympathetic and parasympathetic systems frequently mediating opposing effects. Resting tone is proportional to the dominance at specific effector sites, which varies with the age of the patient. There is increased parasympathetic tone in children particularly under the age of 2 years and most pronounced in the newborn. This has numerous clinical and interventional implications and these children are more prone to the five Bs:

- bradycardia
- bronchospasm
- bronchial and lacrimal secretions
- bowel activity
- bladder activity.

The sympathetic response and its effect on heart rate, systemic vascular response and to a smaller extent, on cardiac output and stroke volume, lead to the state of compensated shock, which will be discussed later.

The body is comprised of solids and water, the proportions of which vary with age. The largest change occurs during the first 2 years of life. At birth, a higher percentage of water is found in the extracellular fluid compartment, unlike older children where the higher proportion is in the intracellular compartment. This is relevant when looking at the metabolic requirements of the patient under a year and the clinical assessment and correction of the fluid status of a child. The renal function of the neonate is reduced compared with adult values. The glomerular filtration rate at birth is only 25–30% that of an adult but in the term neonate increases rapidly in the first extra-uterine month and reaches almost 80% of adult values by a year of age (Stoelting and Dierdorf 2002). Neonates have a limited ability to increase their urine volume following a fluid load but have a reduced ability to concentrate urine. A healthy newborn will therefore tolerate a mild to moderate fluid overload much better than moderate dehydration. Decreased renal function, along with decrease phase 2 hepatic metabolisms, can also delay metabolism and excretion of drugs dependent on hepatic metabolism and renal clearance for elimination. Neonates and infants are vulnerable to the development of hypothermia particularly during periods of stress, for example: illness and perioperative periods. This is related to large body surface area relative to body weight, reduced subcutaneous fat, and less ability to produce heat.

Approach to pathophysiology

The pathological conditions that can occur in children, can either be:

- congenital
- hereditary
- temporal (age-related)
- incidental.

'Classic' signs are often missed at the extremes of age. Common conditions occur commonly but clinicians must be careful of conformational bias. Certain conditions and situations may be particularly elusive and difficult to resolve, for example.

- pyrexia of unknown aetiology especially between 3 and 36 months
- intussusception
- meningitis.

As clinicians it is vitally important to listen to mother, caregiver, community/paediatric nurse. Experience (theirs, yours) and 'gut feelings' are invaluable. Remember that medicine is a matter of degrees and very little is 'black or white' or absolute. So never say never!

Systematic assessment, 'warning signs' and management

Within the scope of this chapter, those symptoms and signs that indicate deterioration in cardiovascular, airways, and pulmonary and neurological function will be discussed. Following a systematic approach to assessment will help in not overlooking important 'clues' in patients who may have a limited history or who may not be able to communicate clearly how they are feeling and why. There are a variety of scoring systems (for example, the Paediatric Early Warning Score) that may be used to document a combination of organ system dysfunction and its severity (this allocates an accumulated score to a variety of clinical assessments to attempt to illustrate the overall clinical condition of the patient). However, it is often better to follow a more simplistic approach remembering that deterioration occurs in degrees rather then being absolute and one has to use clinical experience to try to anticipate when increasing organ support will be required and to try to intervene early where appropriate to prevent progression to decompensated respiratory and possibly secondary cardiac failure or arrest and to reduce morbidity and mortality. A rapid, reliable, clinical, structured and sequential approach is required and should be easy to follow (ABCDE method): **Airways/Breathing/Circulation/Disability/Evaluation**. The most appropriate individual and/or team should be mobilized to intervene in the most appropriate manner in the particular circumstances for the best possible outcome for the child. Any situation may introduce many variables and guidelines should not be adhered to mindlessly, they should be used as basis for action with rational thinking. This illustrates the importance of utilization of appropriate technical and non-technical skills, clearly described by the mnemonic **Knowledge/Understanding/ Skills/Attitudes/Behaviour** (Rogers 2002). The knowledge and skills required will be further described in this chapter in an attempt to introduce an understanding. The non-technical skills required include (Weller et al. 2003):

- know and optimize the environment when possible
- anticipation and planning
- vigilant monitoring, cross-checking, and utilization of available data (situation awareness)
- calling for help early
- prioritization of tasks
- utilization of resources and appropriate distribution of workload

- leadership and team co-ordination
- appropriate and effective communication (sharing mental models).

Three possible approaches:

- A disease-based approach, e.g. diabetes, cardiac, sepsis (including meningococcal), trauma (including burns). With disease recognition and management, which may limit spectrum of skills including initial stabilization.
- A generic approach with application of first principles, which requires development, and updating of generic skills but may forget important components of treatment for specific conditions.
- A combination of the both by taking a generic approach (with early stabilization of the airways, breathing, and circulation) but taking into account treatments for specific aetiologies (for example: insulin in diabetes, antibiotics and steroids for meningitis or refractory shock, antidotes for specific toxin ingestion). In our opinion this third option is best as illustrated with the modern management for meningococcal infection (Pollard *et al.* 1999).

Most children will do badly if hypoxia and/or hypovolaemia are not recognized. Death in children is most likely going to be due to hypoxaemia and/or hypovolaemia. This 'cardiopulmonary failure' is a poorly defined concept and doesn't emphasize other organ dysfunction that may have an impact on outcome, for example: hypoxic ischaemic encephalopathy. The mortality and possibly outcome does seem to have been influenced by the introduction of the life-support courses possibly due to improved airways management and pattern recognition. However, the outcome after out of hospital arrest is still dismal (Schindler 1997), particularly if the resuscitation is longer than 20 minutes and/or there are fixed dilated pupils, where less than 2% of patients will have a satisfactory outcome. Cardiopulmonary arrest in paediatrics is rarely a sudden event but is usually the result of progressive deterioration in respiratory and possibly circulatory function. This means that by the time a cardiopulmonary arrest occurs, the child's organs may have already experienced ischaemic effects and those sensitive to hypoxia (brain, renal medulla, heart) may be seriously damaged resulting in a reduce chance of a good outcome even if a cardiac output can be obtained.

The best approach is the early recognition of the child that is deteriorating. This is best done via the ABCDE method:

- **A (Airways)**: to assess the airways one must look, listen, and feel. The airways may be:
  - normal or safe
  - maintainable or at risk where the breathing is noisy (therefore indicating gas movement) and although the level of consciousness (LOC) may be reduced, the child requires and tolerates simple support such as positioning, suctioning and simple devices like a Guedal airway.
  - unmaintainable when airways cannot be obtained to enable oxygenation and ventilation without intubation or a surgical airway.

◆ **B (Breathing)**: one way to assess respiratory insufficiency is to look at the breathing. Increased work of breathing is both a sign of pathology as well as its result. This may be due to: upper airways obstruction, lower airways obstruction, altered pulmonary compliance (related to alveolar, interstitial/parenchymal, or chest wall changes) or a combination of all three. This may initially be compensated for by increasing the rate of breathing (tachypnoea) and respiratory effort (an indication of which may be noted with stirtor and stridor, positioning, head bobbing, nasal flaring, grunting, the use of accessory muscles and retractions, wheezing, heart rate, central cyanosis, and skin colour). A reduction in tidal volume and air entry, increasing heart rate and worsening restlessness, hypotonia, and interaction with carers may occur as the child deteriorates, and hypoxia and availability of nutrients worsen with disease progression. Respiratory failure is a clinical state characterized by inadequate oxygenation and/or ventilation and may be due to increased work of breathing or decreased respiratory effort, which may be due to reduced respiratory drive, exhaustion, and due to the effects of respiratory inadequacy. The diagnosis of potential or actual respiratory failure is a clinical one that may be supported with blood gas analysis. This may also be used to assess the child's baseline status and also a response to therapy. Useful parameters include: amount of oxygen required (FiO_2), PaO_2 (hypoxaemia), $PaCO_2$ (hypercapnoea), pH, standard bicarbonate and base excess or deficit.

◆ **C (Circulation)**: shock is a clinical state in which there is inadequate circulation and delivery of oxygen and metabolic substrates to meet the demands of tissues. Hypovolaemia is due to fluid losses or fluid redistribution. The first may be due to conditions such as gastroenteritis, diabetes, or trauma. Distributive shock (as may be found with sepsis, anaphylaxis, anaphylactoid, and spinal conditions) is classically described as being due to vasodilatation, increased capillary permeability or a combination of the both. Cardiogenic components (myopathic or dysrrthmogenic) may be found in isolation or in combination with other pathologies (for example: sepsis) resulting in potential or actual cardiovascular failure. It is obviously very difficult to assess right and left ventricular pre-load, after-load, contractility, and overall cardiac output. Clinical signs may include: heart rate, respiratory rate, capillary refill time, pulse character, core-toe temperature differences, line of coldness, skin colour, LOC, urine output (including wet nappy), response to fluids, worsening metabolic acidosis and lactate production all as an indication of perfusion. This may be preferable to the measuring of blood pressure, which may be initially maintained in the shocked child due to increase in sympathetic outflow with increased systemic vascular resistance leading to a compensated state. More invasive monitoring may be possible in the appropriate settings but this is used in conjunction with all the above clinical signs. As the pathophysiology progresses, then the compensatory mechanisms may fail resulting in a state of decompensation as indicated by systolic hypotension and further decreasing organ perfusion.

The importance of recognizing altered LOC, as a significant element in recognition of critical illness in children cannot be over emphasized. This may prove difficult, as

Table 2.3 Blood pressure limits to maintain cerebral perfusion pressures

Age	Mean arterial pressure (mmHg)
<3 months	40–60
<1 year	45–75
1–5 years	50–100
6–11 years	60–90
12–14 years	65–95

Source: Miles (2004).

conscious level may not be easy to assess. The Glasgow Coma Scale and some of the modifications (Adelaide, Glasgow, others) may be particularly difficult to use. Possibly an easier tool, utilized by the 'life-support' courses, is the AVPU system (Table 2.4), which may be used in conjunction with other signs such as pupils and posture. Secondary brain injury is a consequence of ischaemic injury resulting from hypoxia and hypotension and may be associated with poorer neurological outcome. Cerebral resuscitation aims to provide sufficient supply of oxygenated blood to the brain to meet demand. Both hypoglycaemia and hyperglycaemia should be avoided as may worsen acidosis, reperfusion injury, and lead to cellular death. Balancing supply and demand may be achieved with the delivery of increased amounts of oxygen with increased oxygen carrying capacity in the blood (as discussed), increased cerebral perfusion and decreased oxygen requirements (including control of factors such as hyperthermia, pain, and seizures).

$$CPP = MAP - ICP$$

Where CPP is cerebral perfusion pressure, MAP is mean arterial pressure and ICP is intracranial pressure. This is further influenced by $PaCO_2$ that may either cause increased ICP if too high or vasoconstriction and decreased perfusion if too low. To maintain a CPP ≥20–25 mmHg (minimum required) one needs to maintain MAP at the higher end of normal.

Potential and actual (compensated and decompensated) respiratory and cardiac failure may initially present as distinct entities. However, they often progress to a state of

Table 2.4 Potential neurological failure

	Conscious level
A	Alert
V	responds to Voice
P	responds to Pain
U	Unresponsive

Source: Chameides (1997).

cardiopulmonary failure. Early recognition is the first step in the management of these children.

Stabilization of the critically ill child includes adequate resuscitation, initiation of supportive therapies, monitoring, and prevention of further deterioration. Initial priority is given to the airways, oxygenation, and ventilation, if circulation and perfusion then fail to improve rapidly, circulatory support should be initiated. This is well described in paediatric life-support courses approach with variations of the acronym (Eaton 1999):

- ◆ **D** exclude any **d**anger to carers and patient (this may be **d**ynamic)
- ◆ **R r**esponse of patient and call for help, **r**eassure where appropriate and **r**elationships, which may indicate a mechanism of injury if trauma related.
- ◆ **Ac a**irway: assessment, positioning and maintenance of a clear airway (head tilt, jaw lift and thrust or recovery position to intubation if truly required and appropriate skill/risk/benefit ratio) always considering the **c**ervical spine
- ◆ **B b**reathing: assessment with appropriate level of support (ranging from supplemental oxygen to the other end of the spectrum with mechanical ventilation)
- ◆ **C c**irculation: pulse check, chest compressions, intravenous/interosseous access if appropriate with fluid administration as required (rehydration, maintenance, replacement, and arrest **h**aemorrhage as appropriate)
- ◆ **D d**isability (e.g.: AVPU, pupils and focal neurology), **d**rugs (including analgesia) and **D**on't **E**ver **F**orget the **G**lucose
- ◆ **E e**xposure to ensure not missing anything initially relevant including other injuries and temperature maintenance (this may be the first requirement for a newborn) and **e**arly **e**vacuation to appropriate setting (e.g. hospital).

Once this has been achieved then a full assessment of the child should be performed. This may include: detailed history, extensive clinical examination and further goal-directed bedside and special investigations if clinical condition allows. Achieving the above may require differing levels of skill and equipment (including the understanding of certain algorithms and availability of certain aids, e.g. resuscitation charts). Ensuring these are available where appropriate is a vital area of human factors previously described. Once this has been achieved then an attempt at diagnosing the causative pathology may be attempted and specific treatment commenced. This does not exclude the requirement for repeated systematic evaluation of the airways, breathing, and circulation.

Ongoing evaluation of cardiopulmonary function is required even if the child's condition appears stable. Evidence for impending deterioration may include:

- ◆ respiratory distress
  - respiratory rate >55/min
  - ongoing tachycardia
  - abnormal chest and abdominal movements and child's adopted position
  - unable to independently maintain airways ± stridor ± history of possible foreign body

- wheeze or other added or reduced breath sounds
- accessory muscles (e.g. sternomastoid leading to head bobbing)
- nasal flaring
- chest recession (intercostals, subcostal, or sternal)
- pallor ± cyanosis (not seen in severe anaemia)
- SaO_2 <94% or PaO_2 <8kPa (on supplemental oxygen)
- $PaCO_2$ >6 or <3.5kPa

  One must always beware of the silent chest. Exhaustion is a pre-terminal event.
- shock
  - heart rate >180 or <80/min
  - absent peripheral pulses
  - cold peripheries and skin colour (pink, pale, blue, mottled)
  - capillary fill time >2 s
  - SBP <70+ (age in years × 2) mmHg (5th centile)
  - urine output <0.5–2 ml/kg per hour (age-dependent)
- deteriorating LOC (agitation, drowsiness, responsiveness, tone, pupils, posturing)
- recurrent seizures
- multiple trauma/burns >10%.

In conclusion, although single observations are useful, it is far better to repeat them on a regular basis so that the trend (improving, deteriorating, or staying the same) in the child's condition can be established. This may be achieved using systems such as 'Paediatric Early Warning Scores' where appropriate, for example in paediatric wards where they may be useful to 'flag-up' patients that may require more attention and one would not want to 'fall between' the gaps during staff hand-over. In other settings it may be more useful to use a more simplistic approach as described by assessing airways, breathing, circulation, and neurological condition. A combination of knowledge, skill, and understanding is required to make the appropriate clinical judgement decisions. However, non-technical skills are also required to optimize patient outcome. These include appropriate attitudes and behaviours including anticipating and planning, effective communication, maintaining situation awareness, and utilizing appropriate personnel and resources. Experience is important in managing these children particularly if there are other factors to be taken into account such as underlying chronic conditions, complex pathology, prolonged resuscitation, and other ethical issues. Calling for help early enough should occur whenever possible. One must never forget that the perspective of the parents, other family members, or other carers may not necessarily be the same as the clinicians and where possible a patient and empathetic approach should be adopted. This may also be the case between differing members of the medical team both during the care of the child and possibly after, depending on the outcome. Finally, one should have a high index of suspicion as children are intolerant of hypoxia, circulatory compromise, and metabolic disturbances and although they can initially compensate they may then rapidly decompensate. If in any doubt then initiate the process to ensure a step-up of care for the patient. Reduction in morbidity and mortality is due to both the early perform-ance of life-saving manoeuvres and the prevention and appropriate treatment of life-threatening pathophysiological events. It is easier to reduce the level of care if not required then to try to attempt to retrieve a situation if the clinical condition has deteriorated too far. It is not what you do, but probably how you do it and the attention to detail that counts.

Remember still kids are ill kids and ill kids are still kids.

Unknown

Wherever the art of medicine is loved, there is also a love of humanity.

Hippocrates

References

Chameides L, Hazinski MF (1997). *Pediatric Advanced Life Support Manual*. American Heart Association. Channing Bete, Maryland.

Davis PD, Parbrook GD, Kenny GNC (2002). *Basic Physics and Measurement in Anaesthesia* (4th ed). Butterworth-Heinemann, Oxford.

Eaton CJ (1999). *Essentials of Immediate Medical Care* (2nd edn). Churchill Livingstone, Philadelphia.

Miles *et al.* (2004). *CATS Guidelines—Head Injury*. London.

Pollard AJ, Britto J, Nadel S, DeMunter C, Habibi P, Levin M (1990). Emergency management of meningococcal disease. *Archives of Diseases in Childhood* **80**: 290–296.

Rogers A (2002). *Teaching Adults* (3rd edn). Open University Press. Milton Keynes.

Schindler, Bohn D, Cox PN, McCrindie BW, Jarvis A, Edmowis J, Barker Geoffrey (1997). Cardiopulmonary resuscitation in children. *New England Journal of Medicine* **336**(18): 1325–1326.

Stoelting RF, Dierdorf SF (2002). *Anesthesia and Co-existing Disease* (4th edn). Churchill Livingstone, Philadelphia.

Weller JM, Bloch M, Young S, Maze M, Oyesola S, Wyner J, Dob D, Haire K, Durbridge J, Walker T, Newble D (2003). Evaluation of the high fidelity patient simulator in the assessment of performance of anaesthetists. *British Journal of Anaesthesia* **90**: 43–47.

West JB (2000). *Respiratory Physiology: the Essentials* (6th edn). Lippincott Williams and Wilkins, Philadelphia.

Chapter 3

Ambulatory paediatrics

Peter Lachman, Fernando Isaza,
and Jackie Bucknall

The concept of 'ambulatory paediatrics' evolved in the USA in the early 1960s. Heller (1994) described the development of paediatricians who could take an overview of children's needs especially those who did not need admission. In this chapter we intend to break down the misconceptions of the terminology and to lead the reader into a clearer understanding of how a modern healthcare service can develop and how this can link into the services provided by the general practitioner. The chapter has two distinct sections—a general overview of this type of health service delivery, and a section on some of the different childhood problems encountered in an ambulatory unit.

Definition of ambulatory care

'General paediatrics' refers to the day to day work of most paediatricians. The arbitrary division of the specialty into hospital and community paediatrics has not been helpful as it fails to reconcile the fact that children who have been admitted to hospital are, at the same time, part of a greater community. 'Child health' is an all embracing term that generally refers to all children in the community including those that are ill. 'Ambulatory paediatrics' relates to a philosophy of health service delivery, which is designed around the needs of the child rather than those of the service. According to Meates (1997) 'ambulatory paediatrics refers to the non-inpatient hospital services and to the provision of care to sick children at home or in their local environment.' She goes on to state that the 'philosophy behind ambulatory paediatrics is that children should not be admitted to hospital unless absolutely necessary and, as much as possible, care should be arranged in their own home.' The term is therefore not restricted to hospital or community paediatrics; neither is it limited to the ill or well child. It follows that the service provided must be flexible in order to adapt to individual needs of the child, based on a growing evidence base of good practice, and delivered by nurses and doctors with appropriate skills.

Types of ambulatory care

One can divide ambulatory paediatrics into a number of categories each defining the type of care provided:

◆ acute emergency care
◆ day care

- community-based care
- outpatients
- child health clinics.

Acute emergency care

Over the past two decades there has been a change in the prevalence of childhood illnesses and the treatments that are required. There has also been a dramatic reduction in the length of stay. Numa and Oberklaid (1991) reported that in Australia at least 65% of all children admitted to a large teaching hospital could be discharged within 12 hours. The Royal College of Paediatrics and Child Health (2002) in its document on new solutions for healthcare delivery noted that while children's attendances at hospitals were increasing, the length of stay was decreasing. There is a large group of children who require hospital type emergency care but who do not require hospitalization beyond a few hours.

The advantages to this approach of care are numerous. Hospital admissions are a source of anxiety for children and their parents, disruptive to family routines, and expensive. The model of care within this philosophical approach can be developed to meet the needs of the local population. While many different models have been proposed to meet individual needs, all share the basic aim of not admitting children to hospital wherever possible.

Treatment modalities

There are several levels of care in an ambulatory unit.

- Resuscitation and stabilization of the collapsed child prior to admission to an inpatient ward or transfer to a more specialized unit.
- Immediate admission of a child to in-patient care if the child's condition is considered to be one that will require more than 24 hours care in hospital.
- Observation for a brief period of time (typically) 6–8 hours will be for children who have acute but self-limiting conditions; assessment with subsequent discharge home will be the outcome for the majority of these children.

The most common types of illness encountered in an ambulatory unit are acute respiratory distress including upper and lower airways obstruction, unexplained fevers, febrile convulsions; diarrhoea, and unexplained rashes. This is similar to the pattern previously seen in an accident and emergency unit (Arnon *et al.* 2001).

Staffing

There is therefore a need for a team of doctors and nurses (along with supportive administrative staff) who are trained to an appropriate level of expertise and who are of sufficient seniority to make effective decisions. The unit can only effectively function if appropriate decisions are made at least every 2 hours and without any unnecessary delay. This eliminates inappropriate investigations and waiting for a second opinion. The essential skills required by the ambulatory team are an ability to come to rapid diagnostic decisions, an ability to assess the outcome of the presenting problem, and an ability to devise a treatment plan in partnership with parents. This role can also be undertaken by experienced nurse practitioners. The role of the nurse practitioner in the ambulatory emergency unit is a key to its success; nurses can assess the severity of illness; commence interventions and be an advocate for the child's needs.

Facilities

Children need to be seen in appropriately designed units that meet their needs and those of their families and that include family rooms, play area, child friendly design, isolation rooms, and resuscitation facilities.

Training

Ambulatory care units provide an ideal setting for the training of nurses, paediatricians, and general practitioners. The paradox is that trainees must not provide the service; they should attend to learn about acutely ill children while the provision of the service is by a highly skilled team. General practice trainees should rotate through ambulatory units to learn at first hand about initial management of the ill child.

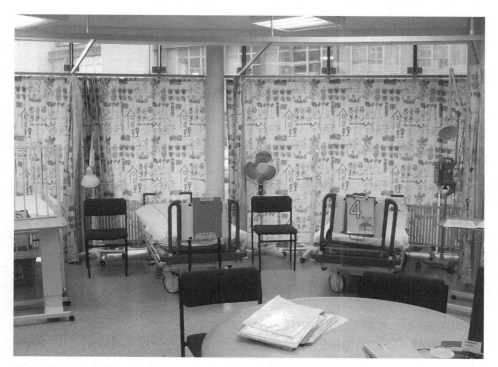

Fig. 3.1 Layout of the room.

Planned care and intervention

Paediatric day care

Paediatric day care refers to the provision of planned interventions in children. These interventions can include:

- phlebotomy
- pain relief
- medication administration for chronic conditions such as oncological disorders, rheumatological and autoimmune disorders
- preparation for procedures such as magnetic resonance imaging under anaesthetic and radiological investigations.

Ideally these services are provided by nurse practitioners in partnership with a lead paediatrician. The service enables children with chronic conditions such as thalassaemia or leukaemia to receive their treatment without being admitted as was in the past.

Paediatric day surgery

Short stay day surgery has become more prevalent over the past few years. A network of support is needed including surgeons, community-based nurses and general practitioners who can support the family once the child has been discharged home.

Planned care in the home: hospital at home

Nurse practitioners provide care for children in the home, where they are most comfortable and secure. Such nurses take on management of pain, provision of chemotherapy, management of tracheotomies, traction for fractures of the long bone, monitoring of postoperative complications, and management of chronic conditions such as eczema and asthma.

Outpatients and child health clinics

Outpatient and child health clinics provide the mainstay of care for children with non-acute problems. This level of secondary care has traditionally been sited in hospitals although there is a move to have such clinics within the community and in areas closer to the homes of children. Outpatients can be streamlined to fit into the continuum of care from telephone, fax, and email consultations, to rapid assessment clinics where a child is seen within a week to routine assessments for children with non-urgent conditions. In all cases close working with the general practitioner is needed. Such services can be provided by paediatric nurse practitioners as well as by paediatricians.

Common clinical conditions to refer to an ambulatory unit

The provision of healthcare to acutely ill children can be a challenge for those in primary care. The majority of children present with fairly simple clinical problems but in children the margin between mild and severe illness is small. We will discuss four key conditions that illustrate the model of care.

The vomiting child

Vomiting is the involuntary expulsion of large, forceful amounts of stomach contents via the mouth. In infants it is important to distinguish from possetting, which is the effortless regurgitation of usually small amounts of milk or food (Sondheim 1996). Vomiting is a non-specific symptom and a frequent feature of many childhood disorders, often being the sole presentation in many illnesses. It occurs as a direct result of gastrointestinal disorders but also as an early sign in many generalized infections, ingested toxins, metabolic disorders, and any disturbance of the central vomiting centre (Silverman 1983). A thorough history and examination are always essential to establish any associated features of concern and the general well-being of the child.

The following features should be considered

- the age of the child
- relationship of vomiting to feeds
- contact and travel history
- recent history of head trauma.

The associated symptomatology of concern

- Disinterest in or reluctance to feed—fluid intake less than half of maintenance requirements
- Fever >38.0°C despite paracetamol elixir at an age appropriate dose
- Abnormal drowsiness or irritability
- Vomiting for more than 6 hours
- Not passing urine for more than 6 hours or urine output less than half of normal (count wet nappies in infants)
- Signs of dehydration—sunken eyes, loose skin, sunken fontanelle
- Continuous abdominal pain in excess of 6 hours, despite appropriate analgesia
- Chronic vomiting for more than 3 weeks with no proven diagnosis
- Weight loss.

Indications for urgent referral

- Bilious vomiting or signs of intestinal obstruction (abdominal distension)
- Gastrointestinal bleeding—haematemesis or malaena
- Signs of acute abdomen
- Severe unremitting abdominal pain
- Dehydration (significant ketonuria +++ on urinalysis)
- Inability to tolerate oral intake

- Lethargy, drowsiness, or irritability
- Signs of meningism
- Electrolyte abnormalities.

Calculation of maintenance fluid requirements

- 0–10 kg body weight: at 4 ml/kg per hour
- 11–20 kg body weight: at 2 ml/kg per hour
- >20 kg body weight: at 1 ml/kg per hour.

Calculate hourly fluid requirement by the above formula using ml/hour for each kilo of body weight; e.g. a 34 kg girl will require:

- (10×4)ml for first 10 kg body weight
- (10×2)ml for second 10 kg body weight
- (14×1)ml for remaining 14 kg body weight
- a total of 74 ml/hour.

Advice on oral rehydration management

- Do not stop breast feeding in an infant
- Stop formula feeds and offer clear fluids for up to 12 hours
- Offer small frequent feeds at 1-hourly volumes (by maintenance calculations as above) via syringe if necessary.

Pineapple or blackcurrant oral rehydration solutions tend to be the most palatable to children.

The crying infant

Crying is a normal physiological response to distress, discomfort, tiredness, or need (hunger, thirst). The average baby of 2 months old cries for up to 3 hours in every 24. Crying becomes abnormal and potentially pathological when it is considered by the child's normal carers to differ in quality (high pitch, shrill, hoarse, or weak) or duration to normal or is inconsolable for more than 2 hours. Excessive crying is defined as in excess of 3 hours per day for more than 3 days per week (Poole 1991). The commonest cause of excessive crying in babies aged 1–4 months is infantile colic. However, it is important to identify a normal range of unsettled behaviour and deviations from this as other pathological problems obviously may arise acutely in an infant with known 'colic'. Also beware of attributing symptoms and signs to teething as there are no objective data to support this. A thorough history and examination is essential in excessive crying but further investigation is only warranted if the history is atypical or examination positive (Corwin 1996).

It is important to establish how urgently assessment is required by

- the frequency of the crying
- any associated symptomology

- general well-being of the child
- the level of parental anxiety or distress.

Parents and carers are often exhausted, distressed, and confused. They have frequently had conflicting advice from health professionals, relatives, and lay public. Remember maternal postnatal depression may also be a factor in presentation. If there is doubt, especially if infantile colic seems unlikely, then the infant should be seen as soon as possible.

Features suggestive of typical infantile colic

- Recurrent episodes
- Diurnal pattern with crying in the late afternoon or early evening
- Crying stops when fed or winded
- Air swallowing and difficult to wind.

The associated symptomology of concern

- Onset after 1 month of age
- Persistent episodes after 4 months of age
- Isolated episode of acute onset with no prior history
- Inconsolability
- Consolation increases crying especially on movement (lifting or rocking)
- History of recent trauma
- Pallor
- Weight loss
- Evidence of neglect
- Reluctance to feed
- Drowsy, poorly responsive, or irritability
- Vomiting especially if under 3 months or bilious
- Fever >38.0 °C.

Key management points

- Identify the ill baby and possible pathological causes of crying.
- Only offer medication for very short periods of time when infantile colic is typical and diagnosis clear.
- Formula milk changes and weaning from breast milk have no proven benefit except in infants with known cow's milk protein or lactose intolerance.
- Empathetic acknowledgement with the family, of the anxiety and stress excessive crying induces, is essential. Offer support to parents and emphasize they should seek further help if they are finding coping difficult.
- Referral for admission should be considered if the infant is felt to be at risk of non-accidental injury, parental exhaustion, or severe maternal postnatal depression.

Upper airways obstruction

Upper airways obstruction can be a frightening condition for the child, parents, and health professional. Several conditions can generate upper airways obstruction:

- laryngotracheitis and laryngotracheobronchitis (croup)
- spasmodic croup
- oesophageal or laryngeal foreign body.

Rarer conditions include:

- diphtheria (*Corynebacterium diphtheriae*)
- epiglottitis (*Haemophilus influenza*)
- retropharyngeal abscess
- bacterial tracheitis (*Staphylococcus aureus, H. influenza*).

Laryngotracheobronchitis (LTB) or viral croup

Croup refers to a group of symptoms that denote upper respiratory airways involvement: barking cough, hoarse voice, inspiratory stridor, and respiratory distress. LTB can be caused by parainfluenza viruses at all ages; respiratory syncytial virus in the under 5 years, and influenza and *Mycoplasma pneumoniae* in children older than 5 years (Denny *et al*. 1983).

The incidence of viral upper airways obstruction is approximately 3%, and accounts for 15% of respiratory tract infections in children (Denny *et al*. 1983). LTB usually occurs in autumn and early winter months. Children present with upper respiratory tract infection for 1 or 2 days and then gradually over several hours develop the barking cough, inspiratory stridor, and hoarse voice; which can last another 1–2 days. Severity is variable; but usually symptoms are benign, although they can increase at night-time or when the child is agitated. Fewer than 2% of children with LTB are admitted to hospital, and of those admitted; only 1–2% require intubation (Osmond 2001).

Anterioposterior and lateral neck X-ray can show subglottic narrowing and the classical 'steeple' sign. This can help differentiating it with epiglottitis, with 93% sensitivity and 92% specificity (Wright *et al*. 2002). However, X ray films are not very popular and the procedure can agitate the child even more, or may waste time in acting on a more ill child like that with bacterial tracheitis or epiglottitis. When the situation goes to the extreme of considering these diagnoses, it is better for the child to be evaluated by a very experienced anaesthetist or ENT surgeon through direct laryngoscopy with a view to intubation.

Spasmodic croup

Spasmodic croup occurs usually in children 1–3 years. It happens usually at night in an otherwise normal child. Viral aetiology, as well as allergies and psychological factors have been advocated. The condition is self-limiting. Fever is usually absent, and symptoms of upper respiratory tract infection are usually not present. Intervention is not needed except for reassurance. These episodes can repeat, leading to the theory of viral antigens generating the symptoms, rather than direct infection (Behrman and Kliegman 2004).

Table 3.1 Croup score

	0	1	2	3
Colour	Normal	Dusky	Cyanotic in room air	Cyanotic on FiO_2: 30%
Air entry	Normal	Mildly decreased	Moderately decreased	Substantially decreased
Retractions	None	Mild	Moderate	Severe
State of consciousness	Normal	Restless	Lethargy (depressed)	Unresponsive
Stridor	None	Mild	Moderate	Severe/absent in presence of severe obstruction

Foreign body

In all cases of upper airways obstruction inhalation of a foreign body must be considered. A careful clinical history usually will differentiate this from the other forms of obstruction.

Key management points if foreign body excluded

Several 'croup scores' have been designed aiming to decide when to treat, and to follow the response to treatment. We recommend the score developed by Taussig *et al.* (1975) (Table 3.1), in which treatment is started with a score of 4 or more.

What to do in primary care

Mist therapy is thought to be beneficial by some researchers (e.g. Schwartz 1999; Wright *et al.* 2002), but randomized control trials have failed to prove its benefit (Osmond 2001; Neto *et al.* 2002). A trial of a warm bath for 10–15 minutes, could benefit the child soothing him/her, producing some relaxation, and eventually generating some anecdotal improvement of the symptoms.

When to refer

Referral to the secondary level should be when the child is distressed or not drinking and the stridor score is above 1 for any of the criteria listed.

Treatment in hospital

Several therapies have been advocated for laryngotracheitis/bronchitis in hospital.

- ◆ Nebulized adrenaline (epinephrine) 1 in 1000 has been tried in the acute phase at a dose of 3–5 ml undiluted, or smaller volumes can be diluted in 3 ml of saline solution. Although this form of treatment produces initial improvement of the symptoms, there is a relapse after 2 hours of treatment (Westley *et al.* 1978; Waisman *et al.* 1992; Osmond, 2001; Royal College of Paediatrics and Child Health 2003).

- ◆ Inhaled budesonide (2 mg nebulized in a single dose) and oral dexamethasone (0.6 mg/kg in a single dose) have shown excellent results in relieving the symptoms of croup as early as 6 hours after treatment. Some authors have found doses of dexamethasone of 0.15 mg/kg in a single dose to be effective, but this low dose needs further evidence. Use of adrenaline (epinephrine) treatments, length of time spent in accident and emergency and inpatient stay in hospital, all have been reduced as a result of these treatments (Milner 1997; Ausejo *et al.* 1999; Ausejo Segura *et al.* 2001; Hay *et al.* 2001; Malhotra and Krilov 2001).

Dexamethasone is probably the drug of choice because of its safety, efficacy, and low cost. In a child who is vomiting nebulized budesonide or IM dexamethasone (0.6 mg/kg) would be preferable to oral dexamethasone.

Rarer causes of upper airways obstruction

Epiglottis is a medical emergency is usually produced by *Haemophylus influenzae* type B, although several other organisms (*Neisseria meningitidis, Streptococcus pneumonia, Streptococcus pyogenes, Staphylococcus aureus*), have been implicated. As a result of *H. influenza* immunization epiglottitis has been eradicated almost completely. Epiglottis usually affects children between 2 and 7 years; generating inflammation and swelling of the supraglottic area (epiglottis and arytenoids folds), compromising the upper airways, leading to a life-threatening obstruction. Symptoms, that usually develop over a few hours, consist of high fever, sore throat, muffled voice (rather than the 'hoarse' voice of the laryngotracheitis/bronchitis), inspiratory stridor, increasing anxiety, drooling, and difficulty swallowing. The child looks 'toxic' and unwell. This is a medical emergency; the child should be referred to hospital by ambulance. Intubation is mandatory showing the classical 'cherry red' epiglottis, and recovery is usually good. Antibiotics covering *H. influenza* (Cefotaxime, Ceftriaxone) should be administered IV.

Bacterial tracheitis is usually produced by *Staphylococcus aureus, Haemophilus influenzae* type b, and *Moxarella catarrhalis*. It is also called pseudomembranous croup, could be defined as a very severe form of laryngotracheitis/bronchitis; and probably is produced by superinfection of the mucosa of the trachea by the above-mentioned bacteria, after a primary viral illness (measles, croup).

This devastating illness should be suspected in the child with an upper respiratory tract infection who is deteriorating, and falling into respiratory failure due to airways obstruction. After few days of 'cold symptoms', the child can develop high fever, toxicity, croupy cough, and copious purulent secretions. Management is as for epiglottitis, adding an antibiotic to cover *Staphylococcus aureus*.

Diphtheria should be suspected in children coming from countries with poor vaccination programmes, presenting with sore throat, fever, hoarseness, and grey/white membranes in the pharynx and nasopharynx. Serosanguinous nasal discharge can be present. This is also a medical emergency; and the child has to be managed in an intensive care unit, with airways support, antibiotics, and antitoxin. Carriers should be identified and treated. Complications (myocarditis, pneumonia, polyneuritis) can arise.

The child with fits

The most common causes of fits in the child under 5 years of age are febrile convulsions, which are defined as convulsions occurring in children aged between 6 months and

5 years of age, associated with fever, in the absence of infection or metabolic disorder affecting the central nervous system, with no previous history of epilepsy, and no abnormality of the central nervous system. (American Academy of Pediatrics 1997). Febrile seizures have a prevalence rate between 2 and 4% being the commonest convulsive disorder in children below 5 years of age.

Types of febrile convulsions

There are two classes of febrile seizures:

- *Simple.* These happen in 70–80% of all cases; are generalized, tonic–clonic, last less than 15 minutes; and do not recur within 24 hours. These have an excellent prognosis, and the risk of developing epilepsy after suffering them is similar to that of the general population not suffering febrile seizures (Nelson and Ellenberg 1976; Verity and Golding 1991).

  - *Complex:*
  - a prolonged seizure lasting more that 15 minutes carried a risk of 3% of recurrent seizures
  - multiple seizures during the same episode of temperature (two or more occurrences within 24 hours of the initial febrile convulsion), has a risk of 4% of recurrent seizures
  - focal seizures rather than generalized, increased the risk of developing epilepsy at the age of 7 to 7% (Nelson and Ellenberg 1976).

The overall risk of developing epilepsy after febrile seizures (including 'simple' and 'complex' seizures), is about 3.4% (Verity and Golding 1991).

The great majority of febrile seizures are generalized (80%), and last less than 6 minutes. It is sometimes difficult to assess the duration of the fit with information from upset parents. Febrile seizures are often familial, and several chromosomes have been implicated: 8q13–21, 19p13.3, 19q13.1, 2q23–24, 5q14–q15 (Panayiotopoulos 2002). There is a fivefold increase in risk in children with parents or siblings with febrile seizures; and they are commoner in monozygotic, than in dizygotic twins.

DPT vaccine has been associated with an increased risk of febrile seizures only on the day of vaccination. Vaccination with MMR has been associated with an increased risk of febrile seizures 8–14 days after vaccination. However, these risks do not appear to be associated with any long-term adverse consequences (Barlow *et al.* 2001). Herpesvirus infection (exanthema subitum-roseola infantum) has also been associated with febrile seizures (Barone *et al.* 1995).

Key management points (Figure 3.2)

The focus of the temperature should be determined and the child observed. Although the overall risk of meningitis associated to febrile seizures is relatively low, it is advisable to have a very low threshold for fully investigating babies below 1 year of age, and being very cautious with children between 1 year and 18 months, or children who are on, or have very recently received antibiotics. In simple febrile seizures with an identified focus

FEBRILE SEIZURES

CRITERIA FOR DIAGNOSIS:
1.- 6 MONTHS TO 5 YEARS.
2.- FEBRILE DURING SEIZURE (Sometimes difficult to prove –try to get evidence).
3.- NOT KNOWN EPILEPTIC (NON FEBRILE SEIZURES).
4.- NOT KNOWN PREVIOUS CNS DISORDER.
5.- NOT KNOWN PREVIOUS METABOLIC DISORDER.
6.- ABSENCE OF CNS INFECTION AT THE MOMENT OF THE SEIZURE.
7.- NORMAL NEUROLOGICAL EXAM.

if above criteria are met, and is the first febrile seizure:

- ADMIT FOR OBSERVATION -

16% may experience a second febrile seizure within first 24 hours.

If it is a second or further febrile seizure,

- ADMIT IF IN DOUBT -

Or if it was accompanied by abnormal signs:
duration >15 min., Todd´s paralysis (0,4%), Focal seizure (4%),
slightest doubt of CNS or systemic infection.

PERFORM TESTS TO CLARIFY ORIGEN OF FEVER (FBC, CRP, MSU, CHEST XRAYS IF INDICATED)
REMEMBER: THERE IS NO EVIDENCE THAT UREA AND ELECTROLYTES, SKULL X RAYS, Ca++,
Mg++, BRAIN CT, BRAIN MRI, GLUCOSE -HELP IN DIAGNOSIS OR MANAGEMENT.

PERFORM THEM IF IN DOUBT, BUT PROBABLY AT THIS POINT YOUR DIAGNOSIS IS NOT FEBRILE
SEIZURE.

IF CHILD IS < 1 YEAR, **STRONGLY CONSIDER LUMBAR PUNCTURE, EVEN IN ABSENCE OF MENINGEAL SIGNS.**

CONSIDER IT TOO IN CHILDREN BETWEEN 1 AND 1 ? YEARS, AND IN CHILDREN WHO HAVE RECEIVED PREVIOUSLY ANTIBIOTICS.

NO NEED FOR Ct (IMAGING), UNLESS INDICATED FOR OTHER REASONS (focal seizure –haemiplegia). Trust clinical findings for raised intracranial pressure (posturing, raised BP, papilloedema {can not be present in early stages}).

IF ANY MINOR CHANGE IN CSF COMPATIBLE WITH MENINGITIS, **TREAT** UNTIL CULTURES ARE BACK.

TAKE BLOOD CULTURE, PCR, GRAM STAIN, AND IF POSSIBLE BACTERIAL ANTIGENS for IDENTIFICATION IN CSF OR IN BLOOD.

FINAL DIAGNOSIS WAS **SIMPLE FEBRILE SEIZURE (UNCOMPLICATED?)** . DISCHARGE -
REASSURE THE PARENTS-Mention 30-50% possibility of recurrence (young age of onset , family history, short duration of fever before the initial seizure, relative low fever at the time of initial seizure.
NO NEED FOR EEG.
NO NEED FOR ANTICONVULSANTS.

Fig. 3.2 Management of febrile seizures.

for the temperature, there is no need to do further investigations such as electrolytes, imaging, and EEG. These are reserved for complex cases, or when there is doubt about other pathology; and in that case probably the diagnosis is not that of a febrile seizure. The risk of having a second febrile convulsion, is about 50% in a child younger than 12 months; and 30% in a child older than 12 months. Those who have a second febrile seizure, have a chance of 50% of having one or more recurrences in the future (Nelson and Ellenberg 1978). Neither continuous nor intermittent anticonvulsant therapy is recommended for children with one or more simple febrile seizures (American Academy of Pediatrics 1999). Antipyretics, although they may improve the comfort of the child, will not prevent febrile seizures. All other children with afebrile convulsions will require a more detailed work-up to determine the cause of the fit (refer to Chapter 19).

Conclusions

In this chapter we have described a model of care for the acutely ill child within the context of a holistic continuum of care for all children. To illustrate the type of emergency care that can be provided we have chosen four common conditions that present to the general practitioner. The close collaboration between primary and secondary care will result in all children receiving a high-quality service appropriate to their needs.

References & Further Reading
Models of service provision

Arnon K, Stephenson T, Gabriel V, Macphaul R, Eccleston P, Werneke U, Smith S (2001). Determining the common medical presenting problems to an accident and emergency department. *Archives of Diseases in Childhood* **84**: 290–292.

Browne GJ (2000). Short stay or 23-hour ward in a general and academic children's hospital: are they effective? *Pediatric Emergency Care* **16**(4): 223–229.

Haggerty RJ, Green M (2003). History of academic general and ambulatory pediatrics. *Pediatric Research* **53**: 188–197.

Heller DR (1994). Ambulatory paediatrics: stepping out in a new direction? *Archives of Diseases in Childhood* **70**: 339–342.

Marks MK, Baskin MN, Lovejoy FH Jr, Hafler JP (1997). Intern learning and education in a short stay unit. A qualitative study. *Archives Pediatric and Adolescent Medicine* **151**(2): 193–198.

Meates M (1997). Ambulatory care—making a difference. *Archives of Diseases in Childhood* **76**: 468–476.

Numa A, Oberklaid F (1991). Can short stay hospital admissions be avoided; a review of admissions less than 24 hours' duration in a paediatric teaching hospital. *Medical Journal of Australia* **155**: 395–398.

Scribano PV, Wiley JF 2nd, Platt K (2001). Use of an observation unit by a pediatric emergency department for common pediatric illnesses. *Pediatric Emergency Care* **17**(5): 321–323.

Shah C, Shahab R, Robb P, Roy D (2001). Role of a home care team in paediatric day-case tonsillectomy. *Journal of Laryngol Otology* (1): 39–43.

Vomiting

Silverman A, Roy CC (eds) (1983). *Paediatric Clinical Gastroenterology* (3rd edn). CV Mosby.

Sondheimer J (1996). Vomiting and regurgitation. In: *Paediatric Gastrointestinal Disease*. CV Mosby, St Louis.

Crying infant

Corwin MJ, Lester BM, Golub HL (1996). The infant cry: what can it tell us? *Current Problems in Pediatrics* **26**(a): 325–334.

Poole SR (1991). The infant with acute unexplained excessive crying. *Paediatrics* **88**(3): 450–455.

Upper airways obstruction

Ausejo M, Saenz A, Pham B., Kellner JD, Johnson DW, Moher D, Klassen TP (1999). The effectiveness of glucocorticoids in treating croup: meta-analysis. *British Medical Journal* **319**: 595–600.

Ausejo Segura M, Saenz A, Pham B *et al* (2003). Glucocorticoids in croup (Cochrane review). *The Cochrane Library*, issue 4. John Wiley & Sons, Ltd, Chichester.

Behrman RE, Kliegman RM (2004). *Nelson: Textbook of Pediatrics*, (17th edn). Saunders-Elsevier Science, p. 1407. Pennsylvania.

Denny FW, Murphy TF, Clyde WA, Collier AM, Henderson FW (1983). Croup. An 11 year study in a pediatric practice. *Pediatrics* **71**: 871–876.

Hay WW, Hayward AR, Levin MJ, Sondheimer J (2001). *Current Pediatric Diagnosis and Treatment*, (15th edn). McGraw-Hill, New York, p. 435.

Malhotra A, Krilov L (2001). Viral croup. *Pediatrics in Review* **22**: 5–11.

Milner AD (1997). The role of corticosteroids in bronchiolitis and croup. *Thorax*; **52**, 595–597.

Neto G, Kentab O, Klassen TP (2002). A randomised controlled trial of mist in the acute treatment of moderate croup. *Academic Emergency Medicine* **9**: 873–879.

Osmond M (2001). Croup. *Clinical Evidence* issue No. 6: 269.

Royal College of Paediatrics and Child Health (2003). *Medicines for Children*, (2nd edn). London.

Schwartz MW (1999). *Clinical Handbook of Pediatrics*, (2nd edn). Williams & Wilkins, Baltimore, p. 586.

Taussig LM, Castro O, Beaudry PH, Fox W, Bureau M (1975). Treatment of laryngotracheobronchitis (croup). *American Journal of Disease of Children* **129**: 790–793.

Waisman Y, Klein BL, Boenning DA, Young GM, Chamberlain JM, O'Donnell R, Ochsenschlager DW (1992). Prospective randomized controlled study comparing L-epinephrine and racemic epinephrine aerosols in the treatment of laryngotracheitis (croup). *Pediatrics* **89**: 302–306.

Westley CR, Cotton EK, Brooks JG (1978). Nebulised racemic epinephrine by IPPB for the treatment of croup. *American Journal of Disease of Children* **132**: 484–487.

Wright RB, Pomerantz W, Luria WJ (2002). New approaches to respiratory infections in children. Bronchiolitis and croup. *Emergency Medicine Clinics of North America* **20**(3): 93–115.

Convulsions

American Academy of Pediatrics (1997). Provisional Committee on Quality Improvement: Practice parameters from the American Academy of Pediatrics. *A Compilation of Evidence Based Guidelines for Pediatric Practice*, p. 71.

American Academy of Pediatrics (1999). Committee on Quality Improvement, Subcommittee on Febrile Seizures. Practice parameter: long-term treatment of the child with simple febrile seizures. *Pediatrics* **103**: 1307–1306.

Barlow WE, Davis RL, Glasser JW, *et al* (2001). The risk of seizures after receipt of whole cell pertussis or measles, mumps and rubella vaccine. *New England Journal of Medicine* **345**: 656–661.

Barone SR, Kaplan MH, Krilov LR (1995). Human herpesvirus-6 infection in children with first febrile seizure. *Journal of Pediatrics* **127**: 95–97.

Nelson KB, Ellenberg JH (1976). Predictors of epilepsy in children who have experienced febrile seizures. *New England Journal of Medicine* **295**: 1029–1033.

Nelson KB, Ellenberg JH (1978). Prognosis in children with febrile seizures. *Pediatrics* **61**: 720–727.

Offringa M, Moyer VA (2001). Evidence based management of seizures associated with fever. *British Medical Journal* **323**: 1111–1114.

Panayiotopoulos CP (2002). *A Clinical Guide to Epileptic Syndromes and their Treatment*. Blandon Medical Publishers, Oxford pp. 50–53.

Verity CM, Golding J (1991). Risk of epilepsy after febrile convulsions: a national cohort study. *British Medical Journal* **303**: 1373–1376.

Chapter 4

Respiratory problems

Jeremy Hull

Respiratory infections and wheezing illnesses in children are very common. Most are easy to recognize and simple to treat. A small proportion are more serious, and can be life-threatening in the acute phase, such as a child with severe croup, or can indicate an underlying problem, such as cystic fibrosis (CF). In this short chapter, I have considered an approach to common respiratory symptoms: wheeze, breathlessness, cough, and stridor, as well as to the more specific problems of the primary care management of a child CF and an infant with apnoea.

Wheeze

Wheeze is a whistling noise loudest in expiration. Its presence implies narrowing of the small airways. In children this is nearly always caused by either bronchospasm or inflammation or a combination of both. In infants, the majority of wheezing illness will be caused by viral respiratory infections. In older children, an increasing proportion will have atopic asthma. The term asthma can reasonably applied to both groups of children, as the same treatments are used, although they are often less effective in the very young. A very small proportion of children who develop wheeze will have other diseases, including CF and congenital lung abnormalities. These rare causes will not be considered further in this section.

Patterns of wheeze

Wheezing can be most usefully categorized according to its frequency. **Infrequent episodic wheeze** can be defined as episodes of wheezing lasting for a few days, occurring not more often than once per month, between which the child is completely well. **Frequent episodic wheeze** describes episodes that occur more frequently than this, but between which the child is still completely well, and **persistent wheeze** is defined as a child who has wheeze on most days.

Clinical assessment

The history should establish the pattern of wheeze. Useful questions to assess impact of wheeze on the child include those that determine the presence of **nocturnal symptoms**, the ability to **exercise,** and in older children, **school attendance**. A dry cough often accompanies wheeze and should be noted. Cough in the absence of wheeze is very unlikely to be asthma. If the child is currently taking medication, close attention to assessing compliance and the use of an appropriate delivery device, such as a large volume valved holding chamber, is essential. It is useful to identify any obvious precipitants, including dust, pollen, grasses, cats, dogs, horses, foods, and fizzy drinks. These precipitants can be avoided, and should be, if they are contributing to the child symptoms. The most common precipitants, however, are viral infections and exercise. The first of these cannot be avoided. Exercise should be encouraged, and the use of pre-exercise bronchodilators should be recommended. In general, tests of specific allergies, such as skin prick tests or RAST tests, are not helpful in the management of asthma, unless there is a particular precipitant the family have identified and wish to confirm.

Treatment

Infants with wheeze generally respond poorly to bronchodilators and steroids. This is most likely because viral-induced inflammation is the predominant cause of airways narrowing. The difficulty in effectively delivering these drugs to small children also contributes to the poor response. In infants over 6 months of age with persistent wheeze it is worth trying inhaled bronchodilators and inhaled steroids but with a low expectation of success. In older children, appropriate levels of treatment can be determined by the pattern of wheeze. Infrequent episodic wheeze needs to be treated only with inhaled bronchodilators as required. Frequent episodic wheeze should be treated with a prophylactic drug such as a leukotriene receptor antagonist, sodium cromoglycate, or more usually inhaled steroids. Persistent wheeze is best treated with inhaled steroids. The British Thoracic Guidelines on the management of asthma in children should be followed.

Outcome

Most infant wheeze does not progress into childhood atopic asthma, and most children with infrequent episodic wheeze before the age of 3 years will not be wheezing by the age of 6 years. Children with more persistent symptoms are likely to be those who continue to wheeze, particularly if there is a family history of atopic disease.

Who should be referred to hospital?

During an acute exacerbation children who fail to respond (that is, they remain very breathless with chest wall recession) after 10–20 puffs of beta-2 agonist via spacer device, or who are needing this level of treatment more often than every 4 hours should be sent to the local hospital emergency department.

In the outpatient setting, referral should be made for children apparently needing high-dose inhaled steroids (more than 600 μg/day) to maintain control, and for children who are on lower doses but with poor control. The outpatient visit provides an opportunity to review the diagnosis, to consider exacerbating factors, to review compliance and inhaler technique, and to consider changes in medication. Children with atypical symptoms should also be referred.

Breathlessness

The appearance of breathlessness can be caused by either an increased respiratory rate or an increased work of breathing, which is usually observed as chest wall recession, and in

Table 4.1 Causes of breathlessness

Cause	Incidence	Clues from history or examination
Infant		
Bronchiolitis	Common	Winter months; crackles on auscultation
Viral-associated wheeze	Common	Wheeze but no crackles
Heart failure	Uncommon	Big liver, heart murmur
Older child		
Asthma	Common	Wheeze
Croup	Common	Stridor, barking cough
Viral pneumonia	Common	Fever, some chest recession. Wheeze and or crackles
Bacterial pneumonia	Uncommon	Fever, chest pain, tachypnoea but no recession
Being unfit	Common	Breathless on exertion only

infants by head-bobbing. In older children breathlessness results in reduced exercise tolerance. In infants the most obvious effect is difficulty in feeding. Common causes of breathlessness are shown in Table 4.1. Asthma, heart failure, and croup are dealt with elsewhere.

Bronchiolitis

In the winter months infants who develop breathlessness are most likely to have a viral respiratory tract infection. Bronchiolitis is a clinical diagnosis based on the presence of an increased respiratory rate, chest wall recession, and the presence of inspiratory crackles on auscultation. Wheezes and fever are also frequently present. **The presence of recession at rest should prompt a referral to hospital.** Occasionally an infant may not have recession but is sufficiently breathless to be unable to feed and this would also be an indication for referral. Particularly care needs to be taken with infants under 1 month of age and infants who were born prematurely, as this group of children have an increased risk of central apnoea associated with bronchiolitis infections. In milder cases, advice to take smaller amounts of fluids more frequently, and regular oral paracetamol may help.

Pneumonia

Children with pneumonia typically present with fever, cough, and breathlessness. Viral pneumonia or mixed viral and bacterial infections are more common than lobar bacterial pneumonia, particularly in pre-school children. Clues to a viral aetiology are the presence of bilateral crackles and the presence of wheeze. Wheeze is almost never caused by a bacterial pneumonia. Both viral and bacterial pneumonias are frequently preceded by a history of an upper respiratory tract infection. Older children with bacterial pneumonia may well be tachypnoeic, but often will not have chest recession. Bronchial breathing on physical examination may be hard to detect, and the diagnosis of lobar pneumonia frequently requires a chest radiograph. Having said that, the British Thoracic society guidelines on community acquired pneumonia suggest that chest radiography should not be performed on children with signs of mild uncomplicated lower respiratory tract infection, as the radiograph is a poor indicator of aetiology. Occasionally children with right lower lobe pneumonia will present with abdominal pain because of irritation to the diaphragm, and in an unwell febrile child this may be misdiagnosed as appendicitis.

There is no specific treatment available for viral pneumonia. Bacterial pneumonias are predominantly caused by *Streptococcus pneumoniae* in all age groups. Amoxycillin remains the first line treatment for this infection. Referral to hospital should be made for all children suspected of having pneumonia if they have in addition noticeable difficulty with breathing, signs of dehydration, or difficulty feeding.

Chronic cough

All children will develop a cough several times a year. The vast majority of coughs will be caused by viral respiratory tract infection. In a smaller proportion the cough will persist. If it is present on a daily basis for more than 3 months, a cause should be sought. For this purpose, it is useful to divide the coughs into those that are dry, and those that sound productive. To some extent this is a matter of judgement, particularly as children under the age of 6 years are unlikely to expectorate sputum even when it is present. The common causes of dry and productive persistent cough are shown in Table 4.2.

Productive sounding coughs

The most important diagnosis to consider in this group of children is CF. **Any child who has a daily productive-sounding cough for more than 3 months should be referred for investigation**. If the history is otherwise unremarkable and the physical examination and chest radiograph are normal, it is reasonable to make a working diagnosis of bronchitis.

Table 4.2 Causes of persistent cough

Cause	Incidence	Clues from history or examination
Productive-sounding		
Bronchitis	Common	Follows a cold. Well child
Cystic fibrosis	Rare	Poor weight gain, abnormal stools
Immune deficiency	Rare	Infections at other sites
Primary cilial dyskinesia	Rare	Recurrent otitis media
Aspirated foreign body	Uncommon	History of choking
Dry		
Asthma	Common	Associated with wheeze
Non-specific post-viral	Common	Intermittent. Well child
Pertussis	Uncommon	Typical paroxysms, usually school age child
Habit	Uncommon	Honking in nature, usually school age children
Gastro-oesophageal reflux	Uncommon	Worse lying flat; waterbrash
Tracheomalacia	Uncommon	Loud cough, worse with colds. Usually pre-school children

If there are any abnormalities, or treatment for bronchitis fails to cure the cough (see below), further investigation, including a sweat test, cilial biopsy, and tests of immune function should be performed.

Bronchitis

Although there is little to be found about this diagnosis in most paediatric respiratory textbooks, bronchitis (chronic endobronchial inflammation) is the commonest cause of chronic productive-sounding cough in our clinic population. It most usually follows an acute viral respiratory tract infection. The cough fails to resolve and is probably exacerbated by further viral and bacterial infection. The bacterial infections are low grade, and limited to the airways mucosa. Repeated infection results in persistent mucus secretion, perpetuating both the cough and the risk of subsequent infection. A prolonged (6-week) course of antibiotics combined with chest physiotherapy is usually sufficient to break the cycle. Once the chest is dry, symptoms resolve. These children have a normal physical examination and a normal chest radiograph.

Aspirated foreign body

This is most likely to cause diagnostic difficulties in pre-school children. The most important part of the assessment is a good history. If the parents report a clear episode of choking, followed by persistent coughing for several minutes, then referral for further investigation is indicated, even if the child subsequently appears well and physical examination is normal. Children in whom this diagnosis is missed may subsequently present with an acute complicated pneumonia, with the risk of destruction of lung tissue, or with chronic productive-sounding cough.

Dry coughs

If a dry cough is associated with polyphonic wheezing, it is most likely due to asthma. On the other hand, **asthma is rarely the cause of an isolated dry cough**, and other causes should be considered. The commonest of these are post-viral and post-pertussis like coughs. These children are otherwise well and their coughs will eventually resolve spontaneously. If these children are treated with inhaled steroids, there will be no immediate benefit, sometimes leading to an increase in the prescribed dose. If the cough subsequently improves, there may then be a temptation to ascribe this to the inhaled steroid, and maintain the dose, with the consequent risk of steroid side-effects. **If a trial of inhaled steroids is used for dry cough, it should be for no longer than 6 weeks**, and no dose escalation should be used. If there is no response, seek an alternative diagnosis.

Stridor

Stridor is the name given to the noise caused by turbulent airflow in the trachea. It arises because of a narrowed tracheal lumen. It is most usually inspiratory, but can be biphasic depending on the location and severity of the narrowing. The common causes of stridor are shown in Table 4.3. Stridor starting soon after birth is most likely to be laryngomalacia, and acute stridor in pre-school children is most likely to be croup.

Table 4.3 Causes of stridor

Cause	Incidence	Clues from history or examination
Chronic		
Laryngomalacia	Common	Present from birth, characteristic stridor
Subglottic stenosis	Uncommon	May be ex-preterm, often biphasic stridor
Tracheal haemangioma	Rare	Often have facial haemangioma
Vascular ring	Rare	Low pitched biphasic stridor. Often just noisy breathing
Acute		
Croup	Common	Pre-school child, barking cough, systemically well
Epiglottitis	Rare	High fever, systemically unwell

Laryngomalacia

This is a common condition affecting about 1% of all babies. It arises because the cartilage supporting the tissue above the tracheal in the larynx is softer than normal, allowing the tissue to prolapse into the tracheal opening on inspiration. It is nearly always a benign condition, whose natural history is one of gradual improvement. Occasionally, the work of breathing required to overcome the upper airways obstruction is sufficient to prevent normal growth and in these infants intervention may be required.

The stridor of laryngomalacia has characteristic qualities. It starts soon after birth, but may not be present in the first few days. It is purely inspiratory. **The presence of an expiratory component of any stridor indicates a fixed narrowing of the trachea and always requires investigation**. On each inspiration the stridor of laryngomalacia has a crescendo quality, increasing in pitch towards the end of inspiration. It can also be staccato in nature, and is frequently variable in loudness and severity. It is almost always absent during sleep.

The severity of any stridor should be judged by the degree of chest wall recession on inspiration, which reflects the amount of work the infant has to do to overcome the obstruction. Infants with mild laryngomalacia will have mild or absent chest wall recession most of the time, with only more marked recession occurring when they are crying. It is usually unnecessary to investigate these infants further. If there is persistent marked chest recession, referral for a specialist opinion is indicated. Careful monitoring of the infant's growth is also an important guide to severity. Infants who are not growing well should also be referred. The stridor from laryngomalacia may get louder as the infant grows and tidal volumes increase. The vast majority will resolve by 18 months of age.

Croup

Croup is a viral infection of the larynx, trachea, and main bronchi. It most usually affects pre-school children. The viral infection causes swelling of the mucosa lining the large airways and consequently narrows the airways lumen. In older children as the trachea grows, the effects of the swelling have proportionately less impact on tracheal diameter.

Usually croup starts with a mild upper respiratory tract infection and a runny nose. Subsequently, a characteristic barking cough develops, and for reasons that are not understood, this typically occurs at night. In a small proportion of children more signifi-cant tracheal narrowing occurs and stridor develops. **Any child with stridor at rest, par-ticularly if it is associated with chest wall recession, should be referred to the nearest emergency department**. Traditional remedies, including the use of steam, are ineffective. Given the potential for steam to cause accidental burns, it is inappropriate to suggest that parents try this therapy. It is essential to avoid distressing children with severe croup, as crying will worsen the obstruction. Throat examination should be avoided. Oxygen should be given and urgent transfer to hospital, via ambulance, should be arranged.

Some children develop recurrent croup. These children may be normal and probably have slightly smaller tracheas that the general population, or there may be an important underlying problem, such as a vascular ring. The most important facts to determine are whether or not the child has any stridor or noisy breathing between episodes of croup, particularly during exercise. If there are no interval symptoms, then further investigation is not required.

Apnoea in infants

Nearly all parents are aware of the phenomenon of cot death. When a parent witnesses an event in which they believe their baby has stopped breathing, it is understandable that this generates considerable anxiety. It is essential that these events are taken seriously by healthcare practitioners and that parental concerns are addressed fully.

Definitions

The term apnoea refers to the temporary cessation of breathing from whatever cause. They are relatively frequent events in infants, where there is immaturity of respiratory control. This can be particularly marked in babies who were born prematurely. Apnoeas can be obstructive, when there is continued respiratory effort but absent or inadequate airflow, or central, when there is no respiratory effort. Apnoeas longer than 15–20 seconds, or those associated with colour change or floppiness, are unusual and require further investigation.

Causes

Apnoea can be a non-specific response by an infant who is generally unwell. The list of potential causes is correspondingly large. The common and important causes are given in the table. Feeding associated events, or those associated with gastro-oesophageal reflux are by far the most common in otherwise well infants. Occasionally parents may be con-cerned by normal periodic breathing that many young infants have during sleep. This is a normal phenomenon and these parents can be reassured.

Approach

It is essential to get a full and detailed history of the event. This must include what the baby was doing beforehand (especially in relation to feeding), whether the baby was awake or asleep, what position the baby was in, what alerted the carer that something was going on, exactly the appearance of the baby (including whether they were responsive, the presence of any vomitus, any abnormal movements, and the baby's colour and tone), what the carer did, and how long it took for the baby to recover. Other details, including gestation and recent health are also vital.

Examination of the baby is often normal, but particular attention to the baby's responsiveness and tone is important. A careful and thorough physical examination looking for other signs of ill-health is essential. All infants who have had an apnoea event should be referred to hospital for assessment, apart from the occasional older infant who has had a clear episode of choking on milk, when simple reassurance is all that is necessary. Investigation of babies who have had apnoeic events will depend on the nature of the event, and may well turn out to be normal. Apnoea events are often frightening for the parents. Some parents believe that their baby is dying. Severe events (with colour change, limpness, and unresponsiveness) are called Apparent Life Threatening Events (ALTEs). Even for these severe events, causes can generally only to be found in about 60%.

Outcome

If no abnormality is found after investigation, the infant's outcome is not predictable. The potential relation between ALTE and sudden infant death syndrome (SIDS) is still unclear, and although ALTEs have been reported in up to 10% for infants who subsequently died from SIDS, the number of ALTE not followed by SIDS is unknown. Thus there can be no certainty that ALTE is a risk factor for SIDS. Home monitoring is not an exact science. SIDS may not be preventable by home monitoring, and deaths have been reported despite the use of monitors. Most simple monitors detect movement rather than breathing, and so will not detect obstructive events, which may precede a terminal central apnoea. The decision to instigate monitoring is a personal one, and may be driven by parental choice. Whether or not monitoring is used, all families should receive frequent help and support. Before leaving hospital, parents of infants who have had an ALTE will be shown how to carry out basic life support suitable for infants.

Cystic fibrosis

CF is an autosomal recessive disease, with an incidence of about 1 in 2500 live births. A general practice serving 10 000 people is likely to have one child with CF on their books. The life expectancy of this severe disease continues to improve and median survival is currently about 34 years. We would expect most children with CF to have normal growth and development and to have only intermittent problems with their chest. Most children will reach adulthood with at least 70% of normal lung function. Others, despite aggressive management, will have more severe disease, and some of these will die before the age of 18 years.

Presentation

About 10% of children with CF will present with neonatal bowel obstruction. The diagnosis in these children is usually straightforward. Thereafter the usual presentation is one

Table 4.4 Causes of apnoea

Cause	Incidence	Type of apnoea	Clues from history or examination
Periodic breathing/delayed maturational control	Common	Central	Preterm baby Under 3 months of age
Laryngeal spasm, + gastrooesophageal reflux	Common	Initially obstructive, may become central	Relationship to feeds History of small vomits
Respiratory infection (especially RSV and pertussis)	Common	Mixed	Coryzal symptoms/cough
Seizure	Uncommon	Usually central but may be mixed	Family history of epilepsy Developmental delay Big head
Occult sepsis e.g. UTI or meningitis	Uncommon	Central	Fever, raised WCC, CRP
CNS structural anomaly (e.g. Arnold Chiari)	Rare	Obstructive or central	
Metabolic disease	Rare	Usually central	Often systemically unwell Acidosis Family history of SIDS
Severe muscular weakness (e.g. SMA type I)	Rare	Mixed	Generalized weakness/floppiness
Central alveolar hypoventilation syndrome	Rare	Central	Usually in first few months Worse during sleep
Smothering (Munchausen syndrome by proxy)	Rare	Obstructive then central	Mother may have odd affect Family history of SIDS

of recurrent respiratory infections, or a respiratory infection which is particularly severe and prolonged. These children will usually also have frequent pale offensive loose stools, and poor growth. The symptoms are usually sufficiently severe to result in diagnosis within the first year of life. A small proportion of patients with CF will have mild disease and present in later childhood, and occasionally even in an adult life.

Management

Routine management of CF is relatively straightforward in principle. The lungs are normal at birth and become damaged by recurrent infection. It is therefore essential that these infections are detected early and treated vigorously. The infections affect only the airways lining and therefore do not cause any symptoms other than cough, and most **frequently there are no abnormal physical findings**. Damaging airways infections can also be asymptomatic. Children with CF will attend the local hospital clinic every 2–3 months. This visit will always include taking a pharyngeal swab after coughing (a so-called cough-swab), which provides a sensitive way of assessing the presence of airways infection. All infections detected by cough-swab culture should be treated with **a minimum 2-week course of antibiotics**. Children who develop a cough, or whose regular cough worsens, should also receive a minimum 2-week course of antibiotics even in the absence of a positive cough-swab. The relatively long duration of the antibiotic courses reflects the difficulty of clearing infections from the CF lung. The range of pathogens that infect the airways in children with CF is limited, and will usually be either *Staphylococcus aureus*, *Haemophilus influenzae*, or *Pseudomonas aeruginosa*. Some children are given long-term prophylactic antibiotics, which may be oral, such as flucloxacillin in the first year of life, or inhaled, such as colomycin or tobramycin for persistent infection with *Pseudomonas aeruginosa*. A useful rule of thumb for managing CF chest problems is, if in doubt, treat with a prolonged course of antibiotics. The other mainstay of the management of chest disease is daily physiotherapy, which is undertaken by the parents. All children with CF should receive annual influenza vaccination. It is particularly important that children with CF, like others with chronic respiratory problems, receive routine immunization with the new conjugate pneumococcal vaccines. After the age of 2 years they should also be given a single immunization with Pneumovax which covers a large number of pneumococcal serotypes than the conjugate vaccines.

Malabsorption in CF is caused by pancreatic insufficiency. This is dealt with by using pancreatic enzyme supplements that the child must take with every meal. In addition the child must receive supplements of the fat soluble vitamins A, D, and E, and increasingly vitamin K as well. Children with CF need to have a high-calorie high-fat diet to maintain normal growth.

The care of the child with CF, even when they are well, places additional strains on family life. These need to be recognized. The family are eligible to receive disability living allowance and invalid care allowance and should receive help in obtaining these financial supplements.

Newborn screening

Newborn screening for CF was introduced nationally in June 2006. The initial part of the screening test measures immunereactive trypsin (IRT) on blood from the heel prick tests already used for screening other childhood diseases. If this level is above 99.5th centile for the population, then a DNA analysis for CF mutations will be carried out, if necessary followed either by a repeat IRT measurement or by a sweat test. It is important to realize that this screening test will fail to detect about 5% of children with CF and clinical awareness of the manner in which this important disease might present will need to be maintained.

Further Reading

British Thoracic Society Guideline on the Management of Asthma: http://www.brit-thoracic.org.uk/sign/index.html

British Thoracic Society Guidelines for the Management of Community Acquired Pneumonia in Childhood: http://www.brit-thoracic.org.uk/docs/paediatriccap.pdf

Cystic Fibrosis Trust: Standards of Care document (including a section of the role of the General Practitioner): http://www.cftrust.org.uk

Silverman M (ed.) (2002). *Childhood Asthma and Other Wheezing Disorders*. Edward Arnold, London.

Chapter 5

Common renal problems

Stephen Marks and Richard Trompeter

Introduction

The aim of this chapter is to concentrate on the range of clinical renal problems that may present to a primary care physician. We will not concentrate on severe childhood renal disease as this is relatively rare and paediatric nephrologists and general paediatricians with an interest in nephrology manage these children. This chapter will deal with the initial management of children with renal disease.

The chapter initially focuses on urinary dipstick abnormalities on screening with evaluation of children who present with proteinuria and/or haematuria. The diagnosis, management, treatment, and investigation of children presenting with urinary tract infections (UTI) continues to prove to be a contentious issue in the twenty-first century. The clinical evaluation of children with nephrotic syndrome (NS) or acute glomerulonephritis will be discussed and the postnatal management after antenatal diagnosis of hydronephrosis will be debated.

Urinary dipstick screening

Many primary care physicians now undertake routine urine dipstick testing when patients join their practice. Some are now extending this to screen all children. This chapter is intended to help the physician in knowing when abnormal urinary dipstick tests should be referred for further investigations. All children with abnormal urine dipstick tests should have family members also tested and ensure that there is no family history of hypertension, renal failure, dialysis, or transplantation.

Proteinuria

- If isolated proteinuria is detected on urinary dipstick testing and is negative on two subsequent occasions then insignificant, transient proteinuria is likely.

- However, if persistent proteinuria exists then orthostatic proteinuria should be considered. This is when consecutive first morning urine samples obtained immediately on rising show either negative or trace of proteinuria on dipstick testing. Orthostatic proteinuria can be a normal phenomenon found in 3—5% of all adolescents and is more precisely excluded by measurement of urine protein excretion in a timed supine overnight urine collection. The maximum normal urine protein excretion is 4 mg/m^2

per hour or 100 mg/m^2 per day with a urine protein/creatinine ratio of 20 mg/mmol. Note that a child with NS has 10 times this level of proteinuria.

◆ If the proteinuria is significant and non-orthostatic, then this necessitates referral to delineate if the proteinuria is of glomerular or tubular origin. Proteinuria due to tubular dysfunction is associated with elevated tubular proteins, glycosuria, aminoaciduria, impaired urine concentration and hypophosphataemia.

Haematuria

◆ Haematuria is defined as the presence of five or more red blood cells (RBCs) per high-power field in all of three consecutive centrifuged specimens obtained at least 1 week apart.

◆ Haematuria may be microscopic, macroscopic, occur on its own or be associated with proteinuria.

◆ Causes of haematuria are:
  • glomerular (glomerulonephritis, benign familial haematuria, hereditary nephropathy (eg. Alport syndrome, which is associated with deafness)).
  • non-glomerular (UTI, urolithiasis, polycystic disease, trauma, menstruation).

◆ In cases of microscopic haematuria, urine sediment microscopy should be undertaken to detect red blood cells and their morphology on phase contrast microscopy as false positives may occur on urinary dipstick testing.

◆ Microscopic haematuria *without* proteinuria or a family history is not suggestive of significant renal disease.

◆ Macroscopic haematuria is more likely to be associated with significant underlying problems (including the possibility of coagulation defects).

◆ Macroscopic haematuria without proteinuria can also be caused by glomerulonephritis (including post-infectious and lupus nephritis), bleeding from the urethra or bladder, papillary necrosis, sickle cell disease, arteriovenous fistula, renal venous thromboses, IgA nephropathy, and bacterial endocarditis.

Urinary tract infections

Childhood UTI represent a significant diagnostic and management challenge. Between 2 and 10% of infants and young children aged between 2 months and 2 years of age will present with an unexplained fever as a result of a UTI. The short-term goals in the management of UTI are to correctly make the diagnosis (which can be difficult not only in the primary care setting, but also in the hospital environment) with early institution of treatment to prevent complications. As symptoms of UTI in small children may be nonspecific, there should always be a low threshold for the investigation to exclude UTI in a febrile child and differentiate between upper and lower UTI. This should always include urine microscopy, culture, and sensitivity because of the risks of false negative results with urinary dipstick tests (including urine nitrites and white cells). Younger children (especially those under 4 years of age) are more likely to have renal damage secondary to vesico-ureteric reflux of infected urine into the upper tracts. It is this group of children for whom a high index of suspicion is required. Unfortunately there is more difficulty in obtaining an appropriate urine sample in this age group.

The long-term goals are to identify those patients in whom we can prevent the complications of chronic renal failure, hypertension, and problems in pregnancy. The main objectives are to identify those children with renal malformations, renal damage, and vesico-ureteric reflux.

The most susceptible groups of children are those in the following categories:

- age 1 year
- recurrent UTI
- bacteraemia
- UTI due to unusual organisms (such as those organisms that are not derived from bowel flora)
- those with clinical signs (including palpable kidneys and poor urinary stream)
- those with a slow response to treatment.

Diagnosis

- Childhood UTI is diagnosed with a pure growth $>10^5$/ml from an uncontaminated specimen of urine, which is sent immediately to the microbiology laboratory.
- Neonates with UTI may only present with prolonged jaundice, septicaemia, poor feeding, pyrexia, or weight loss.
- Non-specific symptoms in infants may include fever, poor feeding, failure to thrive, vomiting, diarrhoea, and irritability.
- Older children are more likely to have urinary symptoms with dysuria, macroscopic haematuria, frequency, urgency, and incontinence.
- Pyelonephritis is suggested in systemically unwell children with pyrexia and loin pain.
- Delay in diagnosis of a UTI should always be avoided in clinical practice with urine culture specimens taken at the earliest opportunity and hopefully prior to the commencement of antibiotics (unless in the case of a very sick child). These specimens can be difficult to obtain and in hospital practice the gold standard of suprapubic aspiration or catheter specimen of urine is not usually employed if uncontaminated specimens are obtained by other techniques and submitted to the microbiology laboratory with minimum delay for microscopy, culture, and sensitivity.
- Urine can be collected in primary care by midstream specimen of urine (MSSU), clean catch urine samples, sterile nappy pads, or with bag urine collections. MSSU samples should always be obtained where possible, but is usually only achievable in older, continent children. There should be no specific cleaning prior to micturition into a sterile container (which can be placed in a potty). If waiting for a clean catch urine sample, then it is imperative that the penis does not rest in the sterile pot prior to collection.

Sterile nappy pads can be used to collect urine in children who are still in nappies as long as the sample is obtained shortly after micturition. The sterile pad is inserted in a nappy, which is turned inside out (to prevent absorption of the urine). Bag urine collections are very convenient but there is a higher false positive rate, which is why the urine bags should not be in place for more than 4 hours (ideally less than 2 hours). The external genitalia should be cleaned prior to the placement of the sterile urine bag, which has a valve mechanism preventing regaining contact with the perineum.

Treatment (Table 5.1)

- Early and adequate treatment of UTI in children is essential with effective antibiotic treatment for at least 7 days.
- *Escherichia coli* and other bowel flora are the commonest cause of childhood UTI with less resistant organisms encountered in primary care, although the sensitivity pattern of the pure growth of organism should always be checked.
- All unwell children should be referred to hospital as the requirement for intravenous antibiotics and high fluid intake is essential in neonates, infants and those with pyelonephritis and/or septicaemia (assuming normal renal function).
- Any child in whom clinical recovery is slow or eradication of the organism on repeated culture has not occurred should be referred for another opinion.

Prevention of recurrent urinary tract infections

Prophylactic antibiotics are often used in clinical practice to prevent recurrent UTI. Indeed, advocating the use of prophylactic antibiotics is advisable awaiting the results of investigations. However, simple hygienic advice should be given to all families including daily showers, avoiding irritant soaps and bubble baths, wearing cotton underwear changed daily, regular and double micturition and wiping front to back after defecation. Clinically, the most important factor to be avoided is constipation with advice on high fluid intake and good nutrition with a high fibre diet, although some children do require

Table 5.1 Antibiotic treatment of urinary tract infection

Antibiotic	Dose (mg/kg/day)	Dose interval (h)	Prophylaxis (dose in mg/kg/day)
Co-amoxiclav	20–40 oral amox content	8	–
	25–45 oral amox content	12 (duo suspension)	–
Amoxicillin	25 oral	8	–
Trimethoprim	8 oral	12	2
Nalidixic acid	50 oral	6	12.5
Nitrofurantoin	3–5 oral	6	1
Cefradine	25–50 oral	8–12	
Cefuroxime	6.25–25 oral	12	

stool softeners with lactulose and sometimes with the addition of senna. The role of circumcision in recurrent UTI should be reserved only for children with additional uropathies.

Investigation

Children with confirmed UTI should be referred to their local paediatrician for further investigations. All children with even one proven UTI require investigation with at least a renal ultrasound to identify those susceptible children with congenital malformations and obstruction, abnormal renal and/or bladder function and those at risk for developing renal scars, damage, calculi, and chronic renal failure.

Micturating cysto-urethrograms (MCUG) should be performed in all infants under 12 months of age presenting with their first UTI to exclude vesico-ureteric reflux. DMSA scans should be performed 6 months after the UTI to exclude evidence of renal scarring. DMSA scans can be performed acutely to help in confirming the clinical diagnosis of pyelonephritis.

Nephrotic syndrome

NS is the commonest chronic glomerular disorder of childhood with an incidence of two to four cases per 100 000 children in the United Kingdom and is characterized by:

- ◆ Heavy proteinuria
  - urine protein excretion exceeding 40 mg/m^2 per hour or 1 g/m^2 per day or
  - spot urine protein/creatinine ratio >200 mg/mmol
- ◆ Hypoalbuminaemia
  - plasma albumin <25 g/l
- ◆ Oedema
  - clinically this is detected by pressure with one finger over a bony prominence for 10 seconds.
- ◆ Hyperlipidaemia.

Although there are many causes of NS in childhood, the majority are idiopathic. Congenital NS corresponds to children presenting with NS under 1 year of age, may be inherited in an autosomal recessive manner or associated with syndromes (Denys–Drash or Nail–Patella syndrome) and all require tertiary paediatric nephrology care. If there is a positive family history of renal disease or deafness in any child with NS, there should be consideration of the diagnosis of Alport's syndrome.

Most cases (80%) of childhood NS are due to minimal change disease (MCD) of which the majority) will respond to corticosteroid therapy. As a result, most children are currently treated empirically at presentation without undergoing a renal biopsy with a course of oral steroid therapy (minimal treatment with oral prednisolone 60 mg/m^2 per day (equivalent to 2 mg/kg per day) total dose not to exceed 80 mg/day for 4 weeks, followed by 40 mg/m^2 on alternate days for at least 4 weeks). Remission of NS is when urinary protein excretion <4 mg/hour per m^2 or negative or trace albustix for three consecutive days. Children who respond to steroid therapy within 28 days of commencing treatment, are said to have steroid-sensitive NS (SSNS). At least 70% of children with SSNS will experience disease relapses, although about 80% will enter long-term remission in later childhood. Relapses of NS is when urinary protein excretion >40 mg/m^2 per hour or albustix +++ or more for three consecutive days having previously being in remission, which is treated with prednisolone 60 mg/m^2 per day (as on first presentation) until remission has been achieved followed by a gradual tapering regimen so that the total treatment period is 12 weeks. Many SSNS children will experience frequent relapsing NS (FRNS) over many years, which is two or more relapses during the first 6 months after the initial episode or four or more relapses within any 12-month period. However, it is the response to steroids, which is the most important factor in determining the future management and prognosis. Children with FRNS require treatment with second-line, steroid-sparing agents such as levamisole, cyclophosphamide, and ciclosporin with significant side-effects. Although the risk of progression to end stage renal failure is extremely rare, there remains a significant morbidity and mortality of acute complications, including infection (especially pneumococcal infection, peritonitis, and sepsis), thromboses (particularly, renal venous, cerebral sinus, and pulmonary arterial thromboses) and hypovolaemia (leading to acute renal failure and occasionally hypertension).

All patients who do not respond to 28 days of oral prednisolone 60 mg/m^2 per day have steroid-resistant NS (SRNS) which necessitates a referral to a paediatric nephrologist for percutaneous renal biopsy as the majority of SRNS will have focal and segmental glomerulosclerosis (FSGS) on histology. Although not characteristic of MCD, microscopic haematuria or hypertension may be found at presentation in approximately 25% of FSGS cases. Children with SRNS due to FSGS have an unpredictable response to cytotoxic immunosuppressive therapy, unlike those patients with SRNS secondary to MCD. Children with FSGS pose a greater therapeutic challenge for paediatric nephrologists as the favourable long-term renal survival associated with sustained remission has revived the enthusiasm to treat SRNS with more aggressive immunosuppressive regimens. Despite this, a significant proportion will progress to end stage renal failure so the benefits of immunosuppressive therapy in SRNS should be meticulously balanced against toxicity. Among children over 10 years of age, there is an increasing incidence of membranous nephropathy and membranoproliferative glomerulonephritis causing NS. Steroid dependence is when two consecutive relapses occur during corticosteroid therapy or within 14 days after its cessation.

Acute glomerulonephritis

The clinical entity of a nephritic syndrome is the onset of haematuria, proteinuria, oliguria, and hypertension caused by glomerular injury and inflammation. The more severe cases will have decreased glomerular filtration rate (with acute renal failure and elevation of the serum creatinine) with sodium and water retention resulting in hypertension and generalized oedema (may have peripheral or pulmonary oedema or congestive cardiac failure). The commonest cause in childhood is a post-infectious glomerulonephritis, usually with group A beta-haemolytic streptococcus cultured from the throat swab or skin lesions, hypocomplementaemia (90% of affected cases will have a low complement C3), elevation of the antistreptolysin O titre and anti-DNAse B (or other streptococcal antigens) and an active urinary sediment on microscopy. The treatment is mainly supportive with fluid and salt restriction, diuretics, antihypertensives and penicillin or erythromycin if streptococcal infection is detected.

Other causes of a hypocomplementaemic glomerulonephritis include systemic lupus erythematosus (75–90% of affected cases will have a low complement C3, often with low complement C4), membranoproliferative glomerulonephritis (50–80% of type I MPGN and 80–90% of type II MPGN will have a low complement C3, respectively), subacute bacterial endocarditis and CSF shunt nephritis (90% of affected cases of both conditions will have a low complement C3).

The other acquired glomerulonephritides are normocomplementaemic and are associated with multisystem diseases (such as Henoch–Schönlein purpura (which is histologically the same as IgA nephropathy), polyarteritis nodosa, Wegener's granulomatosis, and other vasculitides), haemolytic uraemic syndrome, sickle cell nephropathy, infections (hepatitis B and human immunodeficiency viral infections).

Many of the causes listed above can overlap with the presence of clinical features of NS with heavy proteinuria resulting in hypoalbuminaemia and generalized oedema.

Antenatal hydronephrosis

With the advent of ultrasonography, the antenatal detection of childhood renal anomalies has greatly increased. This is due to routine practise of antenatal ultrasounds performed at least once in all known pregnancies between 14 and 20 weeks' gestation to identify severe congenital malformations and allow prospective parents to have informed consent on termination of pregnancy. Most information on the fetal urinary tract is gained from knowledge of the kidneys, bladder, renal and/or ureteric dilatation and amniotic fluid volume. This section is included as primary care physicians are likely to be asked about the future investigations and management of these identified fetal uropathies.

However, obstetric practice has led to increased postnatal investigation of the urinary tract and the realisation that some degrees of 'dilatation' may not equate with either reduced renal function or obstruction. There is no debate that antenatal diagnosis may help some families on one side of the spectrum adjust to the likelihood of a child being born with end-stage renal failure, although less than 5% of all antenatally detected anomalies require any nephrological input. It is only those cases with bilateral or severe unilateral renal disease that have relevant physical signs and some of the bilateral cases will have associated syndromes. The postnatal investigation protocols of antenatally dilated urinary tracts are designed to detect obstructive uropathies in boys and other congenital or structural abnormalities in either sex (such as primary vesico-ureteric reflux or obstruction (pelvi-ureteric or vesico-ureteric junction)) which may require subsequent referral and more detailed investigations. However, the more common scenario of spontaneous resolution of mild antenatal hydronephrosis (in the absence of a family history of reflux nephropathy) in 'normal' children only causes problems with the family in inducing parental anxiety, so accurate counselling with appropriate prognosis is paramount in clinical practice. These 'normal' neonates are physically healthy on clinical examination and have become 'patients' in an unconventional manner.

Many investigative protocols have been formed in various local units. It is common practice to refer for further imaging if there is 5 mm dilatation at the 20 weeks' gestation antenatal ultrasound. If the repeat ultrasound shows dilatation that is 5 mm in size or increasing (usually at a level of 1 mm per month gestation) or non-resolution of the dilatation, then postnatal imaging is required. Postnatal ultrasound scans may be performed in the first 48 hours to detect gross abnormalities, but as the neonate is in a period of relative dehydration, there is underestimation of the degree of dilatation and the scan will need to be repeated.

If there is mild unilateral dilatation with the anteroposterior diameter (AP) <15 mm without ureteric dilatation or bladder abnormality detected antenatally, then postnatal ultrasound is required. If this is confirmed postnatally, then a further ultrasound needs to be repeated at 3 months of age.

If there is antenatally detected renal collecting system dilatation with bilateral renal dilatation without ureteric dilatation or bladder abnormality on postnatal ultrasound, a MCUG needs to be performed to exclude posterior urethral valves or primary vesico-ureteric reflux. If these investigations are normal, then pelvi-ureteric or vesico-ureteric junction obstruction can be diagnosed on MAG3 (mercaptoacetyltriglycine) nuclear imaging (which is also the preferred investigation if there is postnatally confirmed unilateral AP renal pelvis >15 mm without ureteric dilatation or bladder abnormality).

If there is antenatally detected unilateral or bilateral renal dilatation with ureteric dilatation with or without bladder abnormality, then a postnatal ultrasound needs to be performed at 24–72 hours with a subsequent MCUG to detect posterior urethral valves or primary vesico-ureteric reflux, prior to embarking on a MAG3 scan to detect pelvi-ureteric or vesico-ureteric junction obstruction.

Many 'normal' adults may have an unidentified solitary kidney until they have a renal ultrasound (usually for another reason). The solitary kidney may be due to renal agenesis or a previous non-functioning multicystic dysplastic kidney (MCDK), which has involuted. MCDK is becoming increasingly diagnosed on antenatal ultrasound, and may require further investigation as there will be 30% incidence of contralateral kidney abnormalities (such as ureteral stenosis and primary vesico-ureteric reflux).

In essence, only children with progressive or bilateral renal pelvic dilatation without vesico-ureteric reflux, non-refluxing mega-ureters, dilated solitary kidney or moiety of a duplex system, unilateral decreased function or symptoms of pain or UTI that require referral to paediatric urologists.

Further Reading

American Academy of Pediatrics (1999). Practice parameter: the diagnosis, treatment, and evaluation of the initial urinary tract infection in febrile infants and young children. American Academy of Pediatrics. Committee on Quality Improvement. Subcommittee on Urinary Tract Infection. *Pediatrics* **103** (4 part 1): 843–852.

Coulthard MG, Lambert HJ, Keir MJ (1997). Occurrence of renal scars in children after their first referral for urinary tract infection. *British Medical Journal* **11**; 315 (7113): 918–919.

Dillon E, Ryall A (1998). A 10 year audit of antenatal ultrasound detection of renal disease. *British Journal of Radiology* **71** (845): 497–500.

Dodge WF, West EF, Smith EH, Bruce H, III (1976). Proteinuria and hematuria in schoolchildren: epidemiology and early natural history. *Journal of Pediatrics* **88** (2): 327–347.

Dudley JA, Haworth JM, McGraw ME, Frank JD, Tizard EJ (1997). Clinical relevance and implications of antenatal hydronephrosis. *Archives of Diseases in Childhood Fetal and Neonatal Edition* **76** (1): F31–F34.

Gorelick MH, Shaw KN (1999). Screening tests for urinary tract infection in children: a meta-analysis. *Pediatrics* **104** (5): e54.

Grignon A, Filion R, Filiatrault D, Robitaille P, Homsy Y, Boutin H, Leblond R (1986). Urinary tract dilatation in utero: classification and clinical applications. *Radiology* **160** (3): 645–647.

Hodson EM, Knight JF, Willis NS, Craig JC (2003). Corticosteroid therapy for nephrotic syndrome in children. *Cochrane Database Systematic Review* (**1**): CD001533.

Iitaka K, Igarashi S, Sakai T. Hypocomplementaemia and membranoproliferative glomerulonephritis in school urinary screening in Japan. *Pediatric Nephrology* **8** (4): 420–422.

Jakobsson B, Esbjorner E, Hansson S (1999). Minimum incidence and diagnostic rate of first urinary tract infection. *Pediatrics* **104** (2 part 1): 222–226.

Jaswon MS, Dibble L, Puri S, Davis J, Young J, Dave R, Morgan H (1999). Prospective study of outcome in antenatally diagnosed renal pelvis dilatation. *Archives of Diseases in Childhood Fetal and Neonatal Edition* **80** (2): F135–F138.

Kitagawa T (1988). Lessons learned from the Japanese nephritis screening study. *Pediatric Nephrology* **2** (2): 256–263.

Ksiazek J, Wyszynska T (1995). Short versus long initial prednisone treatment in steroid-sensitive nephrotic syndrome in children. *Acta Paediatrica* **84** (8): 889–993.

Nissenson AR, Baraff LJ, Fine RN, Knutson DW (1979). Poststreptococcal acute glomerulonephritis: fact and controversy. *Annals of Internal Medicine* **91** (1): 76–86.

Popovic-Rolovic M, Kostic M, Antic-Peco A, Jovanovic O, Popovic D (1991). Medium- and long-term prognosis of patients with acute poststreptococcal glomerulonephritis. *Nephron* **58** (4): 393–399.

Roy S, III, Pitcock JA, Etteldorf JN (1976). Prognosis of acute poststreptococcal glomerulonephritis in childhood: prospective study and review of the literature. *Advances in Pediatrics* **23**: 35–69.

Vehaskari VM, Rapola J, Koskimies O, Savilahti E, Vilska J, Hallman N (1979). Microscopic hematuria in school children: epidemiology and clinicopathologic evaluation. *Journal of Pediatrics* **95** (5 part 1) 676–684.

Vernon S, Foo CK, Coulthard MG (1997). How general practitioners manage children with urinary tract infection: an audit in the former Northern Region. *British Journal of General Practice* **47** (418): 297–300.

Yeung CK, Godley ML, Dhillon HK, Gordon I, Duffy PG, Ransley PG. The characteristics of primary vesico-ureteric reflux in male and female infants with pre-natal hydronephrosis. *British Journal of Urology* **80** (2): 319–327.

Chapter 6

Neonatal issues in primary care

Richard Nicholl

Introduction

In this chapter I shall attempt to address the common and current issues likely to confront primary care physicians in relation to the term baby and also review some current issues in the management of the preterm newborn baby. It is not my purpose to give a complete review of normal newborn development and pathophysiology. For a guide to common conditions in the first year of life I would refer the reader to Valman (2002) and for a comprehensive atlas of conditions affecting the term and preterm newborn, to Thomas and Harvey (1997).

The full term baby

Neonatal mortality

Every year an estimated 4 million babies die in the neonatal period-the first 28 days of life (Lawn *et al.* 2005). A similar number are stillborn and about 0.5 million woman die from pregnancy related causes. Globally, 38% of all child deaths occur in the neonatal period. Three-quarters of neonatal deaths happen in the first week, with the highest risk of death in the first day. Nearly all (99%) of neonatal deaths occur in low and middle income countries, especially sub-Saharan Africa and south-central Asia. Worldwide, the main attributable causes of neonatal death are preterm birth (28%), severe infections (26%), and asphyxia (26%).

In the year 2000, 189 countries endorsed the United Nations Millennium Declaration (Haines and Cassels 2004). The eight goals in the section on development and poverty eradication are known as the millennium development goals (MDGs). They build on agreements made at previous major United Nations' conferences and represent a commitment to reduce poverty and hunger, to tackle ill health, gender inequality, lack of education, lack of access to clean water, and environmental degradation. The fourth goal (MDG-4) commits to reducing mortality in children younger than 5 years by two-thirds, between 1990 and 2015.

Full term birth is defined as a gestation of between 37 and 42 completed weeks. In the UK neonatal mortality rates (deaths up to 28 days) and infant mortality rates (deaths in infants under 1 year of age) have declined with improvements in population health to an all time low (http://www.doh.gov.uk/HPSSS/TBL_A14.HTM). However, in 2000 the UK still had the third highest infant mortality rate in western Europe at 5.6 per thousand live births. The lowest infant mortality rate was in Sweden at 3.4 per thousand live births (http://www.bliss.org.uk/about/facts.asp). The infant mortality rate is much higher in certain at-risk groups, for example lower social class (social class V had IMR of 8.1 per thousand live births), young age (mothers under 20 years of age had IMR of 8.4 per thousand live births) and country of birth (Pakistan IMR of 12.2 per thousand live births; Caribbean 11.0 per thousand live births).

Infant mortality has been identified by the Department of Health as a health inequality target, with a plan to reduce 'by at least 10% the gap in mortality between manual groups and the population as a whole' by 2010 (http://www.doh.gov.uk/healthinequalities/targetsupdatemar02.pdf).

The newborn exam and 6-week check

All parents are anxious about their baby's well-being after birth. Routine examination of the newborn is accepted as good practice (Maternity Services Advisory Committee to the Secretaries of State for Social Services and for Wales 1985; Hall 1996). Traditionally, in the UK this examination is conducted by a trainee doctor who may have little paediatric (neonatal) experience. There is currently interest in training midwives to perform the routine newborn check. Trained neonatal nurse practitioners may be more effective than trainee doctors at detecting abnormalities in the newborn period (Lee *et al.* 2001). Examination of the newborn by midwives compared with junior doctors may give greater maternal satisfaction. Midwives appear more likely to discuss healthcare issues such as feeding, sleeping, and skin care (Wolke *et al.* 2002).

The purpose of the examination is to detect abnormality, provide reassurance to the parents, and should be an opportunity to discuss educational and preventative health aspects of newborn care. Clinical examination will often reveal minor or insignificant abnormalities that may cause alarm to the parents but that are of little long-term importance. Examples include transient rashes (e.g. erythema toxicum), mild jaundice, cephalhaematoma, umbilical hernia, and pre-auricular skin tags.

Other conditions may be more difficult to detect and may require diligence and experience to detect. Unless actively looked for, congenital cataract, cleft palate, minor hypospadias, and undescended testis may easily be missed.

Parents and examiners need to be ware that many conditions (e.g. cerebral palsy, inherited metabolic conditions, sickle cell disease) will not be detectable on routine examination at birth and may present many weeks or months after hospital discharge. The two conditions that seem to cause most anxiety to those charged with performing newborn examinations are congenital heart disease and congenital dislocation of the hips. Detection of both is problematic.

Congenital heart disease

Most of the serious causes of congenital heart disease will present in the first few days of life either with hypoxia (the 'blue baby') or as heart failure (usually a breathless baby that is feeding poorly). Unfortunately even an experienced examiner may miss cases during either routine examination of the newborn or at the 6-week check. Ainsworth *et al.* conducted a 2-year prospective study of 7204 newborn babies to determine the prevalence and significance of heart murmurs detected at birth after routine examination. The prevalence of murmurs was less than 1%. About half of these were caused by an underlying malformation. The absence of a murmur did not exclude serious heart disease. The same centre reviewed the performance of the neonatal and 6-week examinations to detect congenital heart disease (Wren *et al.*) in a retrospective review of 1590 babies with congenital heart disease. More than half of these abnormalities were missed by the routine neonatal check and more than one-third by the 6-week check. The authors recommend early referral of any newborn with a murmur for paediatric cardiological evaluation.

Developmental dysplasia of the hip (DDH; previously referred to as congenital dislocation of the hip)

The terminology now includes hips that are clinically unstable at birth and also hips that appear to be stable at birth but later become unstable in infancy (about 0.6% of cases). Variations in screening programmes and differing definitions of what is meant by 'clinically significant' make it difficult to compare the published incidence in different populations. DDH has been reported as being very infrequent in African and Asian populations. This low prevalence has been attributed to the way in which newborns are carried with the hips in abduction, in these traditional societies.

The incidence of DDH is probably about 1 per 1000 live births in Western countries that routinely screen for the condition. Between 5 and 20 hips per thousand may be unstable on clinical examination but not all will be dislocated or require treatment. The natural history of the condition is that most clinically unstable hips will resolve spontaneously in the first few weeks of life.

Certain factors have been shown to increase the risk of the condition: female infants, a positive family history of DDH in a first-degree relative and breech presentation in the third trimester all make the condition more likely. Oligohydramnios and other conditions where there is lack of space for the fetus in the womb are also associated (large for dates, fixed foot deformity: talipes equinovarus). However, these factors, singly or in combination, are only present in 40% of cases.

There has been debate and conflicting evidence as to the value of screening programmes and the contribution of ultrasound. In the UK a national screening programme was introduced in 1966 to detect those infants at risk of developmental dysplasia of the hip (Standing Medical Advisory Committee 1966). All infants are examined using Barlow's and Ortolani's tests to detect hip instability or dislocation. Concern has been expressed about the difficulty in training staff to adequately carry out the screening examination. There are wide variations in the numbers of cases detected with no good evidence that screening leads to reduced morbidity (www.nelh.nhs.uk/screening). Screening for DDH by clinical examination alone can lead to false-positive results and unnecessary over treatment as well as failure to identify those affected with DDH (false negatives). Because of these problems with clinical examination to screen for DDH there has been increasing interest in the use of ultrasound scanning to improve the performance of the test (Dezateux *et al.* 2003). Although practice may vary, usually all babies are examined clinically and then ultrasound is used selectively. Risk factors that would indicate the use of ultrasound include those babies in whom the hip was clinically dislocated or unstable or in who there are known risk factors (see above).

The results of this approach are still debated as treatment rates are high, suggesting overdiagnosis and unnecessary treatment. The increased costs of secondary screening using ultrasound in the at-risk population is offset by the reduced treatment costs of treating children with DDH diagnosed at a later age (Boere-Boonekampe and Verkerk 1998).

Signs of illness in newborn babies

The febrile infant is a common problem in the primary care setting. Signs of serious illness in the newborn may be subtle and non-specific. It is impossible to clearly distinguish between a viral or bacterial cause by simple clinical examination. Also, babies may present with serious bacterial infection and no fever. Although the majority of febrile illness in this age group will be due to viral causes and self-limiting, if bacterial infection is not detected and treated promptly, then the baby will have a serious outcome. The most common invasive organisms are those that colonize the birth tract during pregnancy: group B streptococcus, *Escherichia coli*, *Listeria monocytogenes*, and other less common Gram-negative organisms. The likelihood of bacterial infection in a neonate with fever is higher (about 13%) than in infancy (about 8%) and highest (about 25%) in babies less than 2 weeks old (Chiu *et al.* 1994; Baker *et al.* 1999). Therefore, one should have a higher index of suspicion for the possibility of serious illness when presented with a neonate who is unwell with a fever, as neonates are a higher risk population compared with older infants or children. If the mother reports a change in the baby's alertness, feeding pattern, crying or simply that the baby 'does not seem right' then it is unwise to dismiss this opinion. It is far better to review the baby after a few hours, than to miss serious bacterial illness. As the signs of illness are not specific it is difficult to be precise.

When parents report that their baby has a fever (axillary or tympanic temperature or simply assessed by touching the baby's skin) they or usually correct. If they report that the baby does *not* have a fever, then this is not reliable and you cannot exclude the possibility of fever and/or bacterial infection based on this assessment (Duce 1996). While the neonate may have a variable breathing rate depending on the state of wakefulness, a respiratory rate greater than 60 per minute is very likely to indicate a serious underlying condition such as pneumonia, sepsis, or congenital heart disease. In two studies from developing countries (Palafox *et al.* 2000; Rajesh *et al.* 2000) the presence of tachypnoea had sensitivity of about 80% and specificity of about 70% for detecting pneumonia and/or hypoxia. Therefore the absence of tachypnoea means that serious respiratory disease is unlikely. It is also worth noting that approximately 1 in 5 hypoxic infants will be missed by using tachypnoea alone as indicator of illness. Any neonate with tachypnoea should be examined carefully and referred for secondary assessment urgently.

Similarly, a rising heart rate is a worrying sign. In the term neonate a resting heart rate greater than 160 beats per minute may be a sign of imminent septic shock.

Confirmation of resting tachycardia or a rising heart rate should lead to urgent secondary assessment of the baby.

Respiratory disorders

NHS maternity statistics for 1998–2001 (http://www.doh.gov.uk/public/sb0211/sb0211.pdf) showed that:

◆ Over 21% of deliveries were induced

◆ Over 21% of deliveries were by caesarean section and over half of these were emergency caesarean sections.

◆ About 11% were instrumental deliveries.

The most commonly reported conditions affecting newborn babies were respiratory disorders: intra-uterine hypoxia in 6% of births, birth asphyxia in 1%, and respiratory distress in 3%.

The high rate of deliveries by caesarean section contributes to and explains much of the respiratory morbidity in full-term babies. The prevalence of neonatal respiratory distress syndrome (RDS) or transient tachypnoea of the newborn (TTN) in full-term babies can be considerably reduced if caesarean section is performed at 39 + 0 to 39 + 6 weeks of pregnancy and not earlier. In a prospective, single centre study over 9 years (Morrison *et al.* 1995) the prevalence of respiratory morbidity (need for admission to neonatal intensive care) was established in relation to the timing of delivery between 37 and 42 weeks gestation. The incidence RDS and TTN was significantly higher for the group delivered by caesarean section before the onset of labour (35.5/1000) compared with caesarean section during labour (12.2/1000; odds ratio, 2.9; 95% CI 1.9–4.4), and compared with vaginal delivery (5.3/1000; odds ratio, 6.8; 95% CI 5.2–8.9). The relative risk of neonatal respiratory morbidity for delivery by caesarean section before the onset of labour during the week 37 + 0 to 37 + 6 compared with the week 38 + 0 to 38 + 6 was 1.74 (95% CI 1.1–2.8) and during the week 38 + 0 to 38 + 6 compared with the week 39 + 0 to 39 + 6 was 2.4 (95% CI 1.2–4.8) (see Table 6.1).

Early onset group B streptococcal infection

Group B streptococcal disease (GBS) is the most common cause of severe neonatal sepsis in developed countries. A recent surveillance study in the UK (Heath *et al.* 2004) looked at the incidence, clinical presentation and mortality of GBS disease. The minimum

Table 6.1 Outcome and prevalence of GBS by gestational age.

Gestation	Outcome	Prevalence	95% confidence interval
Delivery at 37 weeks	RDS/TTN	7.3% (27/366)	5–10%
Delivery at 38 weeks	RDS/TTN	4.2% (45/1063)	3–5.6%
Delivery at 39 weeks	RDS/TTN	1.8% (9/505)	0.8–3.3%
Delivery at 40 weeks	RDS/TTN	0.4% (1/243)	0.02–2.6%
Delivery at 41 weeks	RDS/TTN	0.6% (1/164)	0.03–3

incidence in the UK is 0.6/1000 live births, with a mortality of 11%. Two-thirds of cases present within the first week of life and especially within 48 hours of birth. Half of cases presented with sepsis, the remainder with either meningitis or pneumonia.

Various strategies to prevent GBS disease are in use. These rely either on mass screening of women for carriage of GBS during pregnancy or selectively administering intrapartum antibiotics on the basis of known risk factors for GBS. These risk factors include preterm labour, prolonged rupture of membranes and known GBS carriage. Neither strategy is ideal, as a policy of mass screening using vaginal swabs, if rigorously applied, would mean administering penicillin to 16% of all women in labour (Oddie and Embleton 2002), whereas a selective policy based on risk factors will likely only prevent about 50% of cases.

With increasing early hospital discharge, babies with GBS disease may present in the community to the visiting midwife or general practitioner with difficulty in breathing and/or tachypnoea or non-specific signs of sepsis.

Neonatal jaundice

Neonatal jaundice is reported in 6% of births.

Early jaundice (jaundice appearing in the first 14 days of life): the identification of which babies to investigate may be difficult. In a blinded comparison (Moyer *et al.* 2000) of clinicians' visual observations of jaundice with serum bilirubin results, clinical assessment of bilirubin levels was not reliable or accurate. If jaundice does *not* extend below the nipple line, serum bilirubin is unlikely to be high enough to require investigation or treatment with phototherapy (Moyer *et al.* 2000). The level of serum bilirubin that is dangerous is not known. There are many nomograms and practice guidelines available (http://www.ngc.gov/summary/phototherapy). If the serum bilirubin level is high enough to require phototherapy, then minimum investigations should include blood group and direct Coombs' test (to exclude haemolytic jaundice due to blood group incompatibility), urine for culture (to exclude urinary tract infection), and urinary reducing sugars (to exclude rare but treatable galactosaemia).

Late jaundice

Although most cases will be attributed to breast milk jaundice, persistence of jaundice after 14 days of age in term infants (prolonged jaundice) may be a sign of underlying liver disease or other pathology and *always* requires referral to a paediatrician for clinical examination and investigation. A minimum set of investigations includes total and unconjugated serum bilirubin, packed cell volume, glucose-6-phosphate dehydrogenase level, urine for culture, and inspection of stools to confirm the presence of pigment that should normally be present (Hannam *et al.* 2000).

Neonatal encephalopathy

While the mortality of very low birthweight babies has continued to improve, this has not been accompanied by a decline in mortality due to neonatal encephalopathy in term infants. Moderate to severe encephalopathy occurs in 3.8/1000 term live births (Badawi *et al.* 1998). The neonatal fatality is 9.1%. Many of the survivors will develop severe neurodisability. There is emerging evidence that the causal events may be antenatal and therefore may not be preventable (Edwards and Nelson 1998). The long-held assumption that cerebral palsy is 'caused' by 'birth asphyxia' is now being questioned in a number of important epidemiological studies. The debate has centred about how much of the neurological impairment in these babies can be attributed simply to perinatal hypoxia and ischaemia and how much to other factors that may be infective, inflammatory, endocrine, or genetic in their origin.

There is currently much research interest into controlled hypothermia of the infant brain and/or whole body in order to facilitate neural rescue and alleviate the devastating effects of brain hypoxia (Azzopardi *et al.* 2000). Currently a multicentre randomized trial of cooling such babies is underway to evaluate this strategy (http://www.npeu.ox.ac.uk/toby/index.php).

Sudden unexplained death in infancy (SUDI; previously 'cot death')

Unexplained death in infancy will occur in about 1 in 2000 live births. In the UK, SUDI is the most common cause of death in babies over 1 month of age. It is more common in the winter months. SUDI is uncommon before 1 month of age, with a peak incidence at about 1–2 months of age. 90% of cases occur by 6 months of age, and it is very uncommon after 1 year. Typically, the baby is well or with minor symptoms of an upper respiratory infection and is later found dead. SUDI can happen to any family although is more common in areas of social deprivation or where there is exposure to cigarette smoke. Advice aimed at reducing the risk of SUDI includes reducing or stopping smoking in pregnancy, not exposing the baby to cigarette smoke (DiFranza and Lew 1995; Anderson and Cook 1997) and placing the baby on his/her back to sleep. The baby should sleep in his/her own cot, in the parents' bedroom during the first 6 months. The baby should not be allowed to get too hot, or to wriggle under the covers. The baby should be placed with his/her feet at the foot of the cot. It is inadvisable to share a bed with the baby, especially if either partner is a smoker, has been drinking alcohol, or is very tired. It is especially dangerous to sleep with the baby on a sofa or armchair. Excellent information and advice is available from the Foundation for the Study of Infant Deaths (FSID) (http://sids.org.uk).

In September 2004, following a number of high profile criminal cases where mothers had been wrongly convicted for causing the death of their babies, a working group convened by the Royal Colleges of Pathologists and Paediatrics and Child Health produced a multi-agency protocol for the investigation of cases of SUDI (http://www.rcpch.ac.uk/publications/recent_publications/SUDI).

This document sets out the recommended procedures that should be followed in such cases and sets the standards and tasks that are expected of individuals and agencies who work together in this often complex and controversial area.

The importance of breast feeding

Breast feeding should always be encouraged. The UK has one of the lowest rates of breast feeding in Europe (defined as the proportion of babies who were breast fed initially): 70% at birth, falling to about 40% at 6 weeks of age and 20% at 4–6 months of age.

Young mothers, single mothers and those from deprived areas are least likely to initiate and maintain breast feeding. Breast feeding provides the baby with a nutritionally complete formula, and strengthens the immune system. There is good evidence from studies in many countries and in diverse populations that breast feeding protects against gastrointestinal infection, otitis media, and necrotizing enterocolitis (Bick 1999). Maximal benefit is achieved if exclusive breast feeding is maintained until 4 months of age. Other benefits include protection against urinary tract infection, lower respiratory infection, childhood diabetes, SUDI (McVea *et al.* 2000), allergies, lower systolic blood pressure in adulthood (Martin *et al.* 2005), and a possible intellectual advantage.

Health benefits for the mother include reduction of mother's blood loss after birth, a natural method for delaying and spacing pregnancies and a reduction in the incidence of ovarian and breast cancers and of later osteoporosis. Breast feeding is also free. See also www.babyfriendly.org.uk

There is clear evidence for the effectiveness of breast feeding support, whether by trained lay people or health professionals. Advice seems effective if given face to face and both before and after the pregnancy (Sikorski *et al.* 2004).

The preterm baby
Epidemiology

Premature birth is the leading cause of neonatal mortality and morbidity in Western society. Premature birth affects not only the baby and his/her family but puts an extra demand on health care resources that are already limited. About 75% of deaths in the perinatal period occur in preterm infants, with over two-thirds of these in the 30–40% who are born before 32 weeks gestation.

In developed countries about 5–10% of all births are premature (i.e. less than 37 weeks completed duration). The UK has the highest preterm birth rate in western Europe. The overall frequency of preterm birth appears to be increasing (Goldenberg and Rouse 1998). This has been attributed to multiple factors such as increased obstetric intervention, assisted reproduction, multiple order births, substance misuse in pregnancy and adverse social environment. About 1–2% will be born at less than 32 weeks gestation and just 0.5% at less than 28 weeks gestation.

In the UK, data is routinely collected in relation to birth-weight, as there may be uncertainty over the length of gestation. This may be misleading when comparing outcome data as it can include babies of higher gestational age with intrauterine growth restriction. The definitions by birthweight are:

* low birthweight <2500 g
* very low birthweight <1500 g
* extremely low birthweight <1000 g.

Babies of higher gestation may be classified as 'low birthweight' because they have experienced in-utero growth restriction (IUGR). In developed countries this is commonly due to poor placentation and pregnancy-induced hypertension (PIH). Babies are often defined as small for gestational age ('SGA') if their birthweight is less than the 10th percentile compared with the normal distribution of birthweights for those babies of the same gestation.

Preterm babies can also be growth restricted, adding to their problems. IUGR, if not secondary to pregnancy induced hypertension and an unhealthy placenta may be caused by maternal factors such as smoking, chronic illness, or substance misuse. IUGR may be a sign that the baby has a chromosomal abnormality or less commonly a congenital infection. Commonly no cause is found in spite of detailed investigation.

Neonatal medicine has made huge advances in a relatively short time. Babies who were previously thought not viable because of their prematurity are now routinely resuscitated, nurtured in intensive care and discharged to their families with a more than fair to good prospect of a healthy future. In the UK the legal limit for abortion was lowered in 1992 from 28 weeks gestation to 24 weeks gestation to reflect this. Although these improvements in survival have been welcomed they bring with them difficult ethical decisions at the margins of viability. This debate will continue.

The widespread implementation of evidence based therapies such as antenatal steroids, the early use of naturally derived surfactants and improvements in ventilation techniques combined with a better understanding of neonatal physiology have all played their part. Importantly neonatal medicine has become a specialty in its own right.

Organization of services

With the advances in neonatal care have come greater demands for service provision. The throughput is of low volume but high cost, involving specialist trained staff and expensive equipment. The level of care a baby needs may vary from day to day or week to week. Babies may progress through different levels of care over many months. In the UK, the British Association of Perinatal Medicine (BAPM) has agreed definitions of the levels of care (http://www.bapm.org/documents/publications/hosp_standards.pdf). These are summarized as:

- *Intensive care*. Babies requiring ventilation, surgery, or other complex invasive procedures; babies less than 1000 g or less than 29 weeks birth gestation.

- *High dependency*. Babies in supplemental oxygen or other respiratory support but not ventilated. Babies receiving total parenteral nutrition (TPN); babies having convulsions.

- *Special care*. All other babies who need extra nursing or medical care but who could not be looked after at home by their parents (e.g. nasogastric tube feeding).

Predicting the demand for provision of different levels of care in order to use resources efficiently is difficult. The common current model is based on a network of different neonatal units working together to serve a defined geographical population. This model should benefit from economies of scale and has the potential to use staff and equipment more efficiently while minimizing the distance that parents may have to travel in order to deliver, and then visit, their babies. Hospitals that do not provide long-term intensive care for babies should have in place arrangements to transfer mothers who are in threatened preterm labour, while the baby is still *in-utero*. The peripheral neonatal units provide high dependency and special care. They also need to be able to provide short-term intensive care for sicker babies prior to possible transfer to the regional neonatal unit.

Prediction and prevention of premature birth

The causes of preterm birth are multifactorial. Although there are many associations, in an individual case it usually difficult to ascribe causality. Such factors include preterm pre-labour rupture of the membranes (pPROM), cervical incompetence, shortened cervical length, polyhydramnios, structural abnormalities of the fetus or the uterus, infections and inflammation of the genital tract, lower social class, smoking, and manual labour. This list is not exhaustive and will no doubt be added to.

If one could accurately predict which woman in threatened preterm labour will actually go on to have a preterm delivery then targeted interventions such as antenatal steroids could be used more effectively. Clinical tests such as transvaginal ultrasound to measure the length of the endocervix and the fetal fibronectin test are not in widespread use as although they have a high negative predictive value they are much less good at correctly predicting which woman will imminently give birth prematurely.

The prevention of preterm delivery has been the subject of much debate and research. Tocolytic agents such as beta-sympathetic receptor stimulators are usually tried—if only to allow time for antenatal steroids to be employed (below). Calcium channel blockers and the selective oxytocin receptor blocker atisoban appear to be as useful in preventing uterine contractions, with fewer side-effects. Prostaglandin synthetase inhibitors such as indomethacin may also prevent uterine contractions. There is currently no evidence to show that any of these agents improve outcomes for the preterm baby.

Cervical cerclage can be used in selected cases; however, there have not been large enough randomized trials to demonstrate whether this is of benefit in preventing or delaying preterm birth.

Antibiotics may help to prevent preterm labour or delay its onset, e.g. where there is preterm rupture of the membranes. The presence of asymptomatic bacterial vaginosis has been associated with preterm labour. Some authorities recommend screening and treating for bacterial vaginosis (an overgrowth of anaerobic bacteria in the birth canal). There is emerging evidence for the efficacy of treating women with asymptomatic vaginosis to prevent second trimester miscarriage and preterm birth. One appraisal of current best evidence suggests that 10 women would need to be treated for asymptomatic vaginosis to prevent one extra late miscarriage or preterm birth in a general obstetric population (Ugwumadu *et al.* 2003).

A single course of antenatal steroids (2 doses of 12 mg betamethasone or 6 mg of dexamethasone) is of proven benefit for the prevention of respiratory distress between 24 and 34 weeks of gestation. Multiple doses of antenatal steroids may be harmful to the developing foetus and should be avoided. This is currently the subject of ongoing research.

Obstetric issues

Obstetric complications such as pre-eclampsia may result in adverse outcomes for the mother or baby if not promptly recognized and treated. For the mother this can lead to eclamptic fits, cerebrovascular haemorrhage, haemolysis with elevated liver enzymes (HELLP syndrome), and death. Other underlying maternal illness, such as diabetes or heart disease will influence the timing, place, and mode of delivery.

It is frequently difficult to balance the risks to the mother in continuing the pregnancy versus the risks to the fetus of a preterm birth. Serial ultrasound measurement of abdominal circumference to assess fetal growth may suggest growth restriction if values fall below the normal centile range.

Doppler ultrasound to measure wave form velocity of the umbilical artery has become routine practice in high-risk pregnancies, in developed countries. It is especially useful where there is placental insufficiency secondary to maternal pre-eclampsia. A reduction or reversal in waveform velocity may be an indication to deliver the baby early.

Surfactant

Exogenous surfactant administration has been available in the UK since the mid 1990s and is now universally used in the early management of preterm infants. Its introduction following many well conducted randomized trials remains a milestone in the history of how neonatology has evolved. Surfactant reduces neonatal mortality from RDS by about 40% and reduces other important complications such as pulmonary air leaks by about 30–50% (Soll and Morley 2001). Use of antenatal steroids followed by postnatal surfactant has an additive effect (Jobe *et al.* 1993). Issues that are still under debate include which surfactant manufacturer has the 'best' product, the use of surfactant at the edge of viability (typically 23 weeks gestation), and how early it should be given after birth—although most people agree that earlier is better (Soll and Morley 2001). Future research is likely to look at whether peptide containing synthetic surfactants may confer advantages over the currently used animal-derived surfactants, the use of surfactant in respiratory conditions other than hyaline membrane disease and stricter criteria regarding the administration of repeated doses of surfactant to individual babies.

Chronic lung disease

Although the increased survival of extremely small babies has been welcome, this has been at the expense of increased comorbidity, such as chronic lung disease (CLD) of prematurity. The greatest risk factor for CLD is the degree of prematurity. About 50% of babies born below 1000 g birthweight will still be oxygen dependent at (corrected) full term age (Wood *et al.* 2000). These babies have a higher prevalence of respiratory infections after discharge from the neonatal unit. They are more likely go home in supplemental oxygen, to require readmission to hospital in the first year of life compared with other premature babies without CLD and may be more likely to develop asthma as young children.

Although the cause of CLD (most usefully defined as oxygen dependency beyond 36 weeks corrected gestational age) is multifactorial, specific factors relating to the way in which they have been ventilated are thought to influence its severity and progression. High inspired oxygen concentrations, positive pressure ventilation with high inspiratory pressures, and inflammatory mediators in the lung have all been implicated. This has led to the development of the concept of 'ventilator induced lung injury' or VILI (Clark *et al.* 2001).

As mechanical ventilation and monitoring has become more sophisticated clinicians are currently looking at a variety of ventilatory strategies to minimize VILI. A 'conservative' approach using nasal continuous positive airways pressure (nCPAP) and avoiding intubation with positive pressure ventilation has been advocated (Wung *et al.* 1985). This approach is common in many parts of Europe, the USA, and Australia. The results of a number of randomized trials are awaited. The place of high frequency oscillation ventilation (HFOV) compared with conventional (time cycled, pressure limited) ventilation is still debated, with conflicting evidence. One study from the USA showed a slight reduction in CLD (Courtney *et al.* 2002) but a study from the UK (Johnson *et al.* 2002) found no such difference. These differing outcomes may be explained by differences in study design and methodology. Currently there is not sufficient evidence-based data from large randomized trials to give specific recommendations for best practice. As the technology available to ventilate sick babies continues to develop, clinicians will have greater choice in how they treat these babies. Larger, randomized studies with long-term follow-up are needed to define what is the best ventilation strategy to minimize the incidence of CLD.

There is little evidence for benefit of other therapies such as postnatal systemic steroids, inhaled steroids, or diuretics in influencing the course of CLD. Although they have often been used they are not with out potential adverse effects. Postnatal systemic steroids have been shown in meta-analysis of clinical trials to be associated with reduced brain growth and an increase in the incidence of later neurodisability, as well as other important adverse events (Halliday 2004).

Resuscitation and initial care

Preparation of staff and equipment prior to a preterm delivery is essential and may impact on the baby's outcome. If time permits it is desirable for the paediatricians to speak to the prospective parents in order to gather information and answer any questions they may have about the likely outcome of their baby. The aims of resuscitation follow the same principles as those for older children and adults: airway, breathing and circulation, 'ABC' (Resuscitation Council 2002). A guide to the equipment and skills required for resuscitation of babies at birth is available (Joint Working Party, BMJ publishing 1997). Resuscitation of smaller and sicker babies requires more people and more skill. Babies above 32 weeks gestation may require little help, and may be dried and wrapped and shown to the parents before admitting the baby for special care. Babies between 28 weeks and 32 weeks are likely to need some respiratory support. Those under 28 weeks will very likely need intubation, administration of exogenous surfactant and ventilation (intensive care). If there is no improvement in the baby's circulation in spite of adequate ventilation then chest compressions should be started if the heart rate remains less than 60 beats per minute. Bradycardia may then respond to administration of adrenaline. Correction of acidosis with intravenous sodium bicarbonate may be helpful.

If the heart rate does not improve after 15–20 minutes of adequate ventilation and attempts at circulatory support, then resuscitation should be stopped. Ideally this will be done after discussion with a senior doctor and consultation with the parents.

Occasionally paediatricians will be called at short notice to resuscitate a small baby of unknown gestation. If the baby appears fetal with translucent skin, or is less than 500 g birthweight or makes a poor response to intubation and manual ventilation then most neonatologists in the UK would not administer chest compressions or adrenaline and instead accept that the baby, although showing signs of life, is pre-viable. In this situation both the parents and attending staff will need support and sensitive discussion after the event.

Thermoregulation, fluids, and feeding

The change from *in-utero* to *ex-utero* life is a time of great change in the physiology of the newborn baby. The preterm baby has extra adaptive stresses to cope with. Most of their organs are structurally and functionally immature. They are more vulnerable to heat loss and to insensible fluid loss through immature skin. They are more prone to invasive infection, partly due to an immature immune system. These very small and immature babies will need intensive monitoring and medical and nursing support to get them through this adaptive process.

The neutral thermal environment is the ambient temperature at which oxygen consumption and energy expenditure are minimal. Measures to maintain the baby's neutral thermal environment should begin at birth. The labour ward temperature should be appropriate for the needs of the baby and not the maternity staff. A number of studies have shown that the temperature of very low birthweight babies can be maintained by placing them immediately after delivery into a polyethylene bag (occlusive wrapping), without drying the baby beforehand. The baby should then be assessed and resuscitated under a radiant heater. After admission to the neonatal unit the baby can be nursed in either a closed or an open incubator providing close attention is paid to the baby's clinical condition, serum electrolytes, and urine output.

The preterm infant is also vulnerable to hypoglycaemia because of reduced glycogen stores in the liver, the relative absence of subcutaneous fat, and a reduced shivering reflex. They are also prone to hyperglycaemia especially if growth *in utero* has been restricted by poor placentation, leading to relative insulin resistance. As ever, maintaining the baby's 'milieu interior' is a major goal in the ill preterm baby.

Adequate nutrition after birth is an essential part of the care of preterm babies. There is emerging evidence of the importance of the early postnatal period as a critical time for brain growth and development (Morley and Lucas 2000). The use of human milk, mother's own where possible, is to be encouraged at all times. Where a mother is too ill to express her own milk or unable to provide it for other reasons, then expressed donor milk should be considered for higher risk babies.

Early discussion about the importance of breast feeding (preferably in the antenatal period), written information, skin to skin contact with the baby and ongoing support and education are all likely to help achieve success in providing breast milk for these babies. On occasion no human milk may be available in which case a preterm formula milk may be used. These are mainly modified cow's milk formulae designed to cope with the extra metabolic demands of prematurity. In spite of manufacturers' claims, there is little to choose between the products and all are inferior to human milk.

Very premature babies have reduced gastric emptying and reduced peristalsis and may be slow to tolerate enteral feeds. While enteral feeds are slowly increased the baby's nutrition will require supplementation with parenteral nutrition. This is a glucose and amino acid solution with added minerals, vitamins, and fat. The solution is hyperosmolar and therefore is usually delivered via a peripherally inserted central catheter. This method of nutrition is expensive and not without potential adverse events such as phlebitis, line infection and occasional extravasation into the soft tissues. Parenteral nutrition should be stopped in favour of enteral feeding as soon as this is tolerated.

Infection

Systemic infection of preterm babies is a common cause of morbidity and an important cause of mortality. Clinical and laboratory diagnosis are difficult, which can lead to both a delay in treatment and a possible over use of antibiotics. The single most effective strategy to prevent cross-infection is hand washing (Handwashing Liaison Group 1999).

Early onset infection presents in the first 48–72 hours of life and is acquired before birth or from the birth canal. The principal organisms responsible in UK practice are Group B streptococcus and *Escherichia coli*. Although it is not common, mortality is high, especially in the very premature babies.

Late onset infection is usually hospital acquired and presents after 72 hours of life. This is common, affecting about 15% of very low birthweight babies at some time, but has much lower mortality. About half of cases are due to coagulase negative staphylococci. The risk of infection is increased in smaller and immature babies, those who have had multiple courses of antibiotics and those with indwelling medical devices. Invasive fungal infection is fortunately not common but has a high mortality in preterm babies. The diagnosis needs to be considered in babies who remain unwell in spite appropriate treatment with broad-spectrum antibiotics. Examination of the retina, cardiac echo, renal ultrasound, and urine culture may all give clues to the diagnosis.

The place of adjunctive therapies to prevent or treat infection, such as immunoglobulin, colony stimulating factors, and anticytokines are currently unclear and await the results of clinical trials.

Parents and families

Having a premature baby can be an overwhelming experience for parents. The neonatal environment can seem alien and even threatening for parents. Most neonatal units try to reduce stress by encouraging parents to visit at any time and to make early skin contact with their baby. Facilities for siblings to play and for parents to sleep all contribute to a more 'family friendly' approach. Often other parents, as well as staff, can be a source of emotional support. Charitable organizations such as BLISS (www.bliss.org.uk) can provide useful support and advice for parents whose babies are ill.

Outcomes of prematurity

Advances in obstetric management and neonatal care have led to increased survival of extremely low birthweight infants. Survival at 24 weeks ranges from 17 to 62% and at

25 weeks gestation from 35 to 72% (Hack and Fanaroff 2000). These wide variations are likely due to differing populations, differing policies on initiating resuscitation and in withdrawing care, and differences in follow-up. Morbidity increases with decreasing gestational age and also becomes more apparent the longer and more completely these babies are followed up. At 24 weeks birth gestation the rates of severe neurodisability range from 22 to 45% and at 25 weeks from 12 to 35%. These problems may be multiple and include any or all of cerebral palsy, seizures, hydrocephalus, visual or hearing impairment, learning difficulties and problems in social development and behaviour. Regular and early follow-up by a multidisciplinary team may allow the early identification of problems. Therapy and support can then be focused according to the needs of the child. Although most premature babies will have a good neurodevelopmental outcome and an acceptable quality of life, those babies with a significant disability may have an adverse effect on family life and will create increased demands on health, education, and social services.

References

Ainsworth SB, Wyllie JP, Wren C (1999). Prevalence and clinical significance of cardiac murmurs in Neonates. *Archives of disease in childhood (Fetal and Neonatal Edition)* **80**: 43–45.

Anderson HR, Cook DG (1997). Passive smoking and sudden infant death syndrome: review of the epidemiological evidence. *Thorax* **52**: 1003–1009.

Azzopardi D, Robertson NJ, Cowan FM, Rutherford MA, Rampling M, Edwards AD (2000). Pilot study of treatment with whole body hypothermia for neonatal encephalopathy. *Pediatrics* **106**(4): 684–94.

Badawi N, Kurinczuk JJ, Keogh JM, Alessandri LM, O'Sullivan F, Burton PR, Pemberton PJ, Stanley FJ (1998). Antepartum risk factors for newborn encephalopathy: the Western Australian case-control study. *British Medical Journal* **317**(7172): 1549–1553.

Baker M, Bell L, Avner J (1999). The efficacy of routine outpatient management without antibiotics of fever in selected infants. *Pediatrics* **103**: 627–631.

Bick D (1999).The benefits of breastfeeding for the infant. *British Journal of Midwifery* **7**(5): 312–319.

Boere-Boonekamp, Verkerk PH (1998). Screening for developmental dysplasia of the hip. *Seminars in Neonatology* **3**: 49–59.

Chiu CH, Lin TY, Bullard MJ (1994). Application of criteria identifying febrile outpatient neonates at low risk for bacterial infection. *Pediatric Infectious Disease Journal* **13**: 946–949.

Clark RH, Gerstmann DR, Jobe AH *et al.* (2001). Lung injury in neonates: causes, strategies for prevention, and long term consequences. *Journal of Pediatrics* **139**: 478–486.

Courtney SE, Durand DJ, Asselin JM Hudak ML, Aschner JL, Shoemaker CT (2002). High frequency ventilation versusconventional mechanical ventilationfor very low birth weight infants. *New England Journal of Medicine* **347**: 643–652.

Dezateux C, Brown J, Arthur R, Karnon J, Parnaby A (2003). Performance, treatment pathways, and effects of alternative policy options for screening for delopmental dysplasia of the hip in the United Kingdom. *Archives of Disease in Childhood* **88**(9): 753–759.

DiFranza JR, Lew RA (1995). Effect of maternal cigarette smoking on pregnancy complications and sudden infant death syndrome. *Journal of Family Practice* **40**(4): 385–394.

Duce SJ (1999). A systematic review of the literature to determine optimal methods of temperature measurement in neonates, infants and children, 1996. *Cochrane Library* **2**: 1–3.

Edwards AD, Nelson KB (1998). Neonatal encephalopathies. Time to reconsider the cause of encephalopathies. *British Medical Journal* **317**(7172): 1537–1538.

Goldenberg RL, Rouse DJ (1998). Prevention of preterm birth. *New England Journal of Medicine* **339**: 313–320.

Hack M, Fanaroff AA (2000). Outcomes of children of extremely low birthweight and gestational age in the 1990s. *Seminars in Neonatology* **5**(2): 89–106.

Haines A, Cassels A (2004). Can the millennium development goals be attained? *British Medical Journal* **329**: 394–397.

Halliday HL (2004). Use of steroids in the perinatal period. *Paediatric Respiratory Reviews* **5**(Suppl. A): S321–327.

Hall DMB (1996). *Health for all Children*. Oxford University Press.

Handwashing Liaison Group. Hand washing: a modest measure with big effects. *British Medical Journal* **318**: 686–686.

Hannam S, McDonnell M, Rennie JM (2000). Investigation of prolonged neonatal jaundice. Acta Paediatrica **89**(6): 694–697.

Heath PT, Balfour G, Weisner AM, Efstratiou A, Lamagni TL, Tighe H, O'Connell LA, Cafferkey M, Verlander NQ, Nicoll A, McCartney AC; PHLS Group B Streptococcus Working Group (2004). Group B streptococcal disease in UK and Irish infants younger than 90 days. *Lancet* **363**(9405): 292–294.

Jobe AH, Mitchell BR, Gunkel JH (1993). Beneficial effects of the combined use of prenatal corticosteroids and postnatal surfactant on preterm infants. *American Journal of Obstetrics and Gynecology* **168**: 508–513.

Johnson AH, Peacock JL, Greenough A, Marlow N, Limb ES, Marston L, Clavert SA (2002). High frequency oscillatory ventilation for the prevention of chronic lung disease of prematurity. *New England Journal of Medicine* **347**: 633–642.

Joint Working Party of Royal College of Paediatrics and Child Health and Royal College of Obstetricians and Gynecologists (1997). *Resuscitation of Babies at Birth*. British Medical Journal Publishing Group, London.

Lawn JE, Cousens S, Zupan J; Lancet Neonatal Survival Steering Team (2005). 4 million neonatal deaths: When? Where? Why? *Lancet* **365**(9462): 891–900.

Lee TWR, Skelton RE, Skene C (2001). Routine neonatal examination: effectiveness of trainee paediatrician compared wih advanced neonatal nurdse practitioner. *Archives of Diseases in Childhood Fetal and Neonatal Edition* **85**: F100–F104.

Martin RM, Gunnell D, Smith GD (2005). Breastfeeding in infancy and blood pressure in later life: systematic review and meta-analysis. *American Journal of Epidemiology* **161**: 15–26.

Maternity Services Advisory Committee to the Secretaries of State for Social Services and for Wales (1985). *Maternity Care in Action. Part III: care of the mother and baby (postnatal and neonatal care)*. HMSO, London.

McVea KL, Turner PD, Peppler DK (2000). The role of breastfeeding in sudden infant death syndrome. *Journal of Human Lactation* **16**: 13–20.

Morrison JJ, Rennie JM, Milton PJ (1995). Neonatal respiratory morbidity and mode of delivery at term: influence of timing of elective caesarean section. *British Journal of Obstetrics and Gynaecology* **102**(2): 101–6.

Morley R, Lucas A (2000). Randomized diet in the neonatal period and growth performance until 7.5–8 y of age in preterm children. *American Journal of Clinical Nutrition* **71**(3): 822–828.

Moyer VA, Ahn C, Sneed S (2000). Accuracy of clinical judgment in neonatal jaundice. *Archives of Pediatric and Adolescent Medicine* **154**(4): 391–394.

Oddie S, Embleton ND (2002). Risk factors for early onset neonatal group B streptococcal sepsis: case-control study. *British Medical Journal* **325**(7359): 308.

Palafox M, Guiscafre H, Reyes H, Muñoz O, Martínez H (2000). Diagnostic value of tachypnoea in pneumonia defined radiologically. *Archives of Disease in Childhood* **82**: 41–45.

Rajesh VT, Singhi S, Kataria S (2000). Tachypnoea is a good predictor of hypoxia in acutely ill infants under 2 months. *Archives of Disease in Childhood* **82**: 46–49.

Resuscitation Council (UK) (2002). *Resuscitation at Birth: newborn life support provider course manual.* Resuscitation Council (UK), London.

Sikorski J, Renfrew M J, Pindoria S, Wade A (2004). Support for breastfeeding mothers (Cochrane Review). *The Cochrane Library*, Issue 1.

Soll RF, Morley CJ (2001). Prophylactic versus selective use of surfactant in preventing morbidity and mortality in preterm infants. *Cochrane Database Systematic Review* CD000510.

Standing Medical Advisory Committee (1966). *Screening for the Detection of Congenital Dislocation of the Hip in Infants.* Department of Health and Social Security, London.

Thomas R, Harvey D (1997). *Neonatology Colour Guide.* Churchill Livingstone, Oxford.

Ugwumadu A, Manyonda I, Reid F, Hay P (2003). Effect of early oral clindamycin on late miscarriage and preterm delivery in asymptomatic women with abnormal vaginal flora and bacterial vaginosis: a randomised controlled trial. *Lancet* **361**(9362): 983–988.

Valman WB (2002). *ABC of the first year.* Blackwell, Oxford.

Wolke D, Dave S, Hayes J, Townsend J, Tomlin M (2002). Routine examination of the newborn and maternal satisfaction: a randomised controlled trial. *Archives of Diseases in Childhood Fetal and Neonatal Edition* **86**: F155–F160.

Wood NS, Marlow N, Costeloe K, Gibson AT, Wilkinson AR (2000). Neurologic and developmental disability after extremely preterm birth. EPICure Study Group. *New England Journal of Medicine* **343**(6): 378–384.

Wren C, Richmond S, Donaldson L (1999). Presentation of congenital heart disease in infancy: Implications for routine examination. *Archives of disease in childhood (Fetal and Neonatal Edition)* **80**: 49–53.

Wung JT, James LS, Kilchevsky E et al (1985). Management of infants with severe respiratory failure and persistence of the fetal circulation without hyperventilation. *Pediatrics* **76**: 488–492.

Chapter 7

Paediatric surgery

Daniel Leff and Peter McDonald

Introduction

This chapter aims to give the reader a guide to the variety of common paediatric surgical conditions that may present to the general practitioner and need only the assistance of the local hospital.

There are a number of rarer neonatal life-threatening surgical conditions that may that warrant urgent involvement of specialist paediatric surgical centres.

It is important to appreciate the differences between adult and paediatric anatomy and physiology. Children are not little adults. Their response to injury and illness may differ both physically and psychologically. In this regard both the general practitioner and the surgeon will invariably need the assistance of paediatricians and neonatologists and many of these children will be under joint medical and surgical care.

Paediatric surgery is more often than not the correction of major embryological anomalies or for minor developmental abnormalities. Treatment outcomes, successful and unsuccessful, last a lifetime and many may impact on future growth and development.

The paediatric surgical patient

A child's circulating blood volume is higher per kilogram than an adult's but the overall volume is low and as a consequence even a small amount of blood loss can be critical.

In the infant the stroke volume is relatively small and is of fixed volume. However, cardiac index is high and as cardiac output is a product of stroke volume and heart rate this accounts for the amplified heart rate changes seen in childhood. Systemic vascular resistance increases after birth and continues to do so during childhood and this results in the marked changes in blood pressure observed in early life.

Children who are unwell present problems during hospital care because of difficulties in communicating with them especially if they have no language ability or if they are still developing their speech and understanding. Hence, the importance of picking up verbal and non-verbal clues to their illness or pain.

Children who are unwell in hospital are often afraid of hospital treatment and investigations, this may be because of fearsome concepts or ideas that they have picked up from films and television. Knowledge can allay their fears and it is important to explain things clearly to children in language they can understand. Play can be used to do this and may maintain some degree of normality in a otherwise stressful and strange situation. This combined with a kind and gentle approach will help to allay the child's fears and will help reduce parental anxiety.

Life-threatening neonatal abnormalities

Gastroschisis

Clinical features

This is a protrusion of the gut through a defect in the abdominal wall usually to the right of a normal umbilicus: The defect is caused by the regression of the right umbilical vein. The defect is usually between 2 and 4 cm in size.

It has an approximate incidence of 1/10 000 live births. Unlike in exomphalos, the protruding viscera are uncovered and are exposed to direct injury and associated chromosomal abnormalities are not common. Approximately 25% of infants with gastroschisis have associated bowel injury (atresia, stenosis, and ischaemia).

Most cases of gastroschisis are detected antenatally as a result of raised maternal serum α-fetoprotein, prompting detailed ultrasonography. These patients are managed in a specialist paediatric surgical unit.

Normal vaginal delivery is preferable; however approximately one-third of these patients will require an emergency Caesarean section for fetal distress during labour.

Treatment

Treatment involves placing the loops of bowel in a sterile surgical bag, thereby maintaining the warm temperature, limiting heat loss and keeping the bowel moist. Early surgical closure (within 4–6 hours) can be achieved in up to three-quarters of patients. The protruding intestine is returned to the abdominal cavity at operation.

If this is not feasible a Silastic silo is fashioned and sutured to the abdominal wall. In the subsequent week the intestinal contents are returned to the abdominal cavity and the abdominal wall is closed at a second operation.

The improvement in neonatal critical care in recent years has meant that the majority of these neonates now survive gastroschisis. The most common post operative problem is protracted paralytic ileus resulting in a need for intravenous nutrition.

Exomphalos

Clinical features

This abnormality occurs due to failure of the primitive gut loop to return to the abdominal cavity following physiological herniation into the umbilical cord at about the sixth to the tenth week of life. This condition has an incidence of approximately 2.5/10 000 live births. The protruding structures may also include liver, small and large intestines, stomach, spleen, or gallbladder, and unlike gastroschisis they have a membranous amniotic covering.

The condition is often detected antenatally as a result of high maternal α-fetoprotein, prompting diagnosis with detailed ultrasonography.

Postnatally exomphalos is divided into major and minor varieties. In exomphalos minor, the neck of the defect is defined as being less than 4 cm in diameter. The sac contains only intestine and the defect is relatively easy to repair surgically. Exomphalos major is a relatively severe abnormality. The defect may be up to 10 cm in diameter and can contain liver or spleen.

Exomphalos is strongly associated with other severe malformations, such as cardiac anomalies (50%) and neural tube defects (40%). Chromosomal abnormalities are present in approximately 50 % of liveborn infants with omphalocele.

Treatment

Caesarean section is the preferred mode of delivery to ensure that the exomphalos sac remains intact during the birthing process. Where the defect is small primary surgical closure may be possible, although if the closure is tight abdominal organ ischaemia can ensue.

Staged closure using a Silastic Silo is an alternative and over a period of time the abdominal organs are gradually returned to the abdominal cavity, with the abdominal wall being closed at a second operation. A further treatment option includes painting the sac with flamazine, which dries out the sac, which then granulates and epithelializes; although surgical closure of the gap between the abdominal wall muscles is usually necessary in later life.

The prognosis of exomphalos major is poor with an overall mortality of between 30–80%.

Oesophageal atresia and tracheo-oesphageal fistula

Clinical features

Oesophageal atresia (OA), with or without tracheo-oesophageal fistula (TOF), is one of the most common conditions requiring surgical treatment in the first few days of life. It has an incidence of 1/2000 and 1/5000 respectively. The commonest variety occurring in 85% of cases is a blind ending proximal oesophageal pouch with a fistula from the trachea to the distal oesophagus.

In half of these cases maternal polyhydramnios is noted but antenatal diagnosis is uncommon. Clinical features include excess saliva, choking on feeds, gastric aspiration, and respiratory distress occurring shortly after birth. Patients with a TOF without OA may present in latter childhood with recurrent chest infections.

Approximately 50% of neonates will have associated congenital abnormalities. The VACTERL or VATER associations are the most frequently occurring, (*v*ertebral anomalies, *a*norectal malformations, *c*ardiac abnormalities, *t*racheo-oesophageal fistula, *r*enal anomalies and *l*imb malformations).

The diagnosis is primarily clinical. This may be confirmed by the inability to pass a large-bore nasogastric tube and/or the presence of gas in the abdomen on a plain abdominal radiograph suggesting a concomitant TOF.

Treatment

Management includes maintaining a patent airway and preventing aspiration of saliva. A sump suction drain is often placed in the upper pouch and left on continuous drainage.

Definitive treatment is surgical and includes ligating the TOF and performing an end-to-end anastomosis of the oesophagus through a right lateral thoracotomy.

Complications include anastomotic leak, re-fistulation, oesophageal stricture, and, most commonly, gastro-oesophageal reflux.

Duodenal atresia and stenosis

Clinical features

This may be complete or incomplete, with a ratio of 2:1 and has an approximate incidence of 1/10 000. It is believed that the deformity is caused by the failure of the duodenum to recanalize. The stomach and proximal duodenum are dilated and hypertrophied, while the distal small bowel is collapsed.

The most common site for atresia is the second part of duodenum at a region close to the ampulla of Vater with 60% being postampullary. The stenosis may be a short narrow segment or be represented by a small diaphragm. The biliary tree is usually normal. In 25% there is association with an annular pancreas encircling the second part of the duodenum, which may be atretic or stenotic.

There is a 50% association with polyhydramnios, and antenatal diagnosis is possible using ultrasound to visualize the hypertrophied, dilated stomach and duodenum.

Symptoms are of high gastrointestinal obstruction with copious vomiting. Postampullary stenosis presents with the classical picture of bile-stained vomiting. There is an association with other congenital abnormalities and gastrointestinal anomalies including Down syndrome (30%) and OA.

Treatment

Treatment includes pre-operative insertion of a nasogastric tube and aggressive fluid resuscitation. 40–50 ml of air can be syringed into the nasogastric tube following which abdominal radiographs may demonstrate the classic 'double bubble' sign. If the diagnosis is still in doubt the patient may be sent for an ultrasound.

The mainstay of surgery is a duodeno-duodenostomy following Kocher's manoeuvre to mobilize the duodenum. One layer of absorbable sutures for the anastomosis is usually sufficient. Diaphragms can be incised or excised. An annular pancreas is often left alone.

The vast majority of patients survive this surgery, the overall mortality is approximately 10% and usually relates to complications of other congenital abnormalities.

Meconium ileus

Clinical features

This is the most common cause of neonatal intraluminal intestinal obstruction. It has an 80% association with cystic fibrosis (CF). CF is an autosomal recessive condition with an incidence of 1/2000 live births.

In CF the pancreatic secretions are abnormally thick often causing obstruction within the pancreas itself with subsequent pancreatic autodigestion. This then triggers abnormal composition of meconium, which becomes devoid of proteolytic enzymes and contains more viscid ileal mucus and excess albumin. Putty-like lumps of meconium are therefore able to obstruct the bowel. They most commonly impact in the terminal ileum.

The proximal ileum distends, and there is often collapsed distal ileum and a microcolon. Complications include volvulus, perforation, and atresia.

Clinical features are bilious vomiting, abdominal distension, palpable distended bowel loops and the inability to pass meconium.

Plain abdominal radiographs often have an intraluminal 'ground glass' appearance as result of the abnormal composition of the viscid meconium. Calcification may occur as a result of meconium peritonitis and the development of an inflammatory mass.

Treatment

Treatment options include gastrografin enemas refluxed into the terminal ileum; the gastrograffin contains a wetting agent that helps to free viscid meconium.

If gastrografin enemas are unsuccessful then operative intervention is warranted. The traditional Bishop–Koop operation or vented ileostomy has now been superseded by enterotomy and lavage using either gastrografin or parvolex to unblock the bowel. At surgery any ischaemic bowel can be excised and the colon can be flushed to exclude distal obstruction.

Ninety per cent of these patients will survive the neonatal period. Their long term survival depends on the extent of the CF on the pulmonary system. (median survival is 31years).

Common neonatal conditions

Umbilical hernia

Clinical features

Anatomical abnormalities or discharge from the umbilicus, are common reasons for referral to a paediatric general surgeon.

Anatomical abnormalities, may be gastrointestinal in nature, such as an umbilical polyp an umbilical sinus or cysts. This latter represents an incomplete obliteration of the vitellointestinal duct. This failure of obliteration may also present with obstruction secondary to a fibrous band or due to a Meckel's diverticulum.

A completely patent vitello-intestinal duct is very rare as is a patent urachus, the former might be suspected as a result of feculent umbilical discharge or a prolapsed ileum via the duct, and the latter when there is passage of urine via the umbilicus during the first 3 weeks of life.

Umbilical hernia is common in infants. It has greater incidence among Afro-Caribbean infants, and is associated with congenital abnormalities such as Down syndrome, Beckwith–Wiedemann syndrome as well as an increase incidence among preterm infants.

It represents a delay in closure of the fascial ring resulting in a circular orifice with intact skin and peritoneum. It is worth noting that many of these defects resolve sponta-neously within the first 5 years of life and complications are rare.

Treatment

It is said that it is worth repairing defects that are of the order of 2 cm or more; however, if a child still has an umbilical hernia at 4 years of age a hernia repair is needed.

The operation involves fashioning a curved incision above or below the umbilicus. The hernial sac is identified and opened, the contents inspected and reduced. The excess fascial covering is excised to expose the free edge of the defect, and the defect is repaired with interrupted non-absorbable sutures. The 'vest over pants' Mayo repair is not routinely used in our practice but may be considered for very large defects. Recently the use of mesh to repair the defects is becoming more frequent.

Inguinal hernia

Clinical features

At the third month of gestation a fold of peritoneum termed the processus vaginalis is formed at the internal inguinal ring. The processus vaginalis extends to the scrotum in association with the descent of the testis. It then closes in the last few weeks of term gestation when testicular descent is completed.

Inguinal hernia and hydrocele in infants result from a failure of this obliterative process.

Inguinal hernia is one of the most common surgical conditions of childhood. It affects 1–5% of all children, with an especially high incidence in preterm infants (10% of preterm infants affected, and 35% of infants less than 28 weeks affected.) It is four to 10 times more common in boys than girls and the right side is more commonly involved.

A patent processus vaginalis only becomes a hernia when it contains viscera by definition forming an indirect inguinal hernia.

The presenting symptom is a reducible groin swelling. The diagnosis may be suspected by history alone, as it may not be possible to visualize the hernia in clinic. It is imperative that one listens to the parents to obtain an accurate history as this is often enough to justify groin exploration. It can be possible to feel the silken texture of the cord as it is rolled under the examining finger and this may help to confirm the diagnosis.

There is no place for conservative management of an inguinal hernia in infancy as the incidence of incarceration, which occurs in up to 18% of patients, is highest in the first 3 months of life and even higher in premature infants. Incarceration may result in strangulation and intestinal gangrene or gonadal infarction in the male, or strangulation of the ovary and fallopian tube in the female. Interestingly a hard lump in the groin in a female may indeed be the ovary trapped in an inguinal hernia sac.

Treatment

The operation of choice is a herniotomy as the hernia is due to a persistence of the processus vaginalis. This is performed through a tiny incision above the external inguinal ring followed by exposure and mobilization of the spermatic cord in the male. The hernial sac is then isolated and separated from the spermatic cord, with great care taken during dissection from the vas deferens and testicular vessels. The sac is the opened, it's contents inspected and reduced.

The sac is then twisted to ensure reduction of the contents and then transfixed with help of a Dennis Browne spoon using a non-absorbable suture. The sac is then divided. The distal end being left open to avoid iatrogenic hydrocele and the internal ring then retracts into the inguinal canal. The wound is closed in layers.

If incarceration does ensue and the child remains well, some surgeons advocate a trial of taxis but there is a risk of reduction of gangrenous bowel or *en masse* reduction. Failure of reduction or evidence of strangulation is an indication for emergency surgery, which can be very difficult in the presence of a friable processus vaginalis. Gravity reduction of hernias by elevation of the legs is not advised nowadays.

Hydrocele
Clinical features

A hydrocele results when the narrowly patent processus communicates with the tunica vaginalis and allows fluid to accumulate inside. It occurs more frequently on the right and may be bilateral. A hydrocele will transilluminate brilliantly and unlike a hernia it is not reducible and depending on the type of hydrocele the examiner may be able to get above the swelling.

Treatment

In the majority of infants hydrocele will resolve spontaneously by 1 year of age and operation is necessary only if it persists until this time. The operation consists of a high ligation of the processus vaginalis through a very similar approach for inguinal hernia repair.

Cryptorchidism
Clinical features

By the seventh month of gestation the testes are normally at the internal inguinal ring. True testicular descent begins at 28 weeks and is usually complete by birth. As the testes enters the internal inguinal ring a separate structure the gubernaculus emerges at the superficial ring. When this reaches the scrotum it contracts and draws the testes down into the scrotum. Failure of descent is usually due to either an abnormal hormonal environment or mechanical failure.

In approximately, 3% of male neonates, the testis will not be present in the scrotum at birth. This figure will have reduced to 1% at 1 year of life, and this is the rationale for waiting until the child is at least 1 year of age before performing an orchidopexy. It is important to be aware that many non-scrotal testes are retractile and require no treatment whatsoever.

A testis that has not descended into the scrotum by 1 year of age will seldom do so spontaneously. If it is located in the inguinal canal it will be subject to higher than normal ambient temperature, which impedes development. We advise orchidopexy near the second birthday. There is no convincing evidence that earlier operation preserves testicular function. The undescended testis is small 'ab initio' and remains so even after orchidopexy.

Treatment

Medical therapies with gonodatrophins succeed in causing decent in only a small percentage of children with cryptorchidism so that surgery is usually recommended.

At operation the testis and its spermatic cord are mobilized in the inguinal canal through an inguinal incision, separating the cremasteric muscle fibres. The spermatic cord is dissected up into the retroperitoneal region to obtain enough length of spermatic vasculature and vas deferens to bring the testicle into the scrotum without tension.

A shallow skin incision is then made through the skin and underlying dartos muscle at the base of the scrotum. A pouch large enough to accommodate the testis comfortably is fashioned between the dartos muscle and underlying loose fascia, and the testis is then secured in the 'dartos pouch' in the scrotum.

It is worth remembering that some undescended testes are abnormal and have failed to descend for that reason. In prune belly syndrome for example, the testes are intra-abdominal and demonstrate abnormal development microscopically and orchidopexy will not improve the long-term prognosis for testicular function in such patients.

There is a 10–40-fold increase in the incidence of testicular malignancy in patients with cryptorchidism and this appears to be true irrespective of orchidopexy. Fertility is also impaired in men with cryptorchidism and is reported to be 75% and 50% respectively in men who have undergone successful unilateral or bilateral orchidopexy.

Neonatal circumcision

While circumcision has been practised since ancient times, it is a surgical procedure that is losing popularity among some surgeons because of increased medical and cultural concerns, greater understanding of the natural history of the foreskin and modern treatment alternatives and a several opposing groups (eg. Society for the Preservation of the Foreskin in the USA).

The primary indications for circumcision in our practice are for a persistent complete phimosis (non-retractibility) and balanitis xerotica obliterans, although we also consider circumcision for troublesome ballooning of the glands and on religious grounds.

There is evidence to show that steroid cream (0.05% betamethasone) applied topically three times per day for 6 weeks has proven effective (80% success rate) in the management of uncomplicated childhood phimosis.

Surgical alternatives to circumcision gaining popularity are adhesiolysis for pronounced adhesions between the glands and the foreskin, and preputioplasty, which entails a longitudinal incision of the phimotic band and transverse closure with no tissue resection.

There are several ways of performing circumcision. Our practice involves preputial adhesiolysis, removal of smegma, elevation of the foreskin with artery clips, the use of a bone cutter to mark the inferior border of the glands followed by sharp dissection to remove the excess foreskin. Bleeding points are ligated and the wound closed with fine absorbable suture.

Infant conditions

Infantile hypertrophic pyloric stenosis

Clinical features

This relatively common condition has an incidence of 2/1000 live births in the UK. It tends to present at about 10 days–10 weeks of life, with a peak at 4 weeks. Boys are affected more than girls (4:1) and approximately half the affected individuals are first born children.

The aetiological factors are believed to be multifactoral. There is a familial tendency with 5% of infants affected from a mother who herself had the condition. A seasonal variation exists with more cases being reported in the winter months. There is also a body of evidence demonstrating a link between the condition and maternal exposure to macrolide antibiotics, such as erythromycin.

Several hypotheses have been postulated including increase stress resulting in a hormonal effect involving gastrin. Immunocytochemistry has shown that there appears to be a lower number of nerve fibres containing vasoactive intestinal peptide and encephalin in the pylorus of affected children.

Macroscopically there is an olive-shaped pyloric tumour measuring about 2.5 cm in diameter, causing gastric distension. At the duodenal end the pylorus bulges into the lumen creating a circumferential fornix. Microscopically, massive hypertrophy of the circular muscle as well as some hypertrophy of the longitudinal muscle is evident. The pyloric canal is lengthened and there is often marked mucosal oedema.

The child feeds normally initially then gradually starts to vomit with increasing frequency and force. The vomit is not bile stained; rather it usually contains milk curds and mucus. In time the vomiting becomes projectile. The infant is characteristically hungry and eager to feed again after vomiting. There is a 20% association with haematemesis secondary to associated oesophagitis. The child has often lost weight by the time they present due to dehydration.

Diagnosis

The diagnosis is made by performing a test feed. The baby is held by the mother using her left hand and takes a test feed from the mother's left breast. Visible peristalsis of the hypertrophied stomach may be seen through the anterior abdominal wall. The examiner uses his left hand to feel the pylorus or pyloric tumour. This has been likened to feeling a walnut through a blanket.

Projectile vomiting, weight loss, and a palpable pylorus make the diagnosis certain. If the test feed is negative but the diagnosis is still suspected, the test feed can be repeated 4–6 hours later or the diagnosis may be confirmed with ultrasound with 90% accuracy.

The children have a characteristic hypochloraemic metabolic alkalosis with dehydration and a renal response that results in potassium loss via the kidneys. The patients must be resuscitated prior to their being transferred to the operating theatre. A recommended regimen being 0.5% normal saline in 10% dextrose plus 2 g of KCl per 500 ml bag to avoid hypokalaemia.

Treatment

Over the last decade these patients tend to be managed in specialist centres. However, there is evidence is emerging to suggest that the condition can be treated safely in a district general hospital when appropriately trained surgical, anaesthetic, and paediatric staff deliver the care.

Medical management, with high-dose atropine sulphate has been shown in some patients to lead to clinical recovery with a reduced pyloric thickness on ultrasound and therefore might prevent the need for surgery in some instances.

The surgical operation of choice being a Ramstedt's pyloromyotomy, this is performed through a right upper transverse muscle splitting incision. Laparoscopic pyloromyotomy has gained popularity in recent years as it results in better cosmesis, reduced hospital stay, less postoperative emesis, and carries a lower risk of wound complications versus the open technique. Laparoscopic pyloromyotomy has in several studies been shown to be as safe and efficient as traditional open pyloromyotomy.

A supra-umbilical incision may be as cosmetically friendly as a laparoscopic procedure and may counter balance the cost of laparoscopic training and the financial implications of offering a laparoscopic service.

In the traditional Ramstedt's procedure the pylorus is delivered with its avascular border uppermost. The serosa is incised near the pyloroduodenal junction to at least 2 cm on the antrum. The muscles fibres are spread using a retractor and the mucosa bulges into the defect. Air may be syringed via the nasogastric tube into the stomach and squeezed past the pylorus to exclude leakage. Feeds are withheld for the first 24 hours postoperatively and then reinstated with no need for complex feeding regimens.

Mortality rates are low following surgery (<1%), wound infection and dehiscence still occur and accounts for an overall morbidity of approximately 10%.

Intussusception

Clinical features

This is the most common cause of intestinal obstruction in infants aged 6–18 months. It occurs most commonly in the terminal ileum and can only occur in the presence of mobile partly malrotated caecum and terminal ileum. When a lead point exists in the bowel wall, peristalsis forces that part of the bowel to invaginate and progress along the lumen through the ileocaecal valve and along the colon. Most intussusceptions only reach the transverse colon but if sufficiently mobile it may present at the anus.

Lead points may include an inflamed Peyer's patch, a Meckel's diverticulum, or a polyp (as in Peutz–Jegher syndrome).

The clinical features include attacks of intermittent intestinal colic that last a few minutes, causing high pitch screaming, pallor, and bilious vomiting. This causes the child to draw their knees up or go on all fours. The child tends to be quiet, listless, and anorexic between these bouts.

Rectal bleeding and the classically described red current jelly stool is said to be a late sign and may not always be present.

Examination may reveal a remarkable soft and non-tender abdomen if the child is examined between attacks. A sausage-shaped mass in the right upper quadrant is seen in approximately 30% of cases. A rectal examination may reveal the apex of the intussusception.

A plain abdominal radiograph will demonstrate the absence of caecal gas shadow from the right iliac fossa. An ultrasound will reveal the classic 'doughnut' sign of the intussusception.

Treatment

All children with intussusception require resuscitation prior to definitive treatment as they have third space fluid losses, losing fluid into the ileum itself and secondary fluid loss due to bowel wall oedema.

Reduction by enema should be attempted in all but the sickest children or in those where there is already a suspicion of ischaemic bowel or free intraperitoneal air. Hydrostatic reduction with barium sulphate has been replaced by air insufflation under ultrasonic guidance with an 85% success rate. (The success rates of these techniques are highest in centres treating more than 20 cases per annum.) Air insufflation has the added advantage that if perforation occurs there is no soiling of the peritoneum with irritant barium. Free reflux of air into the terminal ileum is the marker of a successful reduction.

If there is a suspicion of necrotic bowel or if the intussusception is irreducible, laparotomy is warranted, this is achieved through a muscle splitting incision in the right iliac fossa. Reduction is achieved by gently squeezing the mass to reduce the oedema. Any polyp can be removed and necrotic bowel excised.

No matter the method used, there is still a 5–10% recurrence rate. Repeated enemas can be used but at the third recurrence laparotomy is justified.

Emergency surgery

Torsion of the testicle

Clinical features

Torsion of the testicle has remained one of the few true common paediatric surgical emergencies and has been recognized as such since Delaisiauvre described the first case in a child with an undescended testicle in a hotel in Paris in 1839. There is still a relatively high rate of testicular loss, which in today's era carries an increasing risk of litigation.

Torsion may occur at any age but is most common around puberty and is rare after the age of 30 years.

The usual predisposing factor is a high investment of the tunica vaginalis, which allows the testicle to hang like a 'bell clapper' inside and the testicle and spermatic cord to rotate within the tunica.

The diagnosis is made on the basis of history, examination, and a high index of suspicion. This is especially true in young men who present with acute pain and swelling as it has been shown that testicular torsion accounts for 90% of acutely presenting scrotal symptoms in the 13–21-year-old age group.

The patient with torsion may experience nausea and vomiting and the pain may be referred to the groin or iliac fossa (a not uncommon mistake is to misdiagnose as acute appendicitis), hence the scrotum must always be examined.

The testis, is swollen and tender and may have a characteristically high and horizontal lie in the scrotum. It is painful in all planes on examination. The differential diagnosis includes torsion of the testicular appendage of Morgani, orchitis, and idiopathic scrotal oedema. More rarely haemorrhage into a testicular tumour can present with acute scrotal pain.

Investigations should not delay urgent exploration. Doppler ultrasound may be helpful in making diagnosis but can often be misleading especially in cases of so-called 'intermittent torsion' where a reactive hyperaemia may occur after an episode of twisting.

Treatment

Surgery within 4 hours usually allows testicular preservation, some atrophy occurs between 4 and 8 hours, and after 10 hours ischaemic necrosis is virtually inevitable. When the testis does appear viable the redundant tunica vaginalis should be resected and the testis returned to the scrotal cavity and fixed to the scrotal septum and dartos muscle by a row of non-absorbable sutures. Three-point fixation is recommended to reduce the risk of recurrent testicular torsion and the contralateral side should also be fixed at the same time. Orchidectomy is the best course of action if the testis is non-viable.

Acute appendicitis

Clinical features

Appendicitis is the most common acute surgical emergency in childhood. The history may be quite variable but often includes peri-umbilical intermittent colicky pain that classically shifts to become a constant, severe, progressive pain in the right iliac fossa. The pain may be associated nausea, vomiting, and anorexia.

As the inflammatory process develops the oedema and swelling may result in thrombosis of the appendicular artery (this is an end artery), which in turn may preclude to gangrene and subsequent perforation. Perforation is a more common occurrence in appendicitis in children than in adults and tends to occur 36–48 hours after the initial symptoms commenced.

The signs of acute appendicitis includes low-grade pyrexia, foetor oris with dry mucous membranes, and a coating of the tongue indicative of sepsis often with an accompanying tachycardia.

Abdominal signs include localized tenderness, with guarding of the overlying muscles in the right iliac fossa. Rovsing's sign and/or a positive psoas stretch test can be elicited in an older more cooperative child.

The laboratory findings in acute appendicitis are the same as those in the adult, specifically a raised white blood cell count and an elevated C-reactive protein are both markers of acute inflammation. While the diagnosis is made on clinical grounds ultrasonographic features of appendicitis include a visible tender tubular mass in the right iliac fossa with a total transverse diameter of 6 mm or greater. Ultrasound may also be used to distinguish from other pelvic pathology in young girls and to aid in the diagnosis of a para-appendiceal abscess. Although some studies have shown 90% overall accuracy for both ultrasound and computed tomography diagnosis of acute appendicitis, in most units the predictive value of these tests, which often delay decision making, is far lower.

Differential diagnosis

The differential diagnosis is broad and includes, urinary tract infection, testicular torsion, Henoch–Scholein purpura, constipation, mesenteric adenitis, and non-specific abdominal pain.

Mesenteric adenitis is often confused with appendicitis, the former is more often associated with a prodromal viral illness with secondary enlargement of the lymph nodes in the small bowel mesentery. The child is often flushed, and has a high pyrexia. The abdominal pain is commonly more diffuse and less localized although the point of maximal tenderness may be in the right iliac fossa.

Treatment

The treatment of acute appendicitis in children is generally the same as in adults, proceeding to appendicectomy on the basis of clinical suspicion. This involves an incision over the site of maximal tenderness, dissecting through the various muscle layers, incising the peritoneum, delivering the appendix then proceeding to ligate the mesoappendix. The base is then crushed and tied and the appendix is removed and it is our practice to invert the appendix stump using a purse string suture. The wound is closed in layers.

The procedure can be preformed laparoscopically and many advocate its use as a means of both diagnosis and treatment.

Only when there is an established appendix mass in a relatively well child can conservative management with antibiotics be considered in order to avoid a hazardous operation in that circumstance.

Chapter 8

Allergy in childhood

Andrew Clark

Introduction

Allergy in the developed world is common and increasing in prevalence, severity, and complexity resulting in an increased burden on the child, their family, and healthcare providers. Diagnosis is usually straightforward and assessment and treatment is aimed at controlling ongoing symptoms and allergen avoidance. To provide effective advice takes considerable time and an understanding of the natural history of allergy.

'The allergic march'

This term is used to describe the way in which allergic disease evolves throughout infancy and childhood. The first manifestation of allergy is eczema, appearing in the first year of life followed by the development of sensitization (the presence of specific IgE) to food allergens. Clinical allergy to those foods emerges in the pre-school years. The onset of asthma follows and sensitization to indoor (e.g. house dust mite) and then outdoor allergens (e.g. grass pollen) occurs by school age. Allergic rhinitis appears last, usually by about 10 years of age.

Eczema

Eczema is the first manifestation of atopic disease appearing in infancy as an itchy, dry scaly rash on the face, trunk, and legs in infants, spreading to the flexor creases in later childhood.

In infants and toddlers with troublesome eczema it may be worth testing for sensitization to airborne allergens e.g. house dust mite as one could recommend avoidance measures which may have an impact on eczema and any coexisting asthma (Table 8.1). Although it should also be remembered that 50% of those with a positive allergen-specific IgE have no clinical allergy.

Food allergy

Milk, egg, and peanut are the commonest foods to cause allergy in early childhood. Diagnosis is straightforward by means of the clinical history and simple diagnostic tests.

Table 8.1 House dust mite avoidance measures

Consider purchasing a house-dust mite allergen protection cover for the mattress, pillows, and duvet; the mattress cover must completely surround the mattress to seal in the allergen. Alternatively, vacuum the mattress weekly.
Damp dust bedroom weekly
Hoover bedroom weekly
Cuddly toys may be frozen overnight (to kill house dust mite) and then washed
Bedclothes should be washed at 60°C
Avoid bunk beds if possible; if not, occupy upper bed and consider mattress covers

Deciding if its food allergy, or not ... the clinical history

Approximately 30% of the population report that they have a food allergy. In children the prevalence of actual IgE-mediated reactions to food is lower, approximately 4–8%. The gold standard for diagnosis is the double-blind placebo-controlled food challenge, but is time consuming and useful only as a research tool. In clinical practice the history is most informative when deciding whether food allergy is present and combined with demonstration of specific IgE, the diagnosis can be made in most cases. Consideration of the following points will give a good indication of the presence of food allergy. First, almost all children with food allergy have a history of at least one other allergic disease usually eczema or asthma and most also have a family history of atopy (but not necessarily food allergy).

Consider the food implicated in the reaction; families usually have a clear idea of the cause and typical foods tend to be responsible for reactions at particular ages, e.g. egg, milk and peanut in infants; tree nuts or fish for older children. It is rare for minor food ingredients such as preservatives or colourings to be responsible.

Take notice of the nature of the reaction described (Table 8.2). Local symptoms with pruritus, urticaria, and angioedema of the mouth, lips, face, or throat are typical of food allergy. However, in infants with eczema, citrus fruit, tomato, and strawberries are often blamed for apparent allergic reactions, because they may induce a flat erythematous rash around the mouth and chin. This represents an irritant effect of these foods on eczematous skin, rather than a specific allergy.

Table 8.2 Features of a type 1 hypersensitivity reaction

Oral/facial and/or generalized angioedema and/or urticaira
Vomiting, diarrhoea, and abdominal pain
Wheeze (lower airways narrowing)
Tight throat and/or change in voice pitch (laryngeal oedema)
Shortness of breath
Drowsiness and collapse (hypotension)

Timing is important; IgE-mediated reactions usually begin within a few minutes of eating the suspected food, this can be delayed by up to a couple of hours if the allergen is part of a large meal or is in a fatty matrix (e.g. a curry), which may delay absorption. The duration of the reaction should also be considered; type 1 reactions usually resolve by 6 hours. Rashes that occur 'a day after' eating a suspect food or last 'for several days' may be unrelated to IgE-mediated food allergy but may be due instead to idiopathic urticaria. Severe reactions to foods are usually characterized by dominant respiratory symptoms; hypotension being an unusual primary feature.

Allergy tests

Allergy tests can be helpful but results should be interpreted in the context of the clinical history and one should appreciate their limitations. The most useful tests are for detection of specific IgE to a suspected allergen (sensitization). The combination of a typical history of a type 1 reaction (see Table 8.2) to an allergen together with evidence of sensitization is usually sufficient to diagnose allergy in the clinical setting.

Two such tests are commonly available:

1. The 'CAP/RAST' tests measure specific IgE levels in the serum; results are reported in both kU/l and a corresponding 'grade' 0–6 (grade 0 ≤0.35 kU/l, grade 6 ≥100 kU/l). A result of ≥0.35 kU/l (grade 1 and above) is taken to be positive.

2. Skin prick tests (SPT) detect specific IgE on mast cells within the skin. These require a skilled operator who performs the test regularly, and maintenance of a range of allergen extracts. A SPT weal diameter of ≥3 mm is taken to be positive.

Although 'CAP/RAST' are widely available and seem the better option in primary care, they do not have high sensitivity or specificity and need to be interpreted with caution: a negative SPT usually refutes clinical allergy. However, 'CAP/RAST' can produce false negative results; in the case of peanut allergy this occurs in up to 19% where there is a convincing history and a positive SPT. If a negative CAP/RAST is found in the context of a typical history, then skin prick testing may confirm the history.

'Blind' testing where there is no history of a reaction available (e.g. testing a sibling of a peanut allergic child), is not usually helpful as approximately 50% of those with a positive specific IgE test will have no clinical allergy. Additionally, even a 'true' negative specific IgE result does not preclude the child from developing allergy some time later. Therefore it is preferable that the use of tests for specific IgE is limited to situations where there is a history of a typical reaction after definite allergen exposure.

It is important to remember that the amount of specific IgE detected by either test (serum specific IgE grade or SPT weal diameter) does not predict clinical severity. It is possible to have a very high level of specific IgE (CAP grade 6 or SPT >20 mm) and only suffer mild clinical reactions and vice versa. Tests for specific IgE should only be used to confirm a clinical history of allergy and not used to inform on severity or whether to provide injectable adrenaline. The severity of food allergy is best assessed from the clinical history and the presence of asthma (see below).

Individual allergies

Peanut allergy

The prevalence of this condition has risen over the past decade and it now affects 1.5% of 5-year old children. The most frequent age at presentation is 6–24 months, usually after the first apparent exposure but it can occur for the first time in older children. Urticaria around the mouth is common with accompanying lip swelling and angioedema of the eyes. Generalized urticaria also occurs, and in a third of cases there is airways narrowing, usually mild wheeze or laryngeal oedema. Severe reactions occur in about 10% and are usually manifest by severe wheeze and dyspnoea. In the presence of a typical clinical history the diagnosis can be confirmed a positive skin or serum IgE test.

The cornerstone of good management is good allergen avoidance advice, which should concentrate on how to check food labelling and situations when accidents are most likely to occur, usually when the child is out of their parents' direct supervision (e.g. birthday parties for toddlers, or eating out for teenagers). Although it seems straightforward to advise a family to avoid nuts, there are caveats. Food warnings, for example may be in small print, hidden under a flap or use an alternate name for the allergen (e.g. arachis for peanut). Further, labels of the sort 'this product may contain traces of nuts' are often mis-interpreted as meaning that there is a risk of only minor contamination and it is safe to eat the food, especially if it had previously been tolerated. However, the amount of potential contamination is not limited to traces and such products have even been found to contain whole nuts. Therefore we currently advise our nut allergy sufferers to avoid foods labelled as such, especially chocolates, cakes and biscuits. Most supermarkets can supply lists of nut-free foods on request and the anaphylaxis campaign provides essential updates on food warnings (see below). We advise children with peanut and/or nut allergy to avoid all nut types to reduce the risk of developing further allergies. This avoidance information should be disseminated to the entire family and also nursery staff, school catering staff, and teachers—good links with paediatric community services is therefore essential.

Up to 20% of young children with mild peanut allergy may grow out of it; however, it is not known if peanut allergy will recur in these children.

Tree nut allergy

Tree nut allergy is also increasing in prevalence, especially among children with peanut allergy. Allergy to Brazil nut accounts for 16% of reactions to peanut or nuts followed by almond, hazelnut, cashew, and walnut. The clinical features of these allergies are different to those of peanut. First, they occur in mostly in older children or adults, although they can occur in infants. Secondly, Brazil and walnut in particular seems to provoke predominately upper airways symptoms of pharyngeal and/or laryngeal oedema and therefore a greater proportion of reactions are severe. Tree nut allergy also seems to be more persistent than peanut allergy and resolution is rare.

Egg allergy

This begins in infancy and again is almost always accompanied by urticaria, although wheeze and breathlessness can occur uncommonly. The natural history is quite different to that of nut allergy as approximately 50% will begin to grow out of egg allergy by 2 years of age and 80% by 5 years. Egg allergens are heat-labile and well-cooked egg is less allergenic than lightly cooked or raw egg. For those with a history of mild allergic reactions to egg and no asthma, from the age of 3 years, egg can be reintroduced at home in a series of step-wise increases in allergen dose. Initially children may tolerate well cooked egg (e.g. in sponge cake) and some months later tolerate lightly cooked egg (e.g. a hard boiled egg) and finally a soft boiled egg. The pace of reintroduction should be guided by the history of previous reactions but a 6-monthly interval usually works well. Any reactions are usually minor and the previously tolerated form of egg should be continued for a further 6 months. Exceptions occur, where there has been a history of airways narrowing during a reaction or there has only ever been trace exposure (e.g. skin contact) and therefore sensitivity is unknown or where there is asthma, where specialist referral is warranted.

MMR vaccination

All children with egg allergy should receive MMR vaccination, even if the allergy to egg is severe. Current guidelines recommend that children with a history of current asthma, or those with a history of airways narrowing during egg reactions should be vaccinated in hospital. All other children can be safely immunized in primary care, where of course facilities for treatment of anaphylaxis should be available. Influenza vaccination is contraindicated in children with egg allergy.

Milk allergy

A proportion of children with eczema have hypersensitivity to cow's milk protein. This may be associated with immediate-type IgE-mediated response (e.g. facial angioedema) or delayed-type hypersensitivity (e.g. worsening of eczema and/or gastro-oesophageal reflux). Allergy tests for IgE to cow's milk protein will only highlight those with immediate-type responses. The only practical way to demonstrate delayed-type allergy to cow's milk protein is to perform a complete dairy exclusion diet for a period of 3 months followed by milk challenges on at least two occasions. During dairy avoidance a highly hydrolysed or elemental formula is recommended in boys aged less than 6 months. Allergy to soya is common in infants who are allergic to cow's milk protein and goat's milk should not be used due to the risk of further sensitization/allergy and anaemia. For children weaned on to solid foods, dairy products such as cheese and yoghurts should also be avoided.

From the age of 2–3 years cow's milk formula could be reintroduced in mild cases as milk allergy/intolerance will resolve in the majority.

Up and coming food allergens

Allergies to sesame seed and kiwi fruit are seen more commonly now, reflecting increased exposure to these foods. Both can provoke severe allergic reactions and warrant prompt introduction of avoidance advice and availability of appropriate emergency medication. The prevalence of allergy to several types of tree nut appears to be increasing, for example cashew, pistachio and pecan. Pine nut can also rarely cause IgE-mediated reactions. Coconut allergy is rare and we do not advise peanut or tree nut allergic patients to avoid this food (except in foods where cross-contamination with nuts is possible).

Comprehensive management of food allergy: not just 'Who needs an EpiPen?'

Often this question is considered in isolation when a child presents with food allergy, but it needs to be seen in the context of the complete management package that includes detailed allergen avoidance advice, selection of emergency medication, provision of an emergency treatment plan, and training of carers. The use of such management plans in children with food allergy has been associated with a reduction in the number and severity of further reactions.

Good allergen avoidance advice is the cornerstone of management. It should be detailed and available in a written form for the family to refer to later. Advice should be individualized for the child's age, e.g. toddlers are at greatest risk from snacks in situations such as birthday parties and visits to grandparents. In contrast, advice given to adolescents may focus on eating out of the home.

A comprehensive management package should also define the appropriate emergency medication for each individual. Every child with food allergy should have oral antihistamines available at all times and they should be used first in any allergic reaction. We advise that children with asthma or those with a previous history of airways narrowing on exposure to the allergen (e.g. wheeze or laryngeal oedema) should also carry injectable adrenaline which may be prescribed by the general practitioner. This should also be considered if a child has had a mild generalized reaction (e.g. generalized urticaria with no airways narrowing) after only a tiny trace had been ingested and therefore their sensitivity is unknown. An individualized written treatment plan should be provided detailing when and how the different medications are to be administered; this can be adopted by the child's nursery or school. The family should be trained in the use of injectable adrenaline if it is provided, with the aid of a 'dummy' trainer device. For convenience, we recommend that one injector is kept at home and one at school/nursery, with a further one for travelling. It is uncommon to need more than one injector per site, but may be useful for example in a large teenager (e.g. 60 kg) where a single EpiPen (0.3 mg adrenaline) may not provide sufficient dosage. Good control of any concomitant asthma is vital. Networks with community paediatric nurses are essential to ensure school teachers are appropriately trained in avoidance strategies and the use of emergency medication.

Families should be reviewed regularly; this gives the chance to record any accidental ingestion, detect new allergies, repeat and modify the avoidance advice, repeat specific IgE testing and to check technique with the injectable adrenaline device. It is important also to review those who are not provided with injectable adrenaline as they are at risk of developing more severe food reactions if they subsequently develop asthma.

Venom allergy

Children only very rarely have severe allergic reactions to insect venom. Those who have suffered generalized venom reactions usually resolve. Children with food allergy do not seem to be at increased risk of severe venom allergy.

Teenagers

Food allergy in the teenage years presents its own difficulties. In common with many other chronic conditions (e.g. asthma or diabetes) disease control deteriorates at this time. The result is that the majority of severe and near-fatal food allergic reactions occur in teenagers and young adults. Factors include peer pressure and acceptance, embarrassment, deteriorating attention to asthma control, alcohol use, and reactions to meals rather than snacks (dose effect). Adolescents with food allergy require an increased level of support.

Other allergies

Latex allergy

Until recently this was seen mostly in children with spina bifida who had been subjected to high latex exposure through multiple surgical procedures and the use of latex indwelling urinary catheters. It is seen less often in childhood now and is becoming more common among healthcare staff, e.g. nurses. Symptoms vary from mild erythema and itching to anaphylaxis on minimal contact. If it is detected it is important that the patient wears a medic-alert bracelet and receives a letter to pass on to their dentist/doctor regarding the use of latex-free gloves. Cross-reactivity to certain foods should be borne in mind, e.g. avocado, kiwi fruit, and banana.

Penicillin allergy

Not infrequently primary care doctors are faced with a child who was said to have had a rash when given penicillin on a previous occasion. This may be approached by examining the history for typical features of an allergic reaction, including any temporal relationship. Serum-specific IgE or skin tests to the major and minor penicillin determinants may reveal sensitization and confirm the history. If there is a history of severe reaction or if the choice of antibiotics is becoming limited then referral to a specialist for more detailed testing may be worthwhile.

Idiopathic angioedema and urticaria

Some children may present with a single episode of urticaria appearing after a viral infection and never be troubled by it again. In others the condition is recurrent.

Some children have urticaria provoked by physical stimuli, e.g. scratching the skin may induce weals in dermographism, localized cooling may cause weals to appear in cold urticaria, or lesions may be provoked by sweating in cholinergic urticaria.

Otherwise, in patients with symptoms occurring without an obvious cause over a 6-week period the condition is termed chronic urticaria and angioedema. There are several characteristics in the history that help to distinguish this condition from IgE-mediated food allergy. First, the lack of a temporal association with ingestion of a food allergen, e.g. an urticarial rash appearing 24 hours after peanut ingestion is unlikely to be due to peanut allergy. Secondly, there may be no peri-oral urticaria or lip swelling-an uncommon finding in true type-1 food allergy. Thirdly, it happens more commonly in children without an atopic history. Finally, the rash usually lasts for more than 6 hours and can be present for several days at a time.

Underlying conditions are uncommon in childhood but important ones to consider are autoimmune thyroid disease and vasculitis.

Treatment is aimed at limiting symptoms of irritation with oral antihistamines, which may need to be given daily. Oral steroids are reserved for use in pharyngeal/laryngeal oedema, which occurs uncommonly in childhood.

Inherited angioedema

This is a rare condition caused by an inherited deficiency of C1-esterase inhibitor. It typically presents in late childhood with a family history of affected members and episodes of angioedema, usually precipitated by physical trauma. The presence of urticaria is very unusual in this condition and makes the diagnosis unlikely. Patients may suffer repeated bouts of abdominal pain due to bowel oedema. Treatment is with concentrated C1-esterase inhibitor during acute attacks.

Patient support groups

The personal and psychological costs of allergy to the family are considerable. For example, a recent study of children with peanut allergy showed this group had a significantly poorer quality of life score than those with insulin-dependent diabetes mellitus.

The Anaphylaxis Campaign (http://www.anaphylaxis.org.uk/; 01252 373793) is a registered charity that provides up-to-date information and guidance to its members, the media, health professionals, and food companies. They have a strong campaigning role, particularly in the areas of product labelling and development of allergy services. The campaign also conducts research into the cause and care of severe allergies. EpiPen trainer packs including dummy pens are available free of charge to health professionals (www.epipen.co.uk). Dummy pens are available for purchase by parents for £7.50 from ALK-Abello (01488 686016).

Details and locations of your local allergy clinic can be obtained by going to: http://www.bsaci.org and clicking on 'Allergy Clinics'.

Further Reading

Clark AT, Ewan PW (2003). Interpretation of tests for nut allergy in a thousand patients, in relation to allergy or tolerance. *Clinical and Experimental Allergy* **33**: 1041.

Ewan PW (1996). Clinical study of peanut and nut allergy in 62 consecutive patients: new features and associations. *British Medical Journal* **312**: 1074–1078.

Ewan PW, Clark AT (2001). Long-term prospective observational study of the outcome of a management plan in patients with peanut and nut allergy referred to a regional allergy centre. *Lancet* **357**: 111–115.

Ewan PW, Clark AT (2005). Efficacy of a management plan based on severity assessment in longitudinal and case-controlled studies of 747 children with nut allergy: proposal for good practice. *Clinical and Experimental Allergy* **35**: 571–556.

Grundy J, Matthews S, Bateman B, Dean T, Arshad SH (2002). Rising prevalence of allergy to peanut in children: data from sequential cohorts. *Journal of Allergy and Clinical Immunology* **110**: 784–789.

Hourihane JO, Kilburn SA, Dean TP, Warner JO (1997). Clinical characteristics of peanut allergy. *Clinical and Experimental Allergy* **27**: 634–639.

Hourihane JO, Roberts SA, Warner JO (1998). Resolution of peanut allergy: a case control study. *British Medical Journal* **316**: 1271–1275.

House of Commons Parliamentary Select Committee on Health Inquiry in Allergy Services (2004). *Report on the Provision of Care and Treatment for Allergies.*

Royal College of Physicians of London (2003). Allergy: the unmet need. A blueprint for better patient care. A report of the Royal College of Physicians Working Party on the provision of allergy services in the UK. Royal College of Physicians of London.

Sporik R, Hill DJ, Hosking CS (2000). Specificity of allergen skin testing in predicting positive open food challenges to milk, egg and peanut in children. *Clinical and Experimental Allergy* **30**: 1540–1546.

Watura J (2002). Nut allergy in schoolchildren: a survey of schools in the Severn NHS Trust. *Archives of Disease in Childhood* **86**: 240–244.

Chapter 9

Ear, nose, and throat problems in childhood

Pandora Hadfield

Acute otitis media

Incidence

Middle ear infection is common in children. In the United Kingdom 30% of children under the age of 3 years visit their general practitioner with acute otitis media (AOM) each year. Of these 97% receive antibiotics. One in 10 children will have an episode of AOM by 3 months of age.

Symptoms

AOM presents with systemic and local signs (see Table 9.1), it has a rapid onset. Younger children often present with non-specific symptoms, 90% of infants and toddlers have associated rhinitis. On otoscopy a middle ear effusion is present, with reduced mobility on tympanic pneumoscopy (formal tympanometry is not necessary). Local signs of inflammation are seen with a bulging, red (Figure 9.1), yellow or cloudy tympanic membrane. This may burst and discharge leaving a temporary perforation which heals once the infection settles.

Natural history

In about 80% of children AOM resolves spontaneously within 3 days and long-term hearing is unaffected. AOM may be uncomplicated (one or two episodes) or recurrent (three episodes in 6 months or four episodes in a year). Some children are at increased risk of AOM. Predisposing factors include cleft palate or Down syndrome (ICSI 2002), AOM before 6 months of age (ICSI 2002), a family history of AOM in a parent or sibling (ICSI 2002), parental smoking (Strachan and Cook 1998), day care attendance, use of a dummy (Hanafin and Griffiths 2002) and bottle feeding (Williamson et al. 1994). If either parent smokes, a child is at increased risk of recurrent AOM and glue ear. With the evidence to date, it is not possible to quantify the risk. The use of a dummy, especially over 10 months of age, triples the incidence of AOM. Breast feeding protects babies against AOM and against glue ear later in life.

Table 9.1 Symptoms and signs of acute otitis media

Children under 3 years	Children 3 years and over
Irritability	Otalgia
Fever	Otorrhoea
Night waking	Hearing loss
Poor feeding	Ear popping
Coryza	Ear fullness
Balance problems	Dizziness
Hearing loss	
Otalgia/pulling at the ear	

Treatment

Analgesia

One randomized controlled trial (Bertin *et al*. 1996) compared paracetamol, the non-steroidal anti-inflammatory ibuprofen and placebo given thrice daily for 48 hours. Pain control was better with ibuprofen; there was no significant difference between

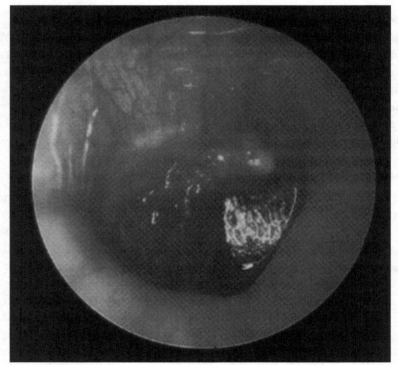

Fig. 9.1 Acute right otitis media. See colour plate 1. Reproduced with permission from: Bingham BJG, Hawke M, Kwok P, *Atlas of Clinical Otolaryngology* 1991, Mosby-Year Book.

paracetamol and placebo. All treatments were equally well tolerated. However, a beneficial effect of paracetamol may have been missed since it is usually given four times a day and the trial numbers were small.

Antibiotics

These do not appear to be indicated for the first or second uncomplicated episode of AOM. Two systematic reviews (Rosenfeld *et al.* 1994; Del Mar *et al.* 1997) showed that at most they may reduce late pain (days 2–7) and reduce the risk of contralateral AOM. However, they had no effect on the first 24 hours of pain (when it is usually at its worst) nor did they reduce subsequent attacks of AOM or deafness 1 month later. The number needed to treat was 20, therefore 20 children had to be treated early with antibiotics to prevent one child from experiencing pain at days 2–7. So 19 of the 20 had antibiotics without benefit. In addition adverse effects (diarrhoea, vomiting, and rashes) were doubled in children taking antibiotics.

In recurrent AOM and in those at increased risk of AOM, antibiotics are indicated.

The commonest causative bacteria are *Streptococcus pneumoniae*, *Haemophilus influenzae*, and *Moraxella catarrhalis*. Guidelines from the Institute for Clinical Systems Improvement (ICIS 2002) are that first-line treatment is amoxycillin 40 mg/kg per day (125 mg tds up to 10 years of age) for 5 days if low risk, 10 days if high risk. As a second-line treatment amoxycillin can be repeated at double the dose, if this is unsuccessful augmentin or a cephalosporin can be used. There is less evidence for trimethoprim, clarithromycin, erythromycin, and azithromycin.

In a systematic review of 33 randomized controlled trials prophylactic antibiotics have demonstrated a modest benefit in preventing recurrent AOM. There was no difference between antibiotics, but a slightly better response if the course exceeds 6 months. A typical regimen would be amoxycillin 20 mg/kg per day (half the normal dose) for over 6 months. This reduces the frequency of AOM by about 50%, but does not abolish it (Williams RL 1993).

Who should be referred?

An ear, nose and throat (ENT) opinion should be sought if medical treatment is unsuccessful or complications are suspected. This includes persistent pain and fever for four or more days after second-line antibiotics or when no benefit is derived from prophylactic antibiotics. Ventilation tubes (grommets) are occasionally recommended if maximum medical treatment has failed. They can be effective in reducing or preventing subsequent AOM; however, the ventilation tubes may become a focus of infection, prolonging episodes of otorrhoea. Complications of AOM are rare but include mastoiditis, venous sinus thrombosis, and meningitis. Symptoms, although often masked nowadays by antibiotic therapy, include fluctuating pyrexia, rigors, headache, neck pain, papilloedema, and visual loss.

Glue ear

What is glue ear?

Glue ear or otitis media with effusion (OME) is a persistent middle ear effusion without the inflammatory signs of AOM. It develops as a result of infection in a child at risk, probably with Eustachian tube dysfunction. An initial viral upper respiratory tract infection is followed by bacterial colonisation of the nasopharynx and ultimately the middle ear becomes infected. Mucosal changes lead to the production of an effusion, this is initially thin and serous but eventually becomes thick and tenacious, hence the term 'glue ear'. It may inhibit the normal developmental pneumatization of the mastoid air cell system. On otoscopy a middle ear effusion with a fluid level and air bubbles (Figure 9.2) may be evident. The tympanic membrane is opaque or yellowish, in a neutral or retracted position (Figure 9.3) with decreased mobility. The diagnosis can be confirmed by pneumatic otoscopy or tympanometry.

How common is it?

Over the next year 42% of 3 year olds may begin an episode of glue ear. Because these episodes are usually short, the prevalence of children with glue ear is less than this, but in the 2–5-year age range 15–20% of children will have glue ear at any time. The prevalence in children older than this falls to less than 5% by 7 years of age (Bandolier 1994). The risk factors are similar to those for AOM: younger age, male sex, cleft palate, Down syndrome, family history, autumn and winter months, day care, and passive smoking. The protective effect of breast feeding lasts for several years.

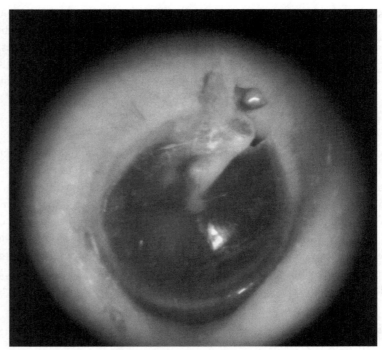

Fig. 9.2 Left middle ear effusion with air bubbles. See colour plate 2. Reproduced with permission from Ian Bottrill.

What effect does it have?

Glue ear is the commonest cause of hearing loss in children. This can have adverse effects on speech acquisition, language, behaviour, cognition, and balance.

When to refer on?

Referral to an ENT surgeon should be made if the effusion persists for three months and the child has difficulty hearing (typically a threshold of 20dB or worse), or if complications are suspected. These include middle ear problems such as tympanic membrane atrophy, a retraction pocket (Figure 9.3), ossicular erosion, or cholesteatoma. A 3-month period of 'Watchful Waiting' after OME has been diagnosed is necessary as a proportion of cases will resolve spontaneously during this time (Effective Healthcare Bulletin 1992).

Treatment options

Most children will have already received antibiotics, if not a trial course of first and, if necessary, second line antibiotics should be given (see recommendations for AOM). Atopic children with rhinitic symptoms should be treated appropriately. The subsequent options are therefore ventilation tubes (grommets), adenoidectomy, hearing aids, and autoinflation. Persistent effusions do not respond to oral decongestants, steroids, or mucolytics.

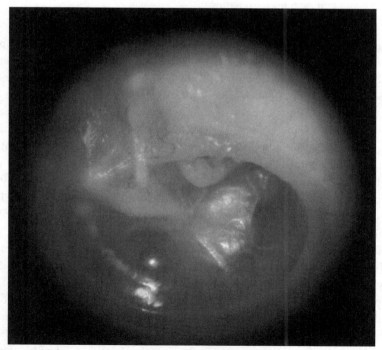

Fig. 9.3 Retracted left tympanic membrane with middle ear effusion. See colour plate 3. Reproduced with permission from Ian Bottrill.

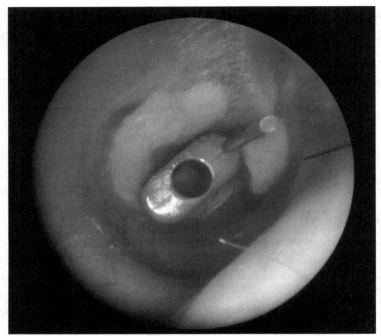

Fig. 9.4 Ventilation tube in tympanic membrane. See colour plate 4.
Reproduced with permission from Ian Bottrill.

The aim of a ventilation tube (Figure 9.4) is to allow equalisation of air pressure between the middle and external ear. This bypasses any Eustachian tube obstruction and allows the middle ear to function normally. It is the most common operation in children in the UK, with a rate of 5/1000 children under 15 years. In children older than 3½ years there is good evidence that the best overall resolution of persistent OME is a combination of ventilation tube insertion and adenoidectomy. Compared with ventilation tube insertion alone, the combined procedure improves hearing for a longer duration and improves physical health. The joint advantages make it seven times more cost-effective than ventilation tubes alone (Haggard 2004). Tonsillectomy does not confer any additional benefit regarding OME resolution compared with adenoidectomy (Maw 1997). In children under 3½ years without gross upper airways obstruction due to adenotonsillar enlargement, ventilation tube insertion alone is sufficient (Maw 1997).

Ventilation tubes are usually inserted as a day case procedure under general anaesthetic. They extrude spontaneously after 12–18 months, once the ear is able to function normally. The risks associated with ventilation tubes are otorrhoea, tympanosclerosis, and tympanic membrane perforation. The otorrhoea is painless (unlike that of AOM) and should be treated with topical antibiotic eardrops. Tympanosclerosis may occur but does not seem to affect hearing adversely. After extrusion of the ventilation tube a tympanic membrane perforation persists in 1–2%, if necessary this can be closed later by a myringoplasty operation. Swimming is not contraindicated but diving and swimming underwater should be avoided. It is more important to protect the ears from soapy bath water or shampoo by using a piece of cotton wool covered with Vaseline in the outer ears during baths and showers.

It is necessary to reinsert ventilation tubes for recurrence of OME in about 30% of cases. Unilateral effusions require a less invasive approach if hearing is normal in the unaffected ear.

A hearing aid avoids the need for surgery or an anaesthetic but does not reventilate the middle ear. It cannot therefore prevent or correct tympanic membrane retraction.

Autoinflation is a technique for optimizing Eustachian tube function by blowing through the nose to inflate a small balloon attached to a plastic tube (Otovent). There is limited evidence that this can be beneficial; however, it is more suitable for older children, who find the device easier to manage (Reidpath 1999).

A downloadable leaflet about glue ear is available from the National Deaf Children's Society (http://www.ndcs.org.uk/information/childhood-deafness/glue-ear).

Sore throat and tonsillitis

How common is it?

In general practice recurrent sore throat has an incidence of 10% of the population per year. It is the sixth most common acute presentation in girls. At all ages the incidence is higher in girls than in boys.

Sore throat or tonsillitis?

Both are associated with fever and cervical lymphadenopathy, both cause throat discomfort, pharyngeal redness and referred pain to the ears. Most sore throats are viral and tend to be associated with coryzal symptoms, whereas in tonsillitis (Figure 9.5) the pain tends to be more severe, the tonsils are usually enlarged, swallowing is difficult and

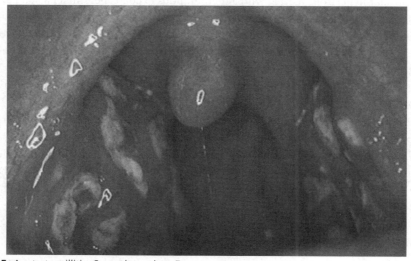

Fig. 9.5 Acute tonsillitis. See colour plate 5.
Reproduced with permission from Bull TR, *Diagnostic Picture Tests in Ear, Nose, and Throat*, 1990, Wolfe.

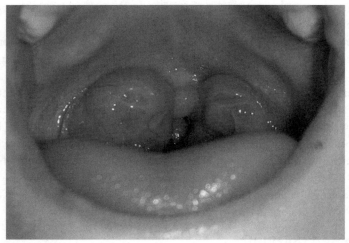

Fig. 9.6 Tonsillar hypertrophy. See colour plate 6.
Reproduced with permission from Pandora Hadfield.

dehydration can occur. The child commonly misses several days from school. Tonsillar hypertrophy may persist between episodes (Figure 9.6), causing the child to be a slow eater, often small for their age and to have apnoeic episodes during sleep.

Other differential diagnoses

Infectious mononucleosis (glandular fever) mainly affects teenagers, occasionally younger children. Symptoms include severe sore throat, prolonged malaise and fever, gross tonsillar hypertrophy, often with a membranous exudate, petechial palatal haemor-rhages, marked cervical lymphadenopathy, and occasionally a transient maculopapular rash on the limbs. Hepatosplenomegaly occurs in about 50% of cases, and occasionally jaundice, hepatitis, and viral myocarditis. Low-grade fever, fatigue, malaise, and tonsillar hypertrophy may persist for several weeks.

Lymphoma may cause unilateral enlargement and ulceration of a tonsil, it may be a dark purple colour, cervical lymphadenopathy occurs.

Acute leukaemia is rare but may cause necrotic ulceration in the pharynx. Purpuric haemorrhages and a leucocytosis of $20-100 \times 10^9/l$ will confirm the diagnosis.

Peritonsillar abscess (quinsy) (Figure 9.7) affects adults more than children. Suppuration behind the tonsil pushes the tonsil medially and causes swelling of the soft palate. It usually follows an episode of tonsillitis, which appears to have settled, then recurs severely on one side with rigors, pyrexia of 40° and a muffled voice.

Are investigations useful?

About 70% of sore throats are viral. The precise diagnosis of viral and bacterial sore throat is not reliable on clinical, serological or microbiological grounds such as throat

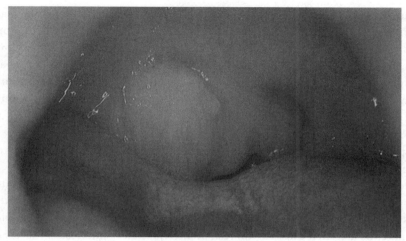

Fig. 9.7 Right peritonsillar abscess. See colour plate 7.
Reproduced with permission from Bull TR, *Diagnostic Picture Tests in Ear, Nose, and Throat*, 1990, Wolfe.

swab or rapid antigen testing. Thus investigation of recurrent sore throat is unproductive and unhelpful in management (Howie 1976; Kellog and Manzalla 1986; White *et al.* 1986; Lewey *et al.* 1998). There is no evidence that bacterial sore throats are more severe than viral ones or that the duration of the illness is significantly different. The most common single identifiable organism is group A beta-haemolytic streptococcus (GABHS). Symptoms however correlate poorly with results of throat swab culture. There is a high asymptomatic carrier rate for GABHS of up to 40% (Caplan 1979) and bacteria cultured from the surface of the tonsil are different to those deep in the tonsillar crypts, which are most likely to be causing the infection. Throat swabs should not therefore be carried out routinely in sore throat.

In suspected infectious mononucleosis, however, the diagnosis can be confirmed by a blood test. A positive Monospot or Paul Bunnel test is diagnostic (the latter may initially show a negative result, becoming positive at day 5). The blood film shows a leucocytosis of $10–20 \times 10^9/l$ with atypical large mononuclear cells.

Treatment

Treatment of sore throat is essentially supportive with bed rest, plenty of fluids and analgesia. Paracetamol is the drug of choice, taking into account the increased risks associated with other analgesics. Non steroidal anti-inflammatory drugs (NSAIDs) have been shown to achieve slightly faster resolution of pain compared with paracetamol or placebo but these effects were short-lived as symptoms tended to resolve spontaneously over 48–72 hours. The risks of gastrointestinal bleeding, nausea, abdominal pain, diarrhoea, and vomiting make paracetamol preferable (Bertin *et al.* 1991). Difflam (benzydamine hydrochloride) oral spray is helpful and can be used in children. In a small study it produced significantly greater relief of pain and dysphagia at 24 hours than placebo (Wethington 1985). Most sore throats are self-limiting within a week whether or not antibiotics are prescribed. There is no convincing evidence of benefit from antibiotics even when culture for GABHS is positive (Del Mar *et al.* 2000). This evidence is backed up by numerous recent studies. In particular no benefit was found from penicillin V in children with acute sore throat. If any streptococcal sequelae occur such as peritonsillar abscess, scarlet fever, impetigo, acute rheumatic fever, or acute glomerulonephritis, it can be started at that stage to good effect (Zwart *et al.* 2003).

A suspected peritonsillar abscess should be referred to an ENT surgeon for aspiration or incision and drainage.

In infectious mononucleosis contact sports should be avoided for several weeks due to the risk of splenic rupture. There is no specific treatment apart from prolonged bed rest, copious fluids, and paracetamol. Antibiotics play no part in the treatment and ampicillin should never be used as it causes a skin rash in infectious mononucleosis. In severe cases hospital admission is indicated. Tonsillar hypertrophy may case upper airways obstruction, in which case corticosteroids are very effective. Tracheostomy is rarely necessary.

In acute tonsillitis, phenoxymethylpenicillin (Penicillin V) is the mainstay of treatment. Bacterial resistance is increasing and clindamycin, vancomycin, or rifampicin can be used as second line treatment. Tonsillectomy is an effective treatment for recurrent tonsillitis. It is one of the most common operations performed on children in the United Kingdom (2.3/1000 children under 12 years of age). Tonsillectomy is no longer primarily an operation for children, young adults comprise one-third of cases and this proportion is rising. Many uncontrolled studies suggest benefit in children who have undergone tonsillectomy. In addition to the reduced frequency of tonsillitis, parents commonly report a major improvement in general health, behaviour, and development. This was shown in the Scottish Tonsillectomy Audit (Blair *et al.* 1996) where patients and parents were overwhelmingly positive about the outcome of surgery and often critical about delay in treatment 'the operation should have been done years ago'. A total of 9773 patients including 5464 tonsillectomies were included. The study reported an extremely high satisfaction rate of 97%. There are limitations in using satisfaction as an outcome measure postoperatively but measures of reduction in time lost at school or work also suggest benefit from surgery. Eighty per cent reported no time off in the 12 months following surgery, and 15% less time off.

Who should be referred for consideration of tonsillectomy?

The Scottish Intercollegiate Guidelines Network (SIGN 1999) recommendations are:

 ◆ sore throats are due to tonsillitis
 ◆ five or more episodes of sore throat per year
 ◆ symptoms for at least 1 year
 ◆ the episodes of sore throat are disabling and prevent normal functioning.

Snoring and obstructive sleep apnoea

Sleep-related upper airways obstruction in children is due to primary snoring or obstructive sleep apnoea (OSA). Snoring occurs in both, apnoea is the temporary cessation of breathing. OSA in children was first described by Guilleminault in 1976. It has subsequently been reported on numerous occasions as a common cause of significant morbidity in children.

Incidence

Approximately 10% of children snore during sleep on most or all nights (Corbo *et al.* 1989; Ali *et al.* 1991; Owen *et al.* 1995), most of these children have primary snoring. Approximately 3% of all children and up to 40% of snoring children who are referred to an ENT surgeon have OSA (Goldstein *et al.* 1994; Carroll *et al.* 1995; Gislason and Benediktsdottir 1995). The highest incidence of OSA coincides with the time of greatest hypertrophy of the tonsils and adenoids, typically between 4 and 6 years of age (Crepau *et al.* 1982).

Predisposing factors

Adenotonsillar hypertrophy (Figure 9.6) is the major predisposing factor in both primary snoring and OSA (Sorensen *et al.* 1980; Fukuda *et al.* 1989). Other contributing causes in snoring and OSA include upper respiratory tract infection, allergy, obesity, passive exposure to tobacco smoke, neurological abnormalities, and nasopharyngeal obstruction (Corbo *et al.* 1989; McColley *et al.* 1997). Children with an anatomic predisposition to OSA include those with craniofacial syndromes, hemifacial microsomia, and Down syndrome. Gastro-oesophageal reflux may be involved in apnoeic episodes (Menon *et al.* 1985; Wennergren *et al.* 1993).

Symptoms and signs

Primary snoring occurs during sleep without associated apnoea, hypoventilation, or hypoxaemia. These children have no associated sleep disturbance or daytime symptoms (Carroll and Loughlin 1995).

Table 9.2 Features of sleep-related upper airways obstruction in children

At night	Daytime
Snoring	Mouth breathing
Increased respiratory effort	Hyponasal speech
Restless sleep	Frequent upper respiratory infections
Sweating	Hyperactivity
Unusual sleeping position	
Enuresis	

Children with OSA demonstrate a variety of symptoms (Table 9.2) at night and during the day (Weider *et al.* 1991; Carroll 1996). Excessive daytime sleepiness is characteristic of adults with OSA, but not children (Brouillette *et al.* 1984; Leach *et al.* 1992; Carroll *et al.* 1995). On the contrary, hyperactivity, and other daytime behavioural problems are more likely (Guilleminault *et al.* 1981; Brouillette *et al.* 1982; Frank *et al.* 1983; Brouillette *et al.* 1984). Obese children with OSA have deficits in memory, vocabulary, and learning when compared with obese children without OSA (Rhodes *et al.* 1995). However, most children with OSA have poor growth and may present with failure to thrive (Guilleminault *et al.* 1981; Brouillette *et al.* 1982).

Complications

Serious complications of childhood OSA, such as pulmonary and systemic hypertension and cor pulmonale (Guilleminault *et al.* 1976; Guilleminault *et al.* 1981; Serratto *et al.* 1981; Brouillette *et al.* 1982) are less common nowadays due to increased understanding of the condition with earlier diagnosis and treatment.

Diagnosis

A careful sleep history should be taken from the parents or caregivers, siblings who sleep in the same room as the child may give additional information. Daytime symptoms should also be elicited. The physical examination should ascertain whether the child is underweight (or occasionally overweight) for age. The pharynx and nose should be examined for space occupying lesions, reduced nasal airflow, and abnormal craniofacial morphology. Abnormalities of neuromuscular tone should be considered.

OSA has been defined as episodes of upper airway obstruction during sleep, usually associated with a reduction in oxyhaemoglobin saturation or hypercarbia, or both (Carroll and Loughlin 1995). The gold standard test for OSA is overnight polysomnography (Leach *et al.* 1992; Goldstein *et al.* 1994; Carroll *et al.* 1995; Suen *et al.* 1995).

Treatment

Treatment is not recommended for children with primary snoring; however, the natural history of the condition is unclear. In OSA treatment is usually surgical, in complex multifactorial cases it may also be non-surgical.

Surgery

Adenotonsillectomy remains the most common treatment for childhood OSA. Rapid relief of obstructive symptoms may be anticipated in children with mild OSA and has been demonstrated on the first postoperative night with polysomnography (Helfaer *et al.* 1996). Adenotonsillectomy can also result in improved growth (Williams EF *et al.* 1991; Marcus *et al.* 1994).

A lack of randomized controlled trials, however, make it difficult to ascertain the exact efficacy of adenotonsillectomy in OSA in children. This is compounded by debate over the validity of polysomnographic criteria and uncertainty about the natural history of the condition (Lim and McKean 2003).

Children with an anatomic predisposition to OSA include those with craniofacial syndromes, hemifacial microsomia and Down syndrome. In addition to adenotonsillectomy they may benefit from a variety of sequential surgical approaches (Cohen *et al.* 1997, Lefaivre *et al.* 1997). Although it is a treatment option for adults who snore, uvulopalatopharyngoplasty (UVPP) is rarely considered for children with OSA. Two small studies using it in conjunction with adenotonsillectomy showed limited improvement in children with neuromotor disease or craniofacial abnormalities (Kosko and Derkay 1995) and residual obstruction in children with Down syndrome (Jacobs *et al.* 1996).

Tracheostomy remains the gold standard for treatment of OSA in complex cases, particularly in dynamic airways problems such as pharyngeal hypotonia.

Non-surgical

Medical treatments include reduction of nasal congestion due to allergies, gastro-oesophageal reflux and weight loss in obese children. Continuous positive airways pressure (CPAP), nasal continuous positive airway pressure (nCPAP) and bilevel positive airways pressure (BiPAP) have been used to treat children whose OSA persists after surgery or in whom surgery is contraindicated (Marcus *et al.* 1995; Waters *et al.* 1995, Massa *et al.* 2002). BiPAP allows independent adjustment of pressure during inspiration and expiration. Nocturnal oxygen supplementation has been used as a temporary measure in severe OSAS with oxygen desaturations pending definitive treatment (Marcus *et al.* 1995; Aljadeff *et al.* 1996). However, this may suppress the hypoxic ventilatory drive and worsen OSA (Gauda *et al.* 1991) so should only be used under monitored conditions (Marcus *et al.* 1995).

A nasal prong or stent may be used to bypass nasopharyngeal obstruction. It requires close monitoring and care to maintain patency and is usually a temporary inpatient procedure.

Who should be referred for polysomnography?

The diagnosis of childhood OSA is difficult as it cannot be distinguished from primary snoring by clinical history and physical examination alone. In one study the majority of parents of both OSA and primary snorers described their child as 'struggling to breathe' at night and said that they were frightened by their child's breathing at night (Carroll *et al.* 1995). As clinical assessment is sensitive but not specific for OSA, it has been suggested that polysomnography should be used in all suspected cases (Goldstein *et al.* 1994; Suen *et al.* 1995). However, the need for polysomnography in all children with suspected OSA and adenotonsillar hypertrophy remains controversial and has enormous cost implications. Moreover, there are no universally accepted or validated criteria for polysomnography (Schechter 2002), making comparison of published series difficult.

Polysomnography is not necessary for children who undergo adenotonsillectomy for non-obstructive indications (such as recurrent tonsillitis) with no other risk factors. It is most helpful in high-risk patients, such as children under 3 years of age, those with craniofacial abnormalities, neuromotor disease, or complications of OSA. Also for children in whom the history and physical examination findings are inconsistent.

Conclusions

Childhood OSA is common and if severe and untreated can lead to cardiopulmonary complications. Overnight polysomnography is the best diagnostic test to differentiate it from primary snoring and establish severity. However, there are no validated polysomnographic criteria. Adenotonsillectomy remains the most common treatment, it is usually curative in otherwise healthy children. Additional surgery in complex cases includes craniofacial procedures and tracheostomy. Non-surgical treatment includes CPAP and weight reduction. Although it is not current practice to offer treatment for primary snoring without OSA, the natural history of this condition is unclear.

References

(1992). The treatment of persistent glue ear in children. *The Effective Health Care Bulletin*, no. 4.

Ali NJ, Pitson D, Stradling JR (1991). The prevalence of snoring, sleep disturbance and sleeprelated breathing disorders and their relation to daytime sleepiness. *American Review of Respiratory Disease* **143**: A381.

Aljadeff G, Gozal D, Bailey-Wahl SL, Burell B, Keens TG, Davidson Ward SL (1996). Effects of overnight supplemental oxygen in obstructive sleep apnea in children. *American Journal of Respiratory Critical Care Medicine* **153**: 51–55.

Bandolier (1994). (Feb) 1–3. Glue Ear—a Sticky Problem. http://www.jr2.ox.ac.uk/bandolier/band1/bl-3.html

Bertin L, Pons G, d'Athis P, *et al.* (1991). Randomized, double-blind, multicenter, controlled trial of ibuprofen versus acetaminophen (paracetamol) and placebo for treatment of symptoms of tonsillitis and pharyngitis in children. *Journal of Pediatrics* **119**(5): 811–4.

Bertin L, Pons G, d'Athis P, Duhamel JF, Mandelonde C, Lasfargues G (1996). A randomized double blind multicentre controlled trial of ibuprofen versus acetaminophen and placebo for symptoms of acute otitis media in children. *Fundamentals of Clinical Pharmacology* **10**: 387–392.

Blair RL, McKerrow WS, Carter NW, Fenton A (1996). The Scottish tonsillectomy audit. Audit Sub-Committee of the Scottish Otolaryngological Society. *Journal of Laryngology & Otology* **110** (Suppl. 20): 1–25.

Brouillette RT, Fernbach SK, Hunt CE (1982). Obstructive sleep apnea in infants and children. *Journal of Pediatrics* **100**: 31–40.

Brouillette RT, Hanson D, David R, Klemka L, Szatkowski A, Fernbach S, Hunt C (1984). A diagnostic approach to suspected obstructive sleep apnea in children. *Journal of Pediatrics* **105**: 10–14.

Caplan C (1979). A case against the use of throat culture in the management of streptococcal pharyngitis. *Journal of Family Practice* **8**: 845–890

Carroll JL (1996). Sleep-related uper-airway obstruction in children and adolescents. *Child and Adolescent Psychiatric Clinics of North America* **5**: 617–647.

Carroll JL, Loughlin GM (1995). Primary snoring in infants and children. In Ferber R, Kryger MH (eds), *Principles and Practice of Sleep Medicine in the Child*. WB Saunders, Philadelphia, pp. 155–161.

Carroll JL, McColley SA, Marcus CL, Curtis S, Loughlin GM (1995). Inability of clinical history to distinguish primary snoring from obstructive sleep apnea syndrome in children. *Chest* **108**: 610–618.

Cohen SR, Lefaivre JF, Burstein FD *et al.* (1997). Surgical treatment of obstructive sleep apnea in neurologically compromised patients. *Plastic and Reconstructive Surgery* **99**: 638–646.

Corbo GM, Fuciarelli F, Foresi A, De Benedetto F (1989). Snoring in children: association with respiratory symptoms and passive smoking. *British Medical Journal* **299:** 1491–1494.

Crepau J, Patriquin HB, Poliquin JF *et al.* (1982). Radiological evaluation of the symptom-producing adenoid. *Otolaryngology Head and Neck Surgery* **90:** 548–554.

Del Mar C, Glasziou P, Hayem M (1997). Are antibiotics indicated as an initial treatment for children with acute otitis media? A meta-analysis. *British Medical Journal* **314:** 1526–1529.

Del Mar C, Glasziou P, Spinks A (2000). Antibiotics for sore throat. *Cochrane Database Systematic Review,* **2000 (2)**, Update in *Cochrane Database Systematic Review* **2000 (4)**.

Frank Y, Kravath RE, Pollak CP, Weitzman ED (1983). Obstructive sleep apnea and its therapy: clinical and polysomnographic manifestations. *Pediatrics* **71:** 737–742.

Fukuda K, Matsune S, Ushikai M, Imamura Y, Ohyama M (1989). A study on the relationship between adenoid vegetation and rhinosinusitis. *American Journal of Otolaryngology* **10:** 214–216.

Gauda EB, Carroll JL, McColley S, Smith PL (1991). Effect of oxygenation on breath-by-breath response of the genioglossus muscle during occlusion. *Journal of Applied Physiology* **71:** 1231–1236.

Gislason T, Benediktsdottir B (1995). Snoring, apneic episodes, and nocturnal hypoxaemia among children 6 months to 6 years old. An epidemiologic study of lower limit of prevalence. *Chest* **107:** 963–966.

Goldstein NA, Sculerati N, Walsleben JA, Bhatia N, Friedman DM, Rapoport DM (1994). Clinical diagnosis of pediatric obstructive sleep apnea validated by polysomnography. *Otolaryngology Head and Neck Surgery* **111:** 611–617.

Guilleminault C, Eldrige F, Simmons FB, Dement WC (1976). Sleep apnea in eight children. *Pediatrics* **58:** 23–30.

Guilleminault C, Korobkin R, Winkle R (1981). A review of 50 children with obstructive sleep apnea syndrome. *Lung* **159:** 275–287.

Haggard M (2004). MRC Multicentre otitis media study group, Addenbrooke's Hospital. Data presented at Royal Society of Medicine, ENT meeting, May 2004.

Hanafin S, Griffiths P (2002). Does pacifier use cause ear infections in young children? *British Journal of Community Nursing* 7(4): 206, 208–11.

Helfaer MA, McColley SA, Pyzik PL *et al.* (1996). Polysomnography after adenotonsillectomy in mild pediatric obstructive sleep apnea. *Critical Care Medicine* **24:** 1323–1327.

Howie JGR (1976). Clinical judgement and antibiotic use in general practice. *British Medical Journal* **2:** 1061–1064.

ICSI Institute for Clincal Systems Improvement (2002). Diagnosis and treatment of otitis media in children. www.isci.org

Jacobs IN, Gray RF, Odd NW (1996). Upper airway obstruction in children with Down syndrome. *Archives of Otolaryngology Head and Neck Surgery* **122:** 945–950.

Kellog JA, Manzalla JP (1986). Detection of group A streptococci in the laboratory or physician's office. *Journal of American Medical Association* **255:** 2638–2642.

Kosko JR, Derkay CS (1995). Uvulopalatopharyngoplasty: treatment of obstructive sleep apnea in neurologically impaired pediatric patients. *International Journal of Pediatric Otorhinolaryngology* **32:** 241–246.

Leach J, Olsen J, Hermann J, Manning S (1992). Polysomnographic and clinical findings in children with obstructive sleep apnea. *Archives of Otolaryngology Head and Neck Surgery* **118:** 741–744.

Lefaivre JF, Cohen SR, Burstein FD *et al.* (1997). Down syndrome: identification and surgical management of obstructive sleep apnea. *Plastic and Reconstructive Surgery* **99**: 629–637.

Lewey S, White CB, Lieberman MM, Morales E (1998). Evaluation of the throat culture as a follow up for an initially negative enzyme immunosorben assay rapid streptococcal antigen test. *Pediatric Infectious Diseases* **7**: 765–769.

Lim J, McKean M (2003). Adenotonsillectomy for obstructive sleep apnoea in children. *Cochrane Database of Systematic Reviews* (1):CD003136.

Marcus CL, Carroll JL, Koerner CB, Hamer A, Lutz J, Loughlin GM (1994). Determinants of growth in children with the obstructive sleep apnea syndrome. *Journal of Pediatrics* **125**: 556–562.

Marcus CL, Ward SL, Maallory GB *et al.* (1995). Use of nasal continuous positive airway pressure as treatment of childhood obstructive sleep apnea. *Journal of Pediatrics* **127**: 88–94.

Massa F, Gonzalez S, Laverty A, Wallis C, Lane R (2002). The use of nasal continuous positive airway pressure to treat obstructive sleep apnoea. *Archives of Disease in Childhood* **87**(5): 438–843.

Maw AR (1997). Otitis media with effusion. In Kerr AG (ed), *Scott-Brown's Otolaryngology, 6/7/1–23. Paediatric Otolaryngology*, (6th edn). Butterworth and Co., Oxford.

McColley SA, Carroll JL, Curtis S, Loughlin GM, Sampson HA (1997). High prevalence of allergic sensitization in children with habitual snoring. *Chest* **111**: 170–173.

Menon AP, Schlefft GL, Thatch BT (1985). Apnea associated with regurgitation in infants. *Journal of Pediatrics* **106**: 625.

Owen GO, Canter RJ, Robinson A (1995). Overnight pulse oximetry in snoring and non-snoring children. *Clinical Otolaryngology* **20**: 402–406.

Reidpath DD (1999). Systematic review of autoinflation for treatment of glue ear in children. *British Medical Journal* **318**, 1177–1178.

Rhodes SK, Shimoda KC, Waid R, O'Neil PM, Oexmann MJ, Collop NA, Willi SM (1995). Neurocognitive deficits in morbidly obese children with obstructive sleep apnea. *Journal of Pediatrics* **127**: 741–744.

Rosenfeld RM, Vertrees JE, Carr J, Cipolle RJ, Uden DL, Gieink GS (1994). Clinical efficacy of antimicrobial drugs for acute otitis media: meta-analysis of 5400 children from thirty-three randomised controlled trials. *Journal of Pediatrics* **124**: 355–367.

Schechter MS (2002). Technical report: diagnosis and management of childhood obstructive sleep apnea syndrome. *Pedaitrics* **109**(4): e69.

Serratto M, Harris VJ, Carr I (1981). Upper airways obstruction: presentation with systemic hypertension. *Archives of Disease of Childhood* **56**: 153–155.

SIGN publication No. 34 ISBN 1899893 66 0 (Jan 1999) Management of sore throat and indications for tonsillectomy. www.sign.ac.uk/guidelines/fulltext/34

Sorensen H, Solow B, Greve E, (1980). Assessment of the nasopharyngeal airway. *Acta Otolaryngology (Stockholm)* **89**: 227–232.

Strachan DP, Cook DG (1998). Parental smoking, middle ear disease and adenotonsillectomy in children. *Thorax* **53**: 50–56.

Suen JS, Arnold JE, Brooks LJ (1995) Adenotonsillectomy for treatment of obstructive sleep apnea in children. *Archives of Otolaryngology Head and Neck Surgery* **121**: 525–530.

Waters KA, Everett FM, Bruderer JW, Sullivan CE (1995). Obstructive sleep apnea: the use of nasal CPAP in 80 children. *Journal of Pediatrics* **125**: 556–562.

Weider DJ, Sateia MJ, West RP (1991). Nocturnal enuresis in children with upper airway obstruction. *Otolaryngology Head and Neck Surgery* **105**: 427–432.

Wennergren G, Bjure J, Gertzberg T, *et al.* (1993). Laryngeal reflex. *Acta Paediatrics* **389** (Suppl. 82): 53–56.

Wethington JF (1985). Double-blind study of benzydamine hydrochloride, a new treatment for sore throat. *Clinical Therapeutics* **7**(5): 641–6.

White CB, Bass JW, Yarnada SM (1986). Rapid latex agglutination compared with the throat culture for the detection of group A streptococcal infection. *Pediatric Infectious Diseases* **5**: 208–2121.

Williams EF, Woo P, Miller R, Kellman RM (1991). The effects of adenotonsillectomy on growth in young children. *Otolaryngology Head and Neck Surgery* **104**: 509–516.

Williams RL (1993). Use of antibiotics in preventing recurrent acute otitis media and in treating otitis media with effusion: a meta-analytic attempt to resolve the brouhaha. *Journal of the American Medical Association* **270**: 1344–1351.

Williamson IG, Dunleavey J, Robinson D (1994). Risk factors in otitis media with effusion. A one year case control study in 5–7 year old children. *Family Practitioner* **11**(3): 271–4.

Zwart S, Roever MM, de Melker RA, Hoes AW (2003). Penicillin for acute sore throat in children: randomised, double blind trial. *British Medical Journal* **327**: 1324–1327.

Chapter 10

Common infectious diseases of childhood

Mainga Hamaluba and Andrew Pollard

Introduction

The incidence, spectrum, and presentation of infections in childhood vary considerably with age as a result of immunological maturation, microbial exposure, and the ability of children of different ages to communicate their symptoms.

Newborns are particularly susceptible to infections as a result of immunological inexperience and immaturity as well as exposure antenatally, to maternal blood-borne infections (e.g. cytomegalovirus, toxoplasmosis, and varicella) and perinatally, to microbes in the birth canal (e.g. HIV, group B streptococci, etc.). A high level of suspicion is required as infection in this age group often presents with non-specific symptoms and signs.

After the risks from infection at birth, the infant up to the age of 6 months, is relatively well protected from infections due to the passive transfer of maternal antibodies. Infants born before 30 weeks gestation do not benefit from placental transfer of antibody and are more susceptible to infection. Immunization in the first 6 months of life, aims to improve infant antibody levels before maternal antibodies wane.

Immunization markedly reduces the risk of life-threatening infections during childhood, such that there are now more deaths in children under the age of 15 in the UK from accidents and cancer than infectious diseases. Routine UK immunization programmes currently protect the paediatric population against diphtheria, tetanus, pertussis, polio, *Haemophilus influenzae* type b, Serogroup C *Neisseria meningitidis*, *Streptococcus pneumoniae*, measles, mumps, and rubella. Immunizations are also available for protection against hepatitis B, tuberculosis (TB), and varicella.

Upper respiratory tract infections
Otitis media

One in four children will have at least one episode of acute otitis media (AOM) by the age of 10 years, with a peak incidence between 2 and 6 years of age. By the age of 3, more than 80% of children will have had at least one episode of AOM (Rothman *et al.* 2003). Differentiating between AOM and otitis media with effusion (OME) is difficult and depends on a thorough history and examination. Studies have suggested that physicians find they are uncertain of the diagnosis in 40% of cases (Rothman *et al.* 2003)

Symptoms of a child presenting with AOM include:

◆ fever, earache, irritability, otorrhoea

◆ lethargy, anorexia, vomiting.

There is often a history of rapid onset of inflammation of the middle ear presenting with local symptoms of pain reflected by rubbing and tugging at the ear. A preceding history of upper respiratory (viral) infection is not uncommon.

Signs on examination of a child with AOM include:

◆ bulging tympanic membranes with red or yellow ear drums

◆ loss of the normal markings on the tympanic membrane.

Note that while a fullness and bulging of the eardrum is pathopneumonic for AOM, this is often not seen.

Risk factors for AOM include; being male, child <2years of age, day care attendance, exposure to cigarette smoke, history of AOM, and autumn and winter seasons. Breast feeding is thought to be protective (Rothman *et al.* 2003) When a diagnosis of a middle ear infection is suspected it is important to enquire about; hearing difficulty, social interactions, behaviour, school, speech and language development or clumsiness and poor balance.

Diagnosis of OME is based on history and otoscopic examination. Children with OME are often asymptomatic or have no localizing symptoms. Earache is uncommon. Clinical findings include tympanic membrane retraction, air bubbles, or fluid levels in the middle ear cleft. Typical pathogens in middle ear infections are: *Streptococcus pneumoniae*, *Haemophilus influenzae*, and, occasionally, *Moraxella catarrhalis* or *Staphylococcus aureus*. In some locations Group A streptococci may be common.

Treatment of acute otitis media

Most cases will settle in 48 hours without antibiotic therapy and antibiotics should not be used routinely. Analgesia should be optimized. Delayed antibiotics can be used for those who do not respond in 48–72 hours. (These can be collected at parents' discretion after 48–72 hours if symptoms have not improved or a prescription provided to be dispensed only if symptoms are not settling.)

A more cautious approach may be necessary for systemically unwell children and infants:

◆ first-line antibiotics: amoxicillin, augmentin

◆ second-line antibiotics: ceflacor, cotrimoxazole, trimethoprim, erythromycin

◆ there is no role for, anticongestants, antimucolytics, or steroids.

It is hard to examine the discharging ear drum in AOM therefore these children should be re-examined in 2 weeks following initial infection. If perforation persists at 2 weeks follow-up is required or referral to an ENT surgeon.

Reasons for referral

In children aged <3 years with bilateral glue ear (OME) and hearing loss of ≤25 dB, but no speech or language problems nor behavioural or developmental problems, it is reasonable to observe only. However, they will need to be re-assessed to exclude persistent hearing loss and alternative diagnoses. Glue ear in children >3 years with speech and language or developmental or behavioural problems should have prompt ENT referral.

Sore throat and recurrent sore throat

The terms, acute pharyngitis, tonsillitis, and exudative tonsillitis all have a similar clinical presentation. There is no agreed definition of recurrent sore throat. Symptoms often seen in these conditions include sore throat for three or more days, loss of appetite, pain, particularly on swallowing and lethargy with or without systemic illness. Some of the physical signs associated with sore throat include; inflamed tonsils or pharynx, purulent exudates on tonsils, fever or anterior cervical lymphadenopathy. Clinical examination does not reliably differentiate between viral and bacterial causes of sore throat and throat swabs lack diagnostic sensitivity and specificity and should not be done routinely (SIGN Guidelines 1999).

In severe cases with systemic features antibiotics should not be withheld. Penicillin is the treatment of choice and should be administered for a 10-day course for presumptive Group A streptococcal tonsillitis/pharyngitis. Antibiotics should not be used routinely to prevent rheumatic fever or acute glomerulonephritis.

Infectious mononucleosis presents in a similar fashion with pharyngitis, exudates, and anterior cervical lymphadenopathy. Ampicillin-based antibiotics including co-amoxiclav should be avoided as they may precipitate onset of an erythematous rash. Peritonsillar abscess (quinsy) is a complication of tonsillitis that presents more commonly in adolescents following severe episodes and is associated with dysphagia and asymmetrical swelling. Retropharyngeal abscess follows bacterial pharyngitis and is uncommon in infants, presenting with stridor, fever, drooling, and lymphadenopathy. Both require intravenous antibiotics and surgical drainage.

Tonsillectomy

Paediatric tonsillectomy is commonly undertaken in the UK. The main indications for tonsillectomy are recurrent tonsillitis and obstructive sleep apnoea syndromes. However, there is poor agreement between ENT surgeons, paediatricians and general practitioners on the definition of 'tonsillitis', the indications for tonsillectomy or the benefits to be expected following tonsillectomy. Consequently there are large variations in tonsillectomy rates. In one study, most doctors chose, 'frequency of tonsillitis' and 'number of days missed from school' as the most important factors in the decision to perform tonsillectomy (Capper and Canter 2001). Several randomized controlled trials have been performed to look at the efficacy of tonsillectomy in recurrent tonsillitis and none have managed to show a clinically significant benefit in terms of frequency of sore throats following tonsillectomy (Paradise *et al.* 1984).

Reasons for referral to ENT for a tonsillectomy The SIGN Guidelines offer a guide on appropriate referral to ENT for a tonsillectomy:

- sore throat due to tonsillitis
- ≥5 episodes of tonsillitis per year

- symptoms for at least 1 year
- episodes are disabling and prevent normal functioning.

Reasons for immediate referral to hospital

- Sore throat accompanied by stridor
- Drooling

Impending upper airways obstruction

- 'Toxic' child
- Lethargy
- Poor perfusion.

Acute laryngotracheobronchitis (croup)

Croup commonly occurs between 6 months and 3 years of age and is rare in children less than 6 months or more than 6 years of age. Viral croup is usually caused by parainfluenza viruses. Another common viral agent is respiratory syncytial virus. Less commonly influenza viruses A and B, adenovirus, and mycoplasma are involved. Symptoms indicate viral replication and the inflammatory response in the larynx, trachea and in some cases the bronchi. Severe croup results from subglottic oedema and represents a medical emergency.

   Clinical presentations include:

- Harsh barking cough
- Hoarse voice with or without coryzal symptoms   } with or without
- Stridor   coryzal symptoms
- Respiratory distress

Symptoms typically worsen at night or when the child is distressed. Croup is usually a mild and self-limiting illness, although it may occasionally cause severe respiratory obstruction.

   In children who appear toxic with high temperature life-threatening alternative diagnoses such as bacterial tracheitis, or epiglotittis should be considered.

   In children less than 4 months of age with a long-standing history of stridor or biphasic stridor the diagnosis of anatomical airways obstruction must be considered (laryngeal cyst, vocal cord paresis, papillomatosis, vascular ring, subglottic haemangioma, etc.)

   The diagnosis is clinical and the presence of severe symptoms including stridor or respiratory distress at rest should be sought, although the most common presentation to primary care is **mild croup**. The child appears happy, playful, will eat and drink and will have mild respiratory symptoms. No treatment is necessary in mild cases.

   Moderate croup presents with stridor at rest, and respiratory distress but the child remains alert and interactive. The child should be treated with oral corticosteroids and monitored carefully for clinical deterioration. Progression of signs indicates need for further treatment and prompt referral.

   Severe croup is marked by the exhausted, agitated child with persistent tachycardia, restlessness and altered conscious level. Excessive pallor and cyanosis are additional indicators of severe croup. Children with severe croup should be admitted to hospital for treatment and observation.

Risk factors for hospital admission after initial steroid treatment include:

- history of severe obstruction prior to presentation
- history of previous severe croup or structural airway anomaly
- <6 months of age
- inadequate fluid intake
- proximity to hospital/transport/social issues
- re-presentation within 24 hours
- poor response to initial treatment
- uncertain diagnosis.

Reasons for immediate referral to hospital:

- stridor or recession at rest
- saturations <92%
- inability to feed.

Unfortunately there are no randomized controlled trials on the use of corticosteroids in the primary care setting. Treating every case of croup with corticosteroids would lead to unnecessary treatment in most cases. However, if any risk factors exist the risk–benefit ratio needs to be considered. For children with moderate to severe croup there is a good evidence base for the use of oxygen, enteral and parenteral corticosteroids and nebulized steroids most often in a hospital setting (Fitzgerald and Kilham 2003).

Epiglottitis

Since universal immunization with a conjugate *Haemophilus influenzae* type b (Hib) vaccine the incidence of the disease has dropped to ≤0.3 cases per 100 000. Seventy-five per cent of cases occur in children aged 1–5 years. Other causal agents include pneumo-coccus and *Staphylococcus aureus*. Clinical features include an unwell, drooling, toxic child. Typically the child will have fever, sore throat, and muffled voice. There is refusal to eat or drink and preferential sitting position with extended neck and open mouth.

Epiglottitis is a medical emergency as a swollen epiglottis can lead to severe airways obstruction. To avoid the risk of obstruction, distress should be avoided. The child should be allowed to adopt a position that they are most comfortable with (maximizes airways opening). Physical examination and stressful procedures should be avoided and the child transferred to the hospital. Management in hospital involves urgent anaesthetic referral with ENT expertise available in case a surgical airway is required. No attempt should be made to place an intravenous cannula, perform X-rays, or examine the child's throat. Once the airway is secure intravenous cefuroxime or cefotaxime are used for treatment. Recovery is typically within 24 hours.

Prevention is by immunization. Household contacts do not require rifampicin prophylaxis if all households contacts are >4 years or <4 years but immunized.

Postexposure prophylaxis is required for all household contacts if there is a contact <1 year even if they are immunized or if there is an immunocompromised child.

Bacterial tracheitis

This is caused by superinfection of the trachea most commonly by *Staphylococcus aureus*. It may complicate laryngobronchitis or occur as a primary infection. Other causal agents include *Haemophilus influenzae* type b, Group A streptococcus, *Moraxella catarrhalis*, and *Streptococcus pneumoniae*. Fortunately this is a rare condition. Children with anatomical abnormalities of the upper airways and Down syndrome are at particular risk.

Clinical presentation is with acute respiratory distress, cough, and stridor. Fever is not always noted on presentation. The child often appears toxic, with shock and agitation, but pharyngitis or tonsillitis is uncommon. Definitive diagnosis is made on intubation by visualization of thick purulent subglottic debris. All children with bacterial tracheitis should be observed on a paediatric intensive care unit and most will need elective intubation and airway toilet. Empirical intravenous antibiotics are used to cover the main pathogens: cefotaxime or ceftriaxone.

Serious complications of bacterial tracheitis include respiratory arrest, anoxic encephalopathy, and death. These can be avoided by early recognition and transfer to hospital. Occasionally toxic shock or septic shock may accompany bacterial tracheitis. The mortality rate is 3–4%.

All children with suspected bacterial tracheitis require urgent hospital referral.

Lower respiratory tract infections

Viruses are the most common cause of acute respiratory symptoms in children and account for 14–35% of childhood community acquired pneumonia (BTS 2002). Furthermore, viral lower respiratory tract infections and 'atypical organisms' are responsible for up to 75% of cases leading to hospitalization (Smyth 2002). Viruses that frequently cause lower respiratory tract infections include (Sinaniotis 2004); respiratory syncitial virus (accounts for 29% of infections), parainfluenza serotypes 1,2,3 (20%, serotypes 1+3 are the commonest), influenza (8%), adenovirus (7%), and rhinovirus (5%). *Human metapneumovirus* (hMPV) accounts for approximately 10% of unexplained respiratory tract infections during the winter.

Streptococcus pneumoniae is the commonest bacterial cause of pneumonia in children, although the incidence is likely to fall following the introduction of the pneumococcal conjugate vaccine into the primary immunization schedule. Mycoplasma and chlamydial pneumonia also cause a significant burden of disease. Other important bacterial causes are Group A streptococci and *Staphylococcus aureus*.

In children ≤3 years of age, a temperature >38.5°C, accompanied by recession and a respiratory rate of ≥50 breaths/min indicates a likely diagnosis of a community acquired pneumonia (BTS 2002). In older children a history of difficulty with breathing is useful. In the pre-school child the presence of wheeze makes primary bacterial infection unlikely. Chest X-rays should not routinely be performed on children with mild uncomplicated acute lower respiratory tract infection. There is no evidence to support microbiological investigation in children being treated for pneumonia in the community.

Reasons for referral to hospital (infants):

- oxygen saturation ≤92%, cyanosis
- respiratory rate >70 breaths/min
- not feeding
- intermittent apnoea/grunting
- 'toxic' child with capillary refill time >2 seconds
- family unable to provide appropriate observation or supervision
- the clinical detection of a para-pneumonic effusion or empyema.

Reasons for referral to hospital (older children):

- oxygen saturations ≤92%, cyanosis
- respiratory rate >50/min
- difficulty with breathing
- grunting
- family unable to provide appropriate level of supervision or observation
- the clinical detection of a para-pneumonic effusion or empyema.

Young children presenting with mild symptoms of lower respiratory tract infection need not get antibiotics (BTS 2002). In those requiring antibiotic treatment amoxycillin is recommended as first-line therapy. Amoxycillin is effective against most of the common pathogens, inexpensive, and well tolerated. Second-line agents include: co-amoxiclav, cefaclor, erythromycin, clarithromycin, and azithromycin. Suspected mycoplasma or chlamydial pneumonia should be treated with macrolides.

Children managed in primary care should be reviewed if there is no improvement after 48 hours of treatment or if there is any deterioration. Parents should also be given information on managing pyrexia, hydration, and how to monitor for deterioration. Agitation may be a sign of hypoxia and children with agitation or low saturations should receive oxygen before and during hospital transfer.

Bronchiolitis

Bronchiolitis is a common viral infection of the lower respiratory tract characterized by moist cough, subcostal/intercostal recession, inspiratory crackles, and expiratory wheeze. It occurs most commonly in early childhood having the greatest burden among infants from the neonatal period to 9 months of age. The clinical history is a preceding coryzal illness for 2–3 days followed by, tachypnoea, recession, and 'bronchiolitic' cough. The cough can last for weeks but the respiratory distress normally abates after 5–7 days. Most children will have mild disease with rhinorrhoea, mild fever, and cough; 2.5% of children will require hospitalization because of mucus obstruction, respiratory distress, and secondary poor feeding. Infants may present with apnoea.

Respiratory syncytial virus accounts for 75–85% of cases of bronchiolitis. Ten to 20% is attributed to rhinovirus or parainfluenzae virus. Rarely adenovirus, influenza or *Bordatella pertussis* is detected; 1.5–8% of cases have been attributed to the recently identified virus, *human metapneumovirus* (hMPV). Co-infection with RSV and hMPV is more common in infants with severe disease (Semple 2005)

Conditions that increase the risk of hospital admission:

- prematurity
- chronic lung disease
- congenital heart disease
- immunodeficiency
- severe neurological abnormalities.

Reasons for referral to hospital:

- history of apnoea
- prematurity
- feeding difficulty
- poor hydration
- cyanosis (saturation <92%)
- respiratory rate >60/min
- family unable to provide appropriate observation or supervision.

Diagnosis is clinical, and chest X-ray is not usually necessary to support the diagnosis, but if performed, will reveal hyperinflation. In a hospital setting if a child is not improving and there is concern of secondary bacterial infection (temperature, raised inflammatory markers) a chest X-ray may be helpful. Management is symptomatic and aims to restore adequate oxygenation. Nasogastric feeding is often necessary for hospitalized children and if this fails intravenous therapy is used. If respiratory failure occurs intensive care is needed and rarely, ECMO.

Genitourinary infections

Urinary tract infections

The diagnosis and management of paediatric urinary tract infections (UTIs) is highly variable and controversial. The incidence of UTIs varies with age, gender, and the presence or absence of a normal renal system. By the age of 11 years, 3% of girls and 1% of boys will have had a UTI. Children may have risk factors predisposing them to infection including congenital renal anomalies, family history, or may even have a reduced risk of UTI (e.g. circumcised boys) (Singh-Grewal 2005). UTIs are important because in children they may represent an underlying congenital anomaly, which increases the chance of recurrent infection and may result in long-term morbidity (renal failure and hypertension). In the past the investigation of UTI was aimed at identification of children with vesicoureteric reflux (VUR) as they were thought to be the children at risk of scarring. However, renal scarring may occur in the presence or absence of VUR (Moorthy *et al.* 2005) and has been associated with hypertension and end-stage renal disease. The risk of renal hypertension and renal failure in children and adolescents with renal damage is controversial. What is thought is that renal damage can be minimized by outpatient follow-up and the institution of appropriate antibiotics where needed.

By definition a UTI is the detection of a pure growth of $>10^8$ bacterial colonies per litre ($>10^5$ bacterial colonies per ml) in the context of a symptomatic child. Long term screening studies using suprapubic aspirates, have identified that some children (2.5% boys, 0.9% girls) before the age of 1 year will have asymptomatic bacteriuria (Zorc *et al.* 2005).

There is also varying practice in the collection of urine in children, particularly in the first 2 years of life. These different collection methods will affect the culture rates in different units. Studies have shown that contamination rates for urine collection bags and Newcastle sterile urine collection pack pads are significantly higher than for clean catch (Alam *et al.* 2005). Although clean catch is possible at any age, it often requires a lot of time and patience and as such is often reserved for the older age groups. The ideal specimen from a child is a clean catch urine, or midstream urine. And certainly in a well child this should be the primary collection method. Alternative methods used by different units include urine pad collection, urine bags, which are used after cleaning the perineum. In a hospital setting suprapubic aspirate and catheter specimens may be local policy.

Depending on local practice, the combined use of appropriate dipstick (nitrites to detect bacteriuria and leucocyte esterase to detect pyuria ± direct microscopy by a trained physician/nurse are rapid diagnostic tests used in the diagnosis of UTIs. If there is going to be delay in specimens reaching the laboratory for culture it is best to store the sample at 0–4°C to avoid the proliferation of contaminants.

The organisms involved in UTIs are mostly gastrointestinal (GI) organisms. In boys there are some suggestions that circumcision should be considered in those with recurrent UTIs or high grade ≥4 VUR. Organisms commonly associated with UTIs include: *Escherichia coli* (65–85% of UTI), *Proteus* species, *Klebsiella* species, other coliforms and enterococci (1–10% of infections) (Davies 2001).

In the older child the clinical presentation is often more straight forward: loin pain, rigors, fever, and dysuria. More commonly the younger child presents with temperature and no other obvious focus and only when a urinalysis is done is the diagnosis apparent. Children may also present with diarrhoea, vomiting, irritability, failure to thrive, or lethargy. In an infant there is a high risk that a UTI will progress to systemic sepsis. Eighty per cent of children <1 year will have temperature, and 2–10% of children between 2 months and 2 years with unexplained fever will have a UTI (Pediatrics 1999).

Who to take urine samples from:

- all children <2 years with unexplained fever
- children with dysuria, frequency, suprapubic pain, loin pain, rigors
- febrile or a febrile children with: diarrhoea, vomiting, irritability, failure to thrive, or lethargy
  The management of UTIs is controversial and like urine collection, practice is variable across different regions. Most children with UTIs will be well and will require oral

antibiotics for a minimum of 7–10 days. Although trimethoprim used to be first line, because of growing resistance patterns a number of units no longer use this as their first-line agent. It is, however, still often used as first line for prophylaxis. For the treatment of UTIs, local resistance patterns should influence choice of antibiotic therapy.

Antimicrobial management of urinary tract infections

Positive urine cultures should be treated with empirical antibiotics until antibiotic sensitivity testing is available. In children, short course treatment should not be used in view of the high rate of relapse and 7–14 days is recommended. After treatment of an acute UTI prophylactic antibiotics should be commenced on all children <5 years of age. The risk of renal damage decreases for children age ≥5 years. If all subsequent investigations are normal, prophylactic antibiotics can be stopped.

All children ≤5 years after a confirmed UTI should be on prophylactic antibiotics.
Lack of clinical improvement after 48 hours may be due to inappropriate antimicrobials or renal tract abnormalities. These children should have repeat urine sample taken and may require renal tract imaging. There is varied practice on when to stop prophylaxis. Some physicians stop prophylaxis sooner if the degree of VUR is mild with no scarring, and continue longer into adolescence if there is persistent VUR in the presence of scarring.

Imaging following urinary tract infection

There is variable practice on postinfective imaging. Children <1 year old should have a renal ultrasound, followed by a static renal isotope scan (DMSA) 3–6 months after acute infection. MCUG (micturating cystogram) should be considered, although there is growing debate on whether this contributes to management (Moorthy *et al.* 2005). Children aged 1–5 years and ≥5 should have an ultrasound and DMSA. Some centres only offer DMSA if there are risk factors. Risk factors include a positive family history and clinical presentation of systemic illness (fever, vomiting, loin pain, and rigors). Renal tract imaging is not without its own risk. Follow up of definite UTIs should be by a paediatrician or nephrologist.

Reasons for referral to hospital:

- unable to tolerate oral treatment
- systemically unwell
- rigors
- poor hydration or perfusion
- poor response after 48 hours oral therapy.

Gastrointestinal infections

Gastroenteritis

Can be defined as the sudden onset of diarrhoea (>3 loose stools/per day), which may be associated with vomiting. The commonest cause of paediatric gastroenteritis worldwide is rotavirus. It is the leading cause of severe gastroenteritis in infants in developed and developing nations. Symptomatic disease occurs most commonly from 3 to 24 months of age and 20% of diarrhoeal deaths are caused by rotavirus in children <5 years worldwide (WHO). By the age of 4 most children have had the infection. Vaccines have now been developed, which are highly effective against this disease, and are now available in the UK. Other viral causes of gastroenteritis include; noroviruses, adenovirus (serotypes 40+41), and astrovirus.

Bacterial infections may present as watery or bloody diarrhoea. *Campylobacter jejuni* is the commonest bacterial cause of GI infections in England and Wales. Bloody diarrhoea is more likely to be caused by; *Campylobacter jejuni*, *Shigella* species, *Salmonella enteritidis*, or enteroinvasive *E. coli* (EIEC) or enterohaemorrhagic *E. coli* (EHEC). Watery diarrhoea is more likely to be caused by enterotoxigenic *E. coli* (ETEC, 'traveller's diarrhoea') or in resource-poor countries *Vibrio cholera*.

Entamoeba histolytica is spread by faecal oral transmission of amoebic cysts. Ingestion of cysts may result in invasive or non-invasive infection of the colon and disease is characterized by bloody diarrhoea. In developing countries it accounts for <3% of cases of bloody diarrhoea. In 2003 there were 131 cases isolated in stool throughout England and Wales compared with 46 178 cases of *Campylobacter jejuni* Health Protection Agency (HPA).

To help determine the likely aetiology of the diarrhoea and vomiting, useful clues in history may be; blood/mucus in stool, length of illness, involvement of other family members, foreign travel, recent ingestion of takeaway food or a previous GI problem. Viral infections are often short lived (2–3 days) and associated with both diarrhoea and vomiting. With bacterial infections diarrhoea predominates. Invasive salmonella is more common in those with sickle cell disease and *Yersinia enterocolitica* is particularly associated with thalassaemia. In the immunocompromised child, pathogens will vary to include all the above as well as; cytomegalovirus, *Cryptosporidium parvum*, *Isospora belli*, microsporidia, and noroviruses.

In children who develop diarrhoea while they are receiving a prolonged course of antibiotics it is important to consider pseudomembranous colitis and look for *Clostridium difficile* toxin in stool. When a child presents with potential gastroenteritis after taking a history it is important to consider surgical causes for their symptoms (e.g. appendicitis) and to assess for non-infective causes of GI upset including signs of chronic disease (e.g. clubbing, mouth ulcers, etc.) All children should be weighed and plotted on a growth chart.

A child with GI symptoms should be assessed for signs of dehydration:

◆ sunken eyes
◆ decreased skin turgor
◆ sunken anterior fontanelle
◆ dry mucous membranes
◆ decreased urine output (determine from history)
◆ weak peripheral pulses/tachycardia (severe dehydration)
◆ poor peripheral perfusion (increased capillary refill time)

- decreased level of consciousness
- low blood pressure (pre-terminal sign of hypovolaemia in children).

  Reasons for referral to hospital:
- severe dehydration (tachycardia and poor peripheral perfusion)
- bilious vomiting (consider surgical causes including intussuception)
- altered level of consciousness
- uncertain diagnosis
- difficult social circumstances.

Management of mild and moderate dehydration in the community consists of oral rehydration therapy (ORT). All children with mild to moderate dehydration should be offered ORT. Once rehydrated (normally over 12 hours, with rehydration achieved in the first 4 hours) with ORT, children may resume a normal diet. Breast-fed babies may continue feeding during ORT (Murphy 1998). There is no role for anti-emetics or antidiarrhoeal agents (RCPCH 2003). There is a limited role for antibiotics. Antibiotics are used in the management of:

- salmonellosis, all species if <6 months of age
- *Salmonella typhi* or *S. paratyphi* at any age
- shigellosis if the child is unwell
- *Entamoeba histolytica*
- giardiasis
- *Campylobacter* in severe infection
- symptomatic *Clostridium difficile*
- enterotoxigenic *E.coli*

Bone and joint infections

Skeletal infection in children is a medical and (often) surgical emergency and can lead to lifelong disability (Choi *et al.*, 1990). Diagnosis can be difficult as early infection often presents in a non-specific manner. Although osteomyelitis and septic arthritis are distinct clinical entities, occasionally they may coexist. This is particularly common in childhood when the metaphysis is intra-articular. As the periosteum in these sites is thin, early drainage of pus at these sites into the joint results in septic arthritis (Davies 2000). Common clinical syndromes include classical haematogenous long-bone osteomyelitis, septic arthritis (acute, subacute, chronic), discitis and osteochondritis, and skeletal infection complicating trauma and puncture wounds.

The majority of cases are caused by *Staphylococcus aureus*. *Haemophilus influenzae* type b is now rare following the introduction of universal Hib conjugate immunization for infants in industrialized nations (Howard *et al.* 1999). *Kingella kingae* may account for a significant number of non-staphylococcal cases but isolation of the organism is more difficult. *Salmonella* osteomyelitis is more common in individuals with sickle cell disease.

Septic arthritis

Septic arthritis typically presents with a short history (<24 hours) of being unwell, pyrexia and severe pain, swelling, and warmth in the affected joint. Septic arthritis is almost twice as common as osteomyelitis (Davies 2000). Pain is an almost universal feature, occurs early and localizes. Infants and young children, however, are unable to describe or clearly localize pain. In this case they may present with history of a limp, reluctance to weight bear, or refusal to walk. Examination of the joint often reveals little or no movement 'pseudo paralysis', and an attempt to move the joint results in severe pain. Classically a red, warm, tender, swollen joint is seen, although these may not all occur simultaneously.

Acute haematogenous osteomyelitis (AHO)

This characteristically occurs slightly later in childhood but >50% of affected children are still <5 years of age. Common features include; bone pain, local tenderness, unexplained fever as an early feature or signs of systemic illness. Children may not be febrile, and local tenderness may not be immediately apparent. In subacute or chronic osteomyelitis the symptoms are much more indolent and the child may be well with no fever at presentation. AHO often affects the lower limbs; femur, tibia or bones of the foot. In neonates and infants signs of septic arthritis or osteomyelitis, may be very difficult to detect. A history of pyrexia of unknown origin, or paucity of movement in an affected limb should alert the clinician of the diagnosis.

Subacute and chronic forms of bone and joint infections by definition have symptoms dating two or more weeks. Generally systemic features are absent and the clinical picture is predominated by local symptoms and signs. The most common differential diagnosis for subacute or chronic osteomyelitis is Ewing's sarcoma, and biopsy may be required to make this distinction. Chronic osteomyelitis may be accompanied by minor ill health with intermittent pyrexia and acute illness. The possibility of TB should be considered.

Discitis

This is an uncommon condition, with characteristic magnetic resonance imaging and clinical features. Older children localize pain to the back, whereas toddlers typically present with refusal to walk or an abnormal posture. Pain affecting the back or hip is not always apparent. Presentation is often delayed by weeks or months. The white blood cell count is usually normal but erythrocyte sedimentation rate may be raised. Blood cultures are often negative (Hambleton and Berendt 2004). Management is usually undertaken by a paediatrician and orthopaedic surgeon and a trial of antibiotic therapy used for empiric therapy. Occasionally a paraspinal abscess may complicate the clinical course. The mainstay of treatment is investigation with appropriate imaging and intravenous antibiotics in a hospital setting. In septic arthritis this represents a surgical emergency at an appropriate centre.

Adverse outcomes after septic arthritis can include; dislocation, ankylosis, permanent stiffness, premature osteoarthritis, growth disturbance, or systemic sepsis. These are most likely after hip joint infections or when there has been a delay in diagnosis (Choi *et al.*, 1990). Growth disturbance may occur after either infection and continued surveillance of skeletal maturity should be undertaken either in a paediatric or orthopaedic clinic.

Refer the following to a paediatric team where joint management with orthopaedics is available:

- septic arthritis or osteomyelitis
- subacute or chronic osteomyelitis, chronic recurrent osteomyelitis
- discitis.

The febrile child

Most children with a fever will have a self-limiting viral infection; 2–10% of children with fever, but no localizing source of infection will have occult bacterial infections (Barraff 2000). The likelihood of invasive bacterial infection rises with higher fevers at presentation. Alternatively, children may present with fever and localizing symptoms (ears, throat, or chest).

The following points from the history may guide diagnosis:

- infectious contacts
- travel history
- animal or insect bites
- immunization status
- evidence of immunocompromise; chemotherapy, immunosuppressants, recurrent infections, multiple infections, high-risk background (e.g. maternal HIV).

Useful signs on examination include:

- rash
- signs of upper respiratory tract infection, including otitis media
- signs of lower respiratory tract infection
- abdominal pain
- meningism
- joint/bone tenderness.

Management

If there are clear localizing signs, investigation and management should be appropriate (e.g. localized crepitations with respiratory signs and symptoms should be treated as a respiratory chest infection). If there are no localizing signs, it is important to consider bacteraemia or UTI. If pyrexia persists for more than 5 days with no cause found, the 'pyrexia of unknown origin' (PUO) should be referred for investigation in most cases.

Although PUO has many causes infections to consider are:

- **viral:** cytomegalovirus, Epstein–Barr virus, human herpesvirus 6, parvovirus, respiratory viruses

- **bacterial:** TB, leptospirosis, brucellosis, spirochaete infections, salmonellosis, subacute bacterial endocarditis, osteomyelitis, abscesses
- **other infections:** malaria, toxoplasmosis, chlamydia, rickettsiae, fungal infections
- **non-infectious causes:** Kawasaki's disease, collagen vascular disorders, malignancies, drugs, inflammatory bowel disease, periodic fever syndrome.

Features associated with a high chance of bacteraemia, which warrant hospital referral include:

- very high temp >39°C
- tachycardia
- pale/mottled skin
- prolonged capillary refill time
- cold peripheries
- depressed level of consciousness.

Central nervous system (CNS) infections
Meningitis/encephalitis

Bacterial meningitis is an important cause of death both in developed and developing countries. The diagnosis may be difficult as in young children symptoms may be non-specific. Symptoms in infants may include: high temperature, poor feeding, vomiting, lethargy, irritability, or dislike of being handled. Clinical signs include; bulging fontanelle, fever, drowsiness/altered mental state, apnoeas, convulsions, or purpuric rash. In older children the more classical signs of headache, neck stiffness, and photophobia are common. The specific signs of Kernig, Brudzinski, and nuchal stiffness are often absent in children (Kaaresen 1995). In adults and children, these signs are poorly sensitive. Both Kernig and Brudzinski have a sensitivity of only 5% while nuchal rigidity has a sensitivity of 30% (Bashir 2003; McCarthy 2005). In view of the non-specific nature of these symptoms a high index of suspicion is required to identify cases in the very young.

Causes of bacterial meningitis vary according to the age of the child:

- **<3 months:** Group B haemolytic streptococcus, *Escherichia coli*, *Listeria monocytogenes*
- **3 months–5 years**: *Neiserria meningitidis*, *Streptococcus pneumoniae*, and *Haemophilus influenzae*
- **>5 years**: *Neiserria meningitidis*, *Streptococcus pneumoniae*

Meningococcal septicaemia has a high mortality, especially when the diagnosis is delayed. Septicaemia without focal infection accounts for 15–20% of cases of meningococcal disease but often coexists with meningococcal meningitis. Isolated meningococcal meningitis presents in the same way as meningitis due to other causes but may be associated with a non-blanching rash. Deaths from meningococcal septicaemia may be prevented by early treatment. Current recommendations include administration of penicillin or ceftriaxone in the community to a patient with a febrile illness and either a petechial or purpuric rash.

Meningococcal disease may be fulminant and cause death within 12 hours or, rarely, chronic and present over weeks. Meningitis is the commonest clinical syndrome accounting for 80–85% of cases. Mortality from meningococcal meningitis is low at 1–5% (Yung 2003); however, meningococcal septicaemia has a 40% mortality rate. Less common syndromes of meningococcal infection include; respiratory tract infection (pneumonia, epiglottitis, otitis media), focal infection (conjunctivitis, septic arthritis, urethritis, purulent pericarditis), and chronic meningococcaemia.

Clinical clues to early diagnosis of meningococcaemia are:

- *A non-blanching rash*. The rash typically begins in the first 24 hours of the illness. The febrile child must be undressed and examined closely for rash in covered areas or on the conjunctivae, sclerae, or oral mucosa.
- *A blanching or maculopapular rash*. This rash may mimic a non-specific viral rash, and may precede evolution into petechiae or disappear. Some children with meningococcal septicaemia have no rash.
- *Rapid evolution of illness*. Previously well children who become suddenly unwell or deteriorate within 24–48 hours or who re-present to a doctor within 24–48 hours of a febrile illness may have an invasive bacterial disease.
- *Concern of parent*. The parents' concern about the child's symptoms should be taken into consideration during the medical assessment.
- *Age*. Risk of infection is highest in children aged 3 months–5 years. There is also an increased rate of meningococcal disease in adolescence and early adulthood.
- *Contact with meningococcal disease*. Secondary cases of meningococcal disease are rare (5% of cases) but any contacts who develop a febrile illness after contact with a case should be investigated in hospital for early meningococcal disease.

The following groups should receive treatment with benzylpenicillin or ceftriaxone BEFORE referral to hospital:

- children with suspected meningococcal septicaemia or meningitis
- children with fever and a non-blanching rash
- any individual with fever and a history of contact with meningococcal disease.

The following should be referred for paediatric assessment:

- A child with fever of unknown aetiology, seen for the second time within 24–48 hours and worsening symptoms.

Suspect invasive bacterial disease such as meningococcaemia and observe closely:

- any unwell child with acute onset of fever and non-specific rash within 12 hours of illness
- a previously well child with febrile illness when the parents are particularly concerned.

Meningo-encephalitis

Although viral infections are common throughout childhood, viral infections of the CNS are uncommon. Viruses can produce a wide variety of manifestations of CNS infection. Some viruses such as mumps and varicella produce a common but relatively benign encephalitic syndrome (mumps is associated with acquired deafness). Herpes simplex virus commonly causes infection but rarely causes encephalitis. Human herpesvirus 6 encephalitis may present with febrile convulsions. Other viruses such as rabies lead exclusively to CNS disease. Measles may cause a postinfectious encephalopathy.

Aetiological diagnosis of viral encephalitis can be difficult using clinical tools alone. Epidemiological features such as season of the year, prevalent diseases within the community, travel, recreational activities, and animal contacts can all be useful. Late summer and early autumn is the season for the presentation of the most common meningo-encephalitis in childhood caused by enteroviruses. Bacterial causes of encephalitis include mycoplasma, *Lepstospira* spp., listeria and TB.

Symptoms of encephalitis include the triad of; fever, headache, and altered level of consciousness. These symptoms may progress to coma, myalgia, altered behaviour, seizures, cranial nerve palsies, ataxia, paresis, and evidence of raised intracranial pressure. Early symptoms may be non-specific and include fever and vomiting. There may also be systemic features such as rash, lymphadenopathy, and pneumonia. There may be an associated meningitic process, presenting with; headache, vomiting, nuchal rigidity, and photophobia.

The postinfectious syndromes are usually preceded by an infectious illness. Varicella usually produces signs of cerebellar dysfunction. Focal seizures are characteristic of herpes simplex encephalitis (one-third of cases occur in children and adolescents) (Whitley *et al.* 2005). Insidious onset of neurological symptoms with minimal systemic upset is typical of acute demyelinating encephalomyelitis. Not all encephalitis is infectious but a good infection history will help guide the diagnosis (travel, exposure to dogs, herpetic lesions, foreign travel, etc.)

Inpatient assessment is required for lumbar puncture and CNS imaging. Treatment is supportive. A few specific treatments are available to treat bacterial meningitis, Lyme disease, mycoplasma and HSV. Vaccines are available for Japanese encephalitis and tick-borne encephalitis.

Refer to hospital all children with:

♦ A febrile illness associated with an altered conscious state, behavioural changes, or focal seizures.

Staphylococcal infections, streptococcal infections, and Kawasaki disease (KD)

Staphylococci are normal commensals of the skin, upper respiratory tract, and GI tract. Up to 40% of individuals are colonized at any one time. Staphylococci are responsible for some skin infections including impetigo and cellulitis and can also cause more serious diseases, including; pneumonia, meningitis, endocarditis, septicaemia, orbital cellulitis, or osteomyelitis. Diseases mediated by toxins produced by staphylococci include scalded skin syndrome, staphylococcal scarlet fever, and toxic shock syndrome (TSS).

Toxic shock syndrome

TSS is caused by *Staphylococcus aureus* (phage group I) exotoxins (TSST-1). In this disease, the source of the Staphylococcal infection is not always apparent or may be related to minor soft tissue injury or tampon use. One third of cases occur in teenagers, and the disease is rare in pre-pubertal children

Diagnostic criteria include:

+ temperature ≥38.5°C

+ hypotension

+ erythematous rash followed by desquamation at 1–2 weeks

+ vomiting and diarrhoea

+ multi-organ involvement

All cases of suspected TSS should be referred to hospital.

Clinical presentation is often non-specific, with 'flu-like' symptoms, including myalgia, chills, and fever. Management is supportive with antimicrobials, cardiovascular support, dialysis, and intubation if required. TSS can also result from toxins released by Group A streptococci. Risk factors include diabetes, HIV, and cardiopulmonary disease. No risk factors are found in 35%.

Scarlet fever

Scarlet fever is caused by Group A beta-haemolytic streptococci producing erythrogenic exotoxin in individuals with no neutralizing antibodies. The incidence is believed to have fallen as a result of the use of antibiotics to treat sore throat. Transmission is by respiratory droplet. Incubation is 2–4 days after streptococcal acquisition.

Clinical features may include: fever, headache, sore throat, and rigors. Other classical symptoms described include; white strawberry tongue, a rash that spreads from the neck downwards, circum-oral pallor, and desquamation after 5 days. ASOT (antistreptolysin O-test) and Anti-DNAse may be useful in diagnosis. Treatment is with penicillin for 10 days. Relapse is common with shorter courses.

Kawasaki disease (mucocutaneous lymph node syndrome)

KD is a vasculitic disease that appears to have an infective aetiology. Patterns of disease are similar to those of an infectious agent with clusters, epidemics, and seasonality, and a suggestion of genetic susceptibility. The incidence in the UK is 3.4/100 000 for typical cases. KD occurs more commonly in boys, and in children under 5 years of age (80% of cases) and there is a higher incidence in children from eastern Asia; Japan, >100/100 000.

If KD is untreated or treated with aspirin alone, coronary artery disease and aneurysms occur in 20–40% of cases (Royle *et al.* 2005). The acute mortality rate was previously reported as 4%, although recent reports show a much lower mortality. KD is currently the leading cause of acquired heart disease in children.

KD is a self-limiting vasculitic illness with resolution of inflammation and apparent complete clinical recovery over several weeks. However, even in cases where there is no evidence of acute coronary damage, histological and conduction abnormalities have been identified and the disease is a risk factor for future coronary artery disease.

Children present with fever as high as 40°C that is unremitting and lasts for 12–15 days when untreated. The child is typically irritable and miserable. Significant morbidity and mortality is caused by the complications following this acute illness including; coronary artery aneurysms, depressed myocardial contractility, heart failure, myocardial infarction, arrhythmias, and peripheral artery occlusion.

The following diagnostic criteria are used for the diagnosis of KD: Fever ≥5 days that is resistant to antibiotics and antipyretics plus the presence of at least four of the features below:

◆ bilateral non-purulent conjunctivitis

◆ cervical lymphadenopathy, unilateral or bilateral, >1.5 cm diameter (50–75% of cases)

◆ polymorphous rash (transient and may only be apparent from history)

◆ changes in extremities: erythema of palms and soles, indurative oedema of hands and feet. in convalescence, desquamation of the skin of the hand, feet, and perineum (may occur earlier in disease)

◆ oral mucous membrane changes: strawberry tongue, diffuse erythema of oral and pharyngeal mucosa, red, dry, cracked lips.

It is believed that many children will present with only a few of the above features and the constellation of clinical symptoms required for the diagnosis often appear over time. As the clinical presentation of KD is similar to many other childhood illnesses it is important to rule out staphylococcal and streptococcal toxin mediated diseases (TSS, scalded skin syndrome, scarlet fever). Other diseases with a similar presentation include; leptospirosis, measles, rubella, enterovirus, and other viral exanthema. In addition inflammatory conditions such as systemic juvenile idiopathic arthritis should be considered.

Atypical Kawasaki disease

Children suspected of having KD who do not fulfil the criteria may have incomplete or atypical KD. Therefore, it is important to include KD in the differential for a prolonged febrile illness with no focus of infection. Infants less than 1 year of age are more likely to present with atypical KD, associated with peripheral oedema and are at greater risk of cardiovascular complications.

Cervical lymphadenopathy is less likely in atypical KD. Ninety per cent of cases have no lymphadenopathy. Rash does not occur in 50% of those with atypical disease compared with 7–10% of those who meet the criteria. 90% of children with either form of the disease will have mucosal membrane changes. Children with atypical disease tend not to have peripheral extremity changes (only 40% of children demonstrate these changes). At least 85% of those with typical disease develop erythema of the extremities or oedema/desquamation.

In KD, systemic inflammation is manifested by elevated acute phase reactants: erythrocyte sedimentation rate, C-reactive protein, and raised white cell count with neutrophilia. In the second week of illness thrombocytosis may occur. Normochromic, normocytic anaemia is common in the first few weeks after onset. Pyuria may be detected on urine microscopy (despite negative dipstick testing) and haematuria or proteinuria is commonly present (Pediatrics 2005). Mild hyperbilirubinaemia or obstructive jaundice associated with hydrops of the gall bladder may occur. Some children will have cerebrospinal fluid pleocytosis or present with joint pain. Echocardiography is used to identify the serious complication of coronary artery disease and should be 6 weeks after presentation as some changes may appear later.

Admission to a paediatric inpatient unit and treatment with intravenous immunoglobu-lin (IVIG) and aspirin reduces the rate of coronary lesions to <5% if administered within 10 days of onset of symptoms (Royle *et al.* 2005). High-dose aspirin is used initially for its anti-inflammatory properties and then reduced to a low dose to produce an antithrom-botic effect once the fever has subsided and acute phase reactants have returned to normal.

Tuberculosis

TB is caused by *Mycobacterium tuberculosis* and occasionally by *Mycobacterium bovis* (about 1.5% of isolates; Davies 2001). Rates of TB are increasing in much of the UK with the highest incidence in inner city areas, particularly London. TB is a notifiable disease under the Public Health (Control of Diseases) Act 1984 and notification triggers contact tracing. In 1994, 9% of cases globally occurred in children (BTS 2000). In the UK in 1998, 56% of cases were people born outside the UK (BTS 2000) and in particular those from the Indian subcontinent and Africa. Transmission is person to person via respiratory droplet from an individual presenting with pulmonary TB.

High-risk groups include:

- immigrants
- children born to immigrant parents
- asylum seekers and refugees
- individuals with HIV infection.

The risk of transmission of TB is increased by overcrowding and appears to be greater in communities with low socio-economic status. There is also a risk of bovine TB from non-pasteurized milk.

TB may present as asymptomatic latent infection (LTBI) or as primary disease. From birth to 8 years of age the risk of acquiring the disease rather than establishing latent infection after recent exposure is inversely related to age. Host and pathogen factors may also be important in determining the outcome.

LTBI is indicated by:

- positive tuberculin skin test (Mantoux) or Gamma interferon assay
- no clinical or radiological evidence of acute TB (except Gohn focus).

These children are presumed to have a small number of dormant tubercle bacilli that do not cause any symptoms.

When disease occurs, clinical manifestations often appear 1–6 months after infection in children. Tuberculous disease has a wide spectrum of clinical presentation: Pulmonary TB accounts for 66% of childhood cases (Davies 2001). This may present as:

- fever, night sweats, chills
- weight loss, growth delay
- unilateral hilar lymphadenopathy ± segmental lung changes.

Phlyctenular conjunctivitis, erythema nodosum, and pleural effusions: should all prompt a differential diagnosis of TB. Extrapulmonary infections include meningitis, disease of the middle ear and mastoid, lymph nodes, bones, joints, and skin. Renal TB or reactivation (adult-type) pulmonary TB are rare in young children but can occur in adolescents.

Diagnosis of both pulmonary and extra pulmonary TB in childhood is difficult but may be associated with a history of exposure to an infectious case, presence of a positive tuberculin skin test and/or an abnormal Chest X-ray. Additional investigations include three sequential early morning gastric washings looking for acid and alcohol fast bacilli and culture. Mycobacterial culture can take 4–6 weeks plus 2–4 weeks for further sensitivities (Mandalakas and Starke 2005). New diagnostic tests that rely on detection of TB-specific T cells in peripheral blood have recently become available and may transform investigation of this disease.

Mantoux testing

Intradermal injection of purified protein derivative of tuberculin of either 10 units (0.1 ml of 1:1000) or 1 unit (0.1 ml of 1:10 000). Ten units should always be used unless there is a risk of hypersensitivity reaction (i.e. children who have had phlyctenular conjunctivitis, erythema nodosum, or BCG immunization within 12 months). Skin tests should be performed on the volar aspect of the forearm and read after 48–72 hours. If the induration after 72 hours increases, the maximum induration should be used as the final reading.

- induration of >5 mm is positive
- if a child has had previous vaccination with BCG induration of >10 mm may suggest infection but >15 mm is more indicative

Only the diameter of the induration should be recorded not the redness.

False positive and negative results do occur. Expert advice should be sought on the choice of drugs and duration of therapy for TB (BTS 1998). Guidance from the National Institute for Clinical Excellence (NICE) will be published soon.

Acknowledgements

The authors are grateful to Kirsten Perrett for critical comments on the final draft of the manuscript.

Table 10.1 Other common childhood infections

Disease	Mode of transmission	Definition of onset	Incubation period	Risk of transmission	Exclusion period	Shedding period
Chickenpox	Physical contact, respiratory droplet, airborne	Skin lesions	11–20 days	Very high, attack rate up to 87% in susceptible children[§]	5 days from start of skin eruption	
Herpes simplex	Oral secretions, physical contact	Gingivosto-matitis	1–6 days	Highly, especially among young children	None	1–8 weeks[‡]

Table 10.1 Other common childhood infections—cont'd

Disease	Mode of transmission	Definition of onset	Incubation period	Risk of transmission	Exclusion period	Shedding period
Impetigo-staphy-lococcal	Physical contact	Skin lesions	No true incubation	? Low	Until lesions healed/ crusted	
Impetigo-strepto-crusted	Skin contact-although broken skin often required for disease development	Skin lesions	Skin carriage 2–33 days before develop-ment	High. During epidemics in house-hold contacts up to 100%	Until lesions skin healed/ coccal	Untreated carriage may persist for weeks
Measles	Respiratory Droplet/ Airborne	Rash	6–19 days	Highly infectious in non-immune. Younger children at higher risk Low risk in vaccinated population	5/7 from onset of rash[†]	−2 to +3 days
Meningo-coccal disease	Respiratory rash, droplet	Petechial meningitis	No true incubation period as organism known to be carried for unknown period before invasive disease	Low. House-holds> nurseries >schools (2.5–75:10[5])	24 hours after starting therapy?	Untreated duration of colonization median 9 months. Treated <2 days from start of chemo-prophylaxis
Molluscum conta-giosum	Direct contact (fomites)	Skin lesions	6–12 weeks	Moderate among family members no data from schools	None—not serious condition and presumably not highly contagious at school	Presumably duration of lesions

Table 10.1 Other common childhood infections—cont'd

Disease	Mode of transmission	Definition of onset	Incubation period	Risk of transmission	Exclusion period	Shedding period
Mumps	Respiratory droplet	Cough	5–21 days	Highly infectious in non-immune population	5/7 if given Erythro-mycin or azithromycin otherwise ?3 weeks*	60% shed-ding at 2 weeks, 20% at 6 weeks, <1 week if treated with macrolide

*Most papers suggest the longer exclusion time. Only one paper (Stocks 1933) has data on 5-day isolation with eryth romycin treatment.

†Exclusion may be ineffective as some transmission occurs before onset of rash up to 2 days before.
Immunocompromised individuals need immunoglobulin.

‡In recurrent infection excreting for about 3 days. After primary infection children intermittently excrete virus in saliva. At any given time-point up to 20% will be shedding virus.

§Infectious from −4 to +5 days. Most usually not infectious before −1 days. Cases often transmit before onset of rash.

References

Alam MT, Coulter JB, Pacheco J, Correia JB, Ribeiro MG, Coelho MF, Bunn JE (2005). Comparison of urine contamination rates using three different methods of collection: clean-catch, cotton wool pad and urine bag. *Annals of Tropical Paediatrics* **25**: 29–34.

Barraff LJ (2000). Management of fever without source in infants and children. *Annals of Emergency Medicine* **36**(6): 602–614.

El Bashir H, Laundy M, Booy R (2003). Diagnosis and treatment of bacterial meningitis. *Archives of Disease in Childhood* **88**: 615–620.

BTS (1998). Chemotherapy and management of tuberculosis in the United Kingdom: recommendations 1998. Joint Tuberculosis Committee of the British Thoracic Society. *Thorax* **53**(7): 536–48.

BTS (2000). Control and prevention of tuberculosis in the United Kingdom: code of practice 2000. Joint Tuberculosis Committee of the British Thoracic Society. *Thorax* **55**(11): 887–901.

BTS (2002). British Thoracic Society guidelines for the management of community acquired pneumonia in childhood. *Thorax* **57** (Suppl. 1): i1–24.

Capper R, Canter RJ (2001). Is there agreement among general practitioners, paediatricians and otolaryngologists about the management of children with recurrent tonsillitis? *Clinical Otolaryngology and Allied Science* **26**(5): 371–378.

Choi IH, Pizzutillo PD, et al (1990). Sequelae and reconstruction after septic arthritis of the hip in infants. *Journal of Bone and Joint Surgery* **72**(8): 1150–1165.

Davies, EG, Monsell F (2000). Managing osteoarticular infection in children. *Current Paediatrics* **10**: 42–48.

Davies EG, Elliman D. A. C, Hart CA, Nicoll A, Rudd PT (2001). *Manual of Childhood Infections*, (2nd edn).

Fitzgerald DA, Kilham HA (2003). Croup: assessment and evidence-based management. *Medical Journal of Australia* **179**(7): 372–377.

Hambleton S, Berendt AR (2004). Bone and joint infections in children. *Advances in Experimental Medicine and Biology* **549**: 47–62.

Howard AW, Viskontas D, et al (1999). Reduction in osteomyelitis and septic arthritis related to Haemophilus influenzae type B vaccination. *Journal of Pediatric Orthopaedics* **19**(6): 705–709.

Mandalakas AM, Starke JR (2005). Current concepts of childhood tuberculosis. *Seminars in Pediatrics and Infectious Disease* **16**(2): 93–104.

McCarthy P (2005). Fever without apparent source on clinical examination. *Current Opinion in Pediatrics* **17**: 93–110.

Moorthy I, Easty M, et al (2005). The presence of vesicoureteric reflux does not identify a population at risk for renal scarring following a first urinary tract infection. *Archives of Disease in Childhood* **90**(7): 733–736.

Murphy MS (1998). Guidelines for managing acute gastroenteritis based on a systematic review of published research. *Archives of Disease in Childhood* **79**(3): 279–284.

Newburger JW, Takahashi M, Gerber MA, Gewitz MH, Tani LY, Burns JC, Shulman ST, Bolger AF, Ferrieri P, Baltimore RS, Wilson WR, Baddour LM, Levison ME, Pallasch TJ, Falace DA, Taubert KA (2004). Diagnosis, Treatment and Long Term Management of Kawasaki Disease: A Statement for Health Professionals from the Committee of Rheumatic Fever, Endocarditis, and Kawasaki Disease, Council on Cardiovascular Disease in the Young, American Heart Association. *Circulation* **110**(17): 2747–71.

Paradise JL, Bluestone CD, et al (1984). Efficacy of tonsillectomy for recurrent throat infection in severely affected children. Results of parallel randomized and nonrandomized clinical trials. *New England Journal of Medicine* **310**(11): 674–683.

Pediatrics AAO (1999). Practice parameter: the diagnosis, treatment, and evaluation of the initial urinary tract infection in febrile infants and young children. American Academy of Pediatrics. Committee on Quality Improvement. Subcommittee on Urinary Tract Infection. *Pediatrics* **103**(4 Pt 1): 843–852.

RCPCH GUIDELINE APPRAISAL Paediatric Accident and Emergency Research Group (2003). Evidence based guidelines for the management of children presenting to hospital with diarhoea, with or without vomiting.

SIGN Guidelines (1999). Management of Sore throat and indications for tonsillectomy.

Singh-Grewal D, Macdessi J, Craig J (2005). Circumcision for the prevention of urinary tract infections in boys: a systematic review of randomised trials and observational studies. *Archives of Disease in Childhood* **90**(8): 853–8.

Smyth, A (2002). Pneumonia due to viral and atypical organisms and their sequelae. *British Medical Bulletin* **61**: 247–62.

Rothman R, Owens T, et al (2003). Does this child have acute otitis media? *JAMA* **290**(12): 1633–1640.

Royle J, Burgner D, et al (2005). The diagnosis and management of Kawasaki disease. *Journal of Paediatrics and Child Health* **41**(3): 87–93.

Sinaniotis CA (2004). Viral pneumoniae in children: incidence and aetiology. *Paediatric Respiratory Review* 5 (Suppl. A): S197–200.

Whitley RJ, Kimberlin DW (2005). Herpes simplex: encephalitis children and adolescents. *Seminars in Pediatric Infectious Disease* **16**: 17–23.

Yung AP, McDonald MI (2003). Early clinical clues to meningococcaemia. *The Medical Journal of Australia* **178**(3): 134–137.

Zorc JJ, Kiddoo DA, et al (2005). Diagnosis and management of pediatric urinary tract infections. *Clinical Microbiology Reviews* **18**(2): 417–422.

Further reading
Resources and useful websites

http://www.sign.ac.uk/guidelines (Guidelines to Management of Otitis Media, Sore Throat,)

http://aapredbook.aappublications.org

http://www.brit-thoracic.org.uk (Guidelines to Community Acquired Pneumonia, Tuberculosis)

http://www.rcpch.ac.uk/publications/clinical_docs.html (Guidelines to management of Gastroenteritis-Paed A&E Research Group, Urinary Tract Infections-American Academy of Pediatrics)

http://www.bhiva.org/chiva (Resources on management of HIV in children)

Chapter 11

Failure to thrive: recognition and management in primary care

Fauzia Khan and Mary Rudolf

When my daughter stopped putting on weight … she was weighed every week and it was over eighteen months of them coming and weighing her every week … and them saying 'oh, she will grow out of it'. After eighteen months she went two weeks without eating, nothing at all, and I packed her bags up one day, took her down to the clinic, and said take her in hospital because I am not doing it anymore. If she got referred after three months instead of eighteen months maybe she wouldn't have been like that and picked up straight away and we wouldn't still have it all three and a half years later.

Failure to thrive has long been viewed as a condition brought about by parental neglect if not abuse, where all that is required is to provide adequate calories for the child to grow and thrive. However, in our experience parents are more often than not desperately concerned about their child, and stressed from their attempts to encourage them to eat.

The following are quotes from mothers seen in our clinic that together with the one above illustrate the emotive nature of failure to thrive, and the failure of healthcare professionals to provide the appropriate help.

It is just my whole life … it sounds like it is you that is doing something wrong.

At one bit I had you coming, the social worker coming, the normal health visitor coming and the doctor coming out, and I was just lost … everyone gives you different advice and then you don't know whose to follow.

The very term *failure to thrive* conjures a sense of doing wrong, or not doing, rather than the situation we commonly see in reality—that of carers trying to do their best in a situation that they believe should be natural and yet has somehow gone wrong.

Failure to thrive occurs in 2–5% of children (Skuse *et al.* 1992). It occurs across all socio-economic groups and in most cases it is responds favourably to straightforward intervention. There are cases when a child's failure to thrive reflects poor or abusive parenting; these are more complicated, usually more resistant to simple approaches and require a coordinated multi-agency plan.

Despite the relatively small numbers of children on a GP's case load at one time who fulfil the strict criteria for failure to thrive there will be many others where there are concerns about weight gain or feeding behaviour. As a worker in primary care this is a condition one is likely to have to manage or give advice on relatively frequently. A study cited in the document 'When Feeding Fails' (2000) found that 64% of health visitors had children on their caseload whose weight was faltering.

As a GP, health visitor, or general paediatrician of a family in this situation you must feel sufficiently informed and capable of making a clinical judgement regarding which children should give concern, which need monitoring over time, and which are within normal limits and simply require reassurance. This chapter aims to provide you with these skills by discussing pointers in the history and examination, the relevance of investigations, and guidance as to who requires onward referral. It also aims to provide you with an action plan in those cases where eating difficulties are the main cause of the weight problem with information to give to the parents that they can start putting into practice immediately.

Defining failure to thrive

Failure to thrive implies both a failure to grow and a failure of emotional and developmental progress. It is usually used in reference to poor weight gain in a toddler or baby, although it may be used in connection with an older child, and may also refer to height. The term is sometimes considered pejorative and is being replaced by growth or weight 'faltering'.

When weight is seen to be crossing down centiles, a decision must be made as to whether there is indeed cause for concern. The child you are presented with may not in fact be failing to thrive. Many small babies are quite normal, and one in six infants cross down centiles in the first year.

Identification of those babies who are born relatively large and are now finding their genetically predetermined centiles involves an assessment of the baby's weight in relation to length and placement within the context of the family's stature (see Figure 11.2).

What causes failure to thrive?

For many years the belief was held that failure to thrive occurred as a result of abuse or neglect on the part of the care-givers. It is now gradually becoming accepted that a pattern of poor weight gain can emerge as a result of a variety of developmental and interactional factors between the child and its carer. For example, a minor illness in the child may lead to a short period of poor feeding. This is usual, and under normal circumstances resolves spontaneously. In some cases, particularly when coupled with increasing anxiety, a negative cycle can be established that leads to stressful mealtimes, an aversion to eating, and a reduction in the child's calorie intake.

The initial difficulty is commonly a period of poor health, unpleasant encounters with eating as a result of reflux, tube feeding or food allergy, or delay in acquisition of oromotor skills. Environmental or stress factors may include a rigid parenting style, attachment difficulties between the child and carer or a lack of a mealtime routine. Problems are often exacerbated or even caused by health professionals worrying unnecessarily about the child's growth pattern and inducing anxiety without being able to provide appropriate input.

The situation is often also compounded by the anxiety that there may be a serious medical cause for failure to thrive, and indeed failure to thrive used to be divided into 'organic' and 'non-organic' aetiologies. This separation is quite unhelpful as medical and non-organic factors may coexist, and it is better to try to view the picture as a whole. The interactional developmental model does not of course exclude abuse or neglect as a factor, and involvement of social services must be considered whenever their presence is suspected. It is also important not to forget that some medical conditions may be instrumental in causing weight to falter (see Table 11.1).

How to assess a child who is suspected of failing to thrive

Problems are often picked up at times of routine child health surveillance, when babies are weighed. Box 11.1 shows growth patterns that are of potential concern.

Table 11.1 Common conditions to identify from the history and examination

Inadequate intake

- Insufficient calories due to:
  - frequent infections and resultant poor appetite
  - unstructured life-style
  - low-fat, high-fibre 'healthy' diet
- Loss of calories due to vomiting or gastro-oesophageal reflux.
- If associated with oesophagitis, pain may lead to aversion to eating
- Delayed oromotor development (delayed biting and chewing skills) as the child is unable to manage the increasingly lumpy food that is offered
- Behavioural eating difficulties—food refusal, extreme fussiness or roaming around the house during the expected mealtime

Problems with absorption

- Intolerance of cow's milk protein or soya milk
- Coeliac disease

Metabolic problems

- Chronic disease, e.g. cystic fibrosis
- Congenital heart disease
- Most cases of congenital hypothyroidism are detected through neonatal screening

IUGR

- The birth history may reveal that the child was born with a low birthweight and may have reduced growth potential

Family history

- The family history and parental heights in particular, may indicate reduced growth potential. However one must bear in mind that the parents may be growth retarded themselves. Many ethnic minority groups show improved growth in subsequent generations.

The presence of a syndrome associated with poor growth maybe indicated by dysmorphic features or abnormal neurological development

- Neurodevelopmental delay
- Turners syndrome
- Foetal alcohol syndrome
- Prader–Willi

Box 11.1   Growth patterns that merit an assessment in primary care

- ◆ sustained fall through two centile spaces
- ◆ height or weight below second percentile
- ◆ a discrepancy of more than two centiles between height and weight.

When poor weight gain is identified, a holistic assessment of the child and their circumstances is required (see Box 11.2). Although 'medical' problems are uncommon as a cause, their exclusion by a doctor early on is important as it is difficult to provide effective input if there are lingering anxieties by either parents or professionals that there is a medical problem. The assessment must not end here, however, and must move to the positive identification of the often complex factors at play.

Box 11.2   Information to gather as part of a holistic assessment

- ◆ history (including dietary, developmental and social history)
- ◆ assessment of growth and full examination (including consideration of child's well-being)
- ◆ any relevant investigations
- ◆ additional information from health visitor, social worker, nursery/alternative carers
- ◆ a home visit
- ◆ observation of a feed or mealtime.

The history

Less than 5% of children who show faltering growth have an occult organic cause (Batchelor and Kerslake 1990). Reassuringly, most pathology can be identified from a thorough history. A study in the 1970s by Sills reviewed children admitted to hospital with failure to thrive. Of the 185 children, only 34 had an organic cause. Half of these were suspected as a result of the history alone, and the remainder were identified through support from physical findings. No diagnosis was made as a result of laboratory studies alone. This study provides an important message for those in primary care—a careful clinical evaluation will exclude a medical cause or will identify those requiring paediatric referral. Table 11.1 shows the common conditions that can be identified by history and examination.

2yr old. ④

FOOD DIARY

Time	THURSDAY 12-4-01 Day 1	FRIDAY 13-4-01 Day 2	SATURDAY 14-4-01 Day 3
6 am			
7 am			WEETABIX
8 am	WEETABIX + WATER	WEETABIX + WATER EATEN ALL	CUP OF WEAK TEA
9 am	WEAK TEA.	CUP OF MILK.	
10 am			
11 am			
12 (mid-day)	POACHED EGG +	BEANS + SAUASE EAT ALL	BEANS + SAUGE EAT ALL
1 pm	WEAK TEA	CUP OF MILK.	CUP OF WEAKTE
2 pm			
3 pm			
4 pm			
5 pm	PIE MASH + BEANS EATEN ALL	SAUASE MASH PEAS GRAVY	MASH BEANS SAUASE GRAVY
6 pm	WEAK TEA	MILK (CUP)	WEAK TEA (ALLSON
7 pm			
8 pm	HALF BAR WHITE CHOCOLATE	HALF BAR WHITE CHOCOLATE	
9 pm			BOTTLE MILK
10 pm	BOTTLE MILK	BOTTLE MILK	ALL GONE.
11 pm	DRANK ALL	DRANK ALL	
12 pm (midnight)			
1 am			
2 am			
3 am			
4 am			
5 am			

Fig. 11.1 A food diary: The diary readily shows that this toddler is only being offered food at main mealtimes and insufficient amounts. The parents can be encouraged for offering home-cooked foods but need to be advised to: (a) provide additional meals midmorning and after-noon; (b) to try larger portions; (c) to increase variety; and (d) to offer puddings and snacks. Advice can also be given regarding the weak tea; a common drink for young children in some communities but it contains few calories and reduces iron absorption.

Taking a dietary history

A dietary history establishes whether the caloric intake is sufficient for the age of the child. It does not take long and can provide information about mealtime routines as well as nutrient intake. The parent is usually asked to recall what the child has eaten the previous day. It is important not simply to ask about meals, as this will give an incomplete picture. Rather, use open questions such as—'Can you tell me everything that Chloe had to eat and drink yesterday and the times that she had them?'

Information can be gleaned about timing and frequency, whether the child is filling up on fluids to the detriment of the food intake, the structure of mealtimes, and what efforts have been made to encourage the child to eat.

It may be helpful to ask the family to keep a diet diary (usually 1–3 days). Figure 11.1 shows an example of a food diary kept by one of our parents.

Examination

A thorough examination should be completed at the first visit complementing the history. In particular care should be taken to obtain a current, accurate height and weight. Mid upper arm circumference is taken by some as being a useful measure of nutrition.

All values should be plotted on a growth chart, correcting for prematurity (babies born before 37 weeks gestation) up to the age of 12 months. Examples of different growth patterns are shown in Figures 11.2–11.4 (see pages 141–143).

Box 11.3   Guidance in weighing and measuring children

Weight

- <2 years should be weighed naked
- aged 2–5 years in their underwear
- >5 years in light clothing.

Length or height

- <2 years measure length using a measuring frame or mat
- <2 years using appropriate equipment.

Head circumference

- up to 2 years.

Mid upper arm circumference

- A normal value is >14 cm between the ages of 1 and 5 years.

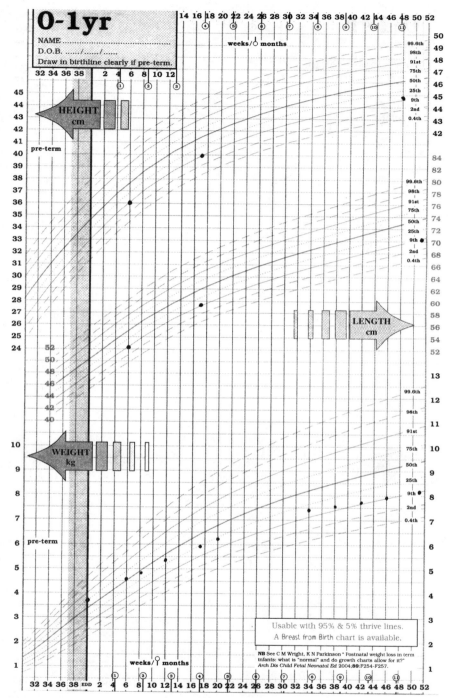

Fig. 11.2 Growth chart 1 – catch down growth.

This child was born with above average weight but below average stature – which is in keeping with the family pattern as both parents are small. Over the first year of life she finds her natural centile position, which is well matched with her length and head circumference. The catch down stops once her weight is established on the ninth centile, where she remains.

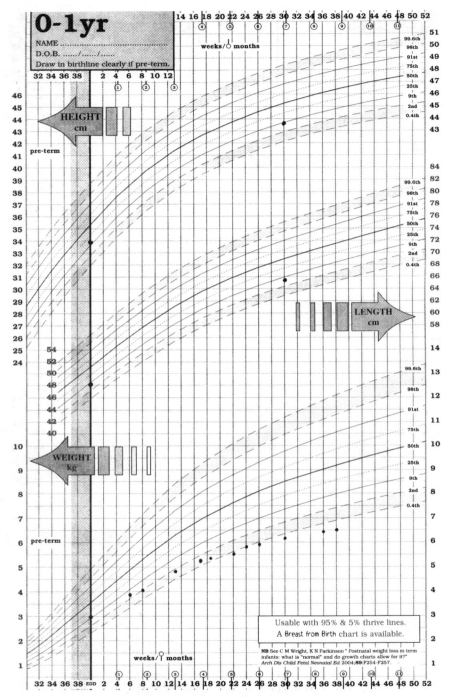

Fig. 11.3 Growth chart 2 – weight falling through the centiles.

This baby's weight starts to falter early on. By the age of eight weeks it has fallen a centile channel and continues to fall below the second centile. In this case a thorough primary care assessment should have taken place at four months looking particularly at his health and dietary intake. If no improvement was seen a paediatric referral should have taken place at that point rather than waiting until 38 weeks of age.

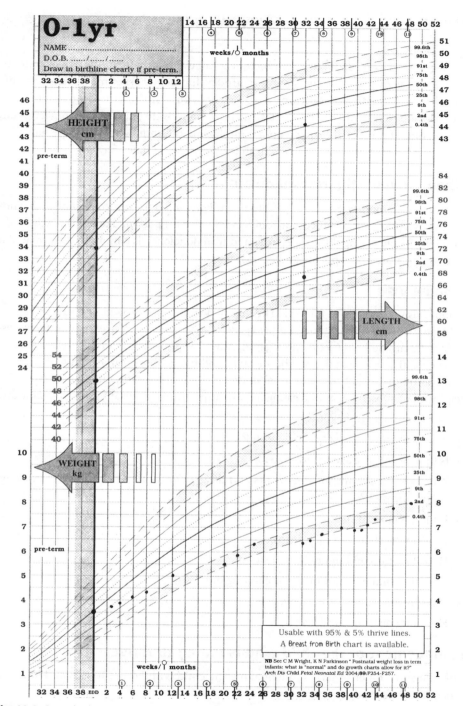

Fig. 11.4 Growth chart 3 – saw tooth pattern.

This boy's weight falters dramatically early in his life. It can be seen that as advice and support were offered to his mother there was an improvement in his weight gain. However, these improvements were not sustained when the level of support decreased. A referral to social services for further assessment of the domestic circumstances and more intensive support was made and a clear improvement in weight gain was seen after 40 weeks of age.

The physical examination should include a full evaluation of all the organ systems, including any dysmorphic signs and a neurodevelopmental assessment. This not only identifies any medical conditions that may account for the growth problems, but provides a baseline of the child's state of health and well-being. Note in particular, any wasting of the muscle bulk; a poor complexion and thin, wispy hair; the nature of the interaction between carer and child, and developmental milestones.

When are investigations indicated?

As previously emphasized, investigations are only required to confirm a clinical diagnosis. The exception is a blood count. Toddlers often have a poor intake of iron-rich foods, especially where eating difficulties exist and iron deficiency is common. If untreated it may compromise both appetite and development.

A home visit

A home visit is essential to fully evaluate the child with failing growth. It is usually carried out by the health visitor, although other agencies such as social services may also have visited the home and hold useful information. As well as providing an opportunity to gather general details regarding the family, life-style, and finances, it is important to include an observation of a mealtime—essential in understanding the difficulties and developing helpful input. Observing a child eating requires experience. Important features to note are:

- Who is present at the meal?
- How is the meal presented to the child?
- Is the portion size age appropriate?
- What are the seating arrangements and do they prevent the child from 'escaping' during the meal?
- Is there a table to sit at?
- How do the child and carer interact?
- How does the child respond to the food?
- Does the child have any biting or chewing difficulties?
- How are any difficulties managed?
- How long does the meal last?

Management of the child who is failing to thrive

There are a number of facets to managing the child with failure to thrive. These can broadly be described as:

- exclusion of a medical cause
- dietary input
- mealtime management
- other family issues.

First and foremost a medical cause must be excluded, as if there are lingering doubts about this it is hard to tackle the root problems. In general this can be done in primary care. Children merit a paediatric referral where there are symptoms or signs indicative of an organic problem such as diarrhoea, vomiting, pallor, persistent respiratory symptoms, dysmorphic signs, congenital abnormalities, or developmental delay. Where there are no concerns by professionals, but there is excessive parental concern, a paediatric opinion may be worthwhile to lay anxieties to rest.

A decision must then be made as to whether there is indeed cause for concern regarding the weight. As already described, many small babies are quite normal, and crossing down centiles can also be normal in the first year. An inability to decide if there is a problem can cause a great deal of harm. Too often in primary care, a baby is repetitively weighed over an extensive period without a full evaluation and appropriate input. Anxiety is generated, with an exacerbation of fruitless attempts to make the child eat. Mealtimes are turned into misery and the negative cycle is perpetuated. If this occurs it needs to be tackled.

What can be done in primary care?

Support and reassurance are cited by parents as one of the most important things a health professional can offer and many cases of faltering growth can be managed well within primary care.

Once a medical diagnosis has been excluded the aim of management is to increase the child's caloric intake and to make mealtimes an enjoyable experience for all. Simple advice can be given on how to increase the calorie density of foods offered and the mealtime set-up. More detailed advice may be offered by a paediatric dietician.

Increasing caloric intake

Some parents feel that 'a good square meal' is what their child needs and in some cases the child is suited to this. However, many children, and in particular those with small appetites and feeding difficulties, respond much better to the opportunity to 'graze'. This

---

Box 11.4   Practical tips for parents on how to increase their child's calorie intake

- High-calorie foods are important for growth in young children; e.g. use full fat milk, cheese, yoghurt, and butter. These can be added to mashed potato, pasta, etc.
- Some children fill up on drinks throughout the day. This can take the edge off their appetite, so offer food first.
- A number of children can find a dummy a comfort, but frequent daytime use can affect food intake and language development.
- If your child is slow at eating, gently encourage but never force-feed.

Box 11.5   Guidance for parents on how to encourage children's eating

- Help your child to become more involved in the feeding process by encouraging touching and playing with food, even if it is very messy.
- Offering meals and snacks frequently will help to stimulate the appetite.
- Start with food that is familiar to the child even if interest is only shown in a limited variety of foods.
- Some children have a small appetite. Offer a small portion of food to start with and if readily eaten, offer more.

---

may be offered as small meals or snacks on a regular basis throughout the day. As long as the calorie and nutrient requirement is met, this is a satisfactory way of approaching mealtimes, although some parents do feel uncomfortable with this advice initially. Protein is present in many foods (e.g. bread, chapattis, potatoes) and parents do not need to worry about it lacking in a diet of a child who eats in this fashion. Calories from fat should be encouraged as these foods are particularly energy dense. Parents should be reassured about the long-term effects of fat on health—these worries are not applicable in young children. If the diet appears to be low in iron, foods such as baked beans, fortified bread and cereals can be recommended if meat is not tolerated.

The most effective intervention is to tailor dietary advice to include food types that the family eats themselves.

Mealtime behaviour

Mealtimes should be an enjoyable and relaxed opportunity for the family to spend time together and the child learns much from the experience. Parents frequently report that

---

Box 11.6   Managing mealtimes

- Try to provide a relaxed, calm atmosphere at mealtimes.
- Encourage the family to eat together as children learn by example.
- Your child may show interest in what others are eating, allow them to share it.
- Limit mealtimes to 30 minutes and remove food without comment. Allowing mealtimes to go on for longer than is necessary rarely results in food being eaten.
- Ignore bad behaviour at mealtime by turning away from the child.
- Praise the child for eating.

Mealtimes should be fun!

their child eats better at friends or relatives and nursery, and certainly most do respond well to the social interaction they find around the table. Appropriate seating is one of the most effective pieces of advice given; once in a high chair a child will usually focus on the meal in front of him or her rather than slipping off a chair or the sofa and being able to wander away. In addition this limits the spread of the inevitable mess a child makes as he or she learns to self-feed and enjoy their food. Some parents do find the issue of mess a challenge and as a result the feeding process becomes controlled and tense and the child is prevented from taking that next, necessary developmental step.

Additional support

Referral routes for additional support include involving social services where there are social concerns or suspicion of neglect or abuse, speech therapy where there are oromotor problems or associated language delay, and a failure to thrive team in areas where they exist. The team will offer additional expertise in intransigent situations and generally include a paediatrician, specialist health visitor, speech therapist, dietician, and psychologist.

Often a referral to a nursery is helpful; it provides support to the carer and regular meals and a peer group to model normal eating behaviour for the child. As knowledge of the child and family grows, the staff become an additional source of information about any difficulties they may be experiencing.

What is the prognosis for an infant with failure to thrive?

Perhaps the most anxiety provoking aspect of having a baby who is failing to gain weight adequately is the concern that their growth and development will be irreversibly stunted. This anxiety is often fed into by health professionals, and parents not infrequently report that they have been told that their baby will be brain damaged if they do not get them to eat. In this circumstance it is hardly surprising that the eating experience becomes a major stressor for the family.

In fact research has shown that the outcomes are nowhere near as severe as previously thought. We carried out a systematic review (Rudolf 2002) on the long-term outcomes of failure to thrive and found that although children are likely to be somewhat thinner and shorter, their growth is unlikely to be outside the normal range by the age of 8. Perhaps more importantly, their IQ is not significantly lower than would be anticipated from their mother's scores.

Of course the poor weight gain shown by some babies is a marker for neurological dysfunction, and in others may reflect neglect or abuse, but the message should be that the majority of babies have a good prognosis. The art is to ensure that eating difficulties are addressed and resolved.

Our experience has led us to believe that the critical factors that contribute to a positive outcome include a thorough evaluation early on to exclude medical problems, and the explicit identification of health, family, and social factors that have contributed to the development of the problem. Too often much time is wasted through professionals simply monitoring the weight and not evaluating the situation fully. As a result the problems become more entrenched and harder to resolve. We have studied the outcomes of children from our own clinic and are pleased to see how well most do with little more than the management we have laid out in this chapter.

References

Batchelor J, Kerslake A (1990). *Failure to Find Failure to Thrive*. Whiting & Birch, London.

Rudolf MCJ (2002). The longterm outcome of failure to thrive: a systematic review. *Archives of Disease in Childhood* **86** (Suppl. 1): A30.

Sills RH (1978). Failure to thrive. the role of clinical and laboratory evaluation. *American Journal of Diseases of Children* **132**: 967–969.

Skuse D, Reilly S, Wolke D (1992). Failure to thrive: clinical and developmental aspects. In Remschmidt K, Schmidt MH (eds), *Developmental Psychopathology*. Hogrefe & Huber, Lewiston, NY, pp. 46–71.

Underdown A (2000). *When Feeding Fails*. The Children's Society, London.

Recommended reading

Recommendations for Best Practice for Weight and Growth Faltering in Young Children. http://www.the-childrens-society.org.uk/media/pdf/info/Best_Practice_For_Weight_And_Growth_Faltering_In_Young_Children.pdf

Underdown A (2000). *When Feeding Fails*. The Children's Society, London.

Chapter 12

Childhood nutrition for primary care

Justine Dempsey

This chapter will look at infant nutrition covering the areas of breast feeding, infant formula, weaning, and look at some of the issues and controversies surrounding these areas. It will also address two of the increasingly common nutritional challenges being faced by health professionals in the community today, iron deficiency anaemia and rickets.

Childhood nutrition

Nutrition has a key role in childhood growth and development and the impacts on health continue through to adulthood. The energy requirements of children are three to four times higher per kilogramme body weight than adults, due to their rapid growth and development especially during infancy.

Breast feeding is the best form of nutrition for the infant. In 2001 the World Health Organization (WHO) issued a global public health recommendation that all infants should be exclusively breastfed for the first 6 months of life to achieve optimum growth, development, and health and that this should continue after the introduction of solids, up until the age of 2 years (WHO Fifty-fourth World Health Assembly 2001). The Scientific Advisory Committee on Nutrition (SACN) 2001 (the government body that replaced the now disbanded COMA (Committee on Medical Aspects of Food Policy) also supported these recommendations.

The WHO recommendations were based on a systematic review of literature from around the world. It concluded that there were benefits of exclusive breast feeding in developing countries e.g. reduction in gastrointestinal and infectious disease.

These recommendations were based on a global population, therefore it is important to remember that each individual's circumstances should be taken into consideration. Parents should be given enough information to make an informed decision. The mothers who choose not to, or the few mothers who cannot breast feed, should be supported in their decision.

The Department of Health then issued a statement in 2003 to support exclusive breast feeding for the first 6 months of life. It stated that breast feeding is the best form of nutrition for infants and can provide complete nutrition for the first 6 months as it provides all the nutrients a baby needs. Although there are conflicting reports in the literature of deficiency of iron and vitamin D when the infant is exclusively breastfed for a prolonged period.

The 2000 Infant Feeding Survey was based on a sample of nearly 9500 mothers of babies born in the U.K. during the year 2000. It reported that 69% of mother's breastfed at birth, but this amount gradually reduced. By the time the infants reached the age of 6 months only 21% of babies were breastfed. In Scotland significant improvements in breast feeding prevalence were seen from the previous infant feeding survey (1995) in all ages up to 8 months. The reasons for cessation of breast feeding varied. In the early weeks baby rejecting the breast, painful nipples were cited as reasons. For mothers who continued for at least a week but gave up by 4 months, insufficient milk was the most important factor. In later months returning to work was the major reason for mothers reducing breast feeding.

Breast feeding also has benefits for the mother as it promotes uterine involution, can delay ovulation and may help the mother to return to her pre-pregnancy weight more quickly.

Mothers should be encouraged to breast feed and given information on the benefits of breast feeding. It should be explained that breast feeding even for a short period of time can be protective for the infant and that this persists beyond the period of breast feeding itself. Studies have reported that breast-feeding exclusively for the first 15 weeks is associated with a significant reduction in respiratory illness during the first 7 years of life (Wilson *et al.* 1998). Other benefits include:

- breast milk contains sufficient energy, protein and nutrients for all the baby's needs
- there is no need to carry around bottles, powdered milk, and sterilizing equipment
- breast feeding and delaying the introduction of solids have beneficial effects on childhood health and subsequent disease.
- Breastmilk is supplied at the right temperature
- breast feeding can also protect against gastrointestinal illness that can confer benefits beyond the initial period of breast feeding
- it can help bonding between the mother and child.

Mothers need to be aware that their own nutritional requirements for certain vitamins and minerals, i.e. vitamin D and calcium increase during lactation. Mothers who are breast feeding need appropriate nutritional advice to ensure that breast milk provides the best nutrition for their babies.

Nutritional content of breast milk

Breast milk has a unique composition and the baby readily absorbs the nutrients, as they are present in a bioavailable form and due to the enzymes present in breast milk.

The breast milk produced for the first few days after birth is called colostrum. It has a lower fat and higher protein content than mature breast milk and is rich in vitamins and minerals growth factor and hormones. The nutritional composition of breast milk varies during a feed and it is also influenced by the stage of lactation. As the breast is emptied the fat content of breast milk increases, which is well absorbed due to its unique structure. This is beneficial for the infant as it means that there are lower levels of free fatty acids in the gut to bind to dietary calcium, and hence there is an efficient absorption of calcium. The amount and variety of fatty acids in breast milk are dependent on the mother's diet. Fat provides more than 50% of the infants total daily energy requirements. Breast milk contains the essential fatty acids, linoleic and linolenic acid and the long chain polyunsaturated fatty acids (LCPUFA) arachidonic acid and docosahexanoic acid. These are important in important in eye and brain development.

Breast milk contains two forms of protein, whey and casein in a ratio of whey to casein of 60% to 40%. The protein is easily digestible and provides an essential source of amino acids for the infant's growth.

Breast milk has a low iron content, but the presence of lactoferrin, an iron-binding protein means the absorption of iron from breast milk is high. The presence of lactoferrin also helps to control the level of intestinal bacteria levels present in colostrum and mature breast milk.

The main carbohydrate source in breast milk is lactose and provides approximately 40% of the energy content. Lactose enhances the absorption of calcium and magnesium. Breast milk also contains Oligosaccharides, which have a prebiotic effect. They are non-digestible carbohydrates and remain in the colon to provide food for beneficial bacteria, e.g. bifidobacteria.

Breast milk also has a lower calcium and phosphate content than cow's milk. The ratio is perfect for maximum calcium absorption and good bone mineralization.

Breast milk also includes nucleotides, these are the building blocks of RNA and DNA which can help to increase the baby's immune response. Women need to be given appropriate information from health professionals and educated about the benefits of breast feeding. In order for the rates of breast feeding to increase, public attitude towards breast feeding needs to change. Women who decide to breast feed need practical advice and support from health professionals, family, and friends to succeed.

Infant formula

If a mother decides not to or is unable to breast feed an infant formula must be used throughout the first year of life. Although breast milk is the best source of nutrition for babies, there are a wide range of infant formula available on the market and this can be confusing for parents. Infant formula can be used from birth, if the mother chooses not to or in rare cases cannot breast feed. There is evidence to suggest that introduction of infant formula instead of breast milk may lead to nutrition-related problems in later childhood and adult life, i.e. increased incidence of asthma, increased systolic blood pressure, and increased gastrointestinal infection.

Composition of infant formulas

Infant formulas can be broadly divided into two categories:

- whey dominant formula: these are more similar in composition to breast milk, with a whey to casein protein ratio of 60:40

- ◆ casein dominant formula: These are more similar to cow's milk in composition with whey–casein protein ratio of 20:80.

The energy content of formula milk is comparable with that of breast milk. Infant formula can provide a sole source of nutrition for the infant for the first 4–6 months of life and should be used throughout the first year of life. The vitamins and minerals are present in higher amounts in formula milk than breast milk. This is to try to compensate for the fact that the absorption rate is less than from breast milk.

Vitamins, minerals, and trace elements are added into the formulas and they comply with the Infant Formula and Follow-on Formula Regulations 1995.

Long chain polyunsaturated fatty acids occur naturally in breast milk and some manufacturers are now adding these into their formulas. They accumulate in the brain and central nervous system and are important in the development of neural cells.

Nucleotides are also added into some manufacturers' formulas.

Follow-on formula can be used from the age of 6 months (in the UK) and up to the age of 2 years as part of the diet. They are generally higher in protein, vitamin D, and iron than infant formula. It is not necessary to change to a follow-on formula at the age of 6 months; however, these can be useful in the child who is a picky eater or vegetarians and those whose diet may be deficient in vitamins and minerals.

Future development of infant formulas

A paper by the ESPGHAN committee on Nutrition entitled Prebiotic Oligosaccharides in Dietetic Products for Infants examined the evidence for adding prebiotic oligosaccharides into dietetic products (Agostoni et al. 2004). It was concluded that addition of prebiotics in infant and follow-on formula has potential to increase the number of bifidobacteria in faeces and soften stools. There is no published evidence of clinical benefits of adding prebiotic oligosaccharides to dietetic products for infants. It concluded that this is an area that will need further research and evaluation.

Other infant formula

If there are concerns that a child may have cow's milk protein intolerance or allergy, this should be discussed with the child's general practitioner. This may necessitate changing to a alternative formula. This chapter does not deal with food allergy.

Soya formula

In March 2003 The Committee on Toxicity of chemicals in Food, Consumer Products and the environment (COT), published a report on phytooestrogens and health. This report included a response from SACN on the use of soya formula. They advised that soya-based formula should only be fed to infants when there is a clinical need. They also stated that mothers who had been advised by their doctor or health professionals to use soya formula for their infants should continue.

The advice was issued due to the findings of two research studies. One study looked at the significant prolonged and painful duration of menstruation in women who had been fed Soya formula as infants (Strom et al. 2001). The other study looked at the suppression of testosterone rise in neonatal marmosets partially fed soya formula (Sharpe *et al.* 2002). The British Dietetic Association Paediatric Group produced a position statement based on available evidence. They recommended as a precautionary measure that the use of soya-based formula, as first-line treatment for cow's milk allergy should be discouraged in the first 6 months of age. Although it was acknowledged that there might be several groups, where soya formula is the only option available, e.g. infants who refuse extensively hydrolysed formula despite perseverance (in cases of cow's milk allergy or intolerance), vegan mothers who cannot, or who do not want to breast feed. There needs to be further research into this area to clarify this issue for the future.

Other mammalian milks such as cow's, goat's, sheep's, and ewe's milk should not be used for the child under the age of 1 year as a main drink. They will not be nutritionally adequate for the infant. These milks could be given to the older child, i.e. over the age of 1 year, if care is taken that that other sources of iron, vitamin A and D are in the diet, or given as a supplement if the diet is of concern. After the age of 1 year, full cream cow's milk can be introduced into the diet as a drink. It can be used in cooking from the age of 6 months.

Semi-skimmed milk can be used from the age of 2 years and fully skimmed milk from the age of 5 years. The use of these milks for children under these ages could decrease the energy content of the diet significantly and impact on their weight gain. These milks will also have a lower content of fat-soluble vitamins.

Weaning

Weaning is the introduction of semi-solid foods into the diet, while continuing to breast feed or use formula milk. The age of introduction of solids has been a matter of debate. The Department of Health COMA Weaning and the Weaning Diet Report 45 (1994) states that introduction of solid foods should occur between the ages of 4–6 months. This report has not yet been updated in light of the new guidance from the WHO and SACN recommending exclusive breast feeding until the age of 6 months, as previously mentioned in this chapter. SACN has replaced the now disbanded COMA and one of the key roles should be the production of updated weaning advice to provide clear guidance for health professionals.

When to wean?

The 2000 Infant feeding survey found that by the age of 3 months 24% of mothers had introduced solid foods. By the age of 4 months 85% of babies had been introduced to solids. By the age of 6 months nearly all of the 9500, babies in the survey were introduced to solids.

Why are solids introduced before the age of 4 months? Reasons given in the survey were advice from family and friends, and parental opinion that they felt that the time was right for their baby.

Early introduction of solids can lead to increased weight, increased percentage body fat, and increased risk of wheezing in childhood (Wilson *et al.* 1998). Late introduction of solids can lead to feeding problems, texture phobic children, and possible undernutrition. It could be argued that in terms of infant health it maybe better to encourage more mothers to breast feed, if only for a few weeks and to discourage solid foods before the age of 4 months than by recommending exclusive breast feeding for 6 months (Fewtrell *et al.* 2003). Another issue for debate is whether the exclusive breastfed infant has different requirements on weaning, compared with the infant who has been fed on infant formula or mixed feeding as their oral experiences will be very different. Should weaning advice differ for infants in whom solids are not introduced until the age of 6 months? Should the progression on to different textured foods be faster? What is the most appropriate age for the introduction of solids? These areas need further research to develop answers to these questions.

Stages of weaning

Weaning should begin with smooth puree textures. The use of foods such as non-wheat cereals, fruit, and vegetable purees are suitable first foods. The textures and variety of solids can be gradually increased over the first 12 months. Food consistency should progress from smooth puree to mashed/minced and to chopped foods. It is important to introduce lumpy foods during age 6–9 months. Failure to introduce lumps at this stage can be associated with faddy eaters at a later stage. Infants need to learn to chew and this can be more difficult if left to a later age to introduce lumpy solids the window of opportunity can be lost.

During the first stages of weaning, breast or infant formula milk will provide the main source of nutrition. The aim is to get the infant used to the feeling of the spoon in the mouth. As weaning progresses and the quantity and variety of solids increase, the milk intake should decrease. By the age of 1 year, the diet should be mixed and varied and the child should be taking three meals a day with two to three snacks.

Each child will progress at its own rate and advice should be tailored to the individual.

A useful resource for the health professional to use when advising parents is the DOH Report 45 Weaning and the Weaning Diet (1994). However, this report has not yet been updated in light of the new weaning advice on the age of introduction of solids into the infant's diet.

Rickets

Nutritional rickets in infancy and childhood is caused by a severe and prolonged deficiency. It can also occur as a result of calcium deficiency (De Lucia MC et al 2003) vitamin D. It causes osteomalacia (soft bones) in older children and adults and rickets in infant and children. Clinical symptoms of rickets can be rickets rosary, muscle weakness, swelling of wrists, bowed legs, and skeletal pain. The main source of vitamin D is from synthesis in the skin in the presence of ultraviolet light. It is converted to an active metabolite, which stimulates the absorption of calcium by the gut and promotes mineralization of the bone. The population groups most at risk of vitamin D deficiency are ethnic groups with dark skin pigmentation and inadequate exposure to sunlight, e.g. groups wearing concealing clothing for religious or cultural reasons. These groups may form less vitamin D via synthesis in the skin. Individuals with darker skin pigmentation can synthesize vitamin D but need longer and more frequent exposure to sunlight because the darker skin pigment can block some of the suns active rays. The amount of vitamin D synthesized also depends on the location we live from the equator. Cloudy skies and pollution can be another factor affecting the amount of sunlight reaching the skin.

Dietary sources are limited, there are small amounts in fatty fish, liver, milk, and eggs, and these are main dietary sources. Foods such as margarines, breakfast cereals, and bread are fortified with added vitamin D. It can be difficult for the diets of young children to be sufficient in vitamin D.

Careful consideration will need to be given to infants following restricted diets, e.g. vegetarian, vegan diets as these can be lacking in essential vitamins and minerals, including vitamin D. The literature shows there can be a significant association between iron deficiency anaemia and poor vitamin D status in children aged 1–2 years in the Asian population (Lawson *et al.* 1998). One study looking at 65 children presenting to four London hospitals with hypocalcaemia and rickets from 1996 to 2001 found they were mostly from black or Asian ethnic groups (Ladhani *et al.* 2004) Of the group 29 had hypocalcaemic symptoms, 17 of these no radiological evidence of rickets. The remaining 48 children had radiological evidence of rickets with or without clinical symptoms. The signs and symptoms reverted to normal with vitamin D supplementation. Studies also show incidences of severe rickets in breast fed Afro-Caribbean children in whom weaning has been unsuccessful and in whom none of the mothers or children had taken vitamin supplements (Hannam *et al.* 2004).

Supplementation of vitamin D should start in pregnancy, especially in at-risk groups to maximize foetal stores.

Table 12.1, from COMA Report 41, shows the daily recommendations for vitamin D intake.

The serum vitamin D concentration of the infant when born, is directly related to maternal vitamin D status. Infants born to mothers that are vitamin D deficient will

Table 12.1 Dietary reference values for vitamin D (μg/day)

Age	Reference nutrient intake
0–3 months	8.5
4–6 months	8.5
7–9 months	7
10–12 months	7
1–3 years	7
4–6 years	0
7–10 years	0
11–14 years	0
15–18 years	0
Pregnancy	10
Lactation	
0–4 months	10
4+ months	10

Table 12.2 Vitamin D content of milks

Vitamin D content of milks	Vitamin D μg content per 100ml
Infant formula	1.0–1.6
Breast milk	0.01
Cows milk	0.02
Follow on formula	1.1–1.9

themselves be deficient in stores of vitamin D, supplementation will need to be given to correct any deficiency. It is important that foetal stores are optimized by supplementation of at risk mothers. Breast feeding mothers should take a supplement of 10 μg (400 IU) a day of vitamin D. Breast milk is low in vitamin D and breast-fed infants will need additional supplementation. Breast milk of mothers who are vitamin D deficient will contain even lower levels of vitamin D than in normal breast milk. The supplement could be started from the age of 1 month if there is concern about the mother's vitamin D status during pregnancy. There are reports in the literature of infants that have been exclusively breastfed for prolonged periods without vitamin D supplementation becoming vitamin D deficient (Mughal *et al.* 1999). Health professionals will be key in deciding at what age to begin supplementation for individuals.

Infant formula milks are fortified with vitamin D and an intake of 500 ml a day of infant formula will provide the infants vitamin D requirements with no need for any additional supplementation. Cow's milk is a poor source of vitamin D and should not be used in a drink for children under the age of 1 year, although it can be used in cooking from the age of 6 months. Other mammalian milks and milks such as rice, oat milk, etc. should not be used as a drink in children under the age of 1 year they are not nutritionally adequate. Vitamin D intake also declines during weaning onto solids as weaning foods can be very low in vitamin D.

Vitamin D content of milks are shown in Table 12.2.

Rickets had previously been eradicated with the introduction of the welfare food scheme, which had provided cheaply available vitamin drops for families (see Table 12.3). There have been problems with the supply of the welfare scheme drops and now it looks as if they will be withdrawn. An alternative product should be used; local policy should be produced so that consistent information is given to parents.

Table 12.3 Welfare Food Scheme Vitamin drops contents

Vitamin A (retinol equivalents)	200 μg
Vitamin C	20 mg
Vitamin D3	7 μg

The COMA Reports 41 and 45 previously referred to specific recommendations for vitamin D supplementation of pregnant and lactating women, infants, and young children. These are not being followed, the consequence is that we can now see an increasing incidence of rickets in this country.

The recommendations are summarized as:

1. Expectant mothers from at risk groups should be supplemented with vitamin D 10 µg (400 IU) a day from 12 weeks of pregnancy.

2. Breast feeding mothers should continue with vitamin D supplements 10 µg (400 IU) a day if the mother is from an at-risk group.

3. All infants should receive vitamin A and D supplements except those receiving at least 500 ml of infant formula milk as this is fortified with vitamin A and D.

4. Vitamin D supplementation of breastfed infants can be delayed until the age of 6 months if the mother is in good vitamin status during pregnancy.

5. Where there is concern about the vitamin status of the mother during pregnancy the breastfed infant should be given vitamin drops from the age of 1 month.

6. Vitamin supplementation should be continued throughout the first 5 years of life for those infants at risk of vitamin deficiency, who have dark skin pigmentation and in whom there are concerns about the diet, i.e. faddy eaters, restrictive or exclusion diets or are born with poor vitamin stores.

The awareness of the need and importance of vitamin D supplementation needs to be raised to prevent the occurrence of rickets Education programmes targeting pregnant women need to be put in place.

All health professionals involved in the care of these women should be aware of the recommendations in the COMA 1994 Report and this advice should be readily available to mothers, pregnant, or lactating women.

Iron deficiency anaemia in childhood

The WHO definition of iron deficiency anaemia is haemoglobin of <110 g per litre for children age 1–2 and <112 g/l in children aged 3–5 years (WHO 1992). Iron deficiency anaemia is one of the commonest nutritional deficiencies in the UK. It is often seen in pre-school children, Asian children living in Britain (Lawson *et al.* 1998) and deprived inner city areas (Daly *et al.* 1996; Childs *et al.* 1997).

The main cause of iron deficiency anaemia is dietary, due to poor dietary intake, faddy eating or restrictive diets, although there are other causes. Symptoms can include tiredness, lethargy, reduced physical activity, susceptibility to infections, and delayed psychomotor development (Booth and Auckett 1997).

There is contradictory evidence in the literature as to whether any delay in psychomotor development is reversible (Morley *et al.* 1999). These symptoms of iron deficiency anaemia in themselves can cause a decreased dietary intake, further compounding the problem.

Infants

The majority of an infant's iron store is laid down during the third trimester of pregnancy. Preterm infants have lower iron stores at birth and increased requirements due to their faster rate of growth. The specific needs of preterm infants will not be addressed in this chapter but a comprehensive review and recommendations of preterm requirements has been written by Tsang *et al.* (1993). The term infant has adequate iron stores for the first 6 months of life. Breast milk has a relatively low iron content; however, the iron is present in a readily bioavailable form called lactoferrin and this is well absorbed. After the infant is 6 months of age, breast milk alone does not have sufficient amounts of iron to keep up with the infants increasing requirements. Iron must be provided by other dietary sources during weaning or additional supplementation at this stage (Pizarro *et al.* 1991). Between the age of 4–6 months and 10–12 months iron requirements double. This is a period of rapid growth and an increased intake of iron is needed to maintain the infant's haemoglobin concentration.

Table 12.4 from COMA report 41 shows dietary reference values for iron.

Infant formulas are fortified with iron, although absorption of iron from formula milk is not as efficient as from breast milk (Booth and Auckett 1997). It is not clear what the absorption rate of iron from formula milk is. To try to compensate for this, iron and other vitamins and minerals are present in higher amounts in formula milk than breast milk.

Follow-on formulas are available on the market and can be used in infants aged 6 months and onwards in the UK. These contain higher levels of iron than standard infant formula. They can be particularly useful in the child who is a picky eater, as a daily intake of approximately 500 ml of follow-on formula milk can provide all of the infants daily iron requirements. It can be useful to continue the use of follow-on formula in children where dietary intake may be of concern (Daly *et al.* 1996).

Table 12.4 Dietary reference values for iron

Age	Iron (μg)
0–3 months	1.7
4–6 months	4.3
7–9 months	7.8
10–12 months	7.8
1–3 years	6.9
4–6 years	6.1
7–10 years	8.7
11–14 years (males)	11.3
11–14 years (females)	14.8
15–18 years (males)	11.3
15–18 years (females)	14.8

Full cream cow's milk can be introduced as main milk drink after the age of 12 months.

Cow's milk is a poor source of iron it contains only 0.05 mg iron per 100 ml compared with follow-on formula, which contains approximately 1.2 mg iron per 100 ml (see Table 12.5).

The calcium and phosphoprotein compounds present in cow's milk, bind to dietary iron and prevents it from being fully absorbed. Early introduction of cow's milk as a main drink before the age of 1 year and large intakes of cow's milk have been linked with development of iron deficiency anaemia. In some cultures there is an emphasis on milk as a staple food, which may be offered in the place of meals. In some families milk consumption is encouraged by adding rusk, baby rice, or sugar to feeding bottles (Lawson et al. 1998). This is something that needs to be discouraged and the reasoning behind limiting cow's milk consumption needs to be explained to families. The prolonged use of bottle-feeding can encourage excessive milk intake. Children should be introduced to a beaker from the age of 6 months and encouraged to drink from a cup by age 12 months to try and reduce their consumption of milk. Some children derive a large amount of their daily calorie intake from milk or squash and therefore have a limited appetite for solid foods. It is common in this group to see children with a bottle that seems to be almost permanently in their hands or mouths. These children are at high risk of iron deficiency anaemia.

Table 12.5 Iron content of milks

Milks	Iron content mg per 100 ml
Breast milk	0.076
Infant formula	0.5–0.8
Follow-on formula	1.2–1.3

Dietary sources

Most foods used during the early weaning period (4–6 months) are generally poor sources of iron, e.g. baby rice, most fruit and vegetables. Weaning is an area that may need to be looked at in light of the Department of Health recommendations promoting weaning from the age of 6 months. More research will need to be done into the age of introduction of solids and the age of introduction of iron-rich solids into infant's diets. Does weaning advice need to be reviewed and iron-rich foods need to be offered sooner in the initial stages of weaning? As we know that the term infant is only born with enough iron stores for the first 6 months of life. It may be necessary to review the weaning literature available to health professionals in light of the new recommendations.

Dietary sources rich in iron include; liver, meat, beans, nuts, dried fruits, poultry, fish, whole grains or enriched cereals, millet and soy bean flour, and most dark green leafy vegetables.

Table 12.6 (page 160) includes the iron content of common foods. The amount of iron absorbed from the diet can vary widely.

Iron is present in the diet in the form of haem and non-haem sources. Haem iron is present in foods such as meat, fish, and poultry. Non-haem iron is derived from plant

Table 12.6 Iron contents of foods

Portion size (g) of foods	Iron content (mg)
Liver 30 g	3–4 mg
Mince beef (stewed) 40 g Lamb mince (stewed) 50 g	1 mg
Chicken (roasted) 100 g	1 mg
1 sausage 50–60 g	1 mg
Brown bread/wholemeal 50 g	1 mg
Fortified breakfast cereal 30 g	2 mg
Sardines/pilchards 100 g	2 mg
Figs 30 g/raisins 25 g/prunes 50 mg/currants100g/sultanas 50 g	1 mg
Spring greens 50 g/spinach 60 g/ broccoli 100 g/peas 60 g/mung beans 70 g/green or brown lentils 30 g/red lentils 50 g/chick peas 50 g/baked beans 80 g	1 mg

sources, e.g. fortified cereals, whole grains, or nuts. Non-haem iron is not as well absorbed from the diet; therefore special care should be taken when advising families who are vegetarian. Vitamin C can help to increase the absorption of iron from non-haem sources. It is present in some fruit, fruit juices, and vegetables. Families should be advised to try to include a source of vitamin C at mealtimes, as well as iron rich foods.

Iron absorption can be inhibited by phytates (present in cereal products), calcium phosphoproteins (present in milk and dairy products), and tannin (present in tea).

Dietary advice around the time of weaning is very important in preventing iron deficiency anaemia. Advice should be given on including good sources of meat, fish, poultry, lentils, and beans.

However, it can be very difficult to advise ways to increase iron intake in the 'picky eater'. It may be useful to suggest three small meals with snacks in between. It may be useful to advise the use of a follow-on milk formula in this group, as 500 ml a day can provide the child's daily iron requirement. Follow-on formula may be also be useful in young vegetarian children who have a poor intake of iron.

Diets of toddlers can be low in iron. The intake of foods low in dietary iron, dislike of chewing foods and excessive milk intake can all contribute to iron deficiency anaemia.

Summary of key points for dietary education

- Dietary iron must be available from 6 months of age.
- The main drink for infants under the age of 12 months should be breast milk or infant formula milk.
- Cow's milk as a main drink under the age of 1 year should be actively discouraged. It may be used in food preparation from the age of 6 months.

- Follow-on formula milks are fortified with higher amounts of iron. They should continue to be used after the age of 12 months if there are particular concerns about the diet.

- Limit full cream cow's milk to 1 pint a day in infants and approximately 350 ml a day in the toddler.

- Encourage use of cup feeding from age 12 months as this may help to limit milk intake.

- Advice should be given on including good dietary sources of iron; fortified cereals, red meat, poultry, fish, whole grains, beans, nuts (whole nuts not under the age of 3 years), green leafy vegetables.

- Tea should be avoided at mealtimes as tannin a compound found in tea decreases iron absorption.

- Include a source of vitamin C and iron at each meal, especially in families who are vegetarian.

To be effective, dietary advice should be tailored to the individual and their dietary/cultural beliefs. Dietary re-education of the whole family must take place. The advice given will need to be followed by all members of the family and all child carers in order for it to be effective. Appropriate resources should be available so that the family can have written information to refer to and this information must contain foods that are familiar to the individual. Review of the child's diet is necessary to ensure that any initial advice has been understood and acted upon.

Community strategies need to be put in place, aimed at primary prevention to prevent the increasing incidence of these preventable conditions. Health professionals must be provided with appropriate training in these areas so they can educate families. It will take combined efforts of health professionals and community-based education programmes to try and reduce the incidence of these condition.

References

Agostoni C, Axelsson I, Goulet O et al (2004). Prebiotic oligosaccharides in dietetic products for infants. A Commentary by the ESPGHAN Committee on Nutrition. *Journal of Paediatric Gastroenterology and Nutrition*. Vol 39 No 5. Nov 2004.

Booth IW, Aukett MA (1997). Iron deficiency anaemia in infancy and early childhood. *Archives of Disease in Childhood* **76**: 549–554.

British Dietetic Association Paediatric Group (2003, June). Position Statement on use of soya protein for infants.

Childs F, Aukett MA, Darbyshire P, Ilett S, and Livera LN (1997). Dietary education and iron Deficiency Anaemia in an inner city *Archives of Disease in Childhood* **76**: 144–147.

Committee on Toxicity of Chemicals in Food, Consumer Products and the Environment. Report on Phytoestrogens and Health Tox/2003/03.

Daly A, MacDonald A, Aukett A et al (1996). Prevention of Anaemia in inner city toddlers by an iron supplemented cows milk formula. *Archives of Disease in Childhood* **75**: 9–16.

Department of Health (1991). COMA report on dietary reference values for food energy and nutrients for the United Kingdom. Report on Health and Social Subjects, 41, London HMSO.

Department of Health (1994). COMA report on weaning and the weaning diet. Report on Health and Social Subjects No. 45. HMSO, London.

De Lucia MC, Munick ME, Carpenter TO. Nutritional Rickets with normal circulating 25-hydroxyvitamin D: a call for re-examining the role of dietary calcium intake in North American infants. *Journal of Clinical Endocrinology and Metabolism 2003* **88:** 3539–45.

Fewtrell M S, Lucas A, Morgan JB (2003). Factors associated with weaning in full term and pre term infants. *Archives of Disease in Childhood Fetal and Neonatal Edition* **88F:** 296–301.

Hannam S, Lee S, Sellars M (2004). Severe vitamin D deficient rickets in black Afro Carribean children *Archives of Disease in Childhood* **89:** 91–92.

Hamlyn B, Brooker S, Oleinikova K. *Infant Feeding 2000.* The stationery office 2002 pp 1–232.

Ladhani S, Srinivasan L, Buchanan C, Allgrove J (2004) Presentation of vitamin D deficiency. *Archives of Diseases in Childhood* **89**: 781–784.

Lawson MS, Thomas M, Hadiman A (1998). Iron status of Asian children aged 2 years living in England. *Archives of Disease in Childhood* **78:** 420–426.

Morley R, Abbott R, Fairweather-Tait S, MacFadyn U, Stephenson T, and Lucas A (1999). Iron fortified follow on formula from 9–18 months improves iron status but not development or growth: a randomised trial. *Archives of Disease in Childhood 1999* **81:** 247–252.

Mughal MZ, Salam H, Greenaway T (1999). Florid rickets associated with prolonged breastfeeding without vitamin D supplementation. *British Medical Journal* **318:** 39–40.

Pizarro F, Yip R, Dallman PR (1991). Iron status with different feeding regimens: relevance to screening and prevention of iron deficiency anaemia. *The Journal of Pediatrics 1991* Vol 118 No 5, 687–691.

Sharpe RM, Marin B, Morris K, Greig I, McKinnell C, McNeilly AS, and Walker M (2002). Infant feeding with soy formula milk: effect on testis and the blood testosterone levels in marmoset monkeys during the period of neonatal testicular activity. *Human Reproduction* **17:** 1692–1703.

Strom BL, Schinner R, Zeigler EE (2001). Exposure to soy based formula in infancy and endocrinological and reproductive outcomes in young adulthood. *JAMA* **286:** 807–814.

Tsang RC, Lucas A Vauy R (1993). *Nutritional Needs of the Pre-term Infant. Scientific basis and practical guidelines.* Calclueus Medical Publishers, New York.

Wilson A, Forsyth F, Greene S, Irvine L, Hau C, and Howe PW (1998). Relation of infant diet to childhood health. *British Medical Journal* **316:** 21–25.

World Health Organization (1992). *Nutritional Anaemias.* WHO Technical Report Series No. 503. WHO, Geneva, p. 972.

World Health Organization (2001). Fifty Four World Health Assembly WHA 54.2 Agenda Item 13.1 *Infant and Young Child Nutrition.* WHO, Geneva.

World Health Organization (2002) *Infant and Young Child Nutrition. Global strategy on infant feeding and young child feeding.* Fifty-fifth World Health Assembly A55/15, 16 April. WHO, Geneva.

Chapter 13

Paediatric cardiology for the primary care physician

Rodney Franklin and Zdenek Slavik

Introduction

Over 90% of cardiac pathology in the paediatric population in the developed world is congenital in origin, in that it is present at birth, even if undetected until older; in contrast, adult heart disease is largely classified as being acquired. In less developed countries, rheumatic fever is still prevalent. This chapter focuses on the role of the primary care physician in the diagnosis and management of congenital heart disease (CHD). It will also consider the commonly encountered problems in primary care which may be attributed to a cardiac abnormality but which are often benign and associated with a normal heart, such as innocent murmurs.

Congenital heart disease

Important general facts concerning CHD are:

1. The incidence of CHD is 6–8 per thousand live births (≈1 in 130–145 live births in the UK), while at 20 weeks gestation this figure is five to 10 times higher, due to associated lethal chromosomal abnormalities. Approximately 25% of congenital heart lesions can be considered complex and one third will require intervention during infancy. These figures do not include the presence of a bicuspid, non-stenotic aortic valve (2%), mitral valve prolapse (3–4%) or the association of a patent arterial duct in those born prematurely. The incidence of the various lesions is detailed in Table 13.1.

2. CHD is the most common congenital malformation, accounting for 10% of infant deaths and 50% of deaths due to a congenital malformation. One-quarter of those with CHD may have other congenital abnormalities (Peterson *et al.* 2003).

3. The diagnosis of CHD can be confirmed in nearly all cases non-invasively by echocardiography. Increasingly, more serious lesions are diagnosed antenatally as a result of routine anomaly screening early in the second trimester or following the finding of an increased nuchal translucency thickness in the first trimester.

4. Improvements over the last 20 years in diagnostic and surgical techniques and pre- and postoperative care have significantly improved the prognosis for even the most complex forms of CHD. Up to 85% of those born with CHD can now expect to survive to adulthood (Perloff and Warnes 2001).

Table 13.1 Frequency of congenital heart lesions (adapted from Hoffman 2005)

Ventricular septal defect	32%
Atrial septal defect	8%
Pulmonary stenosis	7%
Patent arterial duct	7%
Tetralogy of Fallot	5%
Coarctation of the aorta	5%
Transposition of the great arteries	4%
Aortic stenosis	4%
Atrioventricular septal defect	4%
Hypoplastic left heart syndrome	3%
Complex functionally univentricular lesions(double inlet ventricle, tricuspid or mitral atresia)	3%
Pulmonary atresia with intact ventricular septum	2%
Double outlet right ventricle	2%
Common arterial trunk	1%
Totally anomalous pulmonary venous connections	1%
Miscellaneous	12%

5. Surgical risks are highest for neonates who present in poor condition with insufficient tissue perfusion and acidosis. An early, preferably prenatal, diagnosis will facilitate the timely instigation of appropriate medical and surgical therapy.

6. Advances in equipment and techniques have led to many simple congenital heart lesions being amenable to definitive treatment using transcatheter methods, such as balloon valvotomy for valve stenoses and device closure of the arterial duct and secundum atrial septal defect (ASD).

7. In the developed world by 2010, there will be more adults than children with CHD; of these adults, nearly 20% have complex problems with ongoing needs.

Detection of congenital heart disease: the role of the primary care physician

In the UK, population-based studies have shown that the current screening strategies of a hospital based post-delivery and pre-discharge examination, followed by a primary care based examination at age 6–8 weeks, are failing to pick up many cases of serious CHD, who require intervention in the first year of life. This is not surprising knowing that most neonates are discharged 6–48 hours following delivery and that of those neonates with CHD, over 40% will not have a murmur and up to 55% will have a normal cardiovascular examination at this time (Abu-Harb *et al.* 1994; Richmond and Wren 2001). As the arterial duct is unlikely to have fully closed by this time murmurless duct dependent lesions, such as aortic obstruction or pulmonary atresia, can often remain concealed with normal peripheral pulses and four limb blood pressures. In one study, 82% of 1074 neonates with CHD were sent home without a diagnosis being made, half becoming symptomatic prior to their 6-week check and 5% dying at home with undiagnosed duct dependent lesions (Abu-Harb *et al.* 1994). Although improvements in antenatal screening have helped to address this problem, with some centres picking up 50–80% of serious lesions, the current detection rate is very variable due to inadequate ultrasound equipment and training (Bull 1999). At present it remains the responsibility of the primary care healthcare team to be aware of the possibility of CHD, particularly during infancy, and to be vigilant with respect to relevant symptoms and signs, even if unreported by the parents.

Aetiology of congenital heart disease

The heart is formed between 6 and 12 weeks gestation and environmental teratogens during this period may effect cardiac development. However, in up to 80% of cases of CHD, no single factor is identified and the aetiology is considered multifactorial or polygenic. A genetic influence is supported by the known recurrence risks of CHD in siblings (3–4% if one sibling affected, 6–8% if two siblings affected) and in the offspring of those with CHD (5–10%, higher if the mother is affected). Although there is a higher risk of CHD in consanguineous families, there is non-concordance in monozygotic twins. Despite there being a tendency for a particular or related lesion to recur, this often is not the case.

Known aetiological factors and associations are:

- **Major chromosomal abnormalities**. The most common is Trisomy 21 (Down syndrome), 45% of whom have CHD (5% of CHD in liveborn neonates), particularly atrioventricular (AV) septal defect. CHD is found in 20% of those with Turner syndrome (45XO, left heart lesions) and 90% of those with the usually fatal Trisomy 18 and 13 (Edward's and Patau's syndromes). Given these facts, all neonates with these syndromes should be offered early echocardiographic screening irrespective of cardiac signs, as should those with other extracardiac abnormalities with a particular association with CHD (e.g. exomphalos).

- **Single gene defects** account for up to 5% of CHD. The most prevalent is 22q11 microdeletion (DiGeorge sequence, velocardiofacial syndrome), associated with conotruncal defects (common arterial trunk, interrupted aortic arch, tetralogy of Fallot variants). Others include Williams syndrome (7q11 deletion, supravalvar aortic stenosis), Noonan syndrome (PTPN11, pulmonary stenosis), Marfan's syndrome (fibrillin gene defect, aortic root dilation).

- **Maternal illnesses**. Associations include: insulin dependent diabetes (3–4%, if poor control in early pregnancy), infections (rubella: pulmonary stenosis, patent arterial duct; parvovirus: myocarditis) and autoimmune disorders such as systemic lupus erythematosus (congenital heart block).

- **Maternal drug ingestion**. Associations include: lithium (Ebstein's malformation), anti-epileptics (phenytoin, valproate: semilunar valvar stenosis, aortic coarctation), alcohol (fetal alcohol syndrome: septal defects) and Ecstasy (septal defects).

Presentation of heart disease in children

If an antenatal diagnosis has been made of CHD, the appropriate mode and place of delivery, the timing of transfer or referral to a paediatric cardiac centre for confirmatory diagnostic echocardiography and instigation of appropriate initial therapies, will all have been organized. With effective communication between the responsible health care groups, the primary care team would be involved in the care of the child. This includes knowledge of the diagnosis and any planned interventions, the implications to the family, and the need for medications or other care, such as assistance with feeding and the timing of vaccinations. A tertiary centre specialist cardiac liaison nurse would be able to facilitate communication and ensure the child and family receive optimal care and support.

Currently most lesions remain undetected antenatally and the diagnosis of CHD depends upon postnatal detection at primary or secondary care level. Over 75% of CHD is diagnosed within the first year of life, 40–50% by 1 week of age. However, given the evolving status of the cardiovascular system in the first few months of life, with closure of the arterial duct in the first week and fall in pulmonary vascular resistance over the next few months, it is important not to assume that a previously 'normal' postnatal cardiovascular assessment excludes CHD, particularly if the parents are concerned about their child's condition.

The mode of presentation is usually linked to age, particularly cyanosis or collapse in the neonatal period (as the arterial duct closes), heart failure during early infancy (as pulmonary vascular resistance falls) and/or the presence of a murmur at any age. Other presentations include, the finding of absent femoral pulses and arrhythmia-related symptoms. Although a detailed history is important, particularly when assessing systemic illnesses with possible cardiac involvement (e.g. Kawasaki disease), and palpitations or syncope, clinical findings are core to the recognition and management of CHD, as well as the need and timing of further referral.

◆ **Cyanosis**. This is due to either inadequate effective pulmonary blood flow due to pulmonary outflow obstruction or inadequate mixing of systemic and pulmonary venous returns (e.g. transposition of the great arteries). To be recognized clinically it necessitates at least 5 g/100 ml of reduced haemoglobin and is central (tongue or gums; not just the peripheries), equating to under 85% oxygen saturation. It is more difficult to ascertain in the presence of anaemia and can be subtle in newborns, due to the presence of fetal haemoglobin, ductal patency, and oval foramen mixing. It may take a few days before the duct closes and cyanosis becomes evident. The distinction from lung disease is made by placing the infant in a high oxygen environment: the saturation will dramatically increase in lung disease but fail to respond in cyanotic CHD. If there is a suspicion of cyanosis, the oxygen saturation needs to be measured. Some neonatal units have instituted pulsed oximetric screening of all newborns. **Clubbing** will not be apparent until at least a year of age, indicating chronic disease and will be accompanied by loud murmurs if cardiac in origin.

◆ **Hypercyanotic episodes** are characteristic of acute pulmonary outflow obstruction as in tetralogy of Fallot (see under this lesion).

- **Acrocyanosis.** It is common for parents of well, asymptomatic children to report intermittent episodes of 'going blue' around the lips, eyes, and limb peripheries. This is a totally benign phenomenon due to alterations in vascular tone and, in the absence of any other cardiac signs, requires no further investigations or referral. For further parental reassurance, a measured pulsed oxymeter reading is helpful.

- **Heart failure.** This is due to excessive pulmonary blood flow, sustained arrhythmias, or primary myocardial failure. In the infant it is characterized by tachypnoea with recession, tachycardia, and hepatomegaly along with feeding difficulties: inability to take age appropriate volumes in under 20 minutes, always being hungry, awakening at frequent intervals, tiring easily, and sleeping excessively. There may be coughing, frequent chest infections (slow to resolve), and excessive sweating (sympathetic drive). This results in poor weight gain and failure to thrive. Auscultation may reveal accentuation of the pulmonary component of the second heart sound, indicating pulmonary hypertension, or a gallop rhythm. Pathological murmurs, often due to high flow over outflow tracts (ejection systolic murmur, ESM) or AV valves (mid-diastolic murmur) are characteristic. Oedema is unusual except in older patients with right heart failure. In the older child, the dominant complaint will be shortness of breath on exertion.

- **Pulses.** Rate, rhythm, and volume are best assessed from the right radial or brachial pulse, while comparing with lower limb ones for possible aortic arch lesions. Radial-femoral delay will not be discernable until at least 4 years of age, so absent or reduced volume femoral or pedal pulses are to be noted. Reduced volume in all limbs suggests poor cardiac output (e.g. myocarditis) or aortic outflow obstruction (e.g. critical aortic stenosis). Note that with respect to left heart obstructive lesions, newborn pulses may well be normal for up to a few days, until the arterial duct closes. Bounding pulses are found with a large aortic run off, such as a large arterial duct, common arterial trunk or marked aortic regurgitation.

- **Auscultation and heart murmurs.** This is a crucial part of assessing and screening for CHD in children. The assessment of the child with an asymptomatic murmur and findings with respect to common specific heart lesions are dealt with below. Detailed descriptions of standard cardiac auscultatory findings are beyond the scope of this book, being available in standard texts (Archer *et al.*1998).

The asymptomatic child with a heart murmur

This is the most frequent problem facing the primary care physician. Up to 90% of children if carefully screened, will be found to have a murmur at some point during their development. By definition, no more than 1% of these children will have CHD, the others having benign or innocent murmurs. The differential diagnosis is therefore between:

- a haemodynamically significant heart lesion requiring an intervention in the near future and early referral. Usually the child will demonstrate other abnormal signs and, on closer questioning, symptoms that will dictate the urgency of the referral;

- a more minor heart lesion, requiring regular reviews with the possibility of an intervention over the medium term (such as a small ventricular septal defect (VSD) or semilunar valve stenosis), requiring elective referral;

- an innocent murmur.

Currently best practice dictates that a strong suspicion of the presence of any form of CHD requires assessment at an early stage by a paediatric cardiologist or a paediatrician with an interest in this area, who has the facility to perform an echocardiogram. Unfortunately it is increasingly difficult for the primary care physician not to refer on asymptomatic patients with clear-cut innocent murmurs. Parental expectations based on media and internet sourced information, have created an environment in which often only an echocardiogram will provide sufficient reassurance of normality. While the authors are aware it may not reflect best practice, by the time the child reaches the paediatric cardiologist it is often more efficient and effective to perform an echocardiogram and provide parents with an information leaflet explaining the nature of such murmurs, than to explain to the family why an echocardiogram is unnecessary on clinical grounds, particularly when the primary or secondary care physician has led the family to expect this investigation. An electrocardiogram (ECG) in such cases is often too insensitive to be used as an effective screening tool and a chest X-ray is certainly unjustified.

When deciding that a murmur is innocent, the history must confirm a lack of symptoms and the examination must exclude heart failure and cyanosis. Peripheral pulses must be demonstrably normal and equal, with a quiet precordium. Heart sounds should be normal with a non-accentuated pulmonary component of the second heart sound, which moves normally with respiration (best heard when non-supine). An ejection click or gallop rhythm will be absent.

Innocent murmurs are usually soft (I–II/VI intensity), are either systolic or continuous (never diastolic), vary with posture, are accentuated by coexistent fever, infection or anaemia, and tend to be localized. Pathological murmurs are usually loud (>II/VI intensity), may be at any point in the cardiac cycle, may be accompanied by added sounds, and tend to have wide radiation, not varying with posture or respiration. Stenotic semilunar valve murmurs will be apparent soon after birth, while septal defect related murmurs may take months to become apparent. Innocent murmurs become less audible with age, as the chest wall thickness increases, but may still be audible in up to 20% of adolescents. Such murmurs may persist throughout life. They characteristically may be present at one examination but not at another.

There are five main types of innocent murmur that can usually be diagnosed with confidence rather than by exclusion:

- *Infantile pulmonary murmur*. This occurs in the premature and in early infancy. It is due to flow acceleration over the pulmonary bifurcation and is characterized by a soft ESM maximal at the upper left sternal border (LSB) with radiation into the axilla and even the back. It disappears before 1 year of age.

- *Still's murmur*. This common innocent murmur, first described in 1909, is a low-pitched ESM, best audible in the mid to lower LSB, with radiation towards the apex and occasionally upper precordium. It is described as being vibratory, musical, buzzing, or 'twangy' and is louder when supine, due to increased stroke volume. In young infants it tends to be have a more squeaky character. It's aetiology remains uncertain, but vibrations of the semilunar valves or left ventricular (LV) tendons have been implicated. These qualities distinguish it from other lower precordial murmurs. VSD murmurs are harsh, loud, and pansystolic or, if the defect is very small, early systolic and decrescendo in character, with a harsh or high-pitched 'aerosol spray' quality (Figure 13.1). Mitral regurgitation is rare in children and the murmur is pansystolic, apical, high pitched and blowing, with radiation to the axilla and back.

- *Venous hum*. This benign continuous murmur is due to blood cascading down the great veins. It is maximally heard in right infraclavicular region, is accentuated in inspiration and is virtually abolished on lying flat. This contrasts with the harsh, machinery, non-positional left infraclavicular continuous murmur of a patent arterial duct.

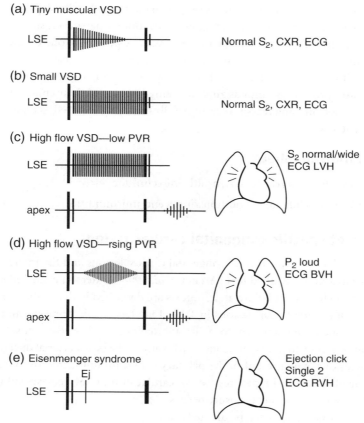

Fig. 13.1 Common murmurs. Characteristic clinical and investigative findings in patients with varying sizes of ventricular septal defects. BVH, biventricular hypertrophy; CXR, chest X-ray; ECG, electrocardiogram; LSE, left sternal edge; LVH, left ventricular hypertrophy; PVR, pulmonary vascular resistance; RVH, right ventricular hypertrophy; VSD, ventricular septal defect.

- *Carotid bruit.* This common harsh, usually short early ESM, is due to flow acceleration from the aortic arch to the brachiocephallic arteries. It is audible in the lower neck and often radiates down to the aortic area, being softer with neck extension or carotid pressure. It should not be confused with aortic stenosis where the murmur is louder below the clavicle.
- *Pulmonary ESM.* This is heard most often in older children or adolescents, is localized to the upper LSB and may be difficult to distinguish from a pathological stenotic murmur (louder with click) or ASD flow murmur (louder).

Ultimately it is the confidence of the primary care physician that will determine whether a child with an innocent murmur is referred for a further opinion and usually an echocardiogram. If in doubt, referral is certainly justified, but even in such cases generous reassurance is required to minimize parental concern while awaiting the appointment. Many parents can be fully reassured by a clear, full explanation, particularly if supported by an explanatory leaflet. Other parents will not rest until a specialist opinion is sought and an echocardiogram performed. The family should be told that their child has a normal heart, requiring no restrictions whatsoever, should be treated entirely as a normal child and that the murmur may be present at one examination, but not at another. A well written explanatory leaflet is particularly useful as parents often find it difficult to retain information when feeling worried or stressed as may be the case in the consulting room. By emphasizing the benign nature of their child's murmur the leaflet will provide ongoing reassurance, hopefully obviating the need to represent for the same reason at a later date.

Innocent murmur sheet

- http://www.rch.org.au/cardiology/health-info.cfm?doc_id=3537
- http://kirkies.net/chdguide/conditions/innocent_murmur.htm

Overview of specific congenital cardiac lesions

This overview does not consider all congenital cardiac lesions and the interested reader should refer to a more detailed text (Archer *et al.* 1998; Anderson *et al.* 2005). Generic presentations such as heart failure and cyanosis are described in detail above and ages of presentation of different heart lesions in Table 13.2. Lesions that present more often in adult life are not covered here (e.g. coronary anomalies, mitral valve prolapse).

It is important to again note that neonates with any of the below arterial duct dependent, obstructive lesions, may present to the primary care team following routine maternity discharge (age 1–2 days) with progressive low cardiac output, severe heart failure, and/or cyanosis, as physiological ductal closure occurs.

Congenital cardiac lesions can be divided into:

1. acyanotic congenital heart lesions with left-to-right shunt, including unobstructed anomalous pulmonary veins;
2. cyanotic congenital heart lesions;

3. obstructive congenital heart lesions;

4. complex cardiac defects.

Table 13.2 Age and mode of presentation of different congenital heart lesions

Age of presentation	Cyanosis	Heart failure
Premature		Patent arterial duct
0–10 days	TGA with intact ventricular septum Pulmonary atresia Obstructed TAPVC (+heart failure) Severe Ebstein's anomaly	Critical aortic stenosis Hypoplastic left heart syndrome Aortic arch obstruction
11–30 days	Severe tetralogy of Fallot Complex CHD with low pulmonary blood flow	TGA + VSD Complex CHD with high pulmonary blood flow Common arterial trunk
Over 1 month	Tetralogy of Fallot (spells) Complex CHD with progressive pulmonary outflow obstruction	Atrioventricular septal defect Large VSD Aortopulmonary window Dilated cardiomyopathy Anomalous LCA from pulmonary artery

CHD, Congenital heart disease; LCA, left coronary artery; TAPVC, totally anomalous pulmonary venous connections; TGA, transposition of the great arteries; VSD, ventricular septal defect.

Acyanotic congenital heart lesions with left-to-right shunt

Ventricular septal defect (VSD)

◆ Most common congenital heart lesion (32%). Often accompany other CHD (e.g. tetralogy of Fallot). May be multiple, 80% are small (<3mm diameter).

◆ High rate of spontaneous closure, especially isolated small defects (90% by age 6 years).

◆ Small isolated defects require infrequent but regular follow-up to determine when closed and if complications develop (e.g. secondary aortic regurgitation in perimembranous VSD). Frequency of follow-up is dependent upon the age, VSD site and size (6–36 monthly).

◆ Significant risk of infective endocarditis until closed.

◆ ECG is useful for monitoring: normal with small defects, LVH with left-to-right shunts without pulmonary hypertension, going on to biventricular hypertrophy with pulmonary hypertension and then pure right ventricular (RV) hypertrophy with pulmonary vascular disease.

Clinical presentation From asymptomatic child with pansystolic or systolic decrescendo murmur at lower LSB (see Figure 13.1), to the infant with severe heart failure and failure to thrive. The larger the defect, the earlier symptoms develop, as the pulmonary vascular resistance drops during early infancy. Large defects, if untreated will eventually develop irreversible pulmonary vascular disease (Eisenmenger's syndrome).

Treatment No treatment required for small defects. Diuretics are prescribed in symptomatic infants. Surgical closure before 1 year of age where significant shunt persists or later if complications develop (e.g. secondary aortic regurgitation, endocarditis). Transcatheter device closure available for a few selected older patients. Once confirmed by a paediatric cardiologist, very small restrictive isolated mid muscular defects could then be followed at primary care level every 2–3 years as once the murmur has gone, the defect will have essentially closed and antibiotic prophylaxis precautions can end with no further follow-up required.

Atrial septal defect (ASD): Secundum (for Primum ASD, see AV septal defect-below)

- Defect in the atrial septum at site of oval fossa (foramen ovale).
- Spontaneous closure of small defects: often stretched patent foramen ovale (PFO).
- Risk of paradoxical emboli, atrial dysrhythmias, and pulmonary hypertension in large defects left untreated until adulthood.
- Do not require endocarditis prophylaxis.
- RSR pattern in the right ECG chest leads.

Clinical presentation Asymptomatic child with fixed splitting of the second heart sound and ESM at upper LSB (due to functional pulmonary stenosis from increased pulmonary blood flow; no murmur over ASD itself). Murmur often not present until after infancy. Shortness of breath on exertion, with reactive airways and frequent chest infections in a few.

Treatment Closure indicated if significant shunt with right atrial and RV enlargement. Transcatheter device closure is feasible in most patients aged 3–5 years or at later presentation, otherwise low risk surgical repair.

Patent arterial duct (patent ductus arteriosus or PDA)

- Part of normal prenatal circulation with high postnatal closure rate in term neonates.
- Patency beyond 1 month is considered significant (3 months in premature).
- With the exception of the murmurless duct ('silent'), all require closure for symptoms or to prevent long-term risk of ductal endarteritis.

Clinical presentation Heart failure and failure to progress in premature neonates. Occasional infant with heart failure; most older children are asymptomatic. Bounding pulses and continuous 'machinery' murmur (often only systolic in infancy) below left clavicle.

Treatment In premature: indomethacin or ibuprofen, going onto surgery in symptomatic cases as required. Diuretics for symptomatic infants. Transcatheter device closure feasible in most, but occasionally low-risk surgery required for large PDAs in infants.

Atrioventricular septal defect (AVSD, AV canal)

- Deficiency of the septum immediately above and/or below the AV valves. Concomitant malformation of AV valves themselves with common AV junction.
- Commonly associated with Trisomy 21 (66%); 33% of T21 children have an AVSD.
- Primum ASD is a partial AVSD with isolated atrial component (deficiency of septum primum).
- Complete AVSD has both atrial and ventricular components with shunting at atrial and ventricular levels.
- Often associated with significant left AV valvar (mitral) regurgitation.
- Characteristic superior ECG QRS axis.

Clinical presentation

- *Primum ASD*: usually asymptomatic child with signs as for secundum ASD but often with additional pansystolic murmur of mitral regurgitation.
- *Complete AVSD*: usually heart failure in early infancy, depending on size of ventricular component. Risk of early increase in pulmonary vascular resistance.

Treatment Diuretics in symptomatic infant followed by early surgical repair at 3–6 months of age. Surgery for complete form involves closure of defects and division of common AV valve into separate orifices. Both forms require AV valve repair to deal with regurgitation.

Common arterial trunk (truncus arteriosus) and aortopulmonary window

- Failure of prenatal septation between ascending aorta and main pulmonary artery.
- Direct communication between systemic and pulmonary circulation with risk of early increase in pulmonary vascular resistance.
- Common arterial trunk associated with 22q11 deletion, especially if coexistent aortic arch obstruction. Truncal valve may be stenotic and/or regurgitant.

Clinical presentation Heart failure in early infancy. In common arterial trunk ESM and early diastolic murmur (EDM) often apparent with ejection click, while aortopulmonary window is characterized by PDA like continuous murmur.

Treatment Diuretics followed by surgical complete repair in early infancy.

Partial or totally anomalous pulmonary venous connection(s)

- One to four pulmonary veins connecting directly into systemic venous vascular bed or right atrium, often with coexistent ASD (e.g. sinus venosus ASD).
- Partial variant can be associated with right lung anomalies (Scimitar syndrome).
- Total variant often associated with obstructed pulmonary venous return and cyanosis.

Clinical presentation Partially anomalous variant similar to ASD: asymptomatic child with ESM. Totally anomalous variant with obstruction: seriously ill neonate or young infant with cyanosis, right heart failure, pulmonary venous congestion, and pulmonary hypertension.

Treatment Anomalous drainage of a single pulmonary vein well tolerated without treatment. Surgical redirection of anomalous veins into left atrium is required for other variants, with timing dependent on clinical symptoms. Emergency surgery is needed if obstruction present.

Cyanotic congenital heart disease

Tetralogy of Fallot and variants

◆ Combination of VSD with overriding aorta, RV outflow tract obstruction, RV hypertrophy.

◆ Severe variant with pulmonary atresia and variable degree of central pulmonary arterial hypoplasia, sometimes with additional aortopulmonary collateral arteries supplying variable segments of the pulmonary circulation.

◆ May be associated with 22q11 deletion, especially if right aortic arch.

Clinical presentation ESM at upper LSB after birth (no murmur from VSD as non-restrictive) with cyanosis if severe pulmonary obstruction, or may be asymptomatic, with balanced pulmonary blood flow ('pink Fallot'). Collaterals cause continuous lung field murmurs. Characteristic are hypercyanotic spells, due to an acute drop in pulmonary blood flow related to muscular spasm of the RV outflow tract, with marked central cyanosis and near disappearance of the ESM. They are common in the early morning on wakening, often with crying, exertion, or feeding and can result in syncope or collapse. Squatting and clubbing observed in older children is now rare, due to early diagnosis and treatment in developed countries.

Pulmonary atresia variant will usually be severely cyanosed and duct dependent, unless major collaterals are present (may even have overgenerous pulmonary flow).

Treatment Surgical complete repair in the first year of life is usual. Preceding palliative systemic-to-pulmonary arterial (SPA) shunt insertion may be required for the small infant (spelling, severe cyanosis or hypoplastic pulmonary arteries).

Treat hypercyanotic spell by positioning (knees pushed to chest), oxygen, intravenous (IV) fluid and IV propranolol (0.1 µg/kg) with morphine bolus; prophylaxis with oral propranolol and generous fluid intake especially in hot environments or with diarrhoea or vomiting. Urgent referral back to the paediatric cardiologist is necessary.

Pulmonary atresia variants will require postnatal IV prostaglandin E to maintain ductal patency (except with collaterals), then SPA shunt. Eventual complete repair (1–2 years of age) with RV to pulmonary arterial homograft conduit.

Pulmonary atresia with intact ventricular septum

◆ Usually pulmonary valvar atresia with variable degree of RV hypoplasia.

◆ Pulmonary blood flow dependent on patency of arterial duct.

- Degree of RV hypoplasia determines suitability for biventricular or univentricular repair.
- May have associated coronary abnormalities.

Clinical presentation Marked cyanosis from birth. Single second heart sound often without a murmur.

Treatment IV prostaglandin E to maintain ductal patency before a SPA shunt. Selected patients with good sized RV suitable for transcatheter radiofrequency perforation and balloon dilation of atretic pulmonary valve, although often still require shunt. Long term may achieve biventricular circulation ± RV to pulmonary arterial conduit or go down univentricular treatment route (see Complex CHD section).

Transposition of great arteries

- Aorta arises from RV and pulmonary artery from LV creating parallel systemic and pulmonary circulations.
- Postnatal survival depends on mixing of blood between systemic and pulmonary circulations, best achieved at atrial level though ASD or large PFO, but also at arterial duct level.
- Frequent association with VSD ± pulmonary outflow obstruction.

Clinical presentation Severe cyanosis from birth in otherwise generally well baby, single heart sounds and no murmurs. Can be extremely sick if atrial septum near intact at birth.

Treatment Initial IV prostaglandin E to maintain ductal patency if unwell usually followed by transcatheter balloon atrial septostomy; both to improve mixing. Surgical repair by aorta and pulmonary arterial translocation to above left and right ventricles respectively and separate transfer of coronary arteries to neoaorta ('arterial switch') in neonatal period.

Obstructive congenital heart lesions

Pulmonary valve stenosis

- Variable degree of valve malformation and stenosis.
- Mild stenosis rarely progresses.
- ECG useful for monitoring progressive RVH if stenosis worsens.

Clinical presentation Usually asymptomatic child with ejection click preceding ESM ± thrill at upper LSB, radiating to lung fields. Critically severe stenosis presents as a cyanosed (due to right to left atrial shunt over PFO), duct dependent neonate.

Treatment Transcatheter balloon valvotomy when stenosis severe (echo Doppler gradient >60 mmHg). Repeat valvotomy occasionally needed for neonatal group, rarely with later presentation.

Aortic valve stenosis

- Variable degree of valve malformation and stenosis. Bicuspid valve present in up to 2% of population (overall rarely presents in children).
- Stenosis usually progresses; may be accompanied by significant regurgitation especially after valvotomy procedure.
- ECG insensitive to severity until very severe.

Clinical presentation Usually asymptomatic child with ejection click preceding ESM at mid LSB and upper right sternal edge, radiating to carotids ± suprasternal thrill. When severe may present with exercise-related syncope and shortness of breath. EDM if aortic regurgitation present. Critically severe stenosis presents as ill infant with low cardiac output, heart failure, an ESM, and low volume pulses.

Treatment In the sick neonate, IV prostaglandin E for ductal patency, inotropic and ventilatory support and rapid transcatheter balloon, or surgical valvotomy. Transcatheter balloon valvotomy when older and stenosis severe (echo Doppler gradient >70 mmHg). If treatment needed, most will later go on to require aortic valve replacement (usually using pulmonary autograft and homograft pulmonary valve replacement: Ross procedure).

Aortic arch coarctation (or interruption)

- Narrowing of distal paraductal aortic arch and/or aortic isthmus.
- If arch interrupted, a segment is absent, the lower body is entirely arterial duct dependent and there will be a coexistent VSD.
- In neonates postnatal arterial ductal closure precipitates symptoms.
- May be associated with other CHD, a bicuspid aortic valve (25%), and Turner syndrome.
- Separate late presentation of coarctation after late childhood with systemic hypertension.

Clinical presentation Critically ill neonate or infant with variable degrees of low cardiac output, heart failure, and absent or low volume lower limb pulses. Older children are usually asymptomatic. There is: right arm systemic hypertension with differential to lower limb BP; often a soft ESM below the left clavicle and/or between the scapulae; and after age 4 years there is usually radial-femoral pulse delay.

Treatment In the sick neonate, IV prostaglandin E for ductal patency, inotropic and ventilatory support, and rapid surgical repair. At present, evidence is in favour of surgical treatment for native coarctation in childhood, while transcatheter balloon angioplasty with stenting is favoured in adolescence. Re-coarctation is treated with balloon angioplasty ± stenting. Short- to medium-term post-procedure antihypertensive treatment is often required, particularly with adolescent presentation (e.g. beta blockade or angiotensin-converting enzyme (ACE) inhibitors).

Hypoplastic left heart syndrome

- Severe underdevelopment of the left heart and aorta: aortic and mitral valvar atresia, stenosis, or hypoplasia with hypoplastic LV, ascending aorta and arch.
- Postnatal arterial ductal closure precipitates symptoms.

Clinical presentation   Critically ill neonate with variable low cardiac output, heart failure, and absent or low volume pulses.

Treatment IV prostaglandin E for ductal patency, inotropic and ventilatory support and rapid high-risk surgical aortopulmonary reconstruction with SPA shunt (Norwood procedure). Thereafter univentricular two stage definitive palliation (see Complex CHD below).

Vascular ring

- Malformation of the aortic arch or its branches encircling and compressing the trachea and/or oesophagus resulting in stridor and occasionally dysphagia.
- Various subtypes with double aortic arch commonest.
- Often coexists with tracheobronchial malacia.
- Diagnosis by barium swallow, echocardiography, and computed tomography or magnetic resonance imaging angiography.

Clinical presentation Stridor in infancy, worse with chest infections and crying.

Treatment Surgical division via left thoracotomy with good outcome but persistent respiratory symptoms dependent upon degree of malacia.

Complex congenital heart defects

- Functionally univentricular hearts.
- Complex CHD with hypoplasia of one ventricle and either absence of an AV connection (tricuspid or mitral atresia) or both AV valves connect to the dominant ventricle (double inlet ventricle). Hypoplastic ventricle connects to dominant ventricle via VSD.
- Characterized by complete intracardiac mixing of pulmonary and systemic venous returns.
- Associated with all forms of ventriculo-arterial connections, outflow tract obstruction, and anomalies of systemic and/or pulmonary venous connections.

Clinical presentation Symptoms dependent on associated lesions: variable degree of pulmonary or aortic outflow obstruction. Thus presentation varies from neonatal severe cyanosis to progressive heart failure as pulmonary resistance falls.

Treatment Initial treatment dependent on associated lesions: IV prostaglandin E followed by SPA shunt in some or diuretics followed by pulmonary artery banding to reduce pulmonary blood flow in others. A univentricular treatment pathway follows with two-stage creation of total cavopulmonary anastomosis (TCPC or Fontan type circulation) to connect the caval veins directly to the pulmonary arteries, bypassing the heart and dividing the systemic and pulmonary venous returns. Note that patients with a TCPC require lifelong anticoagulation to prevent thrombi in the venous circulation.

Double outlet right ventricle

- Spectrum of lesions characterized by both aorta and pulmonary artery arising from the morphological RV.
- Relative position of associated VSD with respect to aorta and pulmonary artery influences clinical presentation and surgical treatment options.

Clinical presentation As with other complex CHD, dependent upon associated lesions (outflow tract obstruction) but also VSD position: subaortic VSD similar to tetralogy of Fallot, subpulmonary VSD similar to transposition of great arteries and VSD.

Treatment Palliative early surgery to optimize pulmonary blood flow, followed by complex surgical procedures to reroute blood flow from LV into aorta where feasible in early childhood. May require univentricular treatment pathway (above).

Acquired heart disease in children

Rheumatic fever

In less developed countries the incidence of acute rheumatic fever still accounts for up to 22 per 1000 school children, particularly in lower income families. Although post-streptococcal in origin, only 3% of those infected will acquire rheumatic fever. The peak incidence is 10–14 years of age, being rare below age 5 years. In primary care the classic features of migratory painful large joint polyarthritis, subcutaneous painless extensor tendon nodules, erythema marginatum rash (10%), and Sydenham's chorea following a proven streptococcal infection may be present. Carditis occurs in up to 60% of cases, usually with signs of mitral regurgitation and/or pericarditis and first- or second-degree AV block on the ECG. The diagnosis is confirmed using the modified Jones criteria. Referral for serological and echocardiographic assessment is indicated. Treatment with penicillin G and aspirin, with glucocorticosteroids if myocarditis or heart failure are evident, follows standard protocols, including the need for long-term penicillin V prophylaxis until at least adulthood. Intramuscular monthly penicillin G is only required if more than one episode occurred, there is significant residual heart disease or with poor compliance. Inadequate early treatment may lead to chronic rheumatic heart disease: mitral regurgitation ± stenosis and aortic regurgitation being most common.

Acquired heart muscle disease

Myocarditis This is usually viral in origin (e.g. Coxsackie, adenovirus) with a poorly functioning LV. Symptoms of heart failure with a gallop rhythm develop acutely or insidiously after an upper respiratory illness, often with dysrhythmias. Early referral is needed as the illness may rapidly progress to death especially in infancy. The ECG will usually be abnormal with T-wave inversion, low voltages, and arrhythmias. Treatment is supportive (diuretics, ACE inhibitors), while some centres advocate immunoglobulin or steroid therapy either empirically or with a positive myocardial biopsy. Roughly one-third will recover, one-third will remain functionally impaired, and one-third will die or require transplant.

Dilated cardiomyopathy This may be difficult to distinguish from myocarditis but tends to have a more insidious onset of heart failure with similar signs and findings. Over 30% have a genetic origin. It may be drug induced (e.g. anthracyclines), due to sustained arrhythmias, due to inborn errors of metabolism or a generalized myopathy, such as Duchenne's, or may be post-myocarditic. Referral is needed, not least to rule out rare but treatable causes, such as carnitine deficiency. Treatment is supportive: diuretics, ACE inhibitors, digoxin (with care as arrhythmogenic) and cautious beta blockade (carvedilol). Some patients require transplantation.

Hypertrophic cardiomyopathy This is usually familial but may be due to infiltrative storage diseases or mitochondrial disorders. More common in older children or adolescents, it may present with sudden death, sometimes with exercise. There may be no symptoms or dyspnoea on exertion, fatigue, anginal chest pain, syncope, or palpitations. Heart failure may occur in infants. Associated progressive LV outflow tract obstruction is characteristic and gives signs of an aortic ESM but without a click but with a fourth heart sound, 'jerky' pulse, and diffusely active apical impulse. The ECG usually shows LVH, often with T-wave abnormalities and inferolateral deep Q waves. Referral is needed for diagnostic investigations. Treatment is targeted at LV outflow obstruction: high-dose beta blockade, disopyramide and possibly surgery.

Kawasaki disease (mucocutaneous lymph node syndrome)

This is an acute self-limiting vasculitis of unknown aetiology, particularly effecting young children and is the leading cause of acquired heart disease in developed countries, occurring in $10-100/10^5$ children under 5 years of age. It is associated with potentially preventable coronary arterial aneurysms. As it is essential that preventative treatment is given before day 10 of the illness, it is important for the primary care physician to be aware of the disease and the requirement for early secondary care referral.

Kawasaki disease is diagnosed when a protracted fever is accompanied by at least four other features (less if coronaries abnormalities are found):

- Fever: high (>38°C), remitting, for at least 4 days (days 1–12 of illness).
- Conjunctivitis/uveitis: bilateral, non-purulent, painless. Days 3–14.
- Upper respiratory tract mucous membrane inflammation: red and cracked lips, strawberry tongue, oropharyngeal injection. No ulcers. Days 2–16.
- Polymorphous rash: extensive maculopapular, urticarial, scarlatiniform, target lesions. On torso. No vesicles. Days 4–12.
- Peripheries. Days 3–10: erythema and oedema; days 10–28: periungual desquamation
- Cervical lymphadenopathy (50–75%): acute, non-suppurative, painless, >1.5 cm. Days 1–14.

- Extreme irritability: especially infants (days 1–21).

- Cardiac: early pancarditis (50–80%), gallop, tachycardia. Days 10–28: coronary aneurysms/ectasia, especially if prolonged fever, male infants, and high inflammatory markers (25% in untreated). Mitral regurgitation (10%). Rarely: myocardial infarction (25% mortality).

- Other manifestations: diarrhoea (early; 50%), urethritis (50%), pauciarticular arthritis (45%, late, older girls), aseptic meningitis (25%).

- Laboratory features: raised C-reactive protein, erythrocyte sedimentation rate, white cell count, platelets (after day 7) and liver function tests, anaemia.

Treatment is aimed at curtailing the vasculitic process using high-dose aspirin therapy (80–100 mg/kg per day) and preventing the development of coronary aneurysms with IV immunoglobulin (IVIG) 2 g as a single dose. Only if IVIG is given before day 10 of the illness will the incidence of coronary aneurysms reduce to below 5%. After IVIG, routine live vaccinations (e.g. MMR and varicella) need to be delayed for at least 11 months to obtain an adequate immune response. Once the inflammatory markers are normal, low-dose antiplatelet aspirin therapy is commenced for 6–8 weeks or until any coronary lesions have resolved (see Prescribing for congenital heart disease, page 185). The presence of large or giant aneurysms (>8 mm diameter) requires more aggressive anticoagulation, usually warfarin (INR 2–2.5) and aspirin long term. Follow-up and management protocols are dependent upon the presence and size of aneurysms, as detailed in the recent AHA guidelines (Newburger *et al.* 2004).

Infective endocarditis and antibiotic prophylaxis

The primary care physician needs to be aware of the risk of endocarditis in nearly all children with CHD, particularly after surgery or dental procedures; although 40% will not have a history of an intervention. It can also occur in those without CHD, particularly the immune suppressed, those with long-tem vascular access catheters or IV drug abuse. Symptoms of a persistent fever, heart failure, fatigue, and poor feeding in a patient with known CHD need to be taken seriously. Anaemia, embolic phenomena, and splenomegaly may be present. Early referral is indicated and antibiotics should not be initiated until several sets of blood cultures have been acquired. Treatment is 4–6 weeks IV antibiotics, with occasional patients being returned home to finish a course under primary care supervision, depending upon the organism, sensitivities, and home circumstances.

Antibiotic prophylaxis is indicated for virtually all children with CHD, whenever they undergo any procedures or invasive dental work which might produce gum bleeding, using the British National Formulary guidelines. The exceptions are: secundum ASD, isolated anomalous pulmonary venous connection(s), closed or silent patent arterial duct, 'physiological' valvar regurgitation or prolapse (usually picked up by chance on echocardiographic screening) and spontaneously closed VSD(s). The primary care physician will often be required to prescribe the appropriate antibiotic for community based procedures, such as dental work.

Paediatric arrhythmias and palpitations

Paediatric ECG, arrhythmia interpretation and treatment protocols are very similar to that in adults and it is beyond the scope of this book to cover this area in detail (Archer *et al.*1998; Anderson *et al.* 2005). Investigations are also similar, with efforts being made to record an ECG both during and when out of an arrhythmic event, the use of prolonged ECG taping and cardio-memo devices. However, certain important differences in children should be noted:

- ECGs are recorded in the same way as for adults but with V_{4R} replacing V_3 in the standard paediatric 12-lead ECG.

- There are physiological changes in heart rate, axis, and ventricular dominance with increasing age: heart rate decreases (100–160 to 70–130 bpm), the QRS axis progressively moves leftward (60–160° to 0–100°) and ventricular dominance shifts from RV dominance to the adult pattern of LV dominance (Lead V_1 R wave to S wave dominant) by age 3 years.

- Although arrhythmias usually occur in isolation with a structurally normal heart, they are particularly associated with congenital lesions with an enlarged atrium (e.g. AV valvar regurgitation) such as Ebstein's malformation of the tricuspid valve.

- Sinus arrhythmia, the normal phasic variation in heart rate with the respiratory cycle (increase with inspiration, decrease with expiration), associated with a regular irregular pulse, is common in children. It is a completely benign phenomenon in the setting of a healthy normal child, requiring no further investigation or treatment.

- 24-hour ECG recordings in normal children may reveal frequent atrial and/or ventricular premature monomorphic beats (abolished with exercise), short episodes of sinus pauses and first-degree or second-degree type I (Wenckebach) AV block. These are all benign and of no consequence in the well child with no other symptoms or signs.

Supraventricular tachycardia (SVT) and palpitations

SVT is the usual tachyarrhythmia in childhood, the mechanism most often being a re-entry circuit, often with an accessory AV pathway, or occasionally an ectopic atrial automatic focus. The tachycardia is usually narrow complex, without the moment to moment rate variation seen in sinus tachycardia. The resting ECG may be normal or show the characteristic short PR interval and pre-excitation slurred delta wave of Wolff–Parkinson–White syndrome.

In infants with sustained tachyarrhythmias symptoms will be those of heart failure with tachypnoea and poor feeding. Conversion may be achieved by vagal stimulation using the diving reflex by an ice-cold flannel to the face or facial immersion in cold water. Referral to hospital is indicated where the drug of first choice will be IV adenosine. Failing this electrical cardioversion may be required. Prophylactic therapy is usually then started with beta blockade or a Class Ic agent (e.g. flecainide) for 6–12 months. Usually the drug can then be stopped without a recurrence but a third of cases relapse in late childhood.

In older children, the dominant symptom is sustained palpitations, sometimes with shortness of breath, irritability, and chest discomfort. Treatment is the same but other vagal manoeuvres can be tried such as the Valsalva or unilateral carotid massage. Eyeball pressure should not be used. Referral for medical therapy and consideration of transcatheter energy mediated ablation is then indicated.

Palpitations are a common complaint in older children as they become aware of their own heart beat while growing up. They are often linked to exercise, are short lived (a few minutes) and spontaneously resolve, being due to benign sinus tachycardia in most cases if no other symptoms or signs are present. They may be provoked by stress, caffeine containing soft drinks, and asthma beta-sympathomimetic therapy. A 12-lead ECG recorded at the time of palpitations will be diagnostic but is often difficult to achieve. If the resting ECG is normal, the symptoms infrequent and short lived, reassurance is all that is needed. Referral is indicated if there are frequent unprovoked or sustained episodes, if there are other symptoms such as syncope or signs and/or the ECG is abnormal. One- to 7-day ECG or cardiac event recording may be required in symptomatic cases to capture an episode or for reassurance that an episode is not associated with an ECG abnormality.

Ventricular arrhythmias

Ventricular arrhythmias are rare in children, except in the context of certain repaired congenital heart lesions such as tetralogy of Fallot, acquired myocardial disease, or long QT syndrome. Symptoms of palpitations with dizziness and syncope or a family history of sudden death require urgent referral to exclude these potentially lethal conditions. A normal ECG will be reassuring.

- **Long QT syndrome:** a group of genetic disorders responsible for prolonged myocardial depolarization and a propensity to polymorphic paroxysmal ventricular tachycardias. It can be associated with deafness. The QT interval on ECG varies with heart rate and a rate corrected QT interval above 440 ms warrants referral. The exact genetic subtype influences treatment and prognosis and should be established; beta blockade is used in the meantime.

- **Brugada syndrome:** a recently described potentially lethal genetic disorder of the sodium channel characterized by right bundle branch block pattern with ST segment elevation in V_{1-3} chest leads with a risk of ventricular fibrillation in the absence of structural heart disease.

Conduction abnormalities and atrioventricular block

These are characterized by impaired conduction within the AV node and bundle of Hiss, which may be benign or give rise to symptoms of syncope or even sudden death.

- Right bundle branch block is quite common after surgery involving VSD closure, particularly tetralogy of Fallot repair. The main risk is the development of complete heart block. It can rarely occur in isolation.

- First degree AV block (prolonged PR interval for age and heart rate) is benign in itself. It can be associated with infection (e.g. rheumatic fever) or with CHD. In isolation it occurs in up to 8% of normal children, requiring no precautions or further investigation in the healthy child.

♦ Second degree AV block occurs in two forms. Type I (Wenckebach) with progressively lengthening PR interval until a QRS is dropped, may occur in normal fit individuals especially at night (vagal tone) and usually benign. Type II with fixed two, three, or four atrial beats to each QRS complex may be a precursor to complete AV block and requires referral.

♦ Third degree or complete AV block may be associated with surgical damage to the AV node, with myocarditis, with complex CHD or be congenital in the setting of maternal connective tissue disease (particularly systemic lupus erythematosus) with positive anti-Ro and La antibodies. Symptoms of syncope or heart failure indicate an inadequate rate for cardiac output and the need for pacing. This may be elective if postsurgical, if 24-hour ECG taping indicates poor variability or a rate below a critical level (e.g. less than 55 bpm in an infant), or if a progressive increase in ventricular size is evident (incipient dilated cardiomyopathy). Pacing is usually endocardial except for infants and generators can be expected to last 5–10 years. A recurrence of symptoms when paced requires urgent referral for pacemaker interrogation.

Syncope in the young

This can be defined as a self-limited loss of consciousness and postural tone, secondary to lack of adequate brainstem perfusion, with variable warning symptoms and complete spontaneous recovery. Syncope is common, effecting 15% of children, particularly adolescent girls. A separate peak at 6–18 months is seen associated with breath-holding attacks (discussed in Chapter 19, Paediatric Neurology). Although alarming, it is usually completely benign. Episodes can be frequent (even daily), disrupting school and sporting activities, and can be associated with fall-related injuries. It is usually a self-limiting condition, lasting some 6–24 months. However, it may be the first indication of a lethal arrhythmia (long QT syndrome) or severe CHD (aortic stenosis or hypertrophic cardiomyopathy). Consequently, the symptom warrants careful evaluation, along with family and past medical history, examination, and usually a 12-lead ECG.

The commonest cause is reflex syncope (also known as neurally mediated, vasovagal, vasodepressor, orthostatic, or neurocardiogenic) and is the result of a paradoxical response of the autonomic nervous system to certain triggers, causing hypotension and/or bradycardia. Triggers include prolonged standing in crowded warm conditions ('church syncope'), pain or injury, after intense exercise, emotional stress (sight of blood), alcohol, or illicit drug use, etc. Prodromal symptoms are usual: dizziness, weakness, dimming or blurred vision, nausea, feeling hot or cold, sweating, and facial pallor with dilated pupils. Myoclonic movements are frequent and occur after falling, in contrast to epilepsy where jerking or tonic–clonic movements begin while standing. Loss of consciousness is usually less than 2 minutes (over 5 minutes with a seizure). Examination during an episode will reveal hypotension and bradycardia (tachycardia and hypertension during a seizure). Other features of epilepsy are usually absent: incontinence, tongue biting and frothing, cyanosis, and a prolonged period of post-ictal confusion, although disorientation and fatigue are common.

Most syncopal episodes with differentiation from epilepsy, can easily be diagnosed from a detailed history. Examination should include cardiac auscultation and lying to standing blood pressures (a fall of greater than 20 mmHg systolic or 10 mmHg diastolic BP within 3 minutes of standing is positive for orthostatic reflex hypotension), as well as neurological assessment. Early referral is warranted when there is a history of CHD (treated or untreated), a pathological murmur, a family history of sudden death, when an injury occurred (no warning) or an episode that occurred during (as opposed to after) exercise. Investigations in most cases can otherwise be limited to a 12-lead ECG to help exclude long QT syndrome, Brugada syndrome, cardiomyopathy, and pre-excitation. Any ECG abnormality or a strong history of associated preceding palpitations would also justify referral to a paediatric cardiologist for further investigations, such as 24–72-hour ECG taping. An echocardiogram is only helpful if there is evidence of structural heart disease.

Assuming all of the above findings are normal and a diagnosis of reflex syncope is made, treatment strategies include reassurance that the episodes are not dangerous and are self-limiting, ensuring an adequate fluid intake (3–4 litres/day for a teenager) and generous salt consumption. A letter to the school can be helpful requesting that s/he be allowed to sit during trigger events such as assembly or if s/he experience prodromal symptoms. Isometric manoeuvres such as leg crossing, tensing abdominal musculature, etc. can also help to prevent a full syncopal episode. Should these manoeuvres fail and the episodes are frequent, referral to a paediatric cardiologist would be appropriate, to consider a Tilt Table Test and therapy such as fludrocortisone or beta blockade.

Chest pain in the young

Chest pain is a frequent complaint in older children and adolescents, giving rise to much anxiety. It is very rarely cardiac and nearly always musculoskeletal or gastrointestinal in origin, especially when it occurs at rest in an otherwise healthy child. It is important to document the characteristics of the pain: precipitating cause, duration, location, frequency, quality, radiation, and changes with posture or breathing, as well as how the pain is relieved. A family history of ischaemic heart disease or recent stress in the family may be an important factor in anxiety associated chest discomfort, particularly if the location and type of pain is variable over time.

If the examination reveals no cardiorespiratory abnormalities and the pain is reproducible by local examination, it is almost certainly of musculoskeletal origin. The pain is usually sharp, intermittent, and short lived, and worse with ventilatory exertion. If there is anterior precordial local tenderness and the pain more sustained, costochondritis is likely. Reassurance and the judicious use of anti-inflammatories are in order. In cases where there is some doubt, a normal ECG will usually be sufficient to further reassure the family.

Factors that would suggest referral and further investigations are an acute severe unremitting pain in an unwell individual, or any abnormal physical findings (e.g. pathological murmur or chest signs). Also a history of pain with syncope, palpitations, during exercise (without local tenderness or reproducibility), or a past history of CHD, Marfan's syndrome, or Kawasaki disease. Investigations usually will include an ECG, echocardiogram, a chest X-ray, and possibly formal exercise testing.

General issues in children with heart disease

Prescribing for congenital heart disease

The primary care physician will be asked to prescribe vaccinations for children with CHD as well as ongoing medications. It is recommended that therapy changes and the prescription of new cardiac drugs for children are only undertaken in liaison with the paediatric cardiac team.

* **Vaccinations.** In general, all routine immunizations should be given at the appropriate times for children with CHD. However, they should be avoided 10 days before, and up to 6 weeks after heart surgery. Children under 2 years of age on medications for heart failure or with other significant CHD may warrant respiratory syncytial virus prophylaxis (palivizumab) injections (monthly from October to March) to prevent viral bronchiolitis. Similarly, influenza and pneumococcal vaccination is recommended for these children with major CHD at any age.

* **Diuretics.** These are used for those with heart failure from whatever cause. The usual regime is furosemide and spironolactone at 1 mg/kg per dose twice daily, the combination being used to maintain potassium homeostasis. Electrolyte levels are not usually required if the doses are balanced. It is common for children post-surgery to be on diuretics for the first few weeks until their first outpatient review.

* **Digoxin.** This is now rarely used in children except as an adjunct for myocardial failure and occasionally in infants with SVT. It is not required for excessive pulmonary flow as there is rarely the need for inotropic augmentation.

* **ACE inhibitors** (captopril, enalapril, lisinopril). These afterload-reducing agents improve cardiac output by decreasing systemic vascular resistance in those with myocardial dysfunction and ameliorating mitral and aortic regurgitation. They are occasionally used as an adjunct in left-to-right shunt mediated heart failure. It is not uncommon to require ACE inhibitors for a few months after major CHD surgery.

* **Beta blockers.** These are a useful for certain arrhythmias (SVT, long QT syndrome), refractory syncope and in Marfan's syndrome to prevent excessive aortic root dilation. Atenolol is often used as it is long acting and relatively β_1 selective, given the frequency of asthma in children. Carvedilol is used as an adjunct in refractory myocardial failure.

* **Anticoagulation.** Antiplatelet dose aspirin (5 mg/kg daily) is prescribed for maintenance of shunt patency and in Kawasaki disease with coronary abnormalities. The risk of Reyes syndrome in children taking aspirin at this dose remains theoretical, as no cases have been reported. It is advised that aspirin should be ceased during any influenzal or varicella illness, until symptoms resolve. Warfarin is used after

mechanical prosthetic valve replacement (INR 3–3.5), in dilated cardiomyopathy (INR 2.5) and after Fontan type operations (INR 2.5), with the need for frequent monitoring in hospital, preferably with additional home kits. Monitoring difficulties in children has lead many centres to switch to a combination of aspirin and clopidogrel, except for mechanical valves.

◆ **Anti-arrhythmic drugs.** The most frequently used are atenolol, flecainide (requiring levels), and amiodarone. Standard adult precautions and restrictions are required.

Congenital heart disease exercise restrictions

In general, no exercise restrictions are required for most children with CHD. However, many patients with more complex lesions, even after repair, will find that they are unable to fully keep pace with their peers. Children should not be restricted but encouraged to do as much as they feel able. A child is more likely to optimize their activity level if sport and energetic break time activities are paced and interspersed with less physically demanding pursuits as necessary.

Competitive sports should be curtailed in patients with severe aortic stenosis, marked hypertrophic cardiomyopathy, established pulmonary vascular disease (Eisenmenger's syndrome), complete AV block, severe unrepaired cyanotic CHD, and those with impaired ventricular function. Usually the timing of an intervention will minimize any such restrictions (e.g. for aortic stenosis). After repair of more complex defects requiring a ventriculotomy, there may be a propensity for cardiac dysrhythmias. Formal exercise testing in such cases is advisable if the child will be involved in competitive sports.

Contact and high impact sports, such as rugby or boxing are restricted in those with a dilated aortic root (Marfan's syndrome), those with pacemakers, for the first 3 months postsurgery and in those on anticoagulation therapy. Isometric exercise (weight training) is discouraged in those with left heart disease such as aortic stenosis, aortic dilation or cardiomyopathy.

Long-term morbidity of congenital heart disease

1. Most of those with CHD have a lifelong risk of infective endocarditis, with 4% of admissions to adult CHD units attributable to this disease.

2. Quality of life assessment in adults with significant CHD have shown reduced physical functioning and general health perception, compared with the general population, especially in those with cyanotic lesions who additionally may have reduced social functioning, energy levels, and mental health, and are more likely to be in pain (Lane *et al.* 2002).

3. Other non-cardiac complications occasionally encountered, particularly with cyanotic CHD, are skeletal deformities (e.g. pectus, scoliosis), renal disease, bleeding dyscrasias, and gall stones.

Altitude and congenital heart disease

Patients with cyanotic CHD will feel the effects of altitude at over 2000 metres due to the fall in atmospheric oxygen tension, particularly if severely cyanosed. Commercial flights are pressurized to about 2500 metres and supplemental oxygen may be required. Patients with unrepaired tetralogy of Fallot are particularly at risk of hypercyanotic spells and require particular care. Patients with established pulmonary vascular disease should avoid flying and altitude where possible but can be formally assessed by a paediatric cardiology or respiratory unit for their fitness to fly, by breathing reduced oxygen content air mixtures. Other lesions with dominantly left-to-right shunts may actually be improved at altitude, due to reactive pulmonary vasoconstriction.

References

Abu-Harb M, Hey E, Wren C (1994). Death in infancy from unrecognised congenital heart disease. *Archives of Disease in Childhood* **71**: 3–7.

Anderson RH, Baker EJ, Macartney FJ, Rigby ML, Shinebourne EA, Tynan M (eds) (2005) *Paediatric Cardiology*, (2nd edn). Churchill Livingstone, London, 2 volumes.

Archer N, Godman MJ, Houston AB, Roxy NS (1998). Cardiovascular disease. In Campbell AGM, McIntosh N (eds), *Forfar & Arneil's Textbook of Paediatrics*: Section 14, (5th edn). Churchill Livingstone, London.

Bull C (1999). Current and potential impact of fetal diagnosis on prevalence and spectrum of serious congenital heart disease at term in the UK. *Lancet* **354**: 1242–1247.

Hoffman J (2005). Incidence, mortality and natural history. In: Anderson RH, Baker EJ, Macartney FJ, Rigby ML, Shinebourne EA, Tynan M (eds), *Paediatric Cardiology*, (2nd edn). Churchill Livingstone, London, Vol. 1, pp. 122–123.

Lane D, Lip G, Millane T (2002). Quality of life in adults with congenital heart disease. *Heart* **88**: 71–75.

Newburger JW, Takahashi M, Gerber MA, Gewitz MH, Tani LY, Burns JC, Shulman ST, Bolger AF, Ferrieri P, Baltimore RS, Wilson WR, Baddour LM, Levison ME, Pallasch TJ, Falace DA, and Taubert KA (2004). Diagnosis, treatment, and long-term management of Kawasaki disease: a statement for health professionals from the Committee on Rheumatic Fever, Endocarditis and Kawasaki Disease, Council on Cardiovascular Disease in the Young, American Heart Association. *Circulation* **110**(17): 2747–2771.

Perloff JK, Warnes CA (2001). Challenges posed by adults with repaired congenital heart disease. *Circulation* **103**: 2637–2643.

Peterson S, Peto V, Rayner M (2003). *Congenital Heart Disease Statistics 2003*. British Heart Foundation Statistics Database. http://www.heartstats.org

Richmond S, Wren C (2001). Early diagnosis of congenital heart disease. *Seminars in Fetal and Neonatal Medicine* **6**: 27–35.

Innocent murmur sheet

http://www.rch.org.au/cardiology/health-info.cfm?doc_id=3537
http://kirkies.net/chdguide/conditions/innocent_murmur.htm

Chapter 14

Paediatric haematology

Shubha Allard and Cecil Reid

The blood count in childhood

Apart from the platelet count, most other haematological parameters are age related and the appropriate normal range for age will be provided by the laboratory. Physiological changes in the haemoglobin and haematocrit are considered below but it is important to note that after the macrocytosis seen at birth, the mean cell volume (MCV) falls rapidly. Most children are microcytic by adult criteria from 3 months of age with adult values only attained at puberty.

A lymphocytosis (both relative and absolute) is normal in infancy and even in children up to 4–6 years of age. Apart from this physiological variation, a marked lymphocytosis may also be seen in pertussis or certain viral infections (e.g. adenovirus) and in infectious mononucleosis. In the latter case the atypical cells have a characteristic appearance and the Paul-Bunnell screen may be diagnostic.

Anaemia

Characterization of the anaemic infant or child must take into account both the age and (in infants) the birth history. The haemoglobin as well as the red cell indices only reach adult values at around puberty.

Physiological anaemia and prematurity

The blood count at birth is not directly affected by maternal deficiencies of iron or other haematinics such as folate or vitamin B12 although the infant's iron stores will be reduced by maternal iron deficiency, by early clamping of the cord and by prematurity. Anaemia at birth has other causes that originate *in-utero*. These include feto-maternal or twin-to-twin blood loss, rhesus haemolytic disease, and rarely inherited haemoglobin disorders such as homozygous alpha-thalassaemia. These conditions are outside the scope of this review and will not be considered further here.

In the normal new-born infant of whatever gestational age the high Hb (19 ± 2 g/dl) and fetal haemoglobin (HbF) levels of 60–90% are both factors that enhance oxygen acquisition from the placenta. With the establishment of normal air breathing and better oxygenation, there is a switch to adult haemoglobin production (HbA) and a temporary reduction in red cell production. This results in a fall in infant Hb levels of about 30% to a nadir of 11 g/dl by 8 weeks of postnatal life (in full-term infants), which is sometimes termed physiological anaemia. Most of the body iron in the new-born is within red cells

Box 14.1 Anaemia from birth to 3 years

- Physiological anaemia appears at 8 weeks in term and at 4–8 weeks in pre-term infants
- Iron deficiency peaks at 18 months (Hb <11 g/dl), is usually of dietary origin and commoner in low birthweight infants who require supplementation from 8 weeks to 1 year
- Iron deficiency anaemia (hypochromic microcytic anaemia, elevated RDW, ferritin < 10 µg/l) is treated with 3 mg elemental iron/kg per day
- Iron deficiency in infancy may affect behaviour and cause developmental delay

(75 mg/kg) and the total mass of red cells determines the likelihood of later iron deficiency. In full-term infants this iron is sufficient for the first 4 months and the Hb rises to 12.5 g/dl by 4 months after which the infant depends upon external sources of iron to maintain a healthy Hb.

In premature infants however, the lower blood volume and faster growth rate means that physiological anaemia occurs earlier (4–8 weeks) and is more severe (6.5–9 g/dl) than in term infants. There is evidence that delayed cord clamping and the administration of recombinant erythropoietin over the early weeks of life may prevent this problem and reduce the need for blood transfusion in very low birthweight infants. Iron stores are exhausted by 2–3 months of age after which time they are at particular risk for developing iron deficiency.

Iron deficiency anaemia in infancy (Box 14.1)

Incidence

Iron deficiency is the commonest cause of anaemia in young children between 6 months and 3 years of age reaching a peak at 18 months. It is currently defined as a Hb less than 11 g/dl between 6 months and 2 years with hypochromic microcytic red cell indices and low iron levels. Unlike in adults the cause is most commonly dietary and the incidence, particularly high in deprived inner cities and in Asian children, is susceptible to adequate public health measures. Thus in America, iron deficiency anaemia in this age group has more than halved over 20 years as a result of education in breast feeding and provision of iron supplemented formulae. In the UK prevalence remains high—in some areas from 12 to 20%, mainly in socio-economically deprived or Asian populations.

Investigation of iron deficiency

In most cases the anaemia and accompanying hypochromic and microcytic red blood cells are clear indications of the nature of the anaemia. There is anisocytosis and this variation in red cell size is reflected in an elevated red cell distribution width (RDW >15). This differentiates the condition from thalassaemia minor (alpha or beta), which may also cause a microcytic anaemia but without elevation of the RDW.

In the presence of such a clear blood picture, iron studies are not mandatory. In doubtful cases, iron status may be estimated in a number of ways. A low serum ferritin (<10 µg/l) reflects depleted iron stores but its elevation in an acute phase response associated with infection or inflammation may cause confusion. A low transferrin saturation (<10%)

or high zinc protoporphyrin (>3 μg/gHb) are other laboratory indicators but are also subject to false positive results like ferritin. The transferrin receptor assay, especially together with ferritin estimation, is the most reliable assay of iron deficiency but is not yet widely available in the UK.

Prevention and treatment

Ensuring adequate maternal nutrition and avoiding immediate clamping of the umbilical vessels (especially in pre-term infants) are ante- and per-natal measures that may minimize later onset of iron deficiency. A full-term infant requires 280 mg of additional iron in the first year of life (1 mg/kg per day after 4 months), which should be met by correct feeding practice. The increased requirements of pre-term and low birthweight infants must be recognized and treated appropriately. In low birthweight infants the iron need is doubled from 2 months of age and is even higher in very low birthweights (3–4 mg/kg/day at birthweights of <1000 g to 1500g). In these infants iron supplementation is necessary from no later than 8 weeks and continued throughout the first year of life.

Sources of dietary iron

Best absorbed is haem iron (25%) but this makes up only up to 10% of the infant diet. Non-haem iron in human and cow's milk (1 mg/l) is variably absorbed. Breast milk iron is uniquely well absorbed: 50% is absorbed compared to only 10% in cows' milk. Cereals that are a staple of infants' diets contain phytates and other factors that can inhibit iron absorption whereas ascorbic acid and orange juice actually enhance absorption.

Prevention

Clearly the dietary measures that will reduce the incidence of iron deficiency in young children are therefore:

- providing breast milk for at least 5–6 months where possible
- non-breast-fed infants should have formula supplemented with 12 mg/l additional iron to 1 year of life
- iron enriched cereal should be provided at weaning.

There is some evidence that whole cows' milk may induce gastrointestinal blood loss and should therefore particularly be avoided. This is not true of infant formula.

Treatment

It is perfectly justifiable to give a therapeutic trial in likely iron deficiency even if not conclusively proven by iron studies. A dose of 3 mg/kg of elemental iron (as 15 mg ferrous sulphate, 9 mg ferrous fumarate, or 26 mg ferrous gluconate) should result in a Hb rise of 1 g/dl after 1 month. It should be continued for 2–3 months but discontinued if no response is seen. Below 3 years non-dietary causes of iron deficiency such as blood loss are rare but may need investigating if therapeutic non-compliance can be excluded.

The clinical significance of iron deficiency in early life should not be underestimated. There is good evidence for behavioural changes and developmental delay in iron deficiency anaemia before 2 years. It is likely that this is related to the anaemia itself and most, though not all studies, show reversibility with treatment.

Iron deficiency in older children

Beyond 2–3 years, dietary iron deficiency is less common and other causes must be considered. These include

- *Gastrointestinal blood loss*. Meckel's diverticulum or hereditary telangiectasia are rare congenital disorders and whole cows' milk may itself induce bleeding as well as being a poor source of iron. Parasites, especially *Ancylostoma* or *Necator* are hookworm infestations prevalent in much of the world. The infections, acquired through the naked feet, are common causes of chronic anaemia world wide and easily excluded by stool studies.
- *Iron malabsorption* is a common presentation of both tropical and non-tropical sprue (coeliac disease). Rarely it may complicate inflammatory bowel disease (Crohn's) or following loss of bowel by surgical excision.

Macrocytic anaemia

Red cells are normally much larger at birth (physiological macrocytosis) however, the mean cell volume falls to below the normal adult range (80–98 fl) by 6 months of life. Thereafter macrocytosis is rare and only occasionally due to deficiencies of folate or vitamin B12. Both haematinics are normal at birth even if there is maternal deficiency; however, pre-term infants are more liable to folate deficiency in the postnatal period. Vitamin B deficiency is rare and may relate to inflammatory bowel disease or a rare congenital inability to absorb the vitamin from the gut (Imerslund–Grasbeck syndrome).

Other causes of macrocytosis include hypothyroidism, cyanotic heart disease, Downs syndrome, and drugs. The latter especially include anticonvulsants, HIV drugs (zidovudine), and trimethoprim–sulfamethoxazole (septrin).

Finally, reticulocytes are large red cells so that macrocytosis may accompany any chronic haemolytic process. Conversely, a stressed bone marrow may also cause a macrocytic anaemia and causes include aplastic anaemia, Diamond–Blackfan (congenital hypoplastic) anaemia and dyserythropoietic anaemias.

Haemolytic anaemias

Destruction of red blood cells may occur acutely, either through an environmental trigger factor such as a drug or infection as in glucose-6-phosphate dehydrogenase (G-6PD) deficiency or through autoimmune haemolysis. It may also be chronic, most commonly owing to a congenital abnormality in the structure of the red cell membrane proteins (hereditary spherocytosis and elliptocytosis) or of the haemoglobin within it (haemoglobinopathies).

Haemolytic anaemias may occur at any age from intrauterine life (severe rhesus haemolytic disesase, α^0/α^0 thalassaemia) through the perinatal and neonatal periods to later childhood. A logical approach to diagnosis takes into account age, ethnicity, symptoms, and family history as well as a range of laboratory investigations (See Box 14.2).

Investigation of haemolysis

Some degree of jaundice is likely as well as the pallor caused by the anaemia, which can be severe. Most important in the history are a record of previous occurrences (including neonatal jaundice), recent administration of drugs or of infections, and a family history. This should include family histories of gall stones, cholecystectomy as well as of anaemia or jaundice. Parents must be asked about the child's urine as discoloration with dark brown, red, or even black urine is tell-tale evidence of intravascular haemolysis. Fever may be present and mild splenomegaly may be found.

The laboratory investigations are both general and specific.

General investigation Full blood count to confirm anaemia, reticulocyte count and blood film inspection looking for characteristic red cell changes (polychromasia, spherocytes, elliptocytes or contracted red cells, 'hemi-ghosts' seen in G-6PD deficiency sickled or target red cells). Bilirubin and lactate dehydrogenase are invariably elevated with increased red cell destruction.

Occasionally, in chronic haemolytic diseases an aplastic bone marrow arrest occurs. This serious and acute event results in a drastic fall in haemoglobin with an accompanying reticulocytopenia. It may be caused by an infection with the parvovirus B19 (an otherwise fairly innocuous agent associated with 'fifth disease' in childhood) or with acute folate deficiency.

Specific investigation

- G-6PD screen and assay to confirm deficiency. This may give an initially spuriously normal result in patients with reticulocytosis as these young cell may express higher levels in some types of G-6PD deficiency.

- Hereditary spherocytosis (HS). Confirmation of the spherocytes seen on the blood film by showing their increased fragility by either osmotic fragility studies or the rapid acidified glycerol lysis test (AGLT). Recently a more specific flow cytometry technique (EMA) has proved of greater specificity. Inspection of parental blood films may also be helpful

- Direct antiglobulin test (DAT or Coombs' test). This identifies immunoglobulin (IgG) or complement products on the red cell surface. A weak DAT (+) may be irrelevant unless accompanied by other signs of haemolysis but a strong DAT (++/+++) for IgG with or without complement suggests a warm antibody autoimmune haemolysis. This may be primary or secondary to another chronic disorder.

- Serum haptoglobin: A fall, often to zero, of this parameter is characteristic of severe intravascular red cell destruction. Once bound to free haemoglobin the complex is renally cleared leading to falling serum values.

- Haemoglobin electrophoresis: to exclude haemoglobinopathy (see section below).

◆ Other tests: the above screening tests are readily performed at the local hospital laboratory. In some cases this proves insufficient and samples may be sent to specialist centres for flow cytometry, red cell membrane analysis (by sodium dodecyl sulphate–polyacrylamide gel electrophoresis), or red cell enzyme studies to exclude rarer causes of inherited red cell disorders such as pyruvate kinase or hexokinase deficiency. Other rare membrane conditions including hereditary pyropoikolocytosis, stomatocytosis, or xerocytosis may need to be excluded in specialist centres.

Clinical presentation and management of haemolytic anaemias

Haemolytic anaemias are not frequently encountered in primary care however, the two most common pathologies are dealt with below.

Hereditary spherocytosis (HS) and elliptocytosis (HE) HS is a dominantly inherited disorder of the red cell membrane though sporadic non-familial cases may occur (10%). It may present in the neonatal period with jaundice but often the first presentation with anaemia, jaundice, and moderate splenomegaly is in childhood or even adult life. The severity is very variable and probably reflects which of the numerous mutations of red cell membrane proteins (spectrin, ankyrin, band 3, protein 4.2) is causing a deficiency.

Manifestations range from a chronic anaemia (Hb 6–8 g/dl) with jaundice and reticulocytosis to being completely asymptomatic. The latter mild cases may suffer from occasional episodes of exacerbated haemolysis (during infections or pregnancy) and these as well as the more severe cases are all prone to develop gall stones. Though a modest reticulocytosis is typical even of well compensated patients with little or no anaemia, an aplastic bone marrow arrest due to parvovirus B19 infection is a feared complication requiring rapid recognition, hospital admission, and transfusion.

All identified individuals should receive folate supplements for life to avoid megaloblastic bone marrow arrest. Chronically anaemic patients and/or those with gall stones benefit from splenectomy, which results in remission of most symptoms. If needed, cholecystectomy is carried out at the same time. The ensuing risk of post-splenectomy sepsis must be considered and adequate prophylactic measures adopted. As the risks are greatest in the very young child, this procedure is not usually considered under the age of 6 years.

HE is characterized by variable numbers of elliptocytes on the blood film. In most cases patients are asymptomatic, the features are identified incidentally and are of little significance. Occasional patients will have acute or compensated haemolysis such as HS. The rare infantile condition of hereditary pyropoikilocytosis is actually a variant of HE presenting with a microcytic anaemia, jaundice, and bizarre red cell fragments in early life.

G-6PD deficiency This X-linked disorder produces instability of the red cell membrane to oxidative stresses that may result from a number of causes (ingestion of fava beans, certain drugs, and infections). Mostly the haemolytic episodes, which may be severe, are acute and self-limiting following one of these 'insults'. However, a deficiency may also be an infrequent cause of jaundice in the new born and rarely lead to a chronic non-spherocytic haemolytic anaemia. The pentose–phosphate shunt, with glucose-6-phosphate as its substrate, is vital to the maintenance of reduced glutathione in the red cell. This 'mops up' hydrogen peroxide generated by free oxygen radicals but its lack in G-6PD deficiency predisposes to red cell destruction, which is largely intravascular.

In an acute episode, the child rapidly becomes pale and jaundiced and with a highly characteristic dark red, brown or even black urine owing to haemoglobinuria. Pale and tachycardic, the child is usually obviously unwell and a blood count shows anaemia, which may be profound. The blood film is highly typical with many small contracted red cells, often with spherocytes, 'bite cells', and cells in which the haemoglobin occupies only a portion of the cell ('hemighosts'). Diagnosis is confirmed by a G-6PD enzyme screen in the laboratory or by assay of the enzyme itself.

It is important to bear two things in mind in this situation. First, the enzyme screen may sometimes be normal in the acute episode as fresh new red cells have higher enzyme levels than do older cells. Reinvestigation when the episode has subsided will then reveal the diagnosis. Secondly, though hemizygous males are most usually affected, females may also be susceptible because of a genetic process called 'imbalanced lyonization' with sufficient numbers of G-6PD deficient cells to cause haemolysis or much more rarely because of homozygosity in the female.

Spontaneous recovery occurs within 3–6 weeks, nevertheless transfusion may be needed. A careful family history should be taken to identify other potential family members and parents counselled about how to avoid such episodes in future. Avoidance of fava beans and of those drugs that induce haemolysis are key and they should be given a list of agents that may or will definitely provoke further attacks.

Other causes of haemolysis Autoimmune haemolytic anaemia is uncommon in childhood and as in adults is usually caused by IgG antibody directed at core red cell antigen giving a positive direct antiglobulin test (DAT or Coombs' test). The blood picture is spherocytic, there is a reticulocytosis and jaundice but splenomegaly, if present, is usually only slight. Though frequently idiopathic and usually responsive to treatment with steroids, it may also be secondary to other disorders, including systemic lupus and lymphomas or, rarely in children, to drugs.

Serious and fortunately uncommon causes of intravascular haemolysis are the related disorders of haemolytic uraemic syndrome and thrombotic thrombocytopenic pupura. Children with these so-called microangiopathic haemolytic disorders develop red cell fragmentation, thrombocytopenia, and accompanying renal failure or neurological abnormalities.

Neutropenia and neutrophilia in childhood

The normal neutrophil count is both age and race related. The normal lower limit in white infants is $1.0 \times 10^9/l$ rising to $1.5 \times 10^9/l$ after 1 year but the range is lower in Afro-Caribbeans. In these children levels may be $0.2–0.6 \times 10^9/l$ lower than in whites. Low white cell counts and specifically neutropenia often give rise to concern though in the majority of cases this is unwarranted. The likelihood of infections caused by the

Box 14.2 Haemolytic anaemia

In the anaemic jaundiced child

History

Ethnicity, family history of anaemia, jaundice, or gall stones
Drug ingestion, foods (broad beans)
Dark, even black urine

Laboratory tests

Film appearances: spherocytes, red cell fragments, hemi-ghosts, reticulocytosis or sickled or target red cells.
Direct antiglobulin test (DAT), osmotic fragility, glycerol lysis test or EMA, bilirubin and LDH.

neutropenia is only substantially increased where counts are $0.5 \times 10^9/l$ or less. In most cases where counts are more modestly reduced the cause is either age or race related or else is temporary and due to concurrent viral infections especially hepatitis, respiratory syncitial virus, or the exanthems. It may last for only 3–6 days and is not of clinical significance. However, if other blood count abnormalities are also present the approach must be more guarded as an accompanying unexplained anaemia or thrombocytopenia are likely to indicate a more serious pathology.

An acute or chronic severe neutropenia ($<0.5 \times 10^9/l$) is much less common and acquired causes include:

♦ Drug induced (especially sulfas, antithyroid, or anticonvulsants—though virtually any drug may be responsible).

♦ Severe sepsis.

♦ Autoimmune (systemic lupus or other connective tissue disorders and sometimes occurring together with idiopathic autoimmune haemolysis or thrombocytopenia).

♦ Felty's syndrome. The triad of splenomegaly, neutropenia, and rheumatoid arthritis is much rarer in children than in adults. The pathology is complex involving suppression of granulopoiesis (by humoral and cellular immunity) as well hypersplenism. Some, though not all children, with severe infectious complications will respond to splenectomy or treatment with granulocyte colony-stimulating factor.

Inherited and congenital causes are:

♦ Kostman's syndrome, which if untreated, is fatal in early life. It may be responsive to treatment with granulocyte colony-stimulating factor though evolution to leukaemia may occur.

♦ Cyclical neutropenia causes 21-day oscillations in white cells and platelets and many individuals suffer fevers and infections at the nadir of neutrophil counts.

◆ Shwachman's syndrome refers to the neutropenia that accompanies the rare multiorgan disease that includes pancreatic failure.

◆ Familial benign neutropenia may be dominantly inherited, is chronic, mild and of little clinical significance.

Malignant disorders of blood in childhood

The diagnosis and management of these conditions are outside the scope of primary care, however, children benefit from prompt referral through recognition of relevant clinical or laboratory findings.

Acute leukaemia

The presence of pallor often accompanied by lassitude or fevers or a purpuric or petechial rash always requires a blood count, which may be diagnostic. In either acute lymphoblastic or myeloblastic leukaemia up to 40% of children may have hepatomegaly or splenomegaly and there may be lymph node enlargement. Bone or joint pain with tenderness is quite a common presentation unlike in adults and the child may develop a limp. Occasionally leukaemic blasts may not be identified right away on the blood film but anaemia with either neutropenia or thrombocytopenia should always raise suspicion and generally warrants bone marrow examination.

Lymphomas

Enlarged lymph nodes are often a cause for parental concern and the decision whether to refer for further investigation can be tricky. Lymphadenopathy will require prompt referral if it is persistent or progressive and especially if painless or accompanied by fevers unrelated to an obvious infectious focus. Lower cervical, supraclavicular, or generalized lymphadenopathy, an abdominal mass or hepatosplenomegaly are all pointers to more serious disease. An Epstein–Barr virus screen may eliminate infectious mononucleosis and a chest X-ray will highlight mediastinal widening or if hilar nodes are affected.

Thrombocytopenia

The normal range for the platelet count in the neonatal period and childhood is similar to that in adults (generally $150–400 \times 10(/l)$. Thrombocytopenia is relatively common and can be found in about 1 % of all apparently normal neonates but is much commoner in unwell infants affecting $\approx 40\%$ of neonates in intensive care.

Causes of thrombocytopenia

In the majority of cases thrombocytopenia in childhood results from increased destruction of platelets due to acquired factors. There are however several uncommon but well recognized inherited thrombocytopenias such as Wiskott–Aldrich syndrome (eczema, immunodeficiency, thrombocytopenia), Bernard Soulier and Chediak Higashi (marked platelet dysfunction).

Destruction of platelets in the neonatal period can be due to maternal factors such as antibodies crossing the placenta in maternal autoimmune thrombocytopenia or in the rarer neonatal alloimmune thrombocytopenia or intrauterine infections such as toxoplasmosis, rubella, cytomegalovirus, parvovirus, or HIV. Consumption of platelets is commonly seen in sick neonates and can be secondary to infection and various hypercoagulable states such as birth asphyxia, respiratory distress syndrome, necrotizing enterocolitis or, haemolytic disease of the newborn.

Disseminated intravascular coagulation in the neonatal period or childhood, resulting in consumption of platelets, can be triggered by many causes including infection, trauma, e.g. burns, liver disease, malignancy, e.g. leukaemia, and acute haemolysis.

Haemolytic uraemic syndrome associated with fever, low platelets, microangiopathic blood film with red cell fragmentation, and renal failure, is usually seen in children in relation to seasonal epidemics of gastroenteritis caused by *Escherichia coli* verotoxin (Strain 0157:H7).

Bone marrow failure syndromes are rare but serious causes of thrombocytopenia in childhood requiring prompt recognition and treatment and include conditions such as acute leukaemia, aplastic anaemia, metastatic neuroblastoma, etc. There is generally reduction of other cell lines with anaemia and neutropenia, i.e. pancytopenia.

Immune thrombocytopenic purpura (ITP)

Childhood ITP has an incidence of between 4.0 and 5.3 per 100 000. Autoantibodies (generally IgG) complex with membrane proteins on platelets and this results in increased and premature removal of platelets from the circulation by the reticuloen-dothelial system, especially the spleen. The normal life span of the platelet is 7 days but in ITP this is reduced to just a few hours.

Acute ITP is the most common type seen in childhood with chronic ITP (lasting >6 months) being the predominant type in adults. In about 75% of affected children there is a preceding trigger such as vaccination or viral infection. ITP may be provoked by the measles, mumps, and rubella (MMR) vaccine, with an estimated risk of 1 in 24 000 doses usually occurring within 6 weeks of vaccination. Children who develop ITP following chicken pox infection need particular scrutiny since in occasional cases more complex coagulation disorders with antibodies directed against proteins S and/or C can occur.

The first signs of bleeding are often easy bruising and petechiae. Adolescents girls can develop troublesome menorrhagia. More serious bleeding such as severe epistaxis or gastrointestinal bleeding occurs only in about 4% of children with ITP. Several studies have confirmed that the incidence of intracranial haemorrhage (ICH) is much less than the 1–3% widely quoted, and is closer to 0.1–0.5%. Antiplatelet drugs such as aspirin or non-steroidal anti-inflammatory drugs, e.g. brufen can further exacerbate risk of bleeding.

The diagnosis of childhood ITP is by exclusion. Apart from bleeding and a low platelet count there should be no other abnormal physical findings and in particular the spleen is not palpable. The haemoglobin and white cell count are typically normal unless the child has developed iron deficiency anaemia due to blood loss. The blood film shows reduced number of platelets and these are often large with normal white cell and red cell appearances (unless iron deficiency). Bone marrow examination is not necessary in children with typical signs and symptoms of ITP described above without any atypical features. Bone marrow examination may be indicated if symptoms persist beyond 6 months, or if treatment with steroids is indicated. In the latter patients with chronic ITP additional laboratory testing is indicated to exclude other autoimmune disease in particular systemic lupus erythematosus and antiphospholipid syndrome.

Bruising and purpura may sometimes be of gradual onset, developing more slowly over weeks or months. In these children particular attention should be paid to the possibility of a congenital disorder, e.g. Wiskott–Aldrich syndrome if presenting within a few months of life or acute leukaemia or aplastic anaemia in the older child.

The presentation of bruising and purpura in a young child for the first time may raise the possibility of non-accidental injury or meningococcal disease. There are likely to be other clinical features in children with infection and generalized purpura is not a typical feature of non-accidental injury.

ITP in childhood is usually a benign disorder that requires no active treatment other than careful explanation and counselling. The majority of children require no treatment and in 80–85% of cases the disorder resolves within 6 months. Bruising and purpura even if extensive, do not indicate a serious bleeding risk on their own and are not *per se* an indication for treatment. It is, however, essential that the parents, and child where able, have an explanation that this is usually a self-limiting benign disorder. About 15–20% of children develop a chronic form of ITP, which can resemble the more typical adult disease. Chronic ITP in childhood has an estimated incidence of 0.46 per 100 000 children per year and is more likely in patients older then 10 years.

Following initial assessment most children do not require hospital admission and can be managed at home. Parents should be advised to watch for other signs of bleeding and be given a 24-hour emergency contact number with advice to avoid as far as possible contact sports or activities with high risk of trauma or head injury. Other activities can be continued as normal, and the child should be encouraged to continue schooling.

Children with clinically important bleeding, such as severe epistaxis or GI bleeding, do require admission and treatment. The options for treatment to raise the platelet count include steroids (either high-dose prednisolone 4 mg/kg per day for a maximum of 4 days or 1–2 mg/kg per day for no longer than 14 days. Intravenous immunoglobulin can raise the platelet count rapidly, but should only be used for emergency treatment of serious bleeding or in children with ITP needing surgical procedures.

Platelet transfusions are only indicated for intracranial haemorrhage or other life-threatening bleeding and in this situation should be given together with high-dose intravenous steroids or intravenous immunoglobulin.

Splenectomy is rarely indicated in childhood ITP. It is very occasionally indicated in children with chronic severe ITP lasting for more than 12–24 months.

There are various ITP support groups, e.g. the ITP Support Association and these can provide useful support and literature to children and their parents.

Coagulation disorders

The normal response to tissue injury relies on interaction between the blood vessel wall (with immediate vasoconstriction), circulating platelets (with formation of primary platelet plug) and blood coagulation factors (with stabilization of the platelet plug by fibrin). This is accompanied by activation of fibrinolysis with digestion of the haemostatic plug, also an essential component of tissue repair.

At birth, the infant's coagulation parameters are significantly different from the adult range reflecting a physiologically immature haemostatic system. The vitamin K-dependent coagulation factors (II,VII, IX, and X) are ≈20% lower then adult values, whereas levels of fibrinogen, factor VIII, and von Willebrand factor (VWF) are similar to adult values. Recognition of these differences is relevant to clinical problems seen in childhood and accurate diagnosis in younger patients.

Haemorrhagic disease of the newborn

Vitamin K-dependent coagulation factors are low at birth and the levels can decrease even further in the first few days after birth in breast-fed babies and this can result in haemorrhage. The prothrombin time (PT) and activated partial thromboplastin time (APTT) are prolonged. The established practice of intramuscular administration of 1 mg vitamin K to all newborns was thrown into controversy by the possible link with increased childhood leukaemia but several well designed studies have now confirmed the safety of this form of prophylaxis. Oral vitamin K can be effective but concerns remain over absorption and compliance.

Disseminated intravascular coagulation

Widespread consumption of coagulation factors and platelets with fibrin deposition can be triggered in the neonatal period and childhood by many conditions with infection probably being the commonest cause, e.g. meningococcal meningitis.

There may be generalized bleeding in particular widespread bruising, oozing from venepuncture sites and bleeding from the mouth, gastrointestinal tract, and urogenital tract. Less commonly formation of microthrombi can result in ischaemic fingers or toes or end organ damage in particular renal failure.

The PT and APTT are prolonged with low fibrinogen levels and low platelet counts and raised fibrinogen degradation products such as D dimer. Treatment includes prompt management of the underlying cause with aggressive supportive therapy including replacement of coagulation factors with fresh frozen plasma, fibrinogen with cryoprecipitate, and platelet transfusion.

Inherited disorders of coagulation

There are several hereditary deficiencies of coagulation factors with haemophilia A, haemophilia B, and Von Willebrand's disease (VWD) being by far the commonest.

Haemophilia A

This is a sex-linked recessive inherited deficiency of the coagulation protein Factor VIII with a prevalence of 30 to 100 per million population. The severity of bleeding relates to the level of Factor VIII and this is used to classify patients as severe, moderate, or mild haemophilia A.

A male infant with severe haemophilia A will have almost no factor VIII and can present with serious bleeding at birth such as cephalhaematoma or even intracranial haemorrhage, particularly if the mother has a long, difficult labour or instrumental delivery, e.g. forceps or vacuum extraction. If a newborn is not suspected of having haemophilia and undergoes circumcision then there is risk of severe bleeding.

As the infant becomes more active and mobile, from about 9 months of age onwards, joint and muscle bleeds may occur following trauma. Prolonged bleeding can occur from tongue and mouth lacerations and following dental extraction. Head injury is of particular concern with risk of intracranial bleeding and needs prompt assessment. Spontaneous haematuria or bleeding from the gastrointestinal tract can also occur.

Soft tissue bruising can be quite marked especially during the first year of life and can trigger concerns regarding non-accidental injury.

As the child gets older, the frequency of falls will decrease but recurrent joint bleeds (haemarthroses) and muscle haematomas may occur in relation to trauma and active sports. Repeated joint haemorrhage can result in synovial inflammation and thickening with spontaneous re-bleeding unrelated to trauma, i.e. the 'target joint'.

If there is a known family history then the diagnosis of severe haemophilia A can be made either prenatally with chorionic villous sampling for genetic testing or at birth from cord blood coagulation testing which will show a markedly prolonged APTT and a very low Factor VIII level (<1%). The absence of a family history cannot exclude a diagnosis of haemophilia due to the high rate of spontaneous mutations and these occur in about a third of newly diagnosed patients.

Women who are carriers may have low Factor VIII levels themselves but accurate carrier detection requires genetic techniques. Detection of carrier status enables appropriate management of pregnancy including prenatal diagnosis together with option for termination if the mother so wishes, and then taking appropriate steps for minimizing bleeding complications in the affected baby, such as avoidance of vacuum extraction or invasive blood sampling, avoidance of intramuscular injections (vitamin K can be given orally) or cord blood assay for prompt diagnosis.

Patients with severe haemophilia A must be treated in specialized haemophilia centres with ready access to multidisciplinary care. Bleeding episodes need prompt replacement treatment with Factor VIII concentrate. Many haemophilic patients became infected with HIV and then hepatitis C from infected plasma-derived concentrate. The use of new techniques for viral inactivation and more recently the use of recombinant Factor VIII concentrate have greatly improved the safety of treatment. The significant complication of factor VIII inhibitor or antibody formation against infused Factor VIII still remains and may require immunosuppressive therapy.

Patients with milder haemophilia may present later in life with bleeding following trauma. In these patients the drug desmopressin (DDAVP) can be used to raise the patient's own Factor VIII levels to control bleeding. The antifibrinolytic agent, tranexamic acid, can be useful in controlling mucosal bleeding from the mouth.

Any patient with haemophilia undergoing surgery or dental extraction should be managed at a specialized centre with appropriate prophylactic measures to minimize the risk of bleeding.

Haemophilia B (Factor IX deficiency, Christmas disease)

The mode of inheritance, clinical presentation and subsequent progress of patients with haemophilia B is identical to that of haemophilia A and only specific assay of coagulation factors can allow the two disorders to be distinguished. Antenatal carrier detection and the principles of treatment of affected patients are similar to those of haemophilia A. Bleeding complications require replacement therapy with plasma derived or recombinant Factor IX concentrate.

Von Willebrand's disease

VWD is a common inherited bleeding disorder with an estimated prevalence of $\approx$1% of the general population to 125 clinically relevant cases per million. In $\approx$80% of cases the disorder is mild, i.e. type I with mild quantitative deficiency of VWF with the remainder having various type 2 forms with qualitative abnormality of VWF and the type 3 form with total absence of VWF is very rare. The coagulation protein VWF promotes platelet adhesion to the damaged endothelium and is also a carrier molecule for factor VIII.

The inheritance of VWD is autosomal dominant but with variable penetrance and the severity of bleeding can be quite variable from very mild to moderately severe. The typical history includes easy bruising and mucosal bleeding such as epistaxis, menorrhagia, bleeding postdental extraction and following operative procedures, e.g. tonsillectomy.

The coagulation screen may show a prolonged APTT, low factor VIII levels, and VWF levels will be reduced. In contrast to haemophilia A or B, the bleeding time is prolonged due to impaired platelet function in VWD.

Options for treatment of bleeding and prophylaxis prior to dental or surgical procedures include tranexamic acid, DDAVP infusion, which is effective in increasing VWF and factor VIII levels in type 1 VWD and replacement therapy with intermediate purity factor VIII concentrate, containing both VWF and factor VIII, for patients with very low levels.

Family testing should be offered though the generally mild nature of bleeding (except type 3) obviates the need the for prenatal diagnosis.

Haemoglobinopathy

The beta globin gene is expressed at low levels in fetal life and therefore the predominant haemoglobin type in the normal infant at birth is fetal haemoglobin (HbF) consisting of two alpha and two gamma globin chains. The main switch to adult haemoglobin occurs at 3–6 months after birth when production of beta chains largely replaces gamma chain synthesis. Haemoglobinopathies are inherited disorders resulting in either synthesis of an abnormal haemoglobin, e.g. sickle cell anaemia or reduced rate of synthesis of alpha or beta globin chains, i.e. alpha or beta thalassaemia

Sickle cell disease

The sickle gene is particularly found in West Africa (1 in 4 of population) but is also seen in the Middle East, Asia, and South America.

The sickle trait (Hb AS) is a carrier status and is not a form of sickle cell disease. Carriers of childbearing age need genetic counselling and partner testing to enable an informed choice regarding future pregnancy.

The term sickle cell disease describes a group of disorders in which the sickle beta globin gene is inherited of which the commonest is homozygous sickle cell anaemia, i.e. HbSS. Other disorders in this group include HbSC (co-inheritance of Hb S and Hb C gene) and sickle beta thalassaemia (co-inheritance of Hb S and beta thalassaemia gene), which are also associated with problems of sickling.

Sickle haemoglobin polymerizes when deoxygenated and forms insoluble crystals causing red cells to take up a sickle shape and these can block small blood vessels resulting in infarction and organ damage. Sickle cells and target cells are seen on the blood film and the diagnosis is confirmed with haemoglobin electrophoresis. Patients with sickle cell disease have a chronic haemolytic anaemia but this is well tolerated due to low oxygen affinity of Hb S and they do not need regular blood transfusion. Folate supplements are recommended particularly if the diet is low in folate and with increased requirement as in pregnancy.

The clinical hallmark of sickle cell anaemia is the painful bony crises, which can be precipitated by infection, dehydration, and conditions associated with deoxygenation such as general anaesthesia, high altitudes, exposure to cold or vigorous exercise. This may first present in childhood with the hand–foot syndrome, which is painful dactylitis caused by infarction of the small bones. Management includes adequate hydration, prompt treatment of infection, and analgesia.

Infection is an important cause of death worldwide in sickle cell anaemia and babies and children are particularly prone to pneumococcal sepsis. All babies diagnosed with sickle cell anaemia should be commenced on prophylactic penicillin. Pneumoccal vaccination is essential for children with sickle cell disease. Splenic sequestration is an alarming complication with rapid enlargement of spleen with rapid onset of severe anaemia requiring prompt transfusion.

Abdominal pain can be a feature of vaso-occlusive crises and may cause diagnostic difficulties with an acute 'surgical' abdomen. The sickle lung syndrome (dyspnoea, pleuritic chest pain, consolidation on chest X-ray, worsening hypoxia) and neurological complications (stroke, transient ischaemic attacks) require exchange transfusion. Other complications of sickle cell anaemia include aplastic crises (rapid fall in haemoglobin and reticulocyte count) leg ulcers, gallstones, priapism, retinopathy, osteomyelitis, and chronic organ damage, including renal failure and pulmonary hypertension. Any surgical procedure requires caution with adequate hydration and oxygenation essential to avoid exacerbation of sickling.

There is now increasing experience with hydroxyurea as an antisickling drug, which reduces the number of painful crises and clinical trials are ongoing in the use of this agent in children.

Thalassaemia

The thalassaemias are the most common gene disorder worldwide, beta thalassaemia occurs particularly in populations from the Mediterranean, Africa, Middle East, Indian subcontinent, and Asia.

Heterozygotes are carriers and are asymptomatic but do have a microcytic anaemia and this needs to be distinguished from iron deficiency anaemia. Carriers do, however, need genetic counselling in relation to pregnancy and partner testing to identify the risk of a fetus with homozygous thalassaemia.

Patients with the most severe forms of homozygous beta thalassaemia present within the first year of life with failure to thrive due to severe anaemia. Regular blood transfusions allow normal early growth and development but result in iron overload which if inadequately treated with iron chelation results in endocrine and pubertal failure and also cardiac and liver damage.

Further reading

Booth IW, Aukett MA (1997). Iron deficiency in infancy and early childhood. *Archive Diseases of Childhood*, **76**, 549–554.

Oski FA (1993). Iron deficiency in infancy and childhood. *New England Journal of Medicine*, **329**, 190–193.

Nathan DG, Oski FA (2004). *Haematology of infancy and childhood*, (6th edn). WB Saunders, London.

Chapter 15

Height: short and tall stature—when to worry and refer

Tim Cole and Michael Preece

Introduction

Adult stature is one of the least variable biological measures, yet an individual's position in the height distribution is important for their self-image. This is particularly true during the growth period in childhood, where different rates of growth can exacerbate differences in height between individuals. Those who enter puberty early are for a time appreciably taller than their late maturing coevals, and a late-maturing short child is doubly disadvantaged. So both a child's height and their growth tempo are important when assessing possible growth problems.

Natural history of stature

Height (length) increases rapidly during infancy, gaining about 25 cm in the first year. The velocity then slows progressively, and may fall to as little as 3 cm per year before puberty; girls are on average 1 cm shorter than boys during this period. The pubertal growth spurt starts 2 years earlier in girls than boys, and for a short time about 12 years girls are typically slightly taller than boys. Peak height velocity varies between 5 and 12 cm per year, slightly greater in boys than girls. It also tends to be greater in those with an early puberty, to compensate for the reduced growth period. After puberty velocity falls to zero and height growth ends, typically by 16 years in girls and 18 years in boys. However, sometimes height continues to increase into the third decade, particularly in ethnic minorities. Tanner's 'Foetus into man' (Tanner 1978), though now rather old, gives a good summary of human growth.

Over the past 150 years there has been a marked secular trend to increased height, with many children ending up taller than their parents, and this has required the height reference charts to be updated periodically. But the secular trend in north Europeans is now only slight, and the current British 1990 height charts are appropriate for the white population (Freeman *et al.* 1995). In the past there were also appreciable social class differences, with the higher social classes being taller—this effect is also now much reduced (Li and Power 2004). Ethnic minorities from South-east Asia are noticeably shorter than Europeans, and within Europe those from the north and east tend to be taller than those from the south. Africans and Afro-Caribbeans are similar in height to whites.

There is a strong familial height correlation, theoretically 0.5 both for parent–child and sibling–sibling correlations. The correlation can be used to predict a child's likely adult height from the parents, but unless there is a growth disorder a better predictor is the child's own height. Broadly speaking a child grows along the same height centile throughout childhood, though this is often disturbed during puberty, so their centile at any age outside puberty is a good predictor of their adult centile. It works less well in infancy, both because infants often cross height centiles either up or down, and because length can be difficult to measure accurately.

Concern about stature

The expression of concern about short stature often comes from a parent, who may or may not be reflecting their child's concern. The child is seen to be shorter than contemporaries in the playgroup or classroom, or shorter for age than their brother or sister or relative. This social pressure applies particularly in puberty when height differences are accentuated. The concern is more likely to be expressed for boys than girls, reflecting the perceived importance of tall stature.

Concern is also more likely to arise in families that are taller than average, where greater stature is expected. But ironically such children are less likely to be detected using the conventional height chart, as the extra height of the family tends to lift the child above the action cut-off (see below).

In short families an unusually short child may not attract so much attention, and here it is the role of the GP or nurse to be concerned. The majority of short children are from short families, reflecting the strong familial determinant of height, so there is a risk that in such cases impaired growth may not be recognized.

Concern about tall stature arises in much the same way as for short stature, but here the concern is much more likely to arise in girls, where tall stature is less socially desirable.

The challenge for primary care is to measure and assess height in a way that recognizes the range of presentations of short and tall stature, e.g. in tall versus short families. Once a growth disorder is suspected and treated, usually in secondary care, the ultimate aim for short stature is to improve height gain and hence adult height, while for tall stature the target is to minimize further growth.

Causes of short and tall stature

The two main disorders leading to short stature are growth hormone deficiency, which has many aetiologies, and, in girls, Turner syndrome. Both conditions are rare, about 1 in 4000 for growth hormone deficiency and 1 in 3500 girls for Turner syndrome. Some other syndromes have short stature as a symptom but growth is not the main issue, for example Down syndrome. In addition short stature can be a symptom of more general disorders, such as asthma, severe renal disease, or inflammatory bowel disease (Voss *et al.* 1992). This emphasizes why height measurement is a valuable part of paediatric clinical assessment.

Disorders leading to tall stature tend to be rarer. Precocious puberty is the most common cause, which is likely to be accompanied by other physical signs. The various syndromes associated with tall stature such as Klinefelter, Marfan, or Sotos are all rarer than Turner syndrome.

The great majority of short children are finally diagnosed with constitutional short stature (which is no more than a description of their presenting symptom) or constitutional delay, meaning that their maturation is delayed and they are likely to catch up once puberty arrives. Like stature the timing of puberty is familially related, so parents or siblings may also report having had delayed puberty.

Assessment

Chart

The first stage of assessment is to measure the child's height. This requires care and attention with the equipment and measuring technique, and should be done by a trained and experienced observer (e.g. the practice nurse) before the doctor sees the child. The equipment ideally consists of a stadiometer or wall-mounted head-board, regularly calibrated with a metre rule or similar. The observer positions the child with heels, buttocks and head touching the wall, places the head in the Frankfort plane (the lower margin of the orbit in a horizontal line with the external auditory meatus), and reads off the height to the nearest 0.5 cm. There is no advantage in 'stretching' the child (Voss and Bailey 1997), but recording the time of measurement is useful as the skeleton 'shrinks' during the day due to vertebral disk compression. Ideally hair ornaments likely to get in the way should first be removed, but if this is not practical their presence should be recorded.

The height measurement fulfils two separate functions—it indicates the child's current height, but in addition it acts as baseline for any future heights to assess height velocity. This is why it needs to be of high quality.

The heights of other genetically related family members who are present, i.e. parent(s) and/or sibling(s), should also be measured at the same time.

The next stage is to plot the child's height on the British 1990 height chart (Freeman *et al.* 1995), for boys or girls as appropriate, and read off the height centile. Heights for siblings should also be plotted and their height centiles recorded. The heights of parents are plotted on a separate chart (see Figure 15.2).

The charts are available via the Harlow Printing website at http://www.healthforall-children.co.uk/. They come in several formats and age ranges, including 0–1, 1–5, and 5–18 years. Figure 15.1 shows the 0–20 year combined height and weight chart for boys, which is part of the 4-in-1 chart. (This assumes a British readership. For North American readers the US CDC 2000 height charts (Kuczmarski *et al.* 2000) can be accessed at http://www.cdc.gov/growthcharts/, and many other countries have their own national height reference charts.)

A height below the British 0.4th centile, the lowest curve on the chart, or above the 99.6th centile (the highest) is clear evidence of short (tall) stature. Only 4 children per

1000 are as short (tall) as this, and it is recommended that such children are referred unconditionally for paediatric assessment.

A height between the 0.4th and 2nd centile may also be of concern, and here the GP should use his/her judgement as to whether or not to refer. About 2% of children—1 in 50—fall into this category, so it is much more common than the 4 per 1000 below the 0.4th centile.

Note that the 0.4th centile is available only on British charts—most other national charts use the 2nd, 3rd, or even 5th centile as the cut-off for short stature. The rationale for the 0.4th centile is that it improves the effectiveness of screening (Cole 1994).

If the family is relatively tall and the concern is short stature, it is worth adjusting for familial height, and similarly for tall stature in a short family. The height chart includes a mid-parent height calculation (Figure 15.1, top right) for this purpose. But in practice it is fiddly to do and hard to interpret, quite apart from the need for both parents' heights, which may not be available. An alternative is the familial height chart (Figure 15.2), which offers a graphical adjustment and works for any available combination of parent(s) and/or siblings (Cole 2000).

The child's height centile, as read off the height chart, is on the left axis in Figure 15.2, and the family height (be it mother, father, and/or sibling(s)) at the bottom. Plot the point(s) where the child and familial heights meet. For parents plot the height, and for siblings the height centile, just as for the index child. The parent heights are converted to centiles using the older Tanner–Whitehouse standard (Tanner *et al.* 1966) to adjust for the secular trend in height.

The action regions on the chart are the triangles to lower right (for short stature) and upper left (tall stature). They correspond to the 4 per 1000 height centile adjusted for family height. If at least half the plotted points lie in a triangle then this is a clear indication to refer. Figure 15.2 shows an example of a child midway between the 0.4th and 2nd centile, plotted against three family members. Two of the three lie in the lower triangle, so the child should be referred.

Height in ethnic minorities

Children from the Indian subcontinent, particularly Bangladeshis, are appreciably shorter than Europeans, and their parents even more so. This can cause problems with the assessment process described above, as it may pick up an Asian child who is no shorter in centile terms than his/her parents yet who still falls below the 0.4th centile. In such situations the familial height chart is more informative than the height chart, as it provides reassurance that the child is not short for their family.

In principle the same argument could be used with short white families, where the short child has similarly short parents. But it is possible that both parents and child have the same growth disorder, and for this reason it would be wrong to dismiss the child's short stature too quickly.

History and examination

Following the height assessment a full history and examination need to be carried out. What is the nature of the concern, who is most concerned, and when did the concern

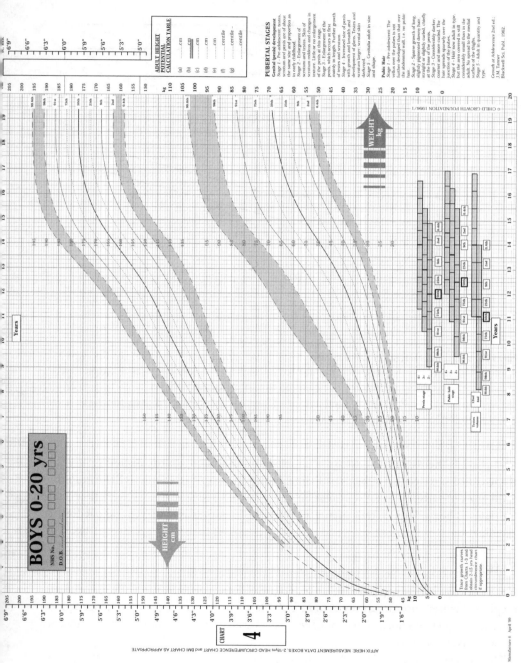

Fig. 15.1 The British 1990 height and weight chart for boys 0–20 years. Refer the child if their height plotted on the chart is below the 0.4th centile or above the 99.6th centile. Reproduced with permission from the Child Growth Foundation.

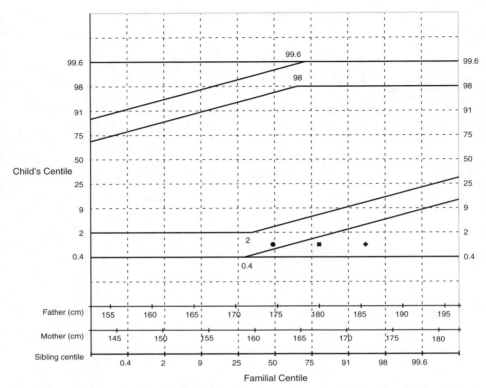

Fig. 15.2 A chart to adjust for familial height. The lower right triangle identifies children whose height is below the 0.4th centile adjusted for family height. The upper left triangle works similarly for tall stature. Plot the child's height on the left axis, and available family heights on the bottom axis (here, from left to right, mother, father and brother). If, as here, the majority of points lie in the triangle, then refer the child.

first arise? Is there a family history of short stature (including more distant relatives)? If the concern is delayed puberty, is there a family history of late puberty? How did the child grow in early life, what was their birth weight and neonatal history, were they light for dates? Then ask for details of any associated ill health, and do a general paediatric examination.

Referral

If the decision is made to refer the child, do provide the paediatrician with the original height measurement (assuming it to be reliable), to shorten the time-scale needed to validly assess height velocity. That said, the paediatrician is likely to repeat the measurement anyway, just to be sure.

The next step in secondary care will depend on the severity of the short stature: if it is mild to moderate, say 2nd–0.4th centile with no other symptoms or signs, the paediatrician will probably just monitor the child for 6–12 months to assess growth velocity.

Conversely if the short stature is moderate to severe, say well below the 0.4th centile, or if there are other associated symptoms or signs, the paediatrician may investigate straight away.

It is worth emphasizing that short stature can be a specific disorder such as growth hormone deficiency, but it can also be a symptom of a more general disorder such as severe renal disease or inflammatory bowel disease (Hindmarsh and Cole 2001). It is a relatively insensitive and non-specific symptom, but it needs taking seriously as if real it can be an index of significant but treatable disease.

Tall stature is much less of an issue except when extreme. It is mostly either untreatable or not needing treatment—the exceptions are Marfan syndrome because there can be significant eye or heart complications; and a growth hormone secreting pituitary tumour, which while very rare in childhood must be treated before the child goes blind.

Conclusions

Concern about possible short or tall stature should be taken seriously. The child's height needs to be measured accurately, plotted on the appropriate chart and interpreted correctly, taking into account the height of the family. Short stature is a marker of a specific growth disorder, but in addition it can be a symptom of more general ill health requiring diagnosis and treatment.

References

Cole TJ (1994). Do growth chart centiles need a face lift? *British Medical Journal* **308**: 641–642.

Cole TJ (2000). A simple chart to assess non-familial short stature. *Archives of Disease in Childhood* **82**: 173–176.

Freeman JV, Cole TJ, Chinn S, Jones PR, White EM, Preece MA (1995). Cross sectional stature and weight reference curves for the UK, 1990. *Archives of Disease in Childhood* **73**: 17–24.

Hindmarsh PC, Cole TJ (2001). Disorders of growth. *Medicine*, **29**: 81–86.

Kuczmarski RJ, Ogden CL, Grummer-Strawn LM, Fegal KM, Guo SS, Wei R, Mei Z, Curtin LR, Roche AF, Johnson CL (2000). *CDC Growth Charts: United States*. National Center for Health Statistics, Hyattsville, MD.

Li L, Power C (2004). Influences on childhood height: comparing two generations in the 1958 British birth cohort. *International Journal of Epidemiology* **33**: 1320–1328.

Tanner JM (1978). *Foetus into Man: physical growth from conception to maturity*. Open Books, London.

Tanner JM, Whitehouse RH, Takaishi M (1966). Standards from birth to maturity for height, weight, height velocity, and weight velocity: British children, 1965 Parts I and II. *Archives of Disease in Childhood* **41**: 454–471, 613–635.

Voss LD, Bailey BJR (1997). Diurnal variation in stature: is stretching the answer? *Archives of Disease in Childhood* **77**: 319–322.

Voss LD, Mulligan J, Betts PR, Wilkin TJ (1992). Poor growth in school entrants as an index of organic disease: the Wessex growth study. *British Medical Journal* **305**: 1400–1402.

Chapter 16

Orthopaedic problems

Benjamin Jacobs and Deborah Eastwood

Orthopaedics means 'straight child' in Greek. When the term was introduced by Nicolas Andry in 1741, the main bone problems were crippling childhood diseases such as rickets and tuberculosis (Andry 1742). Today's orthopaedic surgeon treats children with a wide variety of conditions that range from simple growing pains to congenital malformations, developmental anomalies, inflammatory arthropathies, benign and malignant tumours, and the complications of metabolic diseases. Fractures remain a common problem and infection is a diagnosis that should not be forgotten.

This chapter describes the most common bone problems by age: infants, toddlers, older children, and adolescents. The chapter ends with a description of the method of orthopaedic consultation for children and this is illustrated with a strategy for an important acute orthopaedic problem in primary care; the limping child.

Problems in infancy

Developmental dysplasia of the hip (DDH)

In DDH the baby is born with an unstable hip joint, the hip may be dysplastic or truly dislocated (congenital dislocation of the hip, CDH). DDH is more common in firstborns (decreased intrauterine space) and is six times more common in females. Approximately two in a thousand babies have true hip dysplasia but 10 times this number present as suspicious cases following neonatal screening. A national screening programme (Standing Medical Advisory Committee (1969) was introduced in the UK in 1969 but the evidence for its efficacy is still not conclusive (National Screening Committee Child Health Sub-Group Report 2004).

The current recommendation is that every baby is reviewed within the first week of life for risk factors, and examined by the clinical screening tests of Barlow (dislocation of hip by adduction and backward pressure on the flexed hip with a stable pelvis) and Ortolani (reduction of dislocation). When the flexed hip is noted to have limited abduction, the hip is dislocated and the femoral head can be lifted into joint by the examiner's fingers on the proximal femur). Babies are screened again at 6 weeks of age.

Babies born in Germany, Austria, and Switzerland are now all screened with postnatal ultrasound scans. In the UK, limited ultrasound facilities restrict its use to babies with risk factors (Table 16.1) or clinical suspicion of instability (a feeling of subluxation, or a positive Barlow or Ortolani test) or a frank dislocation.

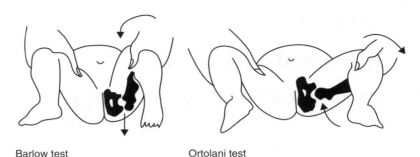

Barlow test   Ortolani test

Fig. 16.1 Tests for CDH.

The first scan should be performed within a month of birth with orthopaedic referral (when necessary) by 6 weeks. An immature hip that is stable may be watched to ensure that the acetabular dysplasia resolves but the hip with instability demands prompt treatment. The treatment at this stage is an abduction/flexion brace such as the Pavlik harness for 2 months with regular monitoring of the child and the hip.

After 3 months of age clinical signs of instability are difficult to elicit, and the diagnosis is made on restriction of motion. In a subluxed or dislocated hip the surrounding musculature shortens. With hips flexed and knees bent a difference in knee height may be evident (Galeazzi sign Figure 16.3). In the fully flexed hip there will then be limitation of abduction unilaterally or bilaterally. The walking child with a dislocated hip leans over the affected hip (dips) with each step (Trendelenburg gait), and in bilateral DDH, a waddling gait may be noted. Only 20% of DDH is bilateral but they account for a disproportionate number of late diagnoses because the clinical clue of asymmetry is not present. Children who present late also have few 'risk factors' because screening programmes tend to pick out the 'high-risk' cases.

As the child grows, the cartilaginous skeleton ossifies limiting the value of ultrasound scans. By 6 months, X-rays are more helpful for hip joint anatomy.

If the hip fails to reduce, or fails to stabilize within the Pavlik Harness or if the hip presents late, a surgical procedure will be required to place the hip in joint and allow normal joint development to resume. The procedure may simply be a closed reduction of

Table 16.1 Risk factors for DDH

DDH risk factors meriting hip ultrasound screening in the UK
Breech (especially if extended legs)
Oligohydramnios (decreased intrauterine space)
Family history (first-degree relative increases risk by factor of 30)
Other 'packaging disorders', such as torticollis and foot deformities
Chromosomal, e.g. Down syndrome
Neuromuscular disorders, e.g. arthrogryposis

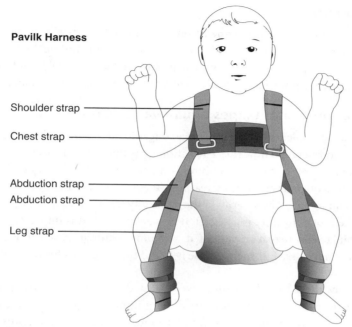

Pavlik Harness

Shoulder strap

Chest strap

Abduction strap

Abduction strap

Leg strap

Fig. 16.2 Pavlik harness.

the joint under a general anaesthetic with a small release of the tight muscles in the groin. However, if the hip has been out for longer and, for example, the child is of walking age, a more aggressive surgical procedure may be appropriate with an open reduction of the joint being performed with the addition of a pelvic and/or femoral osteotomy as necessary. The child may be placed in a plaster cast for several months following such a procedure.

The more work needed to stabilize the hip, the greater the risk of complications. However, even after major surgery an essentially normal hip is the usual outcome meaning that the child will have a comfortable, mobile hip for the foreseeable future.

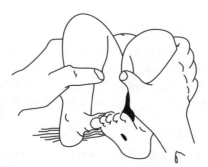

Fig. 16.3 Galeazzi sign in a 4-month-old baby.

Foot deformities

If a baby lies awkwardly *in utero* one of several foot 'deformities' may be apparent at birth. The foot will tend to lie in either calcaneovalgus (up and out) or equinovarus (down and in). The position is usually partially correctable and flexible and the problem resolves completely within a few weeks either spontaneously or with physiotherapy.

Idiopathic congenital talipes equinovarus (CTEV)

CTEV (previously called a 'Club Foot') is a congenital deformity where the toes point downwards and the ankle inwards. The aetiology is unknown. It occurs in about 1 in 1000 children. It is more common in boys and affects both feet in about 60% of cases. The deformity is obvious at birth. Increasingly the diagnosis is made on antenatal scans but it is difficult to judge the severity of the deformity from the scan alone.

At birth the foot deformity is assessed. It is usually 'fixed'. It is important to examine the whole child to ensure that an associated syndrome (arthrogryposis) or neuromuscular abnormality is not missed. If such a cause is found the prognosis for the foot deformity is worse.

Traditionally, these foot deformities were treated by stretching, strapping, and on occasion plastering. If the foot deformity did not improve significantly then a surgical release of the tight soft tissues was performed about the age of 8–12 months so that the foot was in a plantigrade (walking) position by the time the child was ready to walk.

Recently, a more aggressive form of manipulation and casting known as the Ponseti technique has been regaining popularity. The method involves weekly or twice weekly sessions of manipulation followed by the application of an above-knee plaster cast. As the foot corrects there is often some tightness of the Achilles tendon that requires a tenotomy performed under local anaesthesia in the clinic. Usually, a major surgical procedure is avoided but the child does have to wear a system of 'boots and bars' for some time.

The outcome of either treatment regimen is a foot that is comfortable and that functions well but usually a shoe size smaller than the other side and with a smaller looking calf muscle no matter how much running around that the child does.

CTEV *always* presents at birth. A foot deformity that develops later requires urgent assessment for a neuromuscular imbalance.

Congenital vertical talus (CVT)

In CVT the child has a rocker-bottom foot. This is sometimes called a 'flat foot' but it is qualitatively different from the common baby flat foot where the arch is simply taken up by fat in the soft tissues. In the congenital vertical talus the head of talus is the bony lump taking up the arch of the foot. Surgery is usually required for this rare condition.

Congenital toe deformities

Lateral deviation of the second or third toes or inward deviation of the fourth or fifth toes are the most common congenital variations but they are of little clinical significance.

The condition is usually familial and functional impairment rare. The fourth and fifth curly toes are readily treated (if the parents wish) by flexor tenotomy performed as a day-case procedure under a general anaesthetic. Over-riding fifth toes can be corrected simply too. Syndactyly (webbing) is rarely more than a cosmetic problem.

Short limbs

Congenitally short limbs are very rare. If a baby is noted to have a short leg or arm soon after birth, birth injury to the hip or shoulder and DDH must be excluded, as these problems require urgent treatment.

Birth injuries

Difficult births such as shoulder dystocia can result in obstetric brachial plexus palsy (e.g. Erb's palsy) or fractures. Once a fracture of the clavicle or fracture separation of the humeral neck/shaft has been excluded the brachial plexus injury itself does not usually require immediate treatment, other than range of movement exercises to prevent muscle imbalance leading to a joint contracture. Fractures heal very quickly in infants but a sling or bandage may be required for comfort for the first week or 2. If there is severe or persistent neurological deficit at 6 weeks of age, the baby should be referred to a specialist nerve injury service for investigation and surgical management.

Torticollis

Congenital torticollis (wry neck) usually manifests at about 6 weeks of age when the baby's head is noted to be tilted and turned to one side. A swelling (tumour) may be palpable in the sternomastoid muscle on that side. The muscle usually relaxes and the neck straightens over the following months. This may be hastened by physiotherapy and placing interesting objects on the other side of the baby's cot to encourage turning. If it persists at 1 year of age orthopaedic referral is required for consideration of surgery. Torticollis present at birth is likely to be due to an abnormality of the cervical spine and should be referred immediately.

Fractures

Fractures may be considered a normal part of childhood. However, if they occur in the pre-ambulant infant, or without a manifest cause, diseases such as child abuse or osteogenesis imperfecta (OI) must be excluded. These are often mistaken for each other at first. Both are difficult diagnoses and yet the stakes are high. A missed diagnosis of child abuse in a young infant carries a significant mortality risk. A false diagnosis of abuse in a child with OI can destroy doctor–parent trust. A diagnosis of child abuse at this age should be supported by a full medical history and examination together with an ophthalmological examination for retinal haemorrhages, an appropriate radiological skeletal survey, social work, and police assessment. OI is much rarer but is more likely with a family history, physical findings, such as blue sclerae and radiological findings on the skeletal survey such as Wormian bones. In the absence of these it may take several fractures until a diagnosis of OI is confirmed. Genetic diagnosis by DNA analysis is now possible in some cases but is expensive and slow.

Problems in toddlerhood

Delayed walking

Most children start to walk with assistance (e.g. hands held or cruising round furniture) by 1 year of age. If a child is not walking by 18 months of age referral to a paediatrician is indicated. Causes include DDH, cerebral palsy, and muscular dystrophies. If there is a family history of bottom shuffling and the child is mobile by this means specialist referral can be deferred until 2 years of age.

Bow legs/knock knees

The shape of a child's legs often causes considerable concern. It is essential to understand that all children are bowlegged at birth (Do 2001). Most have grown out of it by 18 months of age. They may then become knock-kneed by 3–4 before their legs straighten out again to a normal physiological position of a few degrees of valgus.

The bowed legs often have a slight twist to them as well (tibial torsion) and the combination of 'problems' makes the deformity seem worse.

If the child is younger than 5, of normal proportions and weight, and the deformity is symmetrical with no history of injury or illness then there is no cause for concern no matter how bad the legs look. They are likely to straighten spontaneously. If the history suggests a poor diet, bowel disease, or anticonvulsant drugs that can cause rickets, blood biochemistry should be checked (Singh *et al.* 2003). An X-ray will also exclude rickets, Blount's disease, or other orthopaedic rarity.

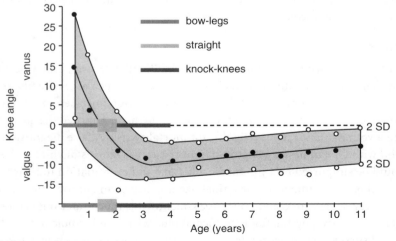

Fig. 16.4 Knee angle by age.

Intoeing

Children often start to walk with their feet pointing towards each other. This twisting may originate in the foot (metatarsus varus), in the tibia (tibial torsion), or in the femur (persistent anteversion of the femoral neck). The cause can be detected easily by assessing the child in the prone position with knees flexed. All these conditions are symmetrical, free of pain, and allow normal mobility. Parents often remark that the toddler frequently trips and falls, but all toddlers do! This is usually more apparent at the end of the day when the child is tired.

The child will get better with growth and maturity. With growth the leg untwists, in the tibia (by 3–4 years) or the femur (by 7–8 years) and with maturity the child learns to control their foot position better so that tripping and falling become less marked. Referral to an orthopaedic surgeon is only indicated if the condition is very asymmetric or progressive. Surgical correction of the deformity is rarely indicated and only in later childhood/ adolescence.

Extoeing

This abnormality of gait is less common than intoeing and tends to present in a younger child. It is often a reason for a child being late to walk—i.e. they are walking but are reluctant to let go of the furniture or their mothers' hand because the externally rotated foot position is associated with an unstable walk. It tends to improve with time in the same way that intoeing does.

Tip-toeing gait

This is a common phase in the development of a mature gait pattern. However, a child who did walk on their heels and becomes a toe-walker may have a neuromuscular cause such as Duchenne muscular dystrophy. Unilateral tiptoeing rings alarm bells for problems such as DDH, limb dysplasia, or hemiplegia. Treatment may be required for the persistent idiopathic toe walker particularly if the Achilles tendon is tight.

Flat foot (pes planus)

A 'flat foot' is one in which the medial longitudinal arch either rests on the ground or appears closer to the ground than the examiner would accept as normal. If the foot is truly flat the heel will be in a valgus position. Flexible flat feet are universal in the infant, very common in the toddler and present in 15% of adults.

The vast majority of flexible flat feet are asymptomatic in both childhood and adulthood. The natural history of the condition is not altered by the use of orthotics. However, if the child is uncomfortable when walking or has a limited walking tolerance and if this is considered to be due to the flat feet then orthotic supports may be beneficial in easing the discomfort. Orthotics will not change the shape of the foot though. If there is true delay in motor development a neurological cause should be sought.

Flat feet are frequently seen in families. They are associated with another inherited condition 'hypermobility' and the simple test of Beighton (see Table 16.2) should be

Table 16.2 Nine-point Beighton hypermobility score

	Right	Left
1. Passively dorsiflex the little finger more than 90°	1	1
2. Oppose the thumb to the forearm	1	1
3. Hyperextend the elbow	1	1
4. Hyperextend the knee	1	1
5. Place hands flat on the floor without bending knees	1	1
Total possible score		9

applied in a child presenting with flat feet, though the wide racial variation must be considered (Cheng *et al.*1991). Jack's test (the great toe extension test) will show if the foot is flexible: When the great toe is extended (or the child stands on tiptoe), the medial arch appears. **Rigid flat feet** are pathological and are due to neurological abnormality or conditions such as an inflammatory arthritis or a tarsal coalition.

Benign joint hypermobility syndrome (BJHS)

Joint laxity is maximal at birth, declining rapidly during childhood, less rapidly during the teens, and slowly during adult life. Women are more lax jointed than men and there is wide ethnic variation. Epidemiological studies have shown that hypermobility is seen in up to 10% of individuals in Western populations (Grahame 1999). The quick clinical test for joint laxity developed by Beighton *et al.* (1973) (Table 16.2) is helpful. A child who scores 5 or more is hypermobile. When hypermobility becomes symptomatic, the 'hypermobility syndrome' is said to exist. Symptoms in children include joint and back pains, occasionally subluxations or frank dislocations, ligament muscle and tendon injuries after mild trauma and fasciitis. On the other hand most children are asymptomatic and violinists, flautists, and pianists (of all ages) with lax finger joints suffer less pain than their less flexible peers (Larsson *et al.* 1993). Symptomatic children can be helped greatly by experienced physiotherapists.

Pulled elbow (subluxation of the radial head)

Children aged 1–5 years can easily sublux the head of the radius at the elbow if pulled suddenly by the hand. They then tend to carry their forearm in a lame position of forearm pronation and elbow flexion. Function is restored and the pain dramatically relieved by supinating the forearm. A click may be felt and heard at the elbow. The arm is then allowed to rest in a sling for a few days. One in five children suffers recurrences but it is very rare beyond the age of 10 years.

Congenital and infantile scoliosis

Congenital scoliosis is the result of anomalous vertebral formation; infantile scoliosis is defined as a spinal curvature that appears before 3 years of age. Both must be referred early to an orthopaedic surgeon for investigation and follow-up.

The older child

Growing pains

Children between the ages of 2 and 10 years commonly complain of leg pains. The pain is usually bilateral, noted in the evening or at night and relieved by massage. As long as there are no physical signs and the pain is short-lived it is safe to label it as 'growing pain'. The aetiology is unclear but the prognosis excellent. Unilateral pain is more concerning, and warrants imaging to exclude a bone lesion. Sympathetic encouragement usually results in resolution of the pain, but if not a more thorough examination of the child and family is required.

Heel pain

There are many causes of pain around the heel varying from Achilles tendinitis to Sever's disease. The latter is the most common in this age group and it is better described as a condition rather than a disease. It is a form of growing pain and usually resolves with time and perhaps some restriction of exercise.

Transient synovitis of the hip

Transient synovitis is also known as irritable hip. It is a common disorder of childhood that presents with acute pain and a limp, sometimes with knee pain and inability to weight bear. The child, usually a boy between 2 and 6 years of age, is otherwise well. The cause is uncertain and the diagnosis, one of exclusion. Minor viral infection and trauma are postulated precipitating factors but evidence for these is usually lacking.

Both hips are affected equally but it is rare for the child to present with bilateral involvement. On examination, the affected leg tends to be held in the position of greatest ease, typically, one of flexion, abduction and slight external rotation. Movement is restricted especially extension and internal rotation, which both increase intracapsular pressure.

Ultrasound may demonstrate an effusion that can be aspirated and cultured to exclude septic arthritis.

The child may need admission to hospital if the diagnosis is in doubt, or if the pain is severe and bed rest is not possible at home. Non-steroidal anti-inflammatory drugs provide relief (Kermond *et al.* 2002), and aspiration of an effusion may dramatically reduce pain temporarily. The child should begin mobilizing once the pain has settled. Symptoms usually resolve within 10 days, although the condition can recur in up to 15% of cases. If symptoms persist at 6 weeks, a follow up X-ray should be taken to exclude Perthes' disease and a diagnosis of juvenile inflammatory arthritis must be considered too.

Perthes' disease

Perthes was a German surgeon a hundred years ago. He was the first to show the X-ray changes of avascular necrosis of the head of the femur in children. This occurs most often in boys aged between 5 and 10 years. The aetiology is not well understood. It is usually unilateral and there is a family history in 12%. The presentation can be either with pain (often referred to the knee) or limp. Clinical examination may be normal

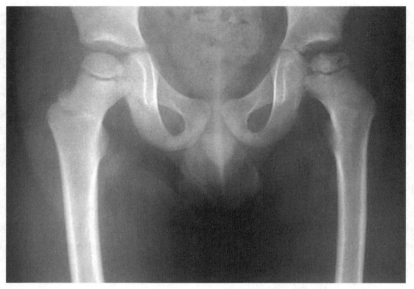

Fig. 16.5 Perthes' disease.

at first. Later limited hip abduction and internal rotation may be found. Anterior–posterior and 'frog lateral' views of the hip often show signs of subchondral fracture, sclerosis, and collapse of the femoral head.

All cases should be referred for early orthopaedic assessment. The prognosis is related to extent of disease as graded by Catterall: the more of the head that is involved the poorer the outlook for the hip (Catterall 1971).

Adolescents

Adolescent idiopathic scoliosis (AIS)

AIS is most common in tall thin girls. They develop a fixed lateral curvature of the spine, with vertebral rotation (the rib hump), around puberty. Spinal anomalies such as congenital hemivertebra, neuromuscular conditions, muscular dystrophies, tumours, neurofibromatosis, and other syndromes need to be excluded for the condition to be labelled idiopathic. Severe pain, a left thoracic curve or an abnormal neurological examination are red flags that point to a secondary cause for spinal deformity.

If there is risk of the scoliosis progressing the orthopaedic surgeon may start treatment with a spinal brace, which can be worn under normal clothing but must be worn day and night. If the scoliosis continues to worsen surgery may be required.

Scheuermann's disease

This presents as backache or a kyphosis (humpback deformity) in the thoracic spine between 12 and 16 years of age. The cause is unclear but there is often a family history. These teenagers may require bracing but rarely surgery.

Table 16.3 Causes of scoliosis

Neurological disorders
  Syringomyelia
  Spinal tumour
  Neurofibromatosis
  Muscular dystrophy
  Cerebral palsy
  Poliomyelitis
  Friedreich's ataxia
  Familial dysautonomia (Riley–Day syndrome)
  Spinal muscular atrophy
  Tethered cord syndrome (spinal cord unable to change positio because of growth related to
    scarring, diastematomyelia or other aetiology)

Musculoskeletal
  Leg length difference (common and commonly missed!)
  Osteogenesis imperfecta
  Klippel–Feil syndrome

Inherited disorders of connective tissue
  Ehlers–Danlos syndrome
  Marfan syndrome
  Homocystinuria

Slipped upper femoral epiphysis (SUFE)

In this condition the head of the femur slips at the epiphyseal growth plate.

The aetiology is unclear but obese boys with delayed secondary sexual development, or tall thin girls, appear particularly susceptible. If it occurs outside the age range of 10–15 years clinical and biochemical investigation is indicated looking for endocrine diseases such as hypothyroidism. It may present with sudden hip pain and limp in which case surgery within 24 hours is most likely to be successful. A slip of less than 50% is treated by pinning *in situ*, but slip of more than 50% may require an osteotomy, with a greater risk of avascular necrosis. Some cases grumble for weeks or even months before presenting but if a chronic slip deteriorates suddenly, urgent surgery may be indicated. The condition is bilateral in 20% and so the teenager should present to an orthopaedic surgeon immediately if the other hip becomes painful. Some surgeons advocate prophylactic pinning of the normal hip.

Osgood–Schlatter disease

This is a specific, uncomfortable and occasionally significantly painful condition associated with tenderness and swelling around the tibial tuberosity (rather than the knee itself). The pain is worse on activity or sometimes after prolonged periods of sitting or rest. It may be precipitated by growth and/or a simple injury. Pain is often bilateral but usually asymmetrical. Conservative treatment consisting of relative rest, reassurance, and analgesia is usually successful.

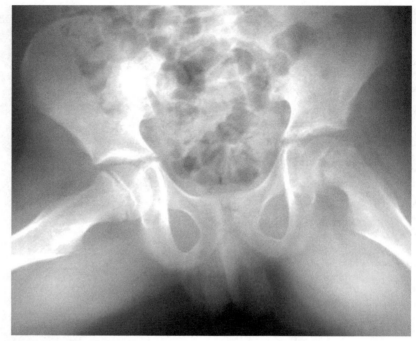

Fig. 16.6 Slipped upper femoral epiphysis.

Anterior knee pain syndrome

Symptoms of ill-defined pain around the front of the knee with giving way and clicking, exacerbated by prolonged sitting or by activity are often present in both knees of teenage girls. Patellofemoral crepitus may be detected on examination.

Recurrent subluxation of the patella (patella maltracking)

This usually presents in adolescent or teenage girls. Treatment is usually conservative with physiotherapy to strengthen the quadriceps muscle. It may be associated with ligamentous laxity and occasionally with Down or Ehlers–Danlos syndrome.

Ingrown toenails (onychocryptosis)

Ingrown toenails are a cause of pain usually in the big toe. They affect adolescents particularly because sweaty feet softens the skin and nails. Basic foot care advice and appropriate footwear often relieves the symptoms. Sometimes, a wedge excision of the lateral edge of the nail is necessary with phenolization of the nail bed to prevent regrowth. This may be performed by chiropodists (Rounding and Hulm 1999).

Bone tumours

Bone tumours present with bone pain and sometimes swelling or limp. They present a diagnostic challenge in primary care, as these are such common symptoms.

An important clinical clue to the diagnosis is nocturnal pain, which is typical of bone tumours. Even benign tumours such as osteoid osteoma typically present with aching pain at night.

Osteosarcoma and Ewing's sarcoma are the most common primary bone cancers. They can occur in children and adults but usually develop in teenagers during the adolescent growth spurt. Boys are affected twice as often as girls. The most common site is around the knee. Leukaemia, lymphoma, and neuroblastoma can present with similar symptoms.

Plain X-ray will usually show a lesion and prompt further urgent investigation. Treatment of malignant tumours involves chemotherapy, radiotherapy, and surgery depending on the biopsy results and staging, but the prognosis has improved steadily over the last generation so that in most cases the limb can be salvaged and 5-year survival is approaching 85%.

Method of orthopaedic consultation for children

With younger children the history should start with the pregnancy and delivery to diagnose packaging problems such as occur with oligohydramnios or developmental concerns due to a traumatic birth. A careful developmental history is needed for toddlers including at least a summary of their gross motor development (sitting, standing, walking, running, hopping).

The other categories of development: social, fine motor (hand function), vision, language, and hearing should be reviewed to allow diagnosis of cerebral palsy and other neuromuscular problems. A family history will elucidate genetic problems and gain insight into family anxieties about relatives with arthritis or orthopaedic problems. Older children should be encouraged to relate their own history and enquiries should include school performance and difficulties in sport.

The clinical examination should be guided by the history. In a minor injury a limited examination of the affected part may suffice, but a full general examination will be needed if the history suggests an underlying medical condition, a developmental or growth problem or the possibility of child abuse. In such cases the child's height and weight should be plotted on a growth centile chart. The orthopaedic examination includes inspection of gait, or (in the infant) observation of gross motor development to assess tone, power and co-ordination. The younger the child the less formal the examination can be. Even children old enough to understand are often not in a mood to co-operate with a full neurological examination and skills need to be developed in opportunistic observation. Toys and activities strategically placed around the consulting room help demonstrate children's abilities and limitations!

The limping child

Children presenting with unexplained limp are a common problem in primary care. Most will be the result of minor trauma that is self-limiting, but it is important to assess limping children quickly to exclude an orthopaedic emergency such as septic arthritis. The hip joint is the most common serious cause of limping and a summary of the

Table 16.4 Common causes of acute limp in childhood

	Septic Arthritis	Transient Synovitis	Perthes' Disease	Slipped Upper Femoral Epiphysis
Age (years)	Any age but most <3 years	3–6	4–9	10–16
Fever	Yes	Mild	No	No
Inflammatory markers (ESR, CRP)	High	Moderate	Normal	Normal
Initial imaging method	X-ray, Ultrasound ± aspiration of effusion for microbiology	X-ray and often ultrasound	X-ray	X-ray
Treatment	Surgical drainage and antibiotics	Rest and anti-inflammatory analgesia	Analgesia ± surgery	Surgery
Prognosis	Depends on early effective treatment	Excellent	Depends on severity and early treatment	Depends on severity and early treatment

important causes is given in Table 16.4. If the child is unwell, or has a fever, a blood count and inflammatory markers must be checked for signs of infection. In the young child it can be difficult to localize the site of a fracture and X-rays may need to include the whole leg. Even if the child is not unwell a blood count and ESR should be checked if the limp remains unexplained for more than a few days as this can be a presentation of arthritis, spinal discitis or malignancies such as leukaemia.

References

Andry N (1742). *Orthopaedia or the Art of Correcting and Preventing Deformities in Children*. Royal College of Medicine, London.

Beighton PH, Solomon L, Soskolne CL (1973). Articular mobility in an African population. *Annals of Rheumatic Disease* **32**: 413–418.

Catterall A (1971). The natural history of Perthes' disease. *Journal of Bone and Joint Surgery* **53**: 37–53.

Cheng JCY, Chan PS, Hui PW (1991). Joint laxity in children. *Journal of Paediatric Orthopaedics* **11**: 752–756.

Do TT (2001). Clinical and radiological evaluation of bowlegs. *Current Opinion in Pediatrics* **13**: 42–46.

Grahame R (1999). Joint hypermobility and genetic collagen disorders: are they related? *Archives of Disease in Childhood* **80**: 188–191.

Kermond S, Fink M, Graham K, Carlin JB, Barnett P (2002). A randomized clinical trial: should the child with transient synovitis of the hip be treated with nonsteroidal anti-inflammatory drugs? *Annals of Emergency Medicine* **40**(3): 294–299.

Larsson L-G, Baum J, Muldolkar GS, Kollia GD (1993). Benefits and disadvantages of joint hypermobility among musicians. *New England Journal of Medicine* **329**: 1079–1082.

National Screening Committee Child Health Sub-Group Report (2004) *Dysplasia of the Hip*. NHS, London.

Rounding C, Hulm S (1999). Surgical treatments for ingrowing toenails. *Cochrane Library* Issue 3.

Singh J, Moghal N, Pearce SHS, Cheetham T (2003). The investigation of hypocalcaemia and rickets. *Archives of Disease in Childhood* **88**: 403–407.

Standing Medical Advisory Committee (1969). *Screening for the Detection of Congenital Dislocation of the Hip in Infants*. Department of Health and Social Security, London.

Chapter 17

Dermatology

Helen Goodyear

This chapter looks at commonly occurring skin disorders in children and their treatment.

The skin often gives valuable information leading to diagnosis with both acutely sick children, e.g. meningococcal disease and chronic conditions, e.g. neurofibromatosis. The skin signs of these conditions have been mentioned in the relevant chapters. History and examination give the clues to skin disorders and as well as asking general questions some specific ones are useful

- History
  - Length of time -When did it start? Does it come and go? Are there crops of lesions?
  - Site—Where did it start? Has it spread?
  - Behaviour—Does it itch? Does it ever blister? How does sunlight affect it?
  - Treatments—What makes it better/worse? What creams/ointments have been used?
  - Family and social history/contacts with a rash
  - Past medical history including drug history in the last 6 months
- Examination
  - In addition to a general examination look at palms of hands and soles of feet, hair, nails, and the mouth
  - Are lesions discrete or confluent?
  - Do lesions follow any particular pattern—linear, annular (ring shaped), following skin dermatomes, hands and feet, generalized distribution
  - Are they impalpable?
  - What is their consistency?—hard/soft/firm
  - Are they tender?
  - Do they feel hot?

If doubt exists about a skin lesion in a child then they should be referred either to a paediatrician with a special interest in dermatology or to a dermatologist. If the diagnosis remains unclear then a skin biopsy will be taken, usually a 3 or 4 mm punch biopsy.

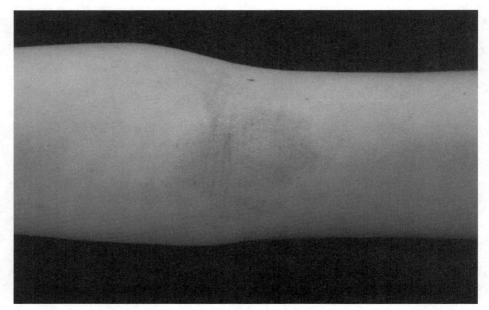

Fig. 17.1 Atopic eczema in flexure of the arm. See colour plate 8.

Child with a red rash

This is the commonest skin complaint in childhood and causes a lot of parental anxiety. The common differential diagnoses are atopic eczema, seborrhoeic dermatitis, urticaria, skin infection, and psoriasis.

Atopic eczema (Figs 17.1 and 17.2)

Key facts

- Affects 10–20% of children in the UK
- It is due to interplay of genetic, environmental, and immunological factors
- Diagnosis depends on the presence of itchy skin (or report of scratching and rubbing) plus ≥3 of the following
  - history of involvement of skin creases
  - history of asthma or hayfever or atopy in a first degree relative if <4 years
  - generally dry skin in the last year
  - onset at less than 2 years of age (not always diagnostic if the child is <4 years)
  - visible flexural eczema (or eczema affecting the cheeks and forehead if <4 years of age)
- Common on the extensor surfaces in infants localizing to flexures after 1 year of age

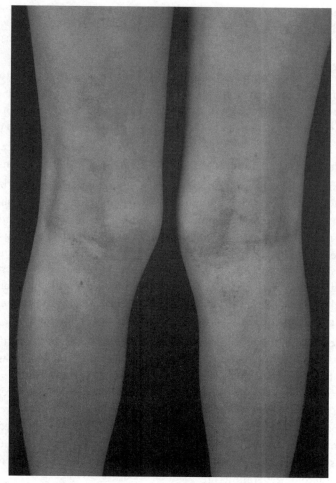

Fig. 17.2 Atopic eczema in flexure of the legs. See colour plate 9.

Treatment

- There is a lack of evidence base for many of the treatments used in atopic eczema.

- It is important that eczema treatments are demonstrated to parents especially the amount to be applied and where and when to apply each treatment prescribed.

- A written treatment plan is recommended.

- Growth should be carefully monitored.

- Many patients have tried alternative therapies such as homeopathy, Chinese herbs and creams. These therapies are not without side-effects and some herbal creams have been found to contain potent topical steroids. Liver and renal function should be monitored 3-monthly if on Chinese herbal products.

Emollients

- Bath daily. There are many emollient bath additives and there is little difference between them. If the skin appears worse after bathing it is usually due to erythema being more visible when the skin is warm. It is worth a change of bath emollient if there are concerns as sensitivity to the preservatives in all emollients can occur.

- Use a soap substitute—many emollients can be used as a soap substitute applied when in the bath or prior to bathing especially if there are multiple excoriations.

- These need to be used liberally and frequently, often every few hours. They provide a surface lipid film that retards evaporative water loss from the skin. They should be supplied as a 500 g tub unless eczema is very mild. There are many products on the market. It is worthwhile starting with generic products using more expensive products if these are not successful. In general, ointments are better for dry skin and creams for when the skin is sore and inflamed. However, compliance is important especially with older children and the key is to find an effective but cosmetically acceptable emollient for the child. Three different emollients may be needed, one for use on the face, one for use during the day and a third greasier emollient for use at night.

Topical corticosteroid preparations   These are safe to use in the long term if appropriate amounts are applied. Many parents are concerned regarding side-effects and underuse these preparations. It is vital to explain how to use topical corticosteroids. Finger tip unit (FTU) application gives a guide to how much should be used (a line of cream from the distal interphalangeal joint to the end of the index finger is sufficient to cover an area the size of both palms and is 0.5 g) as does the number of tubes being requested. Ointments are preferable to creams as they cause less irritation and hypersensitivity reactions, which are usually associated with preservatives in creams. Factor to consider when applying topical corticosteroid preparations are:

- *Age.* In children under 2 years of age use a mild potency topical steroid preparation, e.g. 1% hydrocortisone up to twice daily. Children over 2 years of age whose eczema is not improving may need to use a moderate potency topical steroid ointment, reducing to mild potency when the eczema is better controlled. Potent topical steroid preparations should not be routinely used in primary care.

- Site:
  - *face*—it is preferable to use 1% hydrocortisone as facial telangiectasia may develop with more potent preparations and these are permanent.
  - *eyelids*—beware of long-term use and the possibility of developing glaucoma.
  - *breast, abdomen, thighs, and upper arms in adolescents*—more potent preparations may lead to development of striae.
  - *palms and soles*—potent preparations may be needed to gain control as absorption is reduced on these sites.

Antihistamines

- A sedative antihistamine should be used as a short-term treatment when the eczema has flared up.
- There is no evidence to support the use of non-sedating antihistamines in atopic eczema.

Diet and allergy testing

- Routine exclusion diets are unhelpful as is RAST testing. Only about 40% of children with a positive RAST test are allergic to the food that has been tested.
- Any diet should be supervised by a paediatric dietician and the eczema monitored to see if exclusion of the food substance leads to improvement in the eczema.
- Routine use of soya milk to help atopic eczema in infants should be avoided.
- A trial of dietary manipulation may be warranted if eczema does not respond to first line treatment especially if there is a history suggestive of specific food allergy.

General measures It is important to keep fingernails short, wear comfortable clothing, and to avoid irritants.

Infection This cannot be diagnosed on a skin swab as most eczema is colonized by *Staphylococcus aureus*. Skin swabs should be taken if the eczema is not improving as some children are now colonized with MRSA and a swab will show if Group A beta haemolytic Streptococcus is present as well as *Staphylococcus aureus*.

Key treatment points

- Usually an oral course of antibiotics is needed as infection tends to be widespread. Use flucloxacillin ± penicillin V for a 10-day course. Oral erythromycin can be used but beware of staphylococcal resistance, which is greater in those who are attending hospital. Owing to the taste of the antibiotics compliance can be poor and Augmentin or a cephalosporin are alternatives.
- Antiseptic bath oils such as Dermol 600 and Oilatum plus are often used as is Dermol 500 lotion as a soap.
- Steroid preparations containing clioquinol, e.g. vioform hydrocortisone are useful for infected eczema.
- In eczema herpeticum Fig 17.3, unless it is very mild and localized, children should be referred to hospital for intravenous aciclovir. Topical corticosteroid preparations should be stopped. A delay in diagnosis of eczema herpeticum could be fatal for a child.
- Only use a combined topical antibiotic and corticosteroid preparation for ≤5 days as otherwise bacterial resistance may develop.

Support groups These can be extremely helpful as eczema can cause not only considerable suffering for the child but also for the family. The National Eczema Society (www.eczema.org) produces a number of helpful information sheets for parents and patients as well as information for professionals.

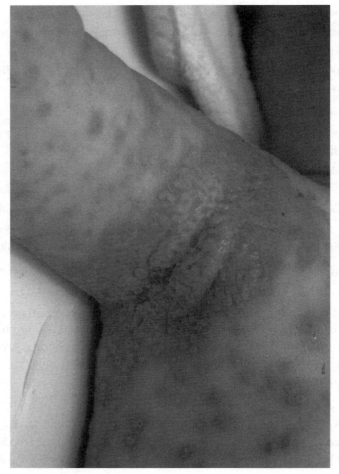

Fig. 17.3 Eczema Herpeticum. See colour plate 10.

Bandages

- Zinc and ichthammol impregnated bandages are useful for chronic lichenified eczema on the limbs. An elasticated bandage, e.g. Coban and actiwrap which are brown and white in colour respectively, helps to keep the impregnated bandage in place. These bandages are changed at 24–72-hourly intervals.

- Wet wraps are made from cotton tubular bandages (Tubifast, Comfifast, and Actifast). Ready made garments are now available in the same cotton tubular material and include vests, leggings, socks, and mittens. Wet wraps have increased in popularity, although there is no evidence to suggest that they are more effective than other treatments. Either an emollient or a weak topical steroid preparation is applied to the skin underneath the wraps and the wrap is made wet either with the preparation applied to the skin or with water.

Topical calcineurin inhibitors There are two licensed products pimecrolimus 1% (Elidel) and tacrolimus ointment (Protopic), 0.03% ointment for use in children ≥2 years and 0.1% tacrolimus for use in children ≥12 years of age.

Key points:

+ They work by immunomodulation of the skin.

+ NICE guidelines (June 2004) are for use in moderate to severe eczema not controlled by conventional therapy or if there is evidence of side-effects of topical corticosteroids.

+ Tacrolimus 0.1% is as effective as potent topical steroids and more effective than 1% hydrocortisone.

+ Pimecrolimus is less effective than potent topical steroids but has not been compared with mild potency ones.

+ Burning and skin irritation occurs in about 10% of cases at the start of treatment.

+ Long-term side-effects are as yet unknown but there have been concerns that use of these agents could predispose to skin cancers.

+ No skin thinning has been observed in studies.

Systemic immunosuppression This should only be used in children who are under the care of a hospital consultant.

+ *Prednisolone*—1–2 mg/kg per day is the starting dose weaning down to the lowest alternate day dose possible to control eczema. Treatment is usually of at least 1–2 years duration and children need close monitoring including growth, urinalysis, and blood pressure measurements.

+ *Ciclosporin* may be prescribed in doses up to 5 mg/kg per day in a short course (3–6 months). Regular monitoring is required including blood pressure and urinalysis and taking blood for a full blood count, renal and liver function, magnesium, and urate. This is usually an unsuitable treatment option for young children due to the need for regular blood tests.

When to refer a child with atopic eczema to secondary care

+ Child not responding to a treatment regimen of appropriate amounts of emollients and topical corticosteroid preparations.

+ A specialist opinion would be useful in counselling the family including a one-off consultation to reinforce the need for continued skin treatments.

+ For bandaging techniques.

+ For use of topical tacrolimus.

+ Children who need potent topical corticosteroids to control their eczema.

+ Children who need a systemic immunosuppressant for disease control.

+ Supervision of exclusion diets.

Differential diagnosis

All causes of an itchy red rash should be considered but especially seborrhoeic dermatitis if the child is less than 1 year of age and scabies at any age.

Seborrhoeic dermatitis

This typically has a very early onset in the first 3 months of life.

Key points

- Typical yellow greasy scaly scalp 'Cradle cap'.
- Affects flexures in the first year, including the napkin area.
- Depigments pigmented skin.
- Babies tend not to be disturbed by the rash and there is much less sleep disturbance than in atopic eczema.
- Usually clear by 12 months of age but may evolve into atopic eczema.

Treatment

- Start with emollients (see Atopic eczema) including the scalp. Olive oil or a greasy emollient, e.g. WSP/LP 50:50 is ideal for the scalp.
- Special and medicated shampoos are best avoided.
- Add in a mild potency topical corticosteroid only if the skin condition does not improve on adequate emollient therapy.

Urticaria

This is a transient erythematous and oedematous rash that may last from a few minutes to usually less than 24 hours. On clearing, there is normal skin. The rash may then appear at a different site. Urticaria that lasts for less than 6 weeks is acute urticaria and is labelled as chronic urticaria if it persists for greater than 6 weeks. In about half of the cases there will be swelling of the subcutaneous tissues (angioedema), often seen on the eyelids

Causes of urticaria

- Idiopathic—50% of cases.
- Infections—streptococcal infections, viral infections and *Toxocara canis*.
- Drugs—penicillin, sulphonamides, non-steroidal anti-inflammatory drugs, aspirin.
- Foods and additives—cow's milk, eggs, nuts, fish, exotic fruits.
- Physical agents—cold, sunshine, heat, water.

Key management points

- Take a detailed history to see if there is an obvious provoking factor and if there have been previous episodes.
- On examination look for other signs of allergy, especially for signs of anaphylaxis such as difficulty breathing and wheezing, shock, and circulatory compromise.

- If acute urticaria alone treat with chlorpheniramine.
- Lesions may become confluent and this is known as giant urticaria, which is often confused with erythema multiforme.
- In chronic urticaria, check a full blood count, renal and liver function, inflammatory markers (erythrocyte sedimentation rate or C-reactive protein) and check stool for threadworms. A long-acting antihistamine should be prescribed and reassurance given. The urticaria may persist for several years.

Urticaria pigmentosa

This is most common in early childhood. Pigmented macules are present, which urticate on rubbing. If there is doubt about the diagnosis a skin biopsy should be taken. Systemic involvement is rare. Antihistamines can be given if needed. The majority resolve spontaneously but may take a number of years to do so.

Infections and infestations

The commonest cause of an erythematous maculopapular rash is one associated with viral infections and these may be itchy. With some viruses there is a distinct pattern of rash, e.g. hand foot, and mouth disease, and further details can be found in the chapter on infectious diseases. In glandular fever a rash occurs in 90–100% of cases who have received ampicillin.

Impetigo

This is a superficially spreading infection which is characterized by a yellow brown honeycomb crust with weeping and erythema. It may be bullous especially in moist sites such as the axillae. It is the commonest infection in children under 5 years of age and tends to peak in the late summer months. Infection is usually due to *Staphylococcus aureus* and less commonly due to Group A beta haemolytic Streptococcus (about 10% of cases).

Key management points

- Check that other family members are not affected.
- Treat localized impetigous rashes with a topical antibiotic.
- If there are multiple patches a systemic antibiotic is indicated, flucloxacillin ± penicillin V or erythromycin.
- If the condition does not improve, take a skin swab for culture and sensitivity to exclude bacterial resistance to the antibiotic prescribed.

Staphylococcal scalded skin syndrome

This is due to enterotoxin producing staphylococci and starts as painful erythema in the flexures associated with fever. Bullae may be present. This is followed by widespread peeling of the skin

Key management points

- Children should be admitted to hospital and treated with intravenous antibiotics and strict fluid balance observation.
- Streptococcal infections can give a similar picture.

Scabies

This tends to cause an itchy skin eruption of variable intensity, usually about 1 month after infestation with the mite *Sarcoptes scabiei humanis*.

Key points

- Always look for a rash in any accompanying adult. The rash is due to an immune response to the mite and there may not be any signs in relatives.
- In infants, the rash is recognized by its distribution rather than burrows. Nodules are usually found in areas that come in frequent contact with adults, e.g. axillae where they are picked up and groins due to napkin changes.
- Secondary bacterial infection may be present and a positive bacterial swab does not exclude scabies.
- Lesions include vesicopustules, bullae, papules, and nodules.
- Secondary eczematization may be present and there is sometimes a transient improvement with eczema therapies.
- Nodules take about 3 months to resolve after successful therapy.
- Previous scabies treatment does not exclude the diagnosis. Always treat lesions on the head if these are present.
- A long history of >6 months may be obtained.

Treatment This should be with an aqueous based preparation of malathion or permethrin. It is important to treat all family members at the same time.

Tinea infections (Fig 17.4)

These are seen on the body as erythematous circular scaly lesions with a clearly defined margin and are known as tinea corporis on the body and tinea capitis in the scalp where there is hair loss associated with erythema and scaling. Patches may be multiple. Most infections in inner cities are due to *Trichophyton tonsurans*, which is spread by human to human contact, whereas *Microsporum canis* is spread by cats and dogs.

Key management points

- Ask about sources of infection and if other family members are affected.
- Check what has been applied to the skin. Steroid application will change the appearance 'tinea incognito' and lesions lose their circular shape, margins are less clearly defined and a pustular folliculitis develops.
- Scalp lesions often become boggy (kerion) and secondary bacterial infection may occur. They need treating with griseofulvin 10 mg/kg per day for at least 6 weeks and often longer. Supply of griseofulvin is often difficult and has to be obtained from abroad. Newer antifungals have been used but are not licensed for this condition. Topical applications will not clear the infection.
- Beware of an Ide reaction in which white papules appear on the trunk, face, and limbs. This is an inflammatory reaction and usually responds to emollients adding in

topical corticosteroids if itching is severe. Antifungal treatment should be continued and is essential for the papules to resolve.

+ A topical antifungal cream can be applied to lesions on the body.

+ To diagnose fungal infection, send skin scrapings or plucked hair for fungal culture. Treatment should be commenced prior to culture results being received for kerions as permanent hair loss may occur with a delay in treatment.

Psoriasis

In 2% of cases onset will be under 2 years of age with 10% of cases beginning at less than 10 years of age. Girls tend to be affected at a younger age than boys (5–9 years compared with 15–19 years). It is typically a relapsing and remitting skin condition with a scaly rash usually affecting the extensor surfaces and scalp.

Key points

+ There is a genetic predisposition with a lifetime psoriasis risk of 0.28 if one parent is affected or 0.65 if both parents are affected, rising to 0.51 and 0.83, respectively, if a sibling is also affected.

+ **Exacerbating factors** include streptococcal infection, psychological factors, drugs such as non steroidal anti-inflammatory drugs, withdrawal of systemic steroids, antimalarials and beta blockers, trauma, and HIV infection.

+ **Guttate psoriasis** classically occurs 2–4 weeks after a streptococcal sore throat and consists of small lesions on the trunk, which may be numerous (raindrop psoriasis).

+ **Nail signs** include pitting, separation of the nail from the nail bed (onycholysis) and subungual hyperkeratosis.

+ **Arthritis** may be severe and may be present prior to skin lesions. There is a higher incidence in patients with nail changes.

Management

+ Avoidance of triggering factors.

+ Use of emollients including a bath oil, soap substitute, and moisturizer.

+ Tar-based products. Crude coal tar is messy and for inpatient use only. Commercial products of distilled coal tar, e.g. Alphosyl and Exorex are less effective. Tar can be combined with salicylic acid in an ointment.

+ Vitamin D analogues such as calcipotriol (Dovonex) can be used if less than 40% of the skin is affected. These give a slow improvement and often need to be continued. They are mildly irritant and use on the face and flexures should be avoided. In children aged 6–10 years a maximum amount is 50 g/week and is 75 g for those aged 10–12 years.

+ Mild potency topical corticosteroids are best reserved for special sites such as the face, flexures, ears, and genitalia and may be combined with tar, e.g. Alphosyl HC.

◆ Dithranol preparations and dithrocream should be used with caution especially in young children with multiple lesions as they cause an irritant dermatitis.

When to refer to secondary care

◆ All children with severe widespread psoriasis including pustular psoriasis.

◆ Children who are not improving on treatment.

◆ Young children.

◆ Any child who requires systemic therapy to control the psoriasis such as methotrexate, ciclosporin, and acitretin.

◆ Doubt over the diagnosis. Differential diagnosis includes pityriasis rosea and lichen planus.

  • *Pityriasis rosea*. There is a herald patch that is oval or round, on the trunk in 45% cases and less commonly on the arms, thighs, and neck. Fine scaly pink plaques or macules appear 1–2 weeks later. There is often a mild prodrome including low-grade fever, headaches, malaise, and anorexia. The lesions of pityriasis rosea usually lasts <3 months.

  • *Lichen planus*. This is characterized by itchy, violaceous hyperkeratotic papules. The fine white scale over the surface, Wickham's striae, may not be present in children. It most commonly affects the flexor surfaces of the upper extremities and uncommonly affects mucous membranes and nails in children.

Viral and yeast infections

Herpes simplex virus infections

These are characterized by a vesicle on an erythematous background and lesions at different stages being present. It is important to take a history to exclude a predisposing dermatosis, e.g. eczema herpeticum and to see if the child is immunocompromised. Aciclovir is the only antiviral agent licensed for use in children.

  Features of primary herpes simplex gingivostomatitis:

◆ malaise/fever

◆ small vesicles develop

◆ multiple lesions

◆ tender cervical lymphadenopathy

◆ halitosis

◆ excessive dribbling in younger children

◆ usually presents late with multiple lesions.

Key treatment points

◆ Children should be treated with adequate and regular oral analgesia.

◆ Fluids will then be tolerated and it is rare to require admission and intravenous fluids.

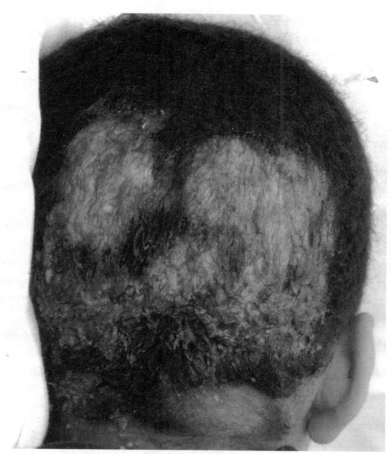

Fig. 17.4 Extensive tinea capitis. See colour plate 11.

◆ Treatment with aciclovir whose mode of action is to prevent further viral replication is usually not applicable as multiple lesions are present.

Herpes simplex virus infections may occur at any cutaneous site and are particularly common on the digits as children suck their fingers and toes. These should be treated promptly with oral aciclovir.

Herpes zoster (shingles)

It is important to ask for a history of chickenpox and to determine if the child is immunocompromised. Children who have had chickenpox <6 months of age are more likely to develop lesions of herpes zoster in childhood. There is a typical herpetic lesion that follows a dermatome(s), usually unilateral but lesions can be bilateral. Pain relief is important and aciclovir should be prescribed if lesions are seen at an early stage. It is important to recognize this condition as other children can catch chickenpox from a child with herpes zoster.

Warts

These are caused by human papillomavirus. They are commonest on the hands and feet (verrucas) but may occur at any site and tend to cause most anxiety when on the face and readily visible.

Key management points

- Treatment can be worse than the condition, which will resolve spontaneously but warts can last for several years.
- Think about child sexual abuse with perianal warts, especially if >2 years of age. The majority have, however, been innocently acquired.
- Refer all children who need treatment for warts on the face and perianal warts.
- Treat with a salicylic acid based wart paint applying daily and rubbing down prior to application with an emery board or pumice stone. This needs to be continued for 6 weeks to 3 months.
- Freezing with liquid nitrogen is poorly tolerated in children <5 years of age. Multiple applications may be needed.
- Imiquimod, applied three times weekly is not licensed for use in children and clinical trials of its use are needed.

Mollusca contagiosum

These are due to a poxvirus and are commonly known as water warts. They are dome-shaped papules with an umbilicated centre.

Key management points

- Reassurance is all that is needed and no treatment is the best option. All treatments are associated with scarring, whereas natural resolution does not leave a permanent scar.
- Mollusca may last for 2–3 years or longer so do not give a time limit on when they will resolve.
- They can be severe in atopic eczema, HIV infection, and Wiskott–Aldrich syndrome.
- When a mollusca contagiosum is looking red, angry, and extruding central cheesy contents, then this is a good sign as lesions usually resolve shortly after this time.

Pityriasis versicolor

This is a yeast infection caused by *Malassezia furfur*, which is part of the normal skin flora. Relapses are therefore frequent. Lesions are scaly and can present as hypo- or hyperpigmented patches usually on the upper trunk and arms. Sometimes lesions are red. Patches often coalesce.

Key management points

+ Lesions often become more noticeable in the summer months when the child gets a suntan.

+ Treatment is with 2.5% selenium sulphide (Selsun), topical imidazoles or ketaconazole shampoo.

Birthmarks and disorders of pigmentation

Strawberry naevi

These are typically not present at birth but develop in the first weeks of life, starting as a flat macular area of erythema which starts to become raised. A growth phase is seen for the first 3–6 months and lesions can become very large. After a stable phase the haemangioma will start to regress and often have a pale centre. Haemangiomas do not usually need treatment and resolve over 3–10 years.

When to refer to secondary care

+ Haemangiomas that are affecting a vital structure, e.g. the eye, which will lead to loss of sight. Treatment includes oral steroids, e.g. prednisolone 2–4 mg/kg per day, intralesional steroid injections, and use of the pulsed dye laser.

+ Ulcerated haemangioma, usually in the napkin area which is not healing.

+ If Kasabach–Merritt syndrome is suspected. The haemangioma is large and platelets become sequestrated leading to thrombocytopenia, haemorrhage, and consumption of clotting factors leading to disseminated intravascular coagulation.

+ Any infant, usually less than 3 months of age with multiple small skin haemangiomas (disseminated neonatal haemangiomatosis) needs careful assessment and referral to hospital. Some of these children will have haemangiomas in internal organs, e.g. liver and these need aggressive treatment with oral steroids. Untreated cases are reported as universally fatal.

+ Resolved haemangiomas that are causing cosmetic concern as plastic surgery can tidy up areas of loose skin.

Salmon patch

A salmon patch ('stork mark') is an area of dull red macular erythema and is present at birth. They are common in the nape of the neck, on the forehead, eyelids, and face. These require no treatment and tend to resolve within the first 2 years. Salmon patches around the hairline at the back of the neck are the most likely to persist. They look worse if the child is hot, e.g. with a temperature or after a warm bath and parental reassurance is often needed.

Port wine stain

These are present at birth as purple/red flat lesions and do not resolve. The majority respond to treatment with the pulse dye laser. The decision on whether or not to treat is a cosmetic one and cosmetic camouflage is an alternative to laser therapy.

- *Sturge–Weber syndrome* occurs typically when there is a port wine stain in the ophthalmic and maxillary divisions of the trigeminal nerve and leptomeningeal angiomas are present. Neurological manifestations include seizures, which may be intractable. Children should be monitored for glaucoma.
- *Klippel–Trenauney–Weber syndrome*. A port wine stain is present on a limb with limb hypertrophy.

Sebaceous naevus

These are usually present at birth and have a yellow greasy appearance. The scalp is the commonest site and hair loss is permanent. They become more prominent in adolescence and nodular in adult life. There is a small risk of malignant change after puberty. The decision to remove these lesions depends on clinical appearance and site.

Melanocytic naevi

- *Acquired naevi* are common and may increase in number at puberty.
- *Halo naevi* (area of pigmentation with a surrounding white ring) are very common in childhood and are entirely benign.
- *Malignant melanoma* is uncommon before puberty except in children with extensive congenital melanocytic naevi (bathing trunk naevus). Any suspicious naevi (sudden increase in size, bleeding, change in pigmentation) should be referred to hospital for evaluation using a dermatoscope.
- *Spitz naevus*. This is a firm reddish brown nodule that develops in childhood. It is benign but if doubt exists about the diagnosis, the naevus should be removed
- *Mongolian blue spot*. This is blue–grey pigmentation found in pigmented skins, often in the lumbosacral area and tends to resolve by the age of 7 years.
- *Naevus of Ito and Ita*, which are similar to Mongolian blue spot, but are permanent and affect skin supplied by the posterior supraclavicular nerve and the ophthalmic and maxillary divisions of the trigeminal nerve respectively.
- *Beckers naevus*. This usually presents in adolescence with hairy macular pigmentation affecting the chest and shoulder area. It is commoner in males.

Disorders of pigmentation

- *Vitiligo*. This affects 1% of the population and is probably autoimmune in aetiology. Spontaneous repigmentation occurs in about 20%. Treatments used include topical corticosteroids and topical tacrolimus ointment and seem to be most effective when applied to a new area of vitiligo. Referral to the skin camouflage service run by Red Cross volunteers can be of great benefit.
- *Albinism*. This is a defect in the gene encoding tyrosinase. There are many clinical and genetic variants with loss of pigment in the skin, hair, and eyes. Careful sun protection is needed as there is a risk of cutaneous malignancies.

◆ *Pityriasis alba.* This is a hypopigmented dermatitis consisting of patches on the cheeks and sometimes shoulders of children and is commoner in those with a history of atopy. The lesions do not have a distinct edge in contrast to vitiligo and blend into the normal coloured skin. If the skin is dry and flaky then an emollient is helpful. It will resolve spontaneously. Sun exposure makes the lesions more obvious.

Neonatal skin disorders

It is important to distinguish transient vesicopustular eruptions in the neonate from infections. Each baby should be assessed to see if they have other symptoms or signs suggestive of infection. Transient vesicopustular eruptions occur in babies who are otherwise well and feeding well.

Milia 'milk spots'

These are 1–2 mm white papules that can occur at any skin site but are often found on the face, especially the nose in newborn babies. They are small keratin retention cysts that usually resolve in the first few weeks.

Transient vesiculopustular eruptions

Miliaria

Miliaria appear due to blockage of the sweat glands leading to a red papular lesions (miliaria rubra). Tiny vesicles (miliaria crystallina) may also be present. It tends to present in the first 2 weeks of life and is worse in hot weather and if the environment is too warm. It usually resolves over the first few months of life.

Erythema neonatorum (toxicum)

This is a blotchy red rash found in 50% of neonates, presenting in the first 2 weeks of life, and often in the first 48 hours. Lesions may be urticarial, macular, papular, or pustular. Pustules are sterile and contain eosinophils. Lesions tend to fade within a few days.

Sebaceous gland hyperplasia

This is seen due to the effect of maternal androgens. Small yellow/white papules are usually most pronounced on the face, especially over the nose and forehead and resolve within a few weeks.

Transient neonatal pustulosis melanosis

This is usually present at birth and presents as vesicles and pustules that may have ruptured *in utero*. When these resolve a brown macule is left, which may persist for many months. It is commoner in Afro-Caribbean children.

Neonatal acne (Fig 17.5)

This must also be included in the differential diagnosis of transient vesiculopustular eruptions in the neonate.

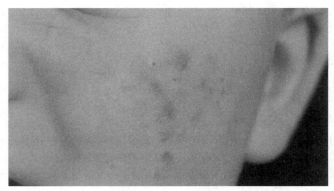

Fig. 17.5 Infantile acne. See colour plate 12.

Epidermolysis bullosa

This is a group of blistering disorders that tend to present at birth or shortly afterwards as areas of skin loss or blistering. The type of epidermolysis bullosa depends on the level of split in the skin whether in the epidermis, junctional, or in the dermis. Most tend to be autosomal recessively inherited with autosomal dominant epidermolysis bullosa simplex tending to present later when the child is beginning to move around and is confined to the hands and feet.

Key treatment point

All children should be referred to a paediatric dermatology and multidisciplinary team specializing in epidermolysis bullosa with specialist outreach nurses. In England there are two teams, based at Great Ormond Street Childrens Hospital and Birmingham Childrens Hospital.

Napkin dermatitis

This is usually due to an irritant contact dermatitis that spares the groins and responds well to the use of a barrier cream. Satellite lesions and skin-fold involvement are seen in *Candida albicans* infection and an antifungal cream with hydrocortisone cream may be needed. It is important to examine any napkin dermatitis that is not resolving carefully as a wide range of skin disorders may present in this way, including atopic eczema, seborrhoeic dermatitis histiocytosis X, acrodermatitis enteropathica, herpes simplex virus, psoriasis, congenital syphilis, and HIV infection.

Acne (Fig 17.5)

Twenty per cent of adolescents will be affected by acne of a severity that leads them to seek medical advice. Lesions found in acne include comedones, papules, pustules, nodules, cysts, and scars. It most frequently begins on the face but also commonly affects the upper back and chest. It is important to think of acne in the differential diagnosis of a skin rash at any age. In neonates it typically presents between 2 and 4 weeks of age and infantile acne is usually seen in children aged 3–6 months. Infantile acne often goes by 1 year of age but may last for 4–5 years. There is often a strong family history of acne and if acne is present when young there is a risk of more severe adolescent acne.

Key management points

- Refer for investigations into an endocrine cause if acne occurs between age 1 and 7 years
- Continuous treatment is essential. Therapy will depend on the severity of the acne.
  - *Mild acne.* Use topical therapy including benzoyl peroxide, antibiotics or a combination of both or a topical retinoid.
  - *Moderate acne.* It is important to continue topical therapy and add an oral antibiotic (tetracyclines but not in children <12 years of age, erythromycin, and trimethoprim are all used).
  - *Severe acne.* Oral isotretinoin (Roaccutane) is indicated. This should be initiated by a dermatologist who regularly treats acne. Screening tests are needed including blood tests (full blood count, renal and liver function test, erythrocyte sedimentation rate, glucose, cholesterol, and triglyceride levels) and a good history regarding possible depression. It is important that patients and parents are counselled about depression occurring as a side-effect of treatment as there have been fatalities. Other side-effects include dryness and cracking of the lips and nasal mucosa (nose bleeds may occur) and dryness of the cornea.

Erythemas

Erythema nodosum

This typically starts as hot red nodules on the shins, although other sites may be affected. Lesions turn to bruising and typically last 4–6 weeks. It is important to recognize as it is associated with underlying disorders, e.g. drugs, tuberculosis, Crohn's disease, and ulcerative colitis.

Erythema multiforme

This is a polymorphic eruption, often composed of distinctive target lesions (skin is abnormal in the centre) particularly on the extremities. There may be involvement of the lips, buccal mucosa, and tongue. Causes are similar to those for erythema nodosum. More severe cases should be referred to hospital as there is an overlap with Stevens–Johnson syndrome in which there is involvement of two or more mucosal surfaces and toxic epidermal necrolysis.

Miscellaneous

Hair disorders

It is important to distinguish the causes of alopecia (hair loss). Tinea capitis, which was discussed earlier, causes redness and scaling of the scalp. Most conditions are non-scarring and scars usually occur if there is underlying skin disorder, e.g. lichen planus or discoid lupus erythematosus, both rare in childhood. An untreated kerion may lead to scarring.

- *Alopecia areata* is a non-scarring disease in which hair loss may occur at any site. There is a family history in 20% of cases. There is usually a coin-shaped area(s) of hair loss. If all scalp hair is lost this is known as alopecia totalis and loss of all body hair as alopecia universalis. Exclamation mark hairs if present are pathognomic. Nail pitting is found in some cases. Key management points:
  - scalp is normal.
  - most cases resolve spontaneously; 50–80% of cases with patchy alopecia areata will show spontaneous regrowth within a year.
  - treatments are of little or transient benefit.
  - wigs can be prescribed.
  - a poorer prognosis is associated with onset in childhood, speed and extent of hair loss.
- *Telogen effluvium* is a disturbance of the hair cycle that occurs after a period of ill health or stress and corrects spontaneously.
- *Traumatic hair loss* may occur unintentionally from hair styling or in trichotillomania where the hair is pulled deliberately.
- *Head lice* (*Pediculosis capitis*). This is an endemic problem that peaks in children aged 4–11 years. Treatment is either mechanical by combing with conditioners or chemical using aqueous malathion or permethrin. If head lice are untreated for long periods of time then secondary bacterial infection may occur requiring treatment with oral antibiotics.

Striae

These occur around puberty and are due to skin distension. They are much commoner in females than males. Exacerbating factors include use of topical as well as systemic treatment with corticosteroids. Initially, lesions are pinkish red but will fade to leave a white linear atrophic area. There is currently no effective treatment and management is based around reassurance that lesions will fade and checking that the patient does not have Cushing's disease or inappropriate use of topical corticosteroid preparations.

Lichen sclerosis et atrophicus

This is a chronic destructive inflammatory condition with a predilection for genital and perianal skin. It has a female to male ratio of 6:1. Symptoms in girls include dysuria, pain on defecation, constipation, pruritus, soreness, and vulval or perianal bleeding. Boys tend to present with recurrent balanitis, fissuring and tightening of the foreskin, phimosis and dysuria. There is extragenital involvement in 10% of cases.

Key management points

- Confirm the diagnosis. Typical signs include erythema, excoriations and lichenification, loss of pigment, an atrophic appearance with 'cigarette paper' wrinkling, purpura, and bruising. It needs to be distinguished from eczema, psoriasis, and sexual abuse.

- There is no curative treatment. The aim of treatment is to keep genitalia as normal as possible. Architectural destruction is irreversible.
- All but the mildest cases should be referred to a local specialist in this condition either paediatrician or dermatologist. Potent topical corticosteroids are needed as well as emollients.
- Childhood lichen sclerosus improves at puberty but complete remission is rare.
- There have been reports of squamous cell carcinoma in adolescents with previously undiagnosed lichen sclerosus.

Dermatitis artefacta

It is important to take a good history, especially past medical history, distribution of lesions and of any worries that the child may have.

Key features

- Pattern of lesions does not correspond with a dermatological disorder.
- Bizarre lesions.
- In accessible sites, e.g. not in the middle of the upper back.
- Often history of other unexplained illness.

Treatment of this condition is usually difficult and needs referral to a paediatric dermatologist widely experienced in childhood disorders.

Juvenile plantar dermatosis

This typically affects the soles of the feet, which are shiny and glazed, slightly scaly, and painful fissures may develop. It is commoner in atopic children. The cause is thought to be due to friction from footwear and sweating is an exacerbating factor. Treatment is based around ensuring footwear fits well, wearing two pairs of cotton socks, and greasy emollients. There is no evidence that topical corticosteroids help this condition.

Further Readings

Harper J, Oranje A, Prose N (2000). *Textbook of Pediatric Dermatology*. Blackwell Scientific; Oxford.

Higgins E, Du Vivier A (1996). *Skin Disease in Childhood and Adolescence*. Blackwell Science Ltd, Oxford.

Atopic eczema

Conroy S (2004). New products for eczema. *Archives of Disease in Childhood Educational Practice* **89**: ep23–26.

Flohr C, Williams HC (1994). Evidence based management of atopic eczema. *Archives of Disease in Childhood Educational Practice* **89**: ep35–39.

McHenry PM, Williams HC, Bingham EA (1995). Fortnightly review: management of atopic eczema. *British Medical Journal* **310**: 843–847.

Santer M, Lewis-Jones S, Fahry T (2005). Childhood eczema. *British Medical Journal* **331**: 497.

Williams HC (2005). Atopic dermatitis. *New England Journal of Medicine* **352**: 2314–2324.

Psoriasis

Leman J, Burden D (2001). Psoriasis in childhood: a guide to its diagnosis and management. *Paediatric Drugs* **3**: 673–680.

Infections

Sladden MJ, Johnston JA (2004). Common skin infections in children. *British Medical Journal* **329**: 95–99.

Sladden MJ, Johnston JA (2005). More common skin infections in children. *British Medical Journal* **330**: 1194–1198.

Neonatal skin disorders

Eichenfield LF, Frieden IJ, Esterly NB (2001). *Textbook of Neonatal Dermatology* WB Saunders Co; Philadelphia.

Van Praag MC, Rooij RW, Folkers E, Spritzer R. Menke HE, Oranje AP (1997). Diagnosis and treatment of pustular disorders in the neonate. *Pediatric Dermatology* **14**: 131–134.

Chapter 18

Gastroenterology problems for primary care

Warren Hyer

It has been estimated that >20% of all paediatric consultations are for gastrointestinal problems in childhood. This chapter will concentrate on a practical approach to those problems most likely to present to general practice.

Recurrent abdominal pain

Chronic abdominal pain is a common cause of parental concern, childhood morbidity, time off school, and hospital referral. Yet if a careful history and examination are performed, and if the nature of the symptoms are typical of functional abdominal pain, many referrals to hospital can be avoided and the child and parents reassured.

A child with functional abdominal pain typically can provide the history—continuous, persistent pain over a period of months, the pain may wax and wane with some days better than others. Functional abdominal pain includes irritable bowel syndrome, functional dyspepsia, functional abdominal pain, and abdominal migraine.

The consultation with the child and parent is an opportunity to identify whether the pain has any features to suggest a significant organic cause. Table 18.1 lists 'red flags' to steer the primary care physician towards a more serious/organic diagnosis. The presence of these symptoms must lead to further investigations or swift referral.

In the absence of 'red flags' the physician can concentrate on whether the symptoms meet criteria of functional abdominal pain. For ease, it is often worth categorizing the pain into one of these functional bowel disorders (Table 18.2).

It will be clear that those children with epigastric symptoms may require an upper endoscopy before a diagnosis of functional dyspepsia is assumed. Similarly those with irritable bowel syndrome may require inflammatory bowel disease (IBD) to be excluded first.

After considering the 'red flags', and the criteria for functional bowel disorders, the physician is in a position to consider whether investigations will contribute or potentially confuse. Urine samples should not be taken without symptoms to suggest an acute urinary tract infection (UTI), e.g. dysuria and frequency. It is common for a child to have a positive urine culture, which is either a contaminant or asymptomatic bacteriuria and then commence renal investigations when there is no suggestion that the urine result has any relevance to the abdominal pain. Those children old enough to describe recurrent abdominal pain should be able to describe dysuria if they have a UTI.

Table 18.1 Red flags in the assessment of chronic abdominal pain

Chronic abdominal pain red flags—signs and symptoms suggesting an organic cause
Age <5 years
Pain further away from the umbilicus
Abdominal mass
Fever
Weight loss
Fall in appetite
Change in bowel habit (although constipation is often associated with functional abdominal pain)
Diarrhoea with tenesmus, urgency or night time defecation
Blood or mucus PR
Mouth disease or mouth ulcers or perianal disease
Joint symptoms
Dysuria or urinary frequency
Family history of inflammatory bowel disease

Children with 'red flags' may require assessment for IBD—either by referral to a hospital specialist or by investigation. The most discriminating blood investigation are inflammatory markers including raised platelet count, anaemia, hypoalbuminaemia, or raised C-reactive protein or erythrocyte sedimentation rate. However, many children with colitis have normal investigations and if the history is suggestive of IBD, then the child should be referred even if the blood investigations are normal. Endoscopy is the investigation of choice in a hospital setting.

Table 18.2 Definitions for functional bowel disorders in children

Rome II criteria for functional bowel disorders
Functional dyspepsia   At least 12 weeks of persistent or recurrent discomfort centred in the upper abdomen, with no evidence of ulcer disease and unrelated to change in stool habit.
Irritable bowel syndrome   At least 12 weeks of abdominal discomfort relieved by defecation, with change in stool habit, but no abnormal biochemical or haematological investigations. There may be mucus PR, abdominal distension, or bloating
Functional or recurrent abdominal pain of childhood   At least 12 weeks of continuous or recurrent abdominal pain, often periumbilical with no other GI symptoms and often some loss of daily functioning
Abdominal migraine   In the past 12 months, 3 or more intense paroxysms of acute onset abdominal pain lasting 2 hours to several days, but symptom free otherwise between spells, often with other migrainous features and headaches.

In those children with principally epigastric symptoms, duodenal ulcer disease should be considered. The investigation of choice in this setting is a gastroscopy, which often necessitates a general anaesthetic. If the epigastric symptoms are mild, variable, and there is no family history of duodenal ulcer disease, then one option is to offer a trial of H_2 receptor antagonist—especially in the older child. If the symptoms fail to settle on this regime, or recur after stopping treatment, then a gastroscopy is required. Measuring *Helicobacter* antibodies is often unhelpful and misleading—the investigation lacks specificity and there is much published data to suggest that presence of *Helicobacter* alone does not cause abdominal pain unless it progresses to either ulcer disease or gastritis.

Similarly constipation should not cause recurrent abdominal pain. It is often associated with functional abdominal pain but the two conditions probably share a common aetiology—dysmotility. Treating constipation may not resolve functional abdominal pain.

The treatment of chronic abdominal pain

If the cause of the pain appears to be anything other than functional abdominal pain, then the cause must be ascertained and choice of treatment depends on the diagnosis. Children with IBD need investigations and the therapy depends on the type. Patients with Crohn's disease are treated with courses of enteral nutrition, or steroids and other immunosuppressants. Those children with ulcerative colitis will need courses of steroids and steroid sparing agents such as azathioprine. Peptic ulcer disease confirmed at gastroscopy necessitates eradication of *Helicobacter*, and a 2-week course of a proton pump inhibitor.

If the child appears to have functional abdominal pain, then much of the treatment depends sharing the benign aspects of the condition and establishing a physician–patient–family relationship. Alleviating symptoms is the main goal, with opportunities to revisit the diagnosis if fresh symptoms arise. There are no specific universally effective therapies for functional symptoms but Table 18.4 lists options.

Constipation

The average prevalence of constipation increases from 2% in childhood to 15% in adults. It is estimated that a general practitioner will see 30 children with constipation per year.

Table 18.3 Significant pathological causes of chronic abdominal pain

Common significant conditions presenting with abdominal pain
Inflammatory bowel disease
Gastritis
Duodenitis
Peptic ulcer disease
Chronic pancreatitis
Gynaecological causes, including mittelschmertz pain
Lead poisoning
Sickle cell disease

Table 18.4 Treatment options for functional abdominal pain in childhood

Treatment options for functional abdominal pain in childhood
Reassurance   Inform the patient that the symptoms are real, explain the nature of the problem, re-establish normal daily life, avoid reinforcing symptoms
Dietary modification   Food-induced symptoms are common in IBS and those with diarrhoea-related IBS symptoms might benefit from an elimination diet, e.g. to lactose or fructose. Data to support high fibre diets in paediatric IBS patients is lacking but might benefit those with IBS symptoms and constipation
Therapies targeted at IBS
Antidiarrhoeal preparations such as loperamide, or antispasmodics such as hyoscine
Serotonin re-uptake inhibitors or serotonin receptor antagonists   Consider options such as paroxetine, fluoxetine but caution should apply to using SSRIs in children. Increased interest in 5-HT$_3$ antagonists and 5-HT$_4$ agonists
Antireflux therapies for functional dyspepsia   Trial of H$_2$ receptor antagonist or proton pump inhibitor for 8 weeks but if fails or symptoms recur, consider gastroscopy
Alternative and complementary therapy and probiotics

Tackling constipation is easy and straightforward and is worth doing well, as this leads to continence and may prevent a megarectum.

To assist the primary care physician tackling constipation, it is worth dividing constipation into different clinical settings, each needing a different approach.

Neonatal constipation including delay in passage of meconium, or failure to pass stool more than once a week in the first month, should lead to a referral to a paediatrician to look for other pathologies presenting as constipation, e.g. Hirschsprung disease or intestinal obstruction.

All children with constipation need to be counselled about toileting habits, dietary fibre intake and adequate fluid intake. Small children under 4 years of age may manifest *stool retaining behaviour*—posturing and buttock clenching. Children may stand and grip furniture, or hide in an attempt to retain stool. They may stain their underclothes as they try hard not to leak stool whilst squeezing tight their external sphincter. These children need both softeners (e.g. lactulose or polyethylene glycol) and stimulants (e.g. senna syrup) to both soften and provide an overwhelming desire to pass stool. Parents need to understand that their children are not truly constipated, but have a fear of defecation. Once the child is confident to use the toilet, then the problem will resolve but this may take months.

Older children with constipation and soiling are often impacted. Even a normal abdominal examination will not exclude an impacted rectum. If the rectum is overfull, then the poor child often soils without any warning and is often surprised to find they have soiled. A sympathetic approach is essential—soiling in a school age child is

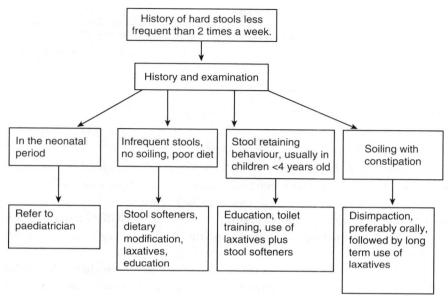

Fig. 18.1 Assessment of childhood constipation.

devastating for child and family and is often not deliberate. Anticonstipation measures are unlikely to work until the rectum is emptied—*disimpaction*. This requires large volumes of polyethylene glycol, occasional sodium picosulphate and rarely enemas. Once disimpaction is achieved, continence will return—with great relief to all. Once the rectum is empty, then it is usually necessary to continue oral therapies, e.g. polyethylene glycol or lactulose and senna for months to prevent reaccumulation in a megarectum.

Table 18.5 lists 'red flags' for primary care physicians' to seek at history and examination—the presence of these findings should lead to a paediatric referral.

Recurrent vomiting and infantile colic in infancy

Gastro-oesophageal reflux (GOR) is a normal process in children—the involuntary passage of gastric contents into the oesophagus. Regurgitation or spitting up refers to gastric contents drooling out the mouth. This is a normal event.

Table 18.5 Red flags/warning issues in assessment of a child with constipation

Failure to improve on laxative therapy
Onset age <1 month
Delay in passage of meconium
Failure to thrive (e.g. hypothyroidism, celiac disease)
Pre-existing psychomorbidity
Anal stenosis or significant abdominal distension
Urinary incontinence (e.g. spinal lesions)

Table 18.6 Serious causes of vomiting in infants

Gastrointestinal obstruction, e.g. pyloric stenosis, intussusception, Hirschsprung disease
Gastrointestinal disorders, e.g. gastroenteritis, food allergy, severe gastro-oesophageal reflux
Neurological, e.g. hydrocephalus, subdural haematoma
Infection, e.g. sepsis, meningitis, urinary tract infection
Metabolic, e.g. galactosaemia, congenital adrenal hyperplasia
Cardiac, e.g. heart failure

Gastro-oesophageal reflux *disease* (GORD) is an issue that needs addressing—this is when the GOR is associated with mucosal damage or the symptoms are so debilitating that they impair the quality of life. The challenge for a primary care physician is to determine whether the vomiting is simply uncomplicated GOR, or GORD or another pathology altogether. Untreated GORD may be associated with oesophagitis, failure to thrive, and stricture formation.

Faced with the vomiting child, the primary care physician must exclude other pathologies first—these are listed in the Table 18.6. Thus the primary care physician must look for the red flags shown in Table 18.7.

Once a more serious problem has been excluded, then the primary care physician can follow the algorithm in Figure 18.2.

Those with warning signs or where the diagnosis includes a disorder listed in Table 18.5 should be referred to the paediatrician.

An infant with uncomplicated GOR (the happy spitter) needs no further tests or investigations. Thickened feeds may have a role to 'buy time' and reduce the inconvenience. Alginate antacids (e.g. Gaviscon) are often offered with no convincing evidence they work in GOR or GORD.

Table 18.7 Red flags or warning signs for a primary care physician to seek when assessing the vomiting child

Bilious vomiting
Gastrointestinal bleeding
Forceful vomiting
Onset of vomiting after 6 months of life
Failure to thrive
Diarrhoea
Constipation
Fever
Lethargy
Hepatosplenomegaly
Bulging fontanelle
Seizures

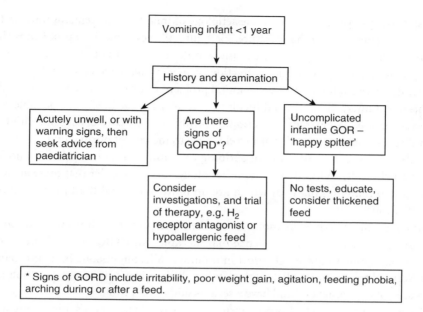

Fig. 18.2 Algorithm for assessing GOR in an infant.

For those where there is a suggestion of GORD with poor weight gain, excessive crying, irritability, disturbed sleep, feeding phobia, agitation on feeding, or respiratory symptoms (including apnoea) then a conservative approach would not be suitable. These infants may require investigations to ascertain the severity of their GORD with 24-hour pH monitoring or manometry, gastroscopy under general anaesthesia or investigations for delayed hypersensitivity to milk. Treatment options include H_2 receptor antagonists, or a trial of hypoallergenic feeds. H_2 receptor antagonists may reduce oesophagitis but do not rectify the underlying disordered motility. Thus prokinetics are often added but some have side-effects, including cardiac electrophysiological effects.

Hydrolysate (hypoallergenic) feeds are useful in infants with GORD with failure to thrive, or atopy. Their use is appropriate when blood investigations support an enteropathy or food allergic process (e.g. low haemoglobin, low albumin, high platelets). Failure to improve on these therapies requires paediatric review, further investigations, or addition of prokinetic agents. Severe GORD with feeding phobia may require an inpatient assessment or a period of nasogastric feeding.

Infantile colic

This is a most troubling complaint, and many mothers may not seek professional help for their screaming or agitated infant. The reported prevalence of infantile colic ranges from 10 to 40% of all children. This describes prolonged crying—crying for at least 3 hours, for at least 3 days of at least 3 weeks.

Despite over 40 years of research, the aetiology of infantile colic remains unclear. Four main causes emerge from the literature. First, infantile colic may be a problem with the gut in which excessive crying is the main symptom. According to this view, excessive crying is the result of painful gut contractions caused by allergy to cow's milk protein, or excess gas. Secondly, it may be a behavioural problem resulting from a less than optimal parent–infant interaction, with a difficult temperament of the infant as a possible explanation for inadequate parental reactions. Thirdly, the excessive crying in a child with infantile colic could be regarded as merely the extreme end of normal crying. Fourthly, infantile colic is just a collection of aetiologically different entities that are not easy to discern clinically. Without a unifying aetiology, it is no wonder that there are a host of suggested remedies many of which are no more beneficial than placebo and the passage of time.

The symptoms described by mothers are often interpreted by clinicians and mothers as possible GOR. There is no evidence that therapies for GOR, e.g. thickeners, or H_2 receptor antagonists have much effect in infantile colic. Simeticone is an antifoaming agent licensed for infantile colic, yet there is very little evidence it works. Anticholinergic drugs are not recommended and have a serious side-effect profile.

A change of formula to hydrolysate formula (thus eliminating cow's milk formula) can have a profound effect on infant crying—the infant must tolerate the taste. However, in a breast-fed infant, changing the feed to a formula must be discouraged as the advantages of breast feeding are overwhelming. In addition, modifying the diet of breast feeding mothers is fraught and often unnecessary. Those formula fed infants presenting with screaming alone (± vomiting) may improve considerably on a change in formula (e.g. to a hydrolysate feed) if they are cow's milk protein intolerant, and there is evidence that this approach may work in the primary care setting.

Any intervention imposed on a child with colic will not be blinded—there is a large placebo effect in treating children with infantile colic and many mothers just require reassurance, and behavioural modification (e.g. less fussing behaviour).

Adverse food reactions and allergy

Faced with a child with a history of an adverse food reactions, the primary care physician should follow the algorithm in Figure 18.3.

Adverse reactions to food may not mediated by immunity—these reactions are not food allergy. These include toxic reactions, e.g. gastroenteritis, carbohydrate malabsorption, and intolerances. It may be possible from history alone to identify whether a reaction is allergic in nature, e.g. a child whose behaviour deteriorates after chocolate is unlikely to be mediated by allergy. While many manifestations of food allergy are immediate and associated with IgE hypersensitivity, in approximately half of young children with challenge—proven food allergy, an IgE-based mechanism cannot be demonstrated. These children often have a delayed manifestation, e.g. atopic eczema, cow's milk induced enteropathy. Table 18.8 classifies gastrointestinal food hypersensitivity reactions.

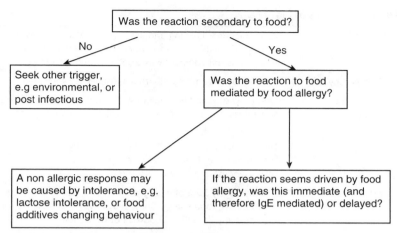

Fig. 18.3 Assessment of adverse food reaction in children.

Food allergy is common—up to 6% of children will manifest food allergy and the prevalence is rising. Cow's milk, egg, wheat, peanut, and soybean account for the majority of food allergy (>90%). Seeds such as sesame seem to be emerging allergens. Severe and fatal reactions can occur at any age and even on first exposure to a food, but those at greatest risk for fatal food-induced anaphylaxis appear to be adolescents and young adults with asthma and a food allergy to peanuts, tree nuts, or milk.

The clinical presentation of food allergy vary according to host factors. Allergic reactions mediated by food-specific IgE antibodies usually result in symptoms that occur soon (within minutes or up to 2 hours) while cell-mediated disorders may present with chronic symptoms or with a delayed onset (e.g. hours). The Table 18.9 lists different manifestations.

Testing for food allergy

History is critical in ascertaining the causal food as the available tests that use IgE antibodies have many false positives, and false negatives. From the description above it will be clear that many responses are neither immediate or associated with positive IgE antibodies. Skin prick tests identify IgE antibodies to a food protein—a positive response

Table 18.8 Classification of gastrointestinal food hypersensitivity

IgE-mediated disorders
   immediate food hypersensitivity
   oral allergy syndrome

Mixed IgE and non-IgE-mediated disorders   allergic eosinophilic oesophagitis, and gastritis
Non-IgE-mediated disorder   dietary protein enterocolitis, proctitis, or enteropathy

Table 18.9 Manifestations of food allergy

Urticaria (and angioedema)	Acute urticaria, flushing and acute cutaneous reactions. These are usually IgE mediated, hence immediate. (Chronic urticaria, however, is not commonly associated with food allergy)
Gastrointestinal anaphylaxis	Nausea, pain, vomiting, diarrhoea, usually IgE mediated
Pollen- food syndrome (oral allergy syndrome)	Oropharyngeal and lip tingling with pruritus to particular fruits/vegetables, e.g. melons, peach, apples) with cross sensitization to pollen proteins
Anaphylaxis	Life-threatening reaction to food mediated by IgE with multiorgan system reaction. In some cases, anaphylaxis occurs only if exercise follows ingestion of the causal food
Atopic eczema	Approximately 30% of young children with moderate to severe eczema have food allergy. Some may have immediate responses, but for many the IgE antibody is not detectable
Food-induced proctocolitis	Infants with mucus and blood in stools, often breast fed. If the colitic symptoms are mild, then this does not require dietary modification
Food protein-induced enteropathy	Diarrhoea, failure to thrive, hypoproteinaemia and anaemia, reflux. Often caused by cow's milk protein in children <2 years old. Coeliac disease, a specific enteropathy caused by immune reaction to gluten associated with HLA DQ2. These disorders are not associated with IgE antibody to causal proteins
Others—e.g. allergic eosinophilic oesophagitis/gastroenteritis, dermatitis herpetiformis	

does not mean a child is allergic to that food, it only infers sensitisation. A weal >3 mm or larger compared with the negative control is significant, i.e. it has detected the presence of an antibody. In older children >1 year, negative skin prick test have a high negative predictive accuracy virtually excluding IgE-mediated food allergy. Of course, the child may still have a non-IgE-mediated disorder, e.g. food induced enteropathy. The positive predictive accuracy is lower, 50% or less. Overall, only approximately 40% of patients with a positive skin prick test will experience allergic symptoms if they ingest the food. The choice of reagents for skin prick testing depends on history—large number of food skin tests applied indiscriminately often leads to confusion. For children with non-IgE-mediated responses, e.g. atopic eczema, then there is a role for patch testing but this test is still seeking its place in the evaluation of food allergy.

In vitro testing (e.g. radioallergosorbent, RAST, tests, or enzyme-linked immunosorbent assays) detect circulating IgE antibody. Unfortunately, the interpretation of this test depends on the assay methodology and it is hard to define positive and negative 'cut-offs'. Families often inquire about 'blood tests'—such assays have false positive and false negative responses. Non-IgE-mediated blood tests, e.g. IgG have not been validated and often add more confusion.

Elimination diet have a major diagnostic and treatment role in the assessment of food allergy—especially in the non-IgE-mediated reactions, e.g. eczema or food induced enteropathy. The type and scope of the elimination depends on the problem. For example, those children fed on a cow's milk infant formula can have a trial of a hypoallergenic formula, e.g. hydrolysate feed. Soy formula is not suitable as a hypoallergenic formula but can be used in children >6 months whose only allergic response was an immediate reaction to milk, e.g. gastrointestinal anaphylaxis to cow's milk.

In an older child, eliminating one or two suspected foods may be appropriate—this must be in conjunction with a dietician and elimination of a large number of foods can lead to unnecessary broad restrictions and subsequent nutritional deficiencies.

Oral food challenges are currently the most effective means to determine whether an individual truly reacts to a food. For investigation of immediate responses, this should be performed in hospital and carries a risk of severe reaction. Children with a history of a severe reaction to a food should not be rechallenged to that food. It may be used to investigate a child with peanut allergy, e.g. to identify whether they also react to tree nuts such as almonds.

Treatment of food allergy

The primary treatment is to avoid the causal food—in some cases even a small amount of the causal protein may trigger a reaction. This requires identifying the causal food by history and testing (perhaps with an oral challenge) and close dietetic support. Alternatives to the causal food should be sought, e.g. the use of hydrolysate feeds in children with cow's milk allergy.

The role of self-injectable adrenaline (epinephrine) is still to be defined. It is valuable in the treatment of severe and potentially fatal food allergic reactions and delayed administration has been associated with poor outcomes. It should not be provided to children and families with food allergy without a package of care including dietetic advice, assessment of likely causal foods, tight control of pre-existing asthma, community nursing, and an emergency plan for school and family. Candidates for self-injectable adrenaline (epinephrine) include those with prior food allergic responses involving the respiratory and cardiovascular system, food allergic children with asthma, children with food allergy to peanuts, or a family history of severe food allergic reactions. The priority must be avoidance of the causal food, hence obligatory dietetic referral. Death from food allergy is still very rare but severe reactions do occur and the child and parent must be educated about avoiding the causal food.

Many children outgrow their allergies. Most children with cow's milk protein intolerance will be able to consume dairy products after age 3 years. It is unclear if children can outgrow their nut allergies. Regular testing, oral challenges, and clinical reviews will help identify those who develop tolerance to foods that previously led to food reactions

Acute onset diarrhoea and vomiting

Gastroenteritis is one of the commonest acute conditions a primary care physician will face in children. It tends to occur in clusters in the winter (rotavirus). It may be bacterial, e.g. salmonella, campylobacter, or *Escherichia coli*. Children with acute onset gastroenteritis may present to a primary care physician with vomiting alone as the first manifestation. Clinicians should be on the guard when faced with a child with vomiting but without diarrhoea—only in time will it become apparent if this will evolve into gastroenteritis and the primary care physician should consider other causes of acute onset vomiting, including sepsis, raised intracranial pressure, and urinary tract infections.

Vomiting and diarrhoea can rapidly lead to dehydration in children. There are many criteria used to assess the degree of dehydration but the best tool is to compare with previous weights, and obtain a history of frequency of diarrhoea and vomiting, and compare this with oral intake in the past 24 hours. The presence of dry nappies confirms significant dehydration.

Those children with cardiovascular compromise including tachycardia, cool peripheries, and reduced urine output are approaching 10% dehydration and should be referred to a paediatrician for rapid oral rehydration. Alternatively, they may be shocked through sepsis. Table 18.10 illustrates clinical findings that suggest the degree of dehydration.

The foundation of treatment for gastroenteritis is rehydration and prevention of further dehydration. Once the degree of dehydration has been estimated, and the child weighed, the volume of rehydration required can be calculated as follows:

Volume of rehydration to overcome deficit (ml) =
(weight of child in kg) × (% dehydration) × 10

Thus a 10 kg child who is 5% dehydrated would require 10 × 5 × 10 = 500 ml. This volume should be replaced over 4 hours orally. Ideally oral rehydration solutions (ORS) should be used, especially in those under 1 year. Children who are not particularly dehydrated may refuse ORS—alternatively water or very dilute juice may be used. Children who fail to tolerate the rehydration or persistently vomit need to be referred to the paediatrician for nasogastric rehydration (or intravenous if older).

Breast-fed infants should continue to be breast fed, using ORS to top up after each diarrhoea or vomit (approximately 10 ml/kg ORS for each big diarrhoea).

After rapid rehydration over 4 hours, all infants and children should be encouraged to eat and drink—topping up with ORS or clear fluids after each diarrhoea. There is

Table 18.10 Assessing the degree of dehydration

	Moderate 5–10%	Severe >10%
Condition	Restless	Drowsy
Eyes	Sunken	Very sunken
Fontanelle	Sunken	Very sunken
Tears	Reduced	Absent
Mucous membranes	Dry	Very dry
Tissue elasticity	Reduced	Absent
Capillary refill time	2–4 seconds	>4 seconds
Pulse	Tachycardia	Thready or very tachycardic
Blood pressure	Normal	Normal or low
Urine output	Reduced	Reduced or absent

no role for routine dilution of formulas after gastroenteritis, use of antidiarrhoeal medication or change in formula (e.g. to soy).

Table 18.11 illustrates red flags that should alert a primary care physician to refer a child with gastroenteritis to a paediatrician urgently.

Chronic diarrhoea

It is not uncommon for the primary care physician to be faced with a child with 'diarrhoea' for >3 weeks. The primary care physician needs to understand what the parent means by diarrhoea. Persistent and severe diarrhoea since birth in a neonate may reflect a congenital diarrhoea and this needs urgent referral. Diarrhoea may persist for up to 14 days after gastroenteritis or courses of antibiotics—beyond that time other causes should be considered. Chronic diarrhoea with weight loss or failure to thrive should be investigated swiftly.

Most children with chronic diarrhoea will require hospital-based investigations (see Table 18.12). Toddlers' diarrhoea is a chronic diarrhoea with loose stools up to six times a day and normal growth and nothing abnormal at examination. The cause is not clearly understood and may be due to abnormal gut transit with colonic bacterial degradation of partially digested foods leading to further diarrhoea. These children and families need reassurance and the condition resolves within 3 years. Some benefit from a diet with increased fat intake, and decreased fibre and fruit juices.

Acute abdominal pain

The first step when assessing a child with acute onset abdominal pain is to identify whether there is an acute emergency, e.g. a surgical abdomen. History and examination are essential to ascertain duration, presence or absence of diarrhoea and vomiting, and presence of fever. It is important to check the hernial orifices and testes and be aware that lower respiratory tract infections (lower lobe pneumonias) may present with abdominal pain alone. It is worthwhile checking the buttocks of children with acute abdominal pain as this may be the first manifestation of Henoch–Schonlein purpura.

Naturally a child with dysuria and frequency may have a urinary tract infection— urine samples should be tested at the bedside to look for leucocytes and nitrites using

Table 18.11 Red flags in gastroenteritis

Assessed to be >10% dehydrated
Failure to tolerate rapid rehydration
Refusal to drink
Relentless vomiting—especially without diarrhoea
Bloody diarrhoea (risk of haemolytic uraemic syndrome)
Pre-existing medical issues, e.g. failure to thrive
Minimal urine output
Diarrhoea that persists >10 days
Home circumstances may preclude rehydration at home

Table 18.12 Assessment of chronic diarrhoea in children

Enteropathy	Look for anaemia, hypoalbuminaemia with diarrhoea and growth failure. Commonest causes are enteropathy driven by cows milk or gluten (celiac disease). Requires small bowel biopsy via gastroscopy
Coeliac disease	Gluten intolerance often presenting with abdominal distension, poor weight gain and pallor—often, but not always with diarrhoea. Diagnosis can be sought by measuring IgA level, IgA antitissue transglutaminase, IgA and IgG antigliadin. Diagnosis must be confirmed by small bowel biopsy via gastroscopy
Inflammatory bowel disease	Abdominal pain, bloody diarrhoea, weight loss, anorexia, mouth ulcers, tenesmus and urgency. full blood count, erythrocyte sedimentation rate, albumin, and C-reactive protein demonstrate raised inflammatory markers. Diagnosis achieved by colonoscopy or gastroscopy and biopsy
Cystic fibrosis	Malabsorption with bronchiectasis. Diagnosis established by sweat test
Persistent infection	Persistent parasites, e.g. giardia. Stool for MCS and parasites. May need aspiration of duodenal juices via gastroscope

testing sticks. However, children with pelvic sepsis, e.g. appendix abscess or pelvic inflammatory disease may present with acute pain and dysuria.

Antibiotic use in children with acute abdominal pain should be avoided, except in urinary tract or respiratory infections, as it may mask evolving peritonitis from an appendicitis. Early appendicitis may be difficult to distinguish from gastroenteritis. These patients need frequent and daily review until their symptoms settle.

It is worthwhile considering the possibility of diabetic ketoacidosis—this endocrine emergency may present with abdominal pain as the only symptom. This can be excluded by urine testing and measuring blood glucose. Mesenteric adenitis is a childhood phenomena with abdominal pain accompanying upper respiratory tract infections, allegedly caused by painfully enlarged abdominal lymph nodes.

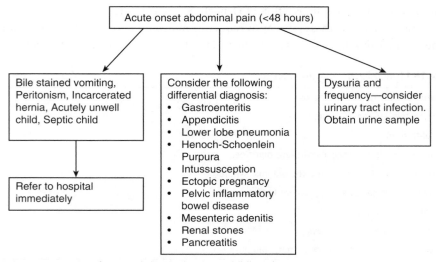

Fig. 18.4 Assessment of acute abdominal pain in childhood.

Figure 18.4 recommends an approach to the child with acute abdominal pain. The presence of tachycardia, fever, and local tenderness is consistent with appendicitis. The clinician should be wary of the young child (<2 years) with abdominal pain, palpable mass, and vomiting—this child may have an intussusception that requires immediate reduction by air enema or surgery. Children with peritonism and bile-stained vomiting need immediate referral to hospital.

Rectal bleeding

In infancy, rectal bleeding may be a presentation of food protein induced enterocolitis as a manifestation of food allergy. Alternatively, children under 1 year are at risk of intussusception—a gastrointestinal emergency with an infant presenting with acute abdominal pain, screaming, and vomiting. As the intussusception fails to resolve, the infant may develop rectal bleeding—classically with red current jelly stool. This is a surgical emergency and requires immediate referral.

An approach to rectal bleeding in children >1 year is shown in Figure 18.5. IBD, typically Crohn's disease or ulcerative colitis, may present with weight loss, fall in appetite, diarrhoea with or without bleeding and mucus from the rectum, abdominal pain, and mouth ulcers. Those with colitic symptoms will present with bloody diarrhoea, urgency, tenesmus, nocturnal defecation, and weight loss. The presence of bloody diarrhoea requires referral for investigation, including colonoscopy and contrast studies.

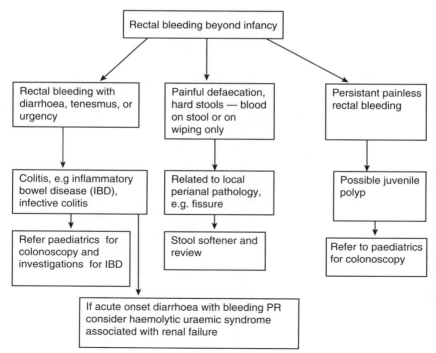

Fig. 18.5 Assessment of rectal bleeding beyond infancy.

Further Reading

1   **Guadalini S** (ed.) (2004). *Textbook of Paediatric Gastroenterology and Nutrition*. Taylor and Francis, Oxford.
2   **Brostroff J, Challacombe SJ** (2002). *Food allergy and intolerance*. Saunders, London.

Chapter 19

Paediatric neurology

Sandeep Jayawant

It is not possible to cover all of paediatric neurology in this short chapter on neurology. Some relevant topics that might be encountered in primary care are discussed briefly. References for further reading are suggested.

Headaches

About 70% of school children experience at least one episode headache per year, with 25% experiencing it more frequently. Migraine and tension headache are the commonest causes of headache in children. Table 19.1 lists various other causes of non-migrainous headaches.

Migraines

Migraine affects 3–10% of children (50/1000 school age children in UK). Mean age at onset is 7.2 years for boys, 8–10.9 years for girls. Twenty per cent of children experience their first attack before the age of 5 years. Incidence increases with age, affecting girls and boys equally before puberty, but girls more commonly thereafter. Migraine, according to the International Headache Society's criteria, can be defined as a recurrent headache that occurs:

- with or without aura
- is usually unilateral
- of moderate to severe intensity
- pulsating in quality
- aggravated by routine physical activity
- accompanied by nausea, vomiting, phonophobia, and photophobia.
- is not attributable to any other cause.

Migraine can occur with or without aura. Migraine with aura occurs in about 10% of cases. There are other atypical and complicated forms of migraine such as familial hemiplegic migraine, opthalmoplegic migraine, and basilar artery migraine. There are other conditions included under a broad umbrella of migraine-like disorders, which includes benign paroxysmal vertigo and benign paroxysmal torticollis.

Episodic tension-type headaches

These are usually bilateral, last from 30 minutes to 7 days, have a pressing or tightening quality and are not aggravated by physical activity, nausea, vomiting. Photophobia and phonophobia are not typical accompaniments.

Table 19.1 Non migraine causes of headaches

Organic headache
    Post-traumatic
    Infections (e.g. otitis media, dental infections, meningitis, sinusitis)
    Postseizure
    Pharmacological (e.g. analgesics, caffeine, food additives)
    Toxic (substance abuse, marijuana, cocaine, carbon monoxide poisoning)
    Arthritis of temporomandibular joint
    Hypertension
    Tumours and other space-occupying lesions
    Raised intracranial pressure (e.g. BIH, hydrocephalus, Chiari malformation)
    Low intracranial pressure (post LP, dural tear)

Vascular headaches
    Cluster headaches
    Intracranial bleed (post-traumatic, ruptured AVM, ruptured aneurysm)
    Various sinus thrombosis
    Vasculitis (e.g. systemic lupus erythematosus)

Non-organic headache
    Chronic episodic tension type
    Chronic daily
    Depression

When these evolve into more continuous headaches occurring on average 15 days of every month for 6 months or more, they are labelled chronic tension-type headaches.

Cluster headaches

There are severe headaches, unilateral, orbital/supra-orbital/temporal in localization, last 15–180 minutes. There is often accompanying conjunctival injection, lacrimation, nasal congestion, rhinorrhoea, forehead and facial sweating, miosis, ptosis, and eyelid oedema on the side of the headache.

Obstructive sleep apnoea

May manifest as early morning headaches with accompanying anorexia in a child who snores at night with nocturnal arousals and daytime somnolence. The possibility of environmental exposure to lead/carbon monoxide and possibility of non-pharmacological drug use or substance abuse should be considered when aetiology of the headaches is unclear.

Raised intracranial pressure

Usually is suggested by recent onset of headaches worsened by lying down, nocturnal vomiting, altered conscious level, papilloedema, hypertension, and increasing head circumference with/without sunsetting eyes and prominent scalp veins. Further pointers to significant intracranial pathology, e.g. brain tumours (which accounts for less than 1% of lifetime prevalence of headaches) include a change in personality or decline in school performance and focal neurological signs such as ophthalmoplegia, weakness, ataxia, nystagmus, dysarthria, and hypotonia.

For the child with long-standing headaches and normal physical examination, no investigation is required. Routine laboratory studies, lumbar puncture, and EEG are not recommended. However, in practice, these are individual cases where it is essential to allay extreme levels of anxiety that maybe responsible for or exacerbate headaches. Imaging in these cases is probably justifiable and 'therapeutic', although there remains a risk of detecting incidental abnormalities such as a Chiari I malformation, which may enhance the anxiety and muddy the waters where clarity of diagnosis is paramount.

Management of headaches

Accurate diagnosis is crucial to successful management. Needless to say careful history and examination is the key to eliminating most differentials in the causation. Various therapies are propounded in the management of headaches, in general and migraines in particular.

Specific dietary exclusions are often used such as chocolates, cheese, coffee, diary products, and gluten-free diets. There is insufficient evidence that any of this helps and often is difficult to identify specific food triggers. Such strict diets tend to be unpopular and difficult to enforce in children.

Stress is often an underlying factor and a clinical psychologist maybe able to identify an underlying factor. Muscle relaxation techniques and stress management programmes may work well in the motivated adolescent. Breakdown of family structures and loss of close personal associates whether pets, family members or friends through separation, bereavement, or illness is often an underlying factor. Complex psychosocial factors play a role at times. Unrealistic academic expectations and bullying in schools can sometimes cause major stress and anxiety. Clinical depression, often underdiagnosed in children can be interwoven inseparably. These factors clearly can exist even with migraines, but are more likely to be present in the tension-type headaches.

Pharmacological treatment of migraine is often resorted to. However, limited data exist on efficacy of drug treatments in migraine. Paracetamol and ibuprofen are often the safest and most useful analgesics. Too much analgesic use can be detrimental and paradoxically may worsen headaches. Other drug therapies include codeine phosphate and ergot derivatives. Triptans (5-HT receptors agonists) are often helpful, but are not licensed for use in children under the age of 16. Agents most commonly used for prophylaxis of migraine attacks include pizotifen, propranolol, flunarizine, and clonidine. There is insufficient evidence about their efficacy. Combinations of analgesics and antiemetics (e.g. migraleve) are often used, again with limited evidence of efficacy. In the chronic tension-type headaches or stress related headaches amitriptyline maybe useful.

Seizures

An intermittent, paroxysmal disturbance of neuronal function is a seizure. This maybe associated with a variety of clinical phenomena. Usually there is a stereotypic disturbance of consciousness, behaviour, emotion, motor function, perception, or sensation. All of these may occur singly or in combination. Epilepsy is a clinical condition characterized by recurrent seizures that are unprovoked. Various cerebral and systemic insults may cause seizures, e.g. fever, hypoxia, hypoglycaemia, hypocalcaemia, drugs, toxins, trauma, hepatic, or renal impairment. These, in themselves, are not epileptic seizures. Sometimes these become recurrent and stereotyped and can then be classed as epileptic seizures, e.g. post-traumatic epilepsy.

Although, an epileptic seizure always causes a transitory disturbance of cerebral function, it may not always be clinically obvious, but may be subtle.

The term 'convulsion' is used to describe an attack in which there is a predominant motor symptomatology.

Febrile convulsions

These occur in about 3% of all children. They occur between 6 months and 6 years of age with a peak at 12 months–3 years. They occur in association with viral infections where there is a rapid rise of temperature, but with no evidence of meningitis or encephalitis.

'Typical' febrile seizures are generalized tonic–clonic seizures lasting less than 20 minutes (usually 1–2 minutes) with no post ictal neurological deficit. There maybe a family history of febrile seizures in first degree relatives. A third of the children who have had one febrile seizure will have another and a further third will go on to have a third seizure. About 15% of children will have a seizure recurrence in the same febrile illness. The risk of a child with febrile seizures developing afebrile seizures (epilepsy) is between 2 and 5%. Atypical febrile seizures carry a greater risk of subsequent epilepsy. This may, however, be purely because the first atypical seizure with fever represents the earliest manifestation of their epilepsy.

The acute management of children with febrile seizures includes ensuring a patients airway, assessment of respiratory and circulation. Facial oxygen may be required. A prolonged seizure needs to be terminated using rectal diazepam, buccal midazolam or intravenous lorazepam. Parents need to be reassured and given information about the condition. They should be taught how to use rectal diazepam or buccal midazolam as well as basic life support measures, with clear instructions about when to access emergency medical services.

In every infant with febrile seizures particularly the first one, especially where the infant is less than 2 years old non-accidental head injury and meningitis/encephalitis must enter the differential diagnosis. Where there is suspicion and/or where the febrile seizure is in any way atypical, hospital assessment would be justified as would cerebrospinal fluid (CSF) analysis, urine analysis, brain imaging, and eye examination. Further consideration may include EEGs, exclusion of cerebral dysgenesis, chromosomal anomalies, neurocutaneous syndromes, and inborn errors of metabolism.

Prophylaxis with oral anti-epileptic drugs such as phenabarbitone or sodium valproate does not reduce the risk of recurrence of febrile seizures or future development of epilepsy.

Epilepsy

Before the diagnosis of epilepsy can be made some basic questions must be addressed:

1. Is it an epileptic seizure (in other words elimination of the differential diagnoses of epileptic seizures)?
2. What are the seizure types?
3. Is it possible to identify an age dependent epileptic syndrome?
4. Is there an underlying aetiology?

Recognition of epileptic seizures

This is primarily based on a meticulous history from the child, carer, parent, or witness of the event. The symptoms at onset of the seizure can give vital clues. Sometimes a home video is very helpful. If unclear, it is better to wait for more information, than to make a hasty and erroneous diagnosis of epilepsy. Investigations such as EEG and imaging should be used to clarify epilepsy syndromes and ascertain aetiology. They should be used as an aid to a diagnosis of epilepsy and not an alternative to a careful history.

Differential diagnosis of epilepsy

Some commonly occurring paroxysmal disorders can mimic epileptic seizures and need to be excluded on the basis of the history.

Some non-epileptic paroxysmal events that maybe misdiagnosed as epilepsy are described briefly:

1. **Benign sleep myoclonus**: repetitive, usually rhythmic jerks of one or more limbs seen in sleep. Episodes are usually easily diagnosed on history of observation.
2. **Non-REM sleep disorders**: usually manifest as night terrors they occur in stage IV NREM sleep, 1–2 hours after sleep onset. These may take the form of simple arousals with some motor automatisms to sleepwalking, talking, and night terrors. There is no recollection of events the following morning. Reassurance, explanation, and improving sleep hygiene helps.
3. **REM sleep disorders**: this usually takes the form of nightmares sometimes accompanied by sleep paralysis. They occur later in the night with a good recollection of the event next morning. Reassurance and behaviour modification is all that is required.
4. **Syncope**: this results from a sudden decrease in cerebral perfusion by oxygenated blood. There is a lot of confusion over the correct terminology of syncope. Broadly they can be divided into:

    *   *reflex anoxic seizures (reflex asystolic syncope)*: often precipitated by intense emotional discharge due to pain or fright, there occurs a brief asystole causing a secondary anoxic seizure. This is essentially a cardiogenic syncope. These resolve spontaneously with time. Very rarely medication or pacing maybe needed.

Table 19.2 Non-epileptic paroxysmal disorders or events

Respiratory/cardiogenic syncope
Cardiac rhythm disturbances (prolonged QT)
Reflex-anoxic seizures
Breath-holding attacks
Gastro-oesophageal reflux (Sandifer syndrome)
Shuddering attacks
Jitteriness
Self gratification
Behavioural stereotypes
Benign sleep myoclonus
Benign paroxysmal torticollis
Benign positional vertigo
Tics and mannerisms
Panic attacks
Night terrors
Pseudo seizures
Hyperekplexia (startle disease)
Paroxysmal dyskinesia's
Episodic ataxia
Cataplexy and narcolepsy
Migraine

- *cardiac syncope*: the commonest example of this is prolonged QT syndrome. Other arrhythmias may also cause syncope. An ECG must be performed in any child with unexplained collapse episodes or seizures especially if precipitated by exercise or if they occur from sleep.
- *breath-holding attacks*: a prolonged expiratory apnoea occurring spontaneously or after emotional upset and crying causes a secondary hypoxic seizure. This is syncope of respiratory origin. This is usually a benign entity that spontaneously resolves. In children with dysmorphism, abnormal neurology and/or development this maybe a result of structural malformations and may need neuroimaging.
- *gastro-oesophageal reflux*: this may result in apnoeic episodes or paroxysmal dystonic episodes called Sandifer syndrome.

5. **Gratification**: pleasurable behavioural stereotypes resembling self-stimulation consisting of rhythmic hip flexion and adduction with a distant expression are commonly seen in pre-school children. They can be misinterpreted as absence seizures.

6. **Non-epileptic paroxysmal events**: usually as a result of anxiety or stress, various events can be seen including panic attacks. Some may be used for secondary gain.

These include conversion reactions and non-epileptic seizure disorder as well as pseudo syncope.

Seizure types

Recognition of the correct seizure types helps in identification of epileptic syndromes as well as the choice of antiepileptic medication.

Generally the following seizure types are recognized; tonic, clonic, tonic–clonic, myoclonic, atonic and absence seizures. Atypical seizure types are sometimes seen especially in premature babies. These are cycling movements, orofacial automatisms, and apnoeas. Infantile spasms are brief characteristic spasms; often occurring in clusters that maybe flexor, extensor, or flexor–extensor involving the limbs often in association with head, neck, and trunk spasms as well. Absence seizures consist of arrest of activity with impaired consciousness often accompanied by eyelid flutter or staring and automatisms including lip smacking that have a prompt onset and offset and last up to an average of 20 seconds (often shorter) and can recur 10s–100s of times a day.

According to the origin of the seizures they may be divided into localization related (partial or focal) and those that are generalized. Partial seizures are further divided into simple (consciousness preserved) and complex (consciousness impaired). Aetiologically they are further divided into symptomatic (cause known), cryptogenic (cause likely), and idiopathic (no cause other than genetic predisposition).

Epilepsy syndromes

Epileptic syndromes are determined by:

- seizure types
- age of onset
- EEG findings
- associated features such as family history and examination findings.

Epilepsy syndrome identification helps in prognostication, choosing the right antiepileptic medication and directing investigations towards identifying aetiology.

Some common epilepsy syndromes:

1. **West syndrome**
   - age of onset 3–12 months (peak 3–7 months)
   - seizure types—infantile spasms
   - EEG—chaotic, large amplitude slow waves with spikes and sharp waves varying in size and site (hypsarrhythmia)
   - aetiology—idiopathic/cryptogenic
   - symptomatic (hypoxic–ischaemic encephalopathy, tuberous sclerosis, metabolic disorders)
   - treatment—vigabatrin, steroids

- prognosis—better if idiopathic/cryptogenic. Poor if symptomatic—often evolve into other epilepsies with severe developmental regression/plateauing (Lennox Gastaut syndrome)
- comment—infantile spasms initially less frequent and mild—often misdiagnosed as infantile colic. Always examine for abnormal neurology, developmental delay and hypo-pigmented macules of tuberous sclerosis (Wood lamp).

2. **Severe myoclonic epilepsy of infancy**
   - age of onset 3–8 months
   - seizure types: febrile clonic seizures followed by generalized or segmental myoclonic seizures. Atypical absences and partial motor seizures with/without secondary generalization
   - EEG—generalized spike/poly spikes-waves discharges often asynchronous, early photosensitivity
   - aetiology—idiopathic
   - treatment—sodium valproate, lamotrigine, benzodiazepines
   - prognosis—poor. Seizures often intractable, developmental retardation/arrest, progressive ataxia
   - comment—initially simulates febrile convulsions. Careful description of event and developmental assessment important.

3. **Childhood absence epilepsy**
   - age of onset—3–12 years (peak 6–7 years)
   - seizure types—absences
   - EEG—generalized, symmetrical 3–3.5 Hz spike wave discharges
   - aetiology—idiopathic
   - treatment—sodium valproate, ethosuximide
   - prognosis—variable seizures remit in 75%. Possibility of developing tonic clonic seizures in adolescence. Subtle cognitive impairment in about 30%
   - comments—periods of inattention often noticed first in school, may be few initially, but frequency rapidly increases to several a day. Hyperventilation for 1–2 minutes in office setting is a useful test to uncover absence seizures.

4. **Benign rolandic epilepsy (benign epilepsy of childhood with centrotemporal spikes)**
   - age of onset—3–12 years (peak 7–9 years)
   - seizures types—unilateral tonic or clonic seizures involving tongue, lips, cheek, larynx, and arm. Secondary generalization common often in early morning seizures
   - EEG—unilateral or bilateral centrotemporal spikes
   - aetiology—idiopathic/genetic
   - treatment—carbamazepine

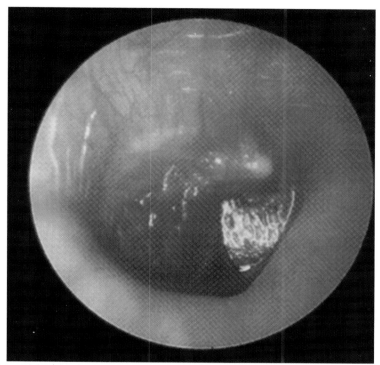

Plate 1 Acute right otitis media. See Fig. 9.1, p 94.
Reproduced with permission from: Bingham BJG, Hawke M, Kwok P, *Atlas of Clinical Otolaryngology* 1991, Mosby-Year Book.

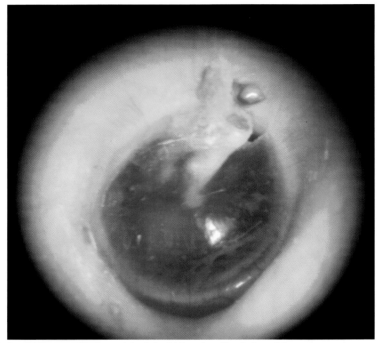

Plate 2 Left middle ear effusion with air bubbles. See Fig. 9.2, p 96.
Reproduced with permission from Ian Bottrill.

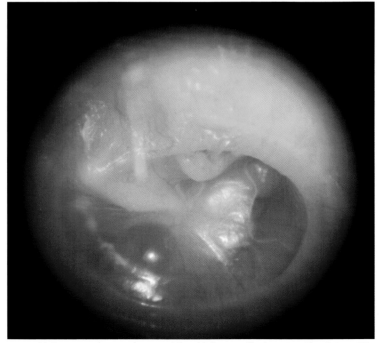

Plate 3 Retracted left tympanic membrane with middle ear effusion. See Fig. 9.3, p 97.
Reproduced with permission from Ian Bottrill.

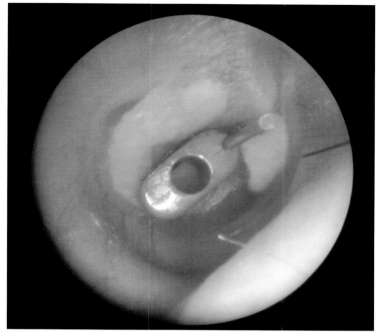

Plate 4 Ventilation tube in tympanic membrane. See Fig. 9.4, p 98.
Reproduced with permission from Ian Bottrill.

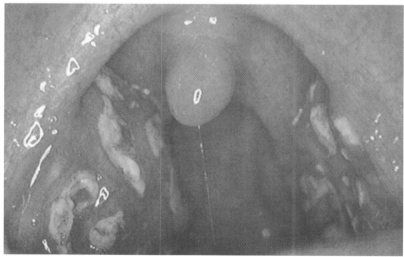

Plate 5 Acute tonsillitis. See Fig. 9.5, p 99.
Reproduced with permission from Bull TR, *Diagnostic Picture Tests in Ear, Nose, and Throat*, 1990, Wolfe.

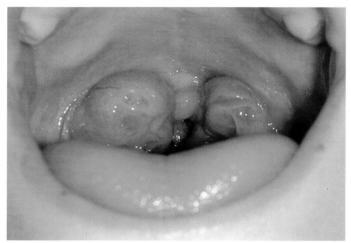

Plate 6 Tonsillar hypertrophy. See Fig. 9.6, p 100.
Reproduced with permission from Pandora Hadfield.

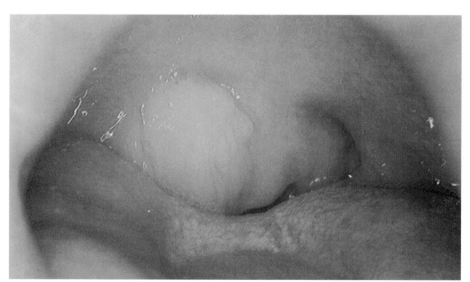

Plate 7 Right peritonsillar abscess. See Fig. 9.7, p 101.
Reproduced with permission Bull TR, *Diagnostic Picture Tests in Ear, Nose, and Throat*, 1990, Wolfe.

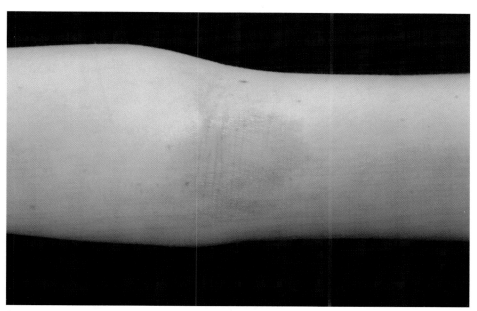

Plate 8 Atopic eczema in flexure of the arm See Fig. 17.1, p 230.

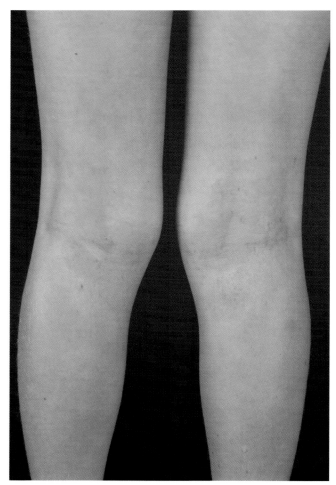

Plate 9 Atopic eczema in flexures of the legs. See Fig. 17.2, p 231.

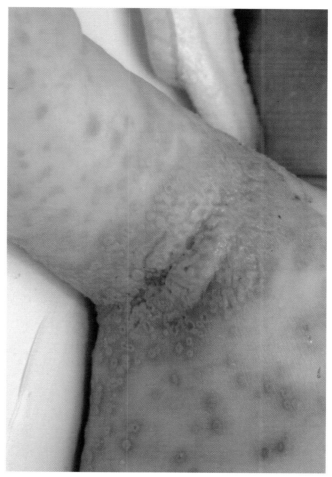

Plate 10 Eczema Herpeticum. See Fig. 17.3, p 234.

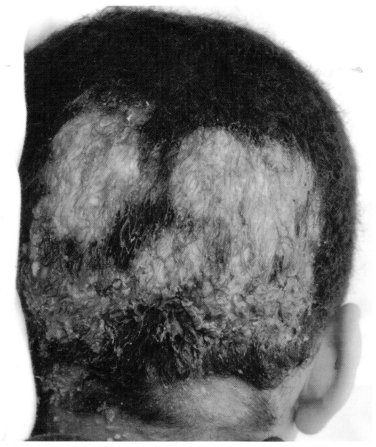

Plate 11 Extensive tinea capitis. See Fig. 17.4, p 241.

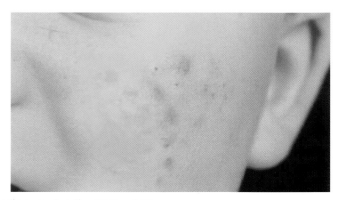

Plate 12 Infantile acne. See Fig. 17.5, p 246.

- prognosis—very good, remit within childhood (usually by puberty). Subtle cognitive difficulties in language if untreated.

5. **Benign epilepsy of childhood with occipital paroxysms**
   - age of onset—1–17 years
   - seizure types—visual symptoms (amaurosis, illusions or hallucinations), vomiting, hemiclonic seizures or automatism and often postictal headache. Consciousness often preserved with vivid description of event
   - EEG—spike waves unilaterally/bilaterally in occipital region on eye closure occasionally spreading to central region
   - aetiology—idiopathic (genetic–family history of migraine) or rarely symptomatic (e.g. cortical dysplasia)
   - treatment—carbamazepine, lamotrigine
   - prognosis—good, remit within childhood small proportion refractory seizures and subsequent generalized seizures
   - comment—vivid descriptions of events may suggest non-epileptic seizure disorder—often misdiagnosed as migraine.

6. **Juvenile myoclonic epilepsy**
   - age of onset—10–18 years
   - seizure types—myoclonic—predominantly in arms—generalized tonic/clonic seizures and absences. Seizures related to sleep deprivation and occurring shortly after awakening or when drowsy
   - EEG—generalized spike and poly-spike wave discharges. Photosensitivity common
   - aetiology—idiopathic (genetic)
   - treatment - sodium valproate, lamotrigine.

Investigations in epilepsy

This can be broadly divided into three main categories.

Electroencephalogram

Often a standard inter-ictal wake EEG is enough for diagnostic purposes. Sometimes ictal EEGs may be needed in which case a video-telemetry or ambulatory EEGs are warranted. Sleep EEGs must be performed if wake EEGs are consistently normal and clinically epilepsy is suspected. EEG should be used as an aid to diagnosis and for identifying epilepsy syndromes. Epilepsy should be a clinical diagnosis, and reliance on EEG to make a diagnosis of epilepsy is inappropriate.

Neuroimaging

Magnetic resonance imaging is the preferred imaging technique. It is not indicated in epilepsies where a syndrome can be diagnosed confidently on clinical/EEG basis. It is particularly useful in neurocutaneous syndromes, developmental regression, early epileptic encephalopathies, and partial seizures (except in some benign partial epilepsy

syndromes). It is also requested in children with persistent seizures difficult to character-
ize and in whom seizures relapse inexplicably following in initial period of good control.

Others

These often include chromosome analysis and CSF, blood, and urine metabolic tests.
DNA analysis is sometimes helpful in mitochondrial cytopathies. Skin fibroblast cultures
may be required as well as muscle biopsy. Where there is doubt about the diagnosis of
epilepsy an ECG should be considered.

Management of epilepsy

Wherever possible correct identification of the epilepsy syndrome and the aetiology
behind it will guide management.

This consists of:

1. *Antiepileptic drugs.* Table 19.3 is a rough guide as regards choice of antiepileptic drugs.
   Changes have to be made to take into account age of child, side-effects and idiosyn-
   cratic drug reactions and the child's life-style as well as preferences of the child the
   family/carers. Drug choices for the common epilepsy syndromes are already mentioned above. Depending on seizure types the following are generally recommended.

   Readers are referred to the NICE guidelines for the diagnosis and management
   of epilepsies in children and young people in primary and secondary care
   (October 2004). Clear guidelines for initial management, investigations, and referral
   to secondary/tertiary care are outlined.

2. *Other drug treatment*:

   - steroids are recommended in the management of infantile spasms and
     Landau–Kleffner syndrome. They are also used in refractory epilepsies with
     frequent episodes of non-convulsive status epilepticus and Rasmussen encephalitis
     (progressive focal epilepsy with brain atrophy);
   - IVIG—intravenous immunoglobulins are used in Rasmussen encephalitis and
     refractory epilepsies;
   - pyridoxine, folinic acid, biotin, pyridoxal phosphate—Epilepsies responsive to
     these vitamins are specific entities. In early onset epileptic encephalopathies and
     infantile spasms they are often tried in the first instance.

Table 19.3 Anti-epileptic drugs

Generalized tonic clonic	Sodium valproate, carbamazepine, lamotrigine
Absence	Sodium valproate, ethosuximide
Myoclonic	Sodium valproate, topiramate, benzodiazepines
Tonic	Sodium valproate, lamotrigine
Atonic	Sodium valproate, lamotrigine, topiramate
Focal	Carbamazepine, lamotrigine, sodium valproate, topiramate, levetiracetam

3. *Ketogenic diet.* High fat, low carbohydrate diets aimed at inducing ketosis as in starvation are often used as an adjunct in refractory epilepsies particularly in myoclonic epilepsies and Lennox–Gastaut syndrome. Careful monitoring and strict diet enforcement is required.

4. *Vagal nerve stimulation.* Implantable devices connected to the vagus nerve in the neck delivers stimulation to increase vagal nerve tone. This is increasingly being used as an adjunct therapy in refractory epilepsies especially partial seizures.

5. *Epilepsy surgery.* In a few carefully selected patients, refractory to antiepileptic drug treatment, after weighing risks and benefits; surgical resection or special surgical treatment maybe of help in controlling seizures. This maybe in the form of lesionectomies, lobectomies, or hemispherectomies. Other surgical interventions include corpus callosotomies and multiple subpial transections. Careful evaluation including detailed and special imaging and neuropsychological evaluation are required prior to considering surgery.

6. *Rescue medication* in children who get frequent, prolonged seizures, rescue medication is often prescribed for use by carers. This is in the form of rectal administration of paraldehyde or diazepam and buccal administration of midazolam. It is recommended that carers are adequately trained in the use of rescue medication, informed about potential adverse effects and given basic life support training.

Floppy infant

Floppiness commonly implies hypotonia. However, ligamentous laxity and weakness may also be called floppiness. These three entities often coexist in the same infant. Floppiness is suggested by abnormal postures (pithed frog posture/rag doll posture). On handling the infant one finds excessive head lag, excessive curvature of the spine in sitting position and hypermobility of the joints. The history is often of delayed motor development. Floppiness can result from:

1. Central causes
   - hypoxic ischaemic encephalopathy
   - benign central hypotonia
   - chromosomal abnormality (Down syndrome)
   - syndromes (Prader–Willi syndrome)
   - hypothyroidism
   - cerebral dysgenesis/malformation
   - iatrogenic/drugs/toxins.

2. Peripheral causes
   - anterior horn cell (spinal muscular atrophy)
   - peripheral nerves (Charcot–Marie–Tooth disease)
   - neuromuscular junction (myasthenia)

- muscular dystrophies
- myotonic dystrophy
- congenital myopathies.

Weakness, paucity of antigravity movements, depressed or absent deep tendon reflexes suggests a peripheral cause (neuromuscular disorder). Hypotonia without weakness, brisk deep tendon reflexes, and upgoing plantar reflexes suggest a central cause. Investigations for a central cause include chromosome analysis and brain imaging as well as blood and urine tests for metabolic abnormalities. Investigations for a peripheral cause include estimation of creatinine kinase enzyme in the serum, an electromyogram, nerve conduction studies, tensilon test, and muscle biopsy.

Muscular dystrophy

By far the commonest muscular dystrophy in children is Duchenne muscular dystrophy. It affects 1:4000 male births. It is inherited as an X-linked recessive disorder, resulting from deletions of exons on the short arm of the X chromosome (Xp21 site). This results in an out of frame deletion causing lack of production of the protein dystrophin. There is a progressive destruction of muscle, which is replaced by fat and connective tissue (dystrophy). Boys present with delayed motor milestones (late walking). There is often a waddling gait and difficulty rising from the floor or climbing stairs. Serum creatinine kinase levels are markedly elevated. DNA testing often confirms the diagnosis without the need for muscle biopsy. Boys get progressively weaker and eventually lose independent ambulation. Hypoventilation and cardiomyopathy may develop. Life expectancy, which was limited to the late teens or early twenties, has significantly improved due to the use of non-invasive ventilation and angiotensin-converting enzyme inhibitors. Scoliosis is another common complication often requiring surgery.

Spinal muscular atrophy

An autosomal recessive disorder resulting in degeneration of the anterior horn cells. This results from deletions of exons on the long arm of chromosome 5 (5q11). Depending on the clinical severity it is divided into

- type 1—never sit independently
- type 2—never stand independently
- type 3—progressive motor weakness.

Extreme weakness, frog leg posturing, tongue fasciculation, absent deep tendon reflexes are some of the features of spinal muscular atrophy type 1 (Werdnig–Hoffman disease). DNA analysis will confirm the diagnosis in most cases. Recurrent respiratory infections, hypoventilation and scoliosis are the main complications.

Neurocutaneous syndromes

Neurofibromatosis

An autosomal dominant inherited condition. Fifty per cent of cases are new mutations. It affects 1:4000 live births. Clinical criteria for diagnosis include:

- more than six café au lait spots greater than 1 cm diameter
- axillary freckling
- subcutaneous plexiform neurofibromas.

There are two types of neurofibromatosis. In the NF-1 (chromosome 17) apart from the cutaneous markers, neurological impairment from involvement of peripheral and cranial nerves may occur. Visual or auditory impairment may occur. Learning difficulties and epilepsy may coexist.

In NF-2 (chromosome 22) bilateral acoustic neuromas are the predominant feature. Sometimes cerebellar ataxia and facial nerve palsy are seen. Other associations include phaeochromocytomas and renal artery stenosis with hypertension. Gliomatous change can occur in the brain lesions. Neurofibromas may rarely change into malignant sarcomas.

Tuberous sclerosis

An autosomal dominant inherited condition, although 80% of cases are de novo mutations. Clinical features include:

- depigmented 'ash leaf' skin macules demonstrated easily on Wood lamp examination (ultraviolet light)
- rough skin patches (Shagreen patches)
- adenoma sebaceum (angiofibromas) in a butterfly distribution over the nose and cheeks.

The tuberous sclerosis complex consists of brain tubers (subependymal calcified nodules), rhabdomyomas of the heart, retinal phakomas, subungual fibromas, and poly-cystic kidneys. Children with brain lesions usually show epilepsy with infantile spasms and developmental regression/plateau; severe learning difficulties often result. Gliomatous change and obstructive hydrocephalus from the brain lesions can occur.

Sturge–Weber syndrome

A sporadic disorder consisting haemangiomatous facial lesions (port wine stain) in the distribution of the ophthalmic division of the trigeminal nerve. These are associated with haemangiomatous pial lesions in the brain that often calcify. It results in intractable focal epilepsy, learning difficulties, and hemiplegia. Hemispherectomy maybe necessary early in intractable focal epilepsy. Glaucoma is often an association. Skin lesions can be treated with laser therapy.

Bell's palsy

A lower motor neurone paralysis of the VIIth cranial nerve leading to facial weakness. In the majority it is unilateral. The aetiology is unclear, although it is postulated that it is a postinfectious immune process. Routine imaging is not indicated. Careful examination must exclude other cranial nerve involvement particularly Vth, VIth, and VIIIth cranial nerves. A full blood count, blood film, and blood pressure monitoring for hypertension and examination of the ear for herpetic lesions is advised. Corticosteroids for 5 days may reduce the oedema and shorten the recovery time. Recovery is complete in the majority. Lubricant eye drops keeps conjunctiva moistened, as eye closure is incomplete.

Hydrocephalus

An imbalance between CSF production and reabsorption or an obstruction to the flow of CSF results in accelerated head enlargement. Main causes are:

- aqueduct stenosis
- posthaemorrhagic
- postinfection
- space occupying lesion/vascular malformation
- cerebral dysgenesis and malformations.

In infants this manifests as irritability, excessive somnolence, feeding difficulty, vomiting, bulging anterior fontanelle, sutural separation, prominent scalp veins, and downward eye deviation (sun setting). Diagnosis is by cranial ultrasound or computed tomography/magnetic resonance imaging scan of the brain. Back should be examined for evidence of spinal dysraphism. Treatment consists of initial sequential ventricular taps to release the fluid and reduce intraventricular pressure or by means of a ventriculoperitoneal shunt. Shunt malfunction due to mechanical obstruction and infection are known complications. This requires antibiotics and revision of the shunt.

Further reading

Appleton R, Gibbs J (1995). *Epilepsy in Childhood and Adolescence*, (1st edn.) Martin Dunitz Ltd, London.

Abu-Arafeh I (ed.) (2002). *Childhood Headache*. Mac Keith Press, London.

Fenichel GM (2001). *Clinical Pediatric Neurology: A Signs and Symptoms Approach*. WB Saunders, Philadelphia.

NICE (2004, October). *The Epilepsies: diagnosis and management of the epilepsies in children and young people in primary and secondary care*. NICE Clinical Guideline 20. NICE, London. www.nice.org.uk/CG020NICEguideline.

Sender P, Jayawant S (2003). Evaluation of the floppy infant. *Current Paediatrics* 13: 345–349.

Wallace SJ, Farrell K (2004). *Epilepsy in Children*, (2nd edn). Arnold Publishers. London.

Chapter 20

Endocrine disorders

Ahmed Massoud

Introduction

Both general paediatricians and healthcare professionals in primary care often think of paediatric endocrine disorders as being rare and rather esoteric. While there is an element of truth in this, it remains a fact that, collectively, paediatric endocrine disorders are common, though, individually, many are rare and may not ever be encountered within the practising lifetime of a primary care health professional. Moreover, endocrinology is not a single organ specialty and therefore the clinical presentation of an endocrine disorder may span many systems within the body. A further unique aspect of endocrine disorders in childhood is the impact they usually have on growth (height and weight). Considering that all healthy children are supposed to grow, one starts to build a picture that the practice of paediatric endocrinology is very much part of every day paediatric practice whether it is in a primary care setting or other.

With that in mind and in an attempt to adhere to the title of the book *Practical Paediatric Problems in Primary Care*, I have attempted to cover in this chapter aspects of paediatric endocrinology that are of practical relevance to the practising primary care physician/healthcare professional. I have used my experience as a paediatric endocrinologist in secondary care (i.e. in a district general hospital, for those familiar with the British national health service) and my interactions with referring primary care physicians to provide the reader with a synopsis of the type of paediatric endocrine problems they are likely to encounter and how to go about dealing with them. I have deliberately steered away from rare endocrine problems. Readers are asked to refer to more comprehensive textbooks of paediatric endocrinology for that purpose.

The chapter is divided into three main sections, reflecting the major and/or important type of endocrine problems that are likely to be encountered in primary care. A large section has been dedicated to 'growth problems' as, in the world of paediatric endocrinology, these constitute the most common reason for parents bringing their child to the primary care physician and for their child being referred to a paediatric endocrinologist. Within this section I have included a synopsis of the two conditions that have been particularly prominent in the paediatric endocrine literature in the last 5 years, namely, children born small for gestational age (SGA) and idiopathic short stature (ISS). Within the section on 'growth problems' I have also touched on the important aspects of hypothyroidism, both congenital and acquired.

The second section deals with pubertal problems, which constitute another major reason for referral. Within this group of disorders I have covered disorders of excessive androgen production, manifesting in the prepubertal child with hirsutism and possibly acne, and the in pubertal girl with both symptoms in addition to menstrual irregularity, usually due to polycystic ovary syndrome.

Childhood diabetes is a chronic, life-long condition that has a major impact on the affected individual and his/her family. Major advances have been made in the field and therefore diabetes has been allocated the third section of this chapter.

Growth disorders

Every individual must grow as he or she progresses from a newborn to an infant to a child to a pubertal young person. Normal growth is regarded as a marker of good health—a child who grows normally is, on the whole, unlikely to have something seriously wrong with him or her. In contrast, a child who is failing to grow adequately is usually suspected of having significant pathology. This hopefully prompts his/her carer to have him/her formally assessed and, where appropriate, investigated and treated.

While most healthcare professionals and society at large regard growth problems as those resulting in short stature, and this entity is indeed the most common problem seen in paediatric endocrine clinics, it is important to remember that tall stature and rapid linear growth are equally important issues, which may have significant underlying pathologies.

Within the larger umbrella of growth problems one should also include disorders of weight, which are a constant worry for parents and therefore make up a significant proportion of non-acute paediatric consultations in primary care. Consequently, many such children get referred for specialist assessments. Infants or children who are significantly underweight are usually and appropriately referred to general paediatricians or paediatric gastroenterologists while those who are overweight find their way to paediatric endocrine clinics. Thankfully, most of these individuals do not have underlying endocrinopathies and are simply suffering from 'simple obesity'.

Short stature

Short stature is defined as being below a certain arbitrarily determined cut-off height percentile (or a number of standard deviations below the mean height for the population of the same gender). The UK cross-sectional reference data growth charts produced and published by the Child Growth Foundation (Freedman et al. 1995) have the upper and lower cut off percentiles as 99.6th and 0.4th, respectively, with the areas between the 98th and 99.6th percentiles and the 0.4th and 2nd percentiles being shaded to indicate the need for closer monitoring of individuals who fall within these areas. Other features of these growth charts are shown in Table 20.1.

It is not sufficient to compare the height of a child to the age- and sex-matched population standard because genetic factors need to be taken into account. From a practical point of view it is always useful to measure the parental heights rather than rely on

Table 20.1 Features of the UK cross-sectional reference data 1996 growth charts

Based on more recent data (late1980s)
Large sample size (approximately 30,000 boys and 30,000 girls)
Wider population base (data sets taken from various parts of the UK)
Nine equidistant (2/3 of a standard deviation) percentile lines
Standards from extreme prematurity (23 weeks gestation) through to 20 years of age
Two main forms (4-in-1 decimal years 0–20 years chart; monthly/quarterly 0–18 years chart)

reported heights. An adjustment for gender needs to be made when plotting the parental heights (for example, when working out a boy's adult height potential, 14 cm is added to his mother's height before plotting it on a male chart; conversely, 14 cm is subtracted from the father's height when plotting his height on a female growth chart when working out his daughter's adult height potential). The mid point of plotted parental heights (having adjusted them as outlined above) is known as the mid-parental height centile (MPH) and the range of normality for the child in question is MPH ± 8.5 cm (known as the target centile range, TCR). This is a vital part of growth assessment, which tells the assessor whether, at that point of time, the child in question is of appropriate height for his/her parents (and also whether the height is normal for the age- and sex-matched general population). Of course this is an assessment at one point in time (cross-sectional data) and does not provide any information about the rate of change of height (height velocity). This requires serial height measurements and provides the healthcare provider with longitudinal data, based on which he/she can decide whether the growth pattern is abnormal and hence the need to investigate further.

Assessment of short stature

When assessing growth problems it is important to interpret the growth data in the context of the child's age/stage of development. Humans grow very fast in infancy, a period that is characterized by a rapid, but a rapidly decelerating, rate of growth (the average length is 50 cm at birth, 75cm at 12 months, and 86 cm and at 24 months), followed by a fairly constant rate of growth during childhood (approximately 5–6 cm per year) until puberty commences. Pubertal growth is characterized by rapid growth, reaching a peak then slowing down as growth comes to an end and the epiphyses fuse. This is commonly referred to in the infancy–childhood puberty model of growth

There are many causes of short stature and/or growth failure (Table 20.2). Some simply cause a child to be short (compared with the normal standards or compared with the TCR) yet grow at a normal rate and end up short as an adult (e.g. Noonan syndrome). The purpose of assessment in this instance is to establish a cause for the short stature that may or may not be amenable to therapy. Other conditions listed in Table 20.2 (e.g. endocrine disorders such as acquired hypothyroidism) lead to inadequate growth rate and eventually cause short stature, unless treatment is instituted at the appropriate time.

As with any medical condition, assessment starts with taking an adequate history and conducting a thorough clinical examination. Salient features in the history include:

Table 20.2 Causes of short stature

Growth hormone deficiency
Turner syndrome
Chronic renal failure
Adult growth hormone deficiency syndrome
Prader–Willi syndrome
Small for gestational age

birthweight (as 10% of all SGA babies fail to catch up, and attain a suboptimal adult height) (Karlberg and Albertsson-Wikland 1995), growth and weight gain in infancy, establishing whether the child has always been short or whether there is a more recent onset of observed/documented growth failure, history of medication that may have impacted on growth (e.g. systemic steroids) and finally any symptoms suggestive of a chronic childhood illness (e.g. chronic diarrhoea, which raises the possibility of inflammatory bowel diseases) or endocrine disorder (e.g. lethargy, constipation, and hair loss, which raises the possibility of hypothyroidism). Past medical history and social history may also give clues as to the cause of short stature

Physical examination should include accurate height and weight measurements of the child and, where possible, measurement of parental heights. The examiner should look specifically for stigmata of chronic illnesses affecting the cardiac, respiratory, gastrointestinal, neurological, or musculoskeletal system. A search for dysmorphic features should be carried out. Signs of endocrine disorders should obviously be looked for. Where appropriate, assessment of pubertal development should be carried out, if only to note whether signs of puberty are present: formal and precise assessment of pubertal staging requires specific training, which very few primary care physicians will have received.

Once the history has been elicited, a physical examination has been carried out and the child's height has been plotted, the physician can start to formulate an opinion as to whether there is indeed a problem or whether reassurance is all that is needed. The above assessments also guide the physician as what (if any) investigations are indicated. If there are clear symptoms or signs of an underlying gastrointestinal disorder then the investigations would be geared towards that system. Generally speaking, children who are short and thin tend to have non-endocrine reasons for their short stature (e.g. inflammatory bowel disease, malabsorption, cystic fibrosis, chronic asthma, congenital heart disease) while those with hormonal problems (e.g. hypothyroidism, growth hormone (GH) deficiency, Cushing syndrome) tend to be short and overweight.

A word of caution. Simply because a child is of normal height for his/her parents and for the general population does not mean that nothing is amiss. If the history is that of a child who is not growing well, one needs to look at previous height data to establish whether there is an abnormality. If no previous height data are available then these need to be accumulated prospectively by measuring the child at 4-monthly intervals over a period of at least 1 year. A decision can then be made whether the child is growing normally or otherwise, and appropriate investigations then performed.

The range of investigations to be performed is clearly wide and will depend on the clinical picture that is giving rise to the growth problem. Some basic routine investigations can be performed in primary care (such as routine haematology and biochemistry, inflammatory markers, thyroid function tests), while others (such as GH stimulation tests) need to be performed in a hospital setting under the close supervision of a paediatric endocrinologist.

Treatment of short stature/growth failure

The treatment of short stature clearly depends on the underlying cause. Those conditions where GH has been used, or at least trialled, are discussed under a separate heading (see below). Endocrine disorders other than GH deficiency require specific intervention (e.g. thyroxine replacement in hypothyroidism, and identifying and treating the cause of glucoroticoid excess in Cushing syndrome). Where the cause of growth failure is due to a chronic childhood illness, optimizing the treatment of the underlying condition (e.g. adequate vitamin D replacement in rickets and adequate inhaled/oral medication in chronic asthma) is the key to restoring normal growth. Identifying psychosocial deprivation as the cause of a child's growth failure may be difficult but this problem will need to be tackled in order to restore normal growth (and also deal with the other associated problems of neglect). The term skeletal dysplasias encompasses a wide range of skeletal disorders, which are largely diagnosed on the basis of radiological features on a skeletal survey. The degree of short stature associated with skeletal abnormalities is highly variable (mild to moderate in hypochondroplasia and severe in achondroplasia). Some of these conditions do respond to GH therapy (Ramaswami *et al.* 1999). Further height can be gained through leg lengthening procedures (Catagni *et al.* 2005).

Growth hormone therapy *GH deficiency* may be congenital (arising from a variety of disorders such GH gene deletion, GH releasing hormone—GHRH—deficiency or developmental abnormalities of the pituitary), or acquired (as a result of tumours of the hypothalamus or pituitary, or secondary to cranial irradiation, head injury or infection). Treatment of GH deficiency, irrespective of the underlying cause, has traditionally been through replacement with exogenous GH. For practical and safety reasons treatment with GHRH analogues or GH releasing peptides (GHRPs) was never established in every day clinic practice.

Recombinant biosynthetic GH became available in 1986 shortly after the cessation of use of human cadaver pituitary-derived GH, which was causally linked to Creutzfeldt–Jakob disease in young recipients. The abundance of recombinant GH meant that this treatment modality was trialled in many disorders of short stature, whether secondary to GH deficiency or otherwise. In the UK there are now a number of licensed indications for the use of GH (Table 20.3). The place of GH treatment in some conditions is well established, the obvious one being GH deficiency. The dwarfism resulting from absolute GH deficiency, whether isolated or part of multiple pituitary

Table 20.3 Licensed indications for use of GH in the UK

Growth hormone deficiency
Turner syndrome
Chronic renal failure
Adult growth hormone deficiency syndrome
Prader–Willi syndrome
Small for gestational age

hormone deficiency, can be avoided by commencing GH replacement therapy in early childhood: normal adult height potential can thus be attained. However, the response to GH treatment in other conditions is not as marked and is much less consistent.

Some children with short stature produce abundant amounts of GH yet they have severe growth failure. This usually arises due to defective GH receptor. The affected individual cannot generate insulin-like growth factor 1 (IGF-1), the protein that mediates GH action on the growth plate and promotes linear growth. This disorder is known as GH insensitivity syndrome. Attempts at treatment with recombinant IGF-1 have been hampered by significant side-effects, mainly severe hypoglycaemia.

Turner syndrome (TS) is one of the most common human chromosome anomalies, occurring in approximately 1:2000 female live births. Approximately 50–60% of TS girls are reported to have a 45,X karyotype, while 30–40% have mosaic patterns such as 45,X/46XX. The remainder have structural abnormalities of the X chromosomes such as rings, isochromosomes of the long arm and partial deletions of the short arm. The TS phenotype consists of lymphoedema in the newborn, cardiac abnormalities, dysmorphic features (epicanthic folds, webbing of the neck, wide carrying angle, low hairline, characteristic nails, and widely spaced nipples), short stature, and gonadal dysgenesis. The latter manifests in delayed or absent puberty, failure of pubertal progression, or premature menopause.

Short stature is the single most common physical abnormality and affects virtually all girls with TS. Untreated TS girls have an average adult height of 144 cm (Sybert 1984). The growth failure starts to manifest in early childhood due to a combination of mild to moderate growth retardation *in utero*, slow growth in infancy, delayed onset of childhood component of growth, and slow growth during childhood. From a practical point of view, any girl who has unexplained short stature should have her karyotype checked. Clinicians all too often rely on the presence of dysmorphic features before considering the diagnosis of TS. Unfortunately, this frequently leads to a delay in diagnosis.

Most studies of GH therapy in TS have not been randomized controlled trials, but as a whole they demonstrate that GH increases growth velocity and improves final height. The magnitude of the benefit has varied tremendously depending on the study design. Earlier studies reported height increments of less than 5 cm, but in these studies GH was started at a relatively late age and given in small doses. Recent studies have documented height increments of 5–16 cm and early diagnosis and initiation of treatment could result in a near normal adult height for most TS girls (Rosenfeld *et al.* 1998; Sas *et al.* 1999). Factors now known to be important in determining the response to GH include age at initiation of treatment, duration of treatment, GH dose, additional therapy with anabolic steroids, and the timing of oestrogen therapy.

As mentioned above, 10% of individuals born **small for gestational age** or following intrauterine growth retardation (IUGR), whether in isolation or part of a syndrome such Russell-Silver, fail to attain their full adult height potential. There are other associated problems with SGA/IUGR, namely, neonatal hypoglycaemia, lower rate of survival in the first year of life (McIntire *et al.* 1999), attenuated intellectual development and later obesity, insulin resistance, and ischaemic heart disease (Godfrey and Barker 2000). The mechanisms leading to IUGR in humans are poorly understood but a variety of factors have been implicated. These include maternal factors, such as maternal malnutrition and infections, placental factors, such as vascular malformations and placental insufficiency, and fetal factors such as chromosomal abnormalities and defects in insulin/IGF-1 gene defects (Woods *et al.* 1996).

Children born SGA who remain short (<2.5 standard deviations—SD—below the mean) during childhood may receive GH therapy. Two large multicentre studies have shown improvement in final height (Hokken-Koelega *et al.* 2004; Dhalgren and Albertsson-Wikland 2005). The criteria for treatment according to the UK license include: birthweight or length <2 SDS (standard deviation scores), current height <2.5 SDS and parental adjusted height <–1 SDS, failure to catch up by age 4 years or later and height velocity <0 SDS during the last year.

The response to GH treatment in children born SGA is dose dependent. High-dose GH therapy increases insulin resistance and leads to variable degrees of impaired glucose tolerance (Cutfield *et al.* 2000). There has therefore been concern about the development of type 2 diabetes and the metabolic syndrome in GH-treated SGA children, who are already predisposed to these complications. However, thus far in the long-term follow-up studies there has been no increase in the prevalence rate of type 2 diabetes (Hokken-Koelega *et al.* 2004).

The world of paediatric endocrinology has recently had a resurgence of interest in *idiopathic short stature* (ISS), a term that has evolved over the years as clinical observation met advances in biotechnology. As hormone assays improved and our understanding of disorders of the GH-IGF-1 axis advanced, it was realized that there remained a significant number of children with short stature who were otherwise normal and had normal stimulated GH levels. These were referred to by a variety of different terms such as 'short-normal children', 'non-GH deficient short stature', and 'ISS'. These terms essentially referred to children with short stature of unknown cause.

The diagnosis of ISS remains controversial, particularly with regard to its definition and the emerging options for its treatment. However, several inclusion criteria are generally accepted: height <2 SD below the mean, absence of an identifiable cause for the short stature, normal weight for gestational age, no evidence of body segment disproportion, normal calorie intake, no psychiatric disorder, and normal GH response on a standard stimulation test. This definition allows for ISS to remain a clinically heterogeneous group rather than being a single clinical entity. Controversies continue to centre on whether the definition should take into account family heights (as it stands, the above definition would include cases of familial short stature), predicted adult height, and assessment of bone maturation (such cases with delayed bone maturation would otherwise be termed 'constitutional delay of growth'). Recent advances in molecular endocrinology have allowed the identification of abnormalities in the GH-IGF-1-bone axis in individuals who were previously thought to have ISS (Abuzzahab *et al.* 2003; Milward *et al.* 2004).

The reason for considering GH treatment in ISS is that GH has been shown to promote growth in other disorders not associated with GH deficiency (e.g. TS). In addition, it has long been known that GH stimulation tests may generate false-positive and false-negative results and cannot therefore categorically discriminate between normality and abnormality. Several studies have documented increase in growth velocity in a high proportion of children with ISS during the first 1–2 years of GH therapy. However, adult height data are unclear. The best response so far reported entailed the use of high-dose GH and this resulted in a height increment of 7 cm (Wit and Rekers-Mombarg 2002).

In 2003 the USA FDA approved GH therapy for children with ISS whose current heights are more than 2.25 SD below the mean for age and sex (or the shortest 1.2% of children), 'with associated growth rates unlikely to permit attainment of adult height in the normal range, in paediatric patients whose epiphyses are not closed and for whom diagnostic evaluation excludes other causes associated with short stature that should be observed or treated by other means'. The heights for those who qualify for treatment correspond to heights of less than 5 ft 3 inches and less than 4 ft 11 inches in adult men and women, respectively (FDA 2003). GH use in ISS is not currently licensed in the UK.

Miscellaneous conditions The use of biosynthetic GH treatment in familial short stature, i.e. individuals who are short (but normal in all respects) and who are of appropriate height for their parental heights (or are predicted to fall within their parental target centile range as adults) failed to result in a significant improvement in adult height (Hindmarsh and Brook 1996).

GH therapy for short stature associated with certain syndromes has also been studied. A UK license has been granted for its use in the Prader–Willi syndrome, where benefits additional to those of improved linear growth may be observed, namely, improved body composition and physical strength (Carrel *et al.* 1999).

Trials in other syndromes such as Noonan have shown improvement in growth velocity but limited data are available on the effect of GH therapy on final height (MacFarlane *et al.* 2001).

Constitutional delay of growth and puberty (CDGP) is a common and important cause of short stature, though strictly speaking it is not a pathological entity. The most frequent treatment modality is pubertal induction using exogenous sex hormones. This will be covered under the section on puberty.

Tall stature

Tall stature is often not regarded by society as a problem and indeed tall stature may confer economic and cultural advantages (Persico *et al.* 2003). While the most common cause of tall stature is familial (i.e. the child in question is the offspring of tall parents), there are obviously a number of pathological conditions that lead to tall stature (Table 20.4). Moreover, excessive rapid growth in childhood requires investigation, as it could indicate precocious puberty (most commonly due to excessive androgen production secondary to certain forms of congenital adrenal hyperplasia, and much less commonly due to gonadotrophin-dependent precocious puberty). Other endocrine causes of rapid growth include thyrotoxicosis, though this usually presents with other features of thyroid overactivity, and the very rare disorder of excessive GH production from a pituitary microadenoma. These conditions should be treated not only on account of the resulting tall stature problem but also because of other associated comorbidities. It is worth pointing out that while congenital adrenal hyperplasia leads to rapid growth and tall stature in childhood, if untreated it will cause premature fusion of the epiphyses leading to eventual short stature in adult life.

Like the assessment of short stature, evaluation of the child with tall stature entails a clinical history and examination as well as accurate measurements of growth parameters. Pubertal assessment is particularly important. Investigations are also dependent on the prevailing clinical findings but almost always entail an assessment of skeletal maturation. Treatment, where possible, is aimed at the underlying cause of the problem (e.g. precocious puberty). In cases of familial tall stature, if the predicted adult height is 'excessive'—an adult height which the child and the parents regard as unacceptable, intervention to limit the adult height can be offered provided the child presents well before the pubertal years. The intervention is usually in the form of cautious induction of early puberty if a girl has not shown signs of developing by the age of 10 years or a boy by the age of 11 years.

Hypothyroidism

Hypothyroidism in childhood has traditionally been divided into two main forms, congenital and acquired. This is indeed a logical way of categorizing hypothyroidism not only because of the clear difference in age of onset but also because of the different symptomatology and underlying aetiologies of the two entities. Central to both types is the detrimental effect thyroxine deficiency has on the growing child.

Congenital hypothyroidism

1 in 4000 infants is born with congenital hypothyroidism (CH). Delay in commencing thyroxine replacement therapy results in short stature and irreversible brain damage. Unfortunately, the early signs of CH are non-specific (umbilical hernia, constipation,

Table 20.4 Causes of tall stature

Familial
Syndromes (e.g. Marfan)
Chromosomal abnormalities (e.g. Klinefelter 47XXY)
Precocious puberty
Endocrine disorders

lethargy, feeding problems, prolonged jaundice) and cannot be relied upon to detect the condition with certainty. Hence, a neonatal screening programme for CH was introduced in the UK in the early 1980s. Mandatory universal neonatal CH screening is now common practice in many countries.

In the UK, the screening programme is based on measuring and detecting elevated levels of thyroid-stimulating hormone (TSH) on dried blood samples collected from newborn babies on day 5 or 6 of life. Once an elevated TSH is detected the baby is referred to his primary care physician or local hospital for formal laboratory measurement of serum TSH and free thyroxine concentration. Based on theses results the diagnosis is confirmed and replacement with thyroxine is commenced as soon as practically possible.

The most common cause of CH is thyroid dysgenesis much may result in athyreosis, or complete absence of the thyroid, leading to severe CH. Other, less severe forms of dysgenesis include ectopic or maldescent of the thyroid gland leading to milder forms of CH. CH may also arise as a result of defects of thyroid hormones biosynthesis, TSH resistance due to TSH receptor mutations, maternal thyrotrophin receptor blocking antibodies and maternal antithyroid medication

The neonatal CH screening programme has been one of the main public health success stories resulting in improved neurodevelopmental outcome and restoration of normal growth. However, follow-up studies showed that those who were severely affected continued to have an IQ deficit of 6–15 points (Tillotson *et al.* 1994), despite early thyroxine replacement. In addition, clumsiness, difficulties with certain motor skills, and behaviour problems may persist (Dattani and Brook 1996). It is suggested that severe antenatal thyroxine deficiency is the reason for the lack of complete normalization of mental function. A higher starting dose of thyroxine (10–15 µg/kg bodyweight, as opposed to the previous practice of giving 6–8 µg/kg bodyweight) may reduce the IQ deficit in severe CH (Dubuis *et al.* 1996) but this remains controversial (Hrytsiuk *et al.* 2002).

Acquired hypothyroidism

This, by definition, is a disease process leading to underactivity of the thyroid gland occurring beyond the neonatal period: it is largely due to autoimmune thyroiditis, which rarely occurs under the age of 3 years but has been described even in infancy. Childhood autoimmune thyroiditis peaks in early- to mid-puberty and has a female preponderance of 2:1.

The presentation of autoimmune thyroiditis may include the development of a goitre with or without disturbance of thyroid function. Hyperthyroidism in children is rare and should be managed a specialist. It will not be discussed further here. Hypothyroidism is not an uncommon condition in childhood and presents usually with growth failure. Because this takes a long time to manifest, the disease often goes unrecognized for 2–3 years, by which time the other features of hypothyroidism have become obvious (lethargy, fatigue, constipation, hair loss, dry and sallow skin, and cold intolerance).

The diagnosis is confirmed by measuring serum TSH and thyroxine concentration together with measurement of thyroid antibodies (thyroglobulin and thyroid peroxidase antibodies). Bone age is classically significantly delayed: the degree of delay of skeletal maturation is often indicative of the duration of the illness. Thyroid scans do not contribute to the management but may be indicated in certain circumstances, e.g. if a solitary nodule is palpated.

Levothyroxine is the replacement of choice. Its long half-life allows convenient once daily administration. Care must be taken when commencing an individual on thyroxine not to give the full replacement dose from the start. The 'hypothyroid brain' needs some time to adjust to the newly initiated thyroxine therapy so it is customary to start with a small dose (25 μg once daily) and build it up at 2-weekly intervals to the desired dose. It is also worth pointing out that if the hypothyroidism is long-standing, commencing thyroxine therapy often results in a complete change in the child's behaviour, manifesting as overactivity, lack of concentration, disturbed sleep, and poor school performance. This occurs despite correct replacement dosage of thyroxine and often takes 12 months before it settles down.

From a practical point of view both congenital and acquired hypothyroidism are relatively straight forward to manage by replacing thyroxine, usually using levothyroxine tablets, adjusted according to the size of the individual as well as the prevailing serum thyroxine and TSH concentrations. Careful attention to growth, neurodevelopmental progress, and puberty is clearly important.

Pubertal disorders

Puberty is an important stage of human development that allows the child's transition into adult life. Puberty requires an intact hypothalamic–pituitary–gonadal axis and the pulsatile secretion of gonadotrophins at sufficiently high amplitudes and frequency. This results in the secretion by the gonads of sex hormones, which bring about the physical changes, and, together with increasing GH pulse amplitude, result in the pubertal linear growth spurt.

The first sign of puberty in a girl is breast development and in a boy testicular enlargement. The cut-off age for precocious puberty in a girl is 8 years and for a boy 9 years, while puberty is said to be delayed if no signs of secondary sexual characteristics are present by the age of 13 years for a girl and 14 years for a boy.

Precocious puberty in girls is much more common than in boys (ratio 10:1) and is usually benign while in boys it is rare and usually pathological. In contrast, delayed puberty in girls is uncommon and usually pathological while delayed puberty in boys is common and usually non-pathological. It follows that precocious puberty in a boy and delayed puberty in a girl need to be promptly and extensively investigated.

While the intricacies of managing precocious and delayed puberty requires specialist knowledge and is best dealt with by a paediatric endocrinologist, it is important for the primary care physician to be aware of these entities and potential for offering treatment where appropriate.

Precocious puberty

The age cut-off for early puberty in boys and girls has already been discussed. Any boy developing sings of puberty below the age of 9 years must be referred for specialist assessment. Early puberty in a boy requires urgent referral so that appropriate investigations are commenced as soon as practically possible. Early puberty in a girl (defined as developing signs of puberty under the age of 8 years), unless occurring at a very young age (under 6 years) is likely to be benign, i.e. due simply to early activation of the normal hypothalamic–pituitary–gonadal axis: the urgency of the referral depends on the age of onset and the prevailing clinical signs.

Possible sources of sex steroids in precocious puberty include the gonads, most commonly driven by pituitary gonadotrophins (luteinizing hormone (LH)/follicle-stimulating hormone (FSH)), either resulting from early activation of a physiological phenomenon or due to a pathological cause (e.g. a hypothalamic or pituitary tumour). Gonadal tumours that secrete sex steroids are very rare as are gonadotrophin-secreting tumours. The adrenal glands are the other source of sex hormones, and the most common cause of sexual precocity here is an enzyme defects (e.g. congenital adrenal hyperplasia due to 21 hydroxylase deficiency). Adrenal tumours are rare but important to exclude. Non-gonadal/non-adrenal tumours that secrete sex steroids are extremely rare.

Investigations of early puberty may include assessment of pituitary function (LH releasing hormone test, magnetic resonance imaging scan of the brain and the hypothalamopituitary area), adrenal function (measurement serum 17hydroxypregesterone, androstenedione, DHEAS (dehydroepiandrosterone sulphate) and testosterone, urine steroid profile, ultrasound/computed tomography scan of the adrenals), testicular function (measurement of serum testosterone, ultrasound testicles), and/or ovarian function (pelvic ultrasound scan) and bone age assessment.

Once the underlying cause of the precocious puberty has been identified, specific treatment can be given (e.g. resection of a brain tumour). Pubertal progression can be halted with pharmacological agents. The type of medication to be used depends on whether puberty is driven by gonadotrophins (i.e., gonadotrophin-dependent precocious puberty, by a hypothalamopituitary mechanism) or directly by sex hormones (i.e., gonadotrophin-independent precocious puberty). The former is treated with monthly or 3-monthly injections of slow-release gonadotrophin-releasing hormone agonists, which work by abolishing the normal pulsatility of endogenous pituitary gonadotrophin secretion (Heger *et al*. 1999). Gonadotrophin-independent precocious puberty is treated using cyproterone acetate (as an anti-androgen) or testolactone and spironolactone (as aromatase inhibitors). Treatment is discontinued once the child reaches an age where it is acceptable for puberty to progress (usually about the age of 10 for a girl and 11 for a boy).

Premature thelarche

This distinct clinical entity, consisting of isolated breast development in a prepubertal girl. It is a common and benign condition, which, for obvious reasons, raises concerns about the affected girl having precocious puberty, as breast development is the first feature of both conditions (Stanhope 2000). Premature thelarche can be differentiated from true precocious puberty by the following features: it usually occurs in the first 3–4 years of life, it never progresses beyond breast stage 2–3, breast development may wax and wane, there are no other signs of puberty, growth velocity remains normal for age, skeletal maturation is not altered and progression to normal puberty occurs at a normal age. The condition is probably due to pulses of FSH resulting in isolated ovarian cyst development. The serum gonadotrophin levels remain at prepubertal levels and the stimulated gonadotrophins (by mean of an LH releasing hormone test) show a prepubertal response. Pelvic ultrasonography shows a prepubertal uterus with no endometrial echo. The condition requires no treatment.

Delayed puberty

Delayed puberty in boys is a common problem and is most commonly due to constitutional delay of growth puberty (CDGP) (see below). However, before this diagnosis can be made a thorough clinical evaluation must be performed to rule out pathological causes. Little in the way of biochemical testing or imaging is usually required. In contrast, delayed puberty in girls requires urgent assessment as it is much less likely to be secondary to simple delay.

A careful history and physical examination, looking for evidence of systemic disease or its treatment (e.g. asthma, inflammatory bowel disease, postradiotherapy/chemotherapy, postcranial surgery, malignancy), eating disorders, hypothyroidism, gonadotrophin deficiency (e.g. postradiotherapy, other features to suggest multiple pituitary hormone deficiency), anosmia (which is seen in Kallman syndrome), pituitary/hypothalamic tumours (e.g. central nervous symptoms and signs) must be performed. Other causes, specific to girls include TS, gonadal dysgenesis, and autoimmune primary ovarian failure (usually part of a polyglandular autoimmune syndrome). Significant features specific to boys include history of undescended testicles, anorchia, testicular torsion, infection or trauma, or features that may suggest an underlying chromosomal abnormality, such as Klinefelter syndrome.

Investigations of delayed puberty depend on the findings from the clinical assessment and may include: full blood count, erythrocyte sedimentation rate, biochemistry profile, coeliac screen, thyroid function tests, prolactin, LH, FSH, bone age assessment, LH releasing hormone test, karyotype, pelvic ultrasound (in girls) and brain imaging. As mentioned above, few of these need to be performed in boys, in contrast with girls who often need to be investigated extensively.

Treatment is aimed at the underlying cause where possible. If not, pubertal induction or full sex hormone replacement therapy may be required.

Constitutional delay of growth and puberty

Individuals with CDGP are healthy and have no underlying organic cause for their pubertal delay. CDGP is a diagnosis of exclusion yet it accounts for more than 60% of causes of delayed puberty in boys and over 20% in girls (Sedlmeyer and Palmert 2002). The clinical characteristics include normal childhood growth, slowing down in growth in the preceding 2 years or so, absence of organic disease, no clinical features of hypopituitarism or hypogonadism, and delayed bone age. There is also usually a family history of delayed puberty.

It is generally accepted that most boys with CDGP will grow to reach a height that is normal for the population and for their parents (Rosenfield 1990). Left alone they will eventually develop and progress through puberty on their accord. However, the delayed puberty or short stature associated with CDGP can be a source of anxiety and emotional stress (Lee and Rosenfeld 1987). These individuals all too frequently come to their primary care physician requesting help and expressing desperation at their lack of progress in puberty.

Treatment of constitutional delay of growth and puberty The aim of therapy is to induce secondary sexual characteristics and growth acceleration without adversely affecting final height or suppressing the maturation of the hypothalamic–pituitary–gonadal axis. The intramuscular administration of low-dose testosterone esters using a dose of 50–100 mg once every 4 weeks for a period of 3–6 months is effective (Richman and Kirsch 1988). Provided the desired effects (increase in height velocity, signs of virilization and enlargement of the testicles) are observed, treatment can be discontinued and the boy reviewed after a further 4–6 months to ensure that he has indeed progressed further into puberty on his own accord.

Oxandrolone, a non-aromatizable anabolic steroid does accelerate linear growth in boys with CDGP without compromising their final adult height. However, it has limited ability to promote physical signs of pubertal maturation.

Testosterone can be given in other forms, e.g. as tablets, skin patches, or gels. Other treatment modalities for CDGP include the use of aromatase inhibitors, which inhibit the conversion of testosterone to oestrogen and thus delay epiphyseal maturation and increase adult height. Initial results of trials have been promising (Wickman et al. 2001) but this mode of therapy requires future large-scale studies to assess the impact on final height and other parameters.

Although CDGP is rare in girls, treatment is on similar lines to that practised in boys. In this instance induction of puberty is by means of administering low dose ethinyloestradiol orally, 2–5 μg once daily for 3–6 months.

Hyperandrogenism in childhood

The clinical manifestation of hyperandrogenism in children is the premature appearance of pubic and/or axillary hair. Other features may include the development of body odour and acne, and, possibly, accelerated growth. By far the most common cause of premature development of pubic and/or axillary hair in childhood is 'premature adrenarche'.

Adrenarche is a normal phenomenon that refers to the maturation of the zona reticularis of the adrenal gland, resulting in increased production of the adrenal androgens DHEA and androstenedione. It normally occurs from the age of 8 years but may develop as early as 6 years. The cause of adrenarche is unknown. It is a separate entity from true puberty and is regulated by a different process (Auchus and Rainey 2004).

The differential diagnosis of premature adrenarche includes simple virilizing congenital adrenal hyperplasia, which tends to present at a younger age than premature adrenarche, and the much rarer conditions of adrenocortical tumours and Cushing syndrome.

It is difficult to differentiate between these conditions early on in the evolution of the disease. Androgen producing adrenal tumours tend to cause more marked and rapidly progressive virilization and lead to accelerated growth. Cushing syndrome has specific features and is usually associated with growth failure.

While premature adrenache is a benign condition that requires neither investigation nor treatment, congenital adrenal hyperplasia, Cushing syndrome, and adrenal tumours must be fully investigated and appropriately treated.

Polycytic ovary syndrome

Polycystic ovary syndrome (PCOS) is a syndrome of variable combination of menstrual irregularity, hirsutism or acne, and obesity. It is the most common endocrine cause of anovulatory infertility and is a major risk factor for the metabolic syndrome and the development of type 2 diabetes in women. Although previously considered a disorder of adult women, an increasing number of teenage women suffer from this condition. PCOS can be documented in perimenarchal girls as young as 10 years of age (Rosenfield *et al.* 2000) but ovarian dysfunction may not manifest till 3 years after menarche (Ibanez *et al.* 1999).

Various criteria have been developed on which the diagnosis can be based. In the absence of other causes of hyperandrogenism, two of the following three are sufficient to make the diagnosis: (1) oligo- or anovulation; (2) clinical and/or biochemical signs of hyperandrogenism; and (3) ultrasonographic evidence of polycystic ovaries. It is worth noting that polycystic ovaries are seen significantly less frequently in hyperandrogenic adolescent girls compared with adults. Also, it has now been recognized that PCOS may be heralded by congenital virilizing disorders, IUGR, premature adrenarche, true precocious puberty, and obesity in mid childhood.

Management of PCOS in the adolescent depends on the specific problem that the individual is troubled by. Weight reduction alone improves almost all the features of the condition. Oligomenorrhoea/amenorrhoea can be managed by using the combined oral contraceptive pill (e.g. Marvelon, which contains a non-androgenic progestogen, desogestrel), Dianette (which contains cyproterone acetate, an antiandrogenic agent with progestogenic properties), or cyclical medroxyprogesterone 5–7 days per month. Hirsutism and acne can be treated using cyproterone acetate (usually in combination with ethinyloestradiol). The combined oral contraceptive pill reduces LH-dependent ovarian androgen production and may have beneficial effects in this respect. Gonadotrophin-releasing hormone analogues also suppress LH production and may therefore reduce androgen production. Infertility in a young teenager is rarely an issue that the paediatric endocrinologist has to address but the primary care physician may be confronted with such a problem. Treatment with clomiphene, gonadotrophin-releasing hormone analogues, and other assisted conception methods can be offered. Other aspects of therapy include cosmetic approaches to treating hirsutism (bleaching, waxing, shaving, creams, electrolysis, and laser hair removal therapy). Psychotherapy may also be an adjunct to the above treatment modalities.

Diabetes

Diabetes is the most common chronic illness in childhood and is associated with significant mortality, morbidity, and long-term complications. The most common form of diabetes in childhood is type 1, which is usually autoimmune in aetiology and invariably requires multiple daily insulin injections. A working classification of diabetes in children is shown in Table 20.5.

The diagnosis of type 1 diabetes in a child or young person has profound effects on the child and the entire family. Adherence to set meals, injection times, and blood glucose measurement all lead to a loss of spontaneity in life. The need to adjust to a life with diabetes is particularly difficult in the very young and the adolescent. There is an additional constant worry about acute medical complications, such as diabetic ketoacidosis and hypoglycaemia, as well as long-term complications (retinopathy, nephropathy, neuropathy, and cardiovascular disease). It is now well established that diabetes is associated with reduced overall life expectancy and increased mortality in early adult life (Edge *et al.* 1999; Laing *et al.* 1999). However, and following the publication of the landmark study, DCCT (Diabetes Control and Complications Trial), in 1993, it now well known that tight diabetic control, currently largely assessed by low HbA1c levels, results in reduction in the risk of long-term diabetic complication (DCCT Research Group 1993).

There have been numerous advances in childhood and adolescent diabetes in the last 10 years, ranging from better understanding about its epidemiology, aetiology, genetics, and immunopathology, to areas of improved treatment and strategies for prevention.

Incidence rates from various parts of the world are now available and show that both type 1 and type 2 diabetes are on the rise (Arsalian 2002; Devendra *et al.* 2004). The exact reason is unknown but environmental factors, such as viral infections, are believed to play an important part. Sedentary life-style is a major contributor to the obesity epidemic and the parallel rise in type 2 diabetes. It is also contributing to the changing pattern of onset of type 1 diabetes at a younger age.

There is now better recognition of the less commonly encountered types of childhood diabetes, such as those associated with syndromes (e.g. Prader–Willi). More recently, the elucidation of the genetics of MODY (maturity onset of diabetes of the young) and the recognition of the different manifestations of its various forms (Owen and Hattersley 2001)

Table 20.5 Working Classification of diabetes in childhood

Type 1 diabetes
Type 2 diabetes
MODY
Neonatal diabetes

Diabetes and a disorder
    Cystic fibrosis related diabetes (CFRD)
    Specific syndrome, e.g. Wolfram, Prader–Willi
    Iatrogenic—steroid therapy
    Insulin resistance syndrome

has resulted in a significant impact both in terms of diagnosis and treatment. Neonatal diabetes, a very rare form of diabetes with an incidence of 1:500 000 live births, may be permanent in 50% of cases. In the latter group, the most common cause has recently been found to be due mutations of the KCNJ11 gene, which codes for the Kir6.2 subunit of the adenosine triphosphate-sensitive potassium channel of the beta cell. The implications of this finding is that affected individuals, who, hitherto, have been treated with insulin injection, could be treatment with sulphonylureas, which restore insulin secretion by binding to the SUR1 subunit of the potassium adenosine triphosphate channel, causing channel closure and membrane depolarization.

Service delivery has likewise been improved and management guidelines have been tightened. This has lead to a family focused approach to managing childhood diabetes and the recognition that input from a multidisciplinary team is of paramount importance. A number of national and international documents have been published outlining the framework under which diabetes services should be provided. These include the ISPAD (International Society for Paediatric and Adolescent Diabetes) consensus statement 2000, NICE (National Institute for Clinical Excellence) guidelines 2004, and the ADA (American Diabetes Association) statement on the care of children and adolescents with type 1 diabetes (Silverstein *et al* 2005). It is perhaps this area of development that has had most impact for families of diabetic children. Recognizing that no single individual professional can provide all aspects of care for a diabetic child has lead to a reform in the way service is delivered. Essential members of a paediatric diabetic team include a diabetes nurse specialist, a paediatric dietician with interest in diabetes, a paediatrician with interest in diabetes, and a child clinical psychologist. Access to podiatry services and input and support from social services is often required.

Among the important new advances are the recently developed insulin analogues that have a much better profile in the circulation and offer a glimpse of hope of mimicking the profile of endogenous insulin secretion. Together with new injection devices, including continuous subcutaneous insulin infusion pumps, and blood glucose monitoring equipment, these developments have made it possible to improve the control of diabetes in the most vulnerable of patients, namely, children and adolescents. As these advances are now increasingly being used in the clinical arena and have implications for the primary care physicians, some detail is provided.

Insulin analogues

Injectable insulin remains the cornerstone of treatment in type 1 diabetes mellitus. Traditionally, most insulin regimens entailed the use of mixtures of short and intermediate acting insulins, in a ready mix preparation (e.g. Mixtard 30:70) or by means of 'free mixing' in an insulin syringe. Injections are usually given twice daily, but more frequent injections are used depending on individual need, blood glucose profile, age and maturity of the child, adequacy of diabetes control, compliance, and practicalities of giving injections at school (e.g. lunchtime injections). The DCCT results suggested that intensification of insulin therapy by means of multiple dose injections (usually four times daily) or by means of continuous subcutaneous insulin infusion (CSII, see below), has beneficial effects on control. Where possible, children are now commenced on so-called basal bolus insulin regimens, or, in some countries, on CSII. The former entails giving a single dose of long-acting insulin and multiple mealtime injections of short-acting insulin.

Advances in recombinant DNA technology in the 1980s allowed biosynthetic insulin production, reducing the likelihood of antibody production, insulin allergy, and lipoatrophy. However, the pharmacokinetic and pharmacodynamic properties of the biosynthetic human insulins were not sufficiently different from the animal-derived insulins to allow for major improvements in control.

Over the last 10 years, modification of biosynthetic insulins has lead to the production of insulin analogues, with improved pharmacokinetic and pharmacodynamic features, including, rapid action, e.g. Lispro (Humalog) and Aspart (NovoRapid), as well as long action, e.g. Glargine (Lantus) and Detemir (Levemir). In contrast to the 'traditional' short- and intermediate-acting insulins (soluble and protophane insulins, respectively), the new insulin analogues have an improved serum profile (see Table 20.6). While it is impossible to reproduce the endogenous insulin serum profile (continuous basal and meal-related acute increase in insulin secretion) even with the most sophisticated of regimens, the new analogues have brought us a step closer towards this ultimate aim.

Insulin Lispro is produced by interchange of a lysine at position 28 and proline at position 29 of the beta chain. This results in decrease non-polar contacts and beta chain interaction. Insulin Aspart is produced by replacing proline with aspart at position 29 of the beta chain. This results in charge repulsion. The monomeric structure and reduced self-association into dimers and hexamers allows rapid absorption and rapid onset of action and less inter-and intra-individual variability. In addition, time from injection to peak serum concentration is independent of dose administered. The practical and clinical benefits include the ability to inject and eat without having to wait (as is the case with soluble insulin), the option of injecting after a meal (in younger children with unpredictable food intake) and less chance of nocturnal hypoglycaemia.

Glargine is produced by two modifications of human insulin: the addition of two positive charges (two arginine molecules) to C terminus of the beta chain and the replacement of an asparagine residue at position 21 in the alpha chain. This shifts the isoelectric point to a pH of 5.4 from 6.7, which reduces solubility at the neutral

Table 20.6 Serum profile of soluble insulin, protaphane insulin and insulin analogues

	Onset	Peak	Duration
Rapid-acting insulin analogues (lispro and aspart)	5–10 mins	0.5–2 hours	3–4 hours
Fast-acting (soluble) insuli	0.5–1 hour	2–5 hours	6–8 hours
Intermediate-acting insulin (isophane, NPH)	1–3 hours	5–8 hours	12–18 hours
Long-acting insulin analogues (glargine and detemir)	1.5–4 hours	None	20–24

subcutaneous pH where it forms a microprecipitate. Detemir is produced by removal of threonine from B30 and acylation of lysine at B29 with a fatty acid. Prolongation of action is due to the self association of the detemir molecule at the site of injection, its ability to remain soluble at neutral pH and the albumin binding via the fatty acid side chain. The advantages of long-acting insulin analogues over protaphane insulin is that they are presented in the form of a solution rather than a suspension that need to be homogeneously mixed, they have a flatter profile and no pronounced peaks over the 24-hour period. This reduces the chances of hypoglycaemia, particularly at night.

Continuous subcutaneous insulin infusion (CSII)

The aim of CSII is to provide background insulin (basal) on a continuous basis and additional insulin (boluses) to cover meals, thus mimicking the endogenous serum insulin profile. Insulin pumps were originally developed in the UK in the 1970s but were subsequently further development in USA, initially in adults and later in adolescents and children. Their use in children was very limited until the mid-1990s mainly because of their relatively large size and their technical limitations, the psychological issues attached to wearing an external device round the clock and, most importantly, because of the lack of commitment of practising physicians to intensive therapy in children. However, following the publication of the DCCT (DCCT Research Group 1993) showing that intensive insulin therapy (multiple dose regimens or CSII) resulted in reduction in HbA1c and dramatic risk reductions in development and progression of complications, data that were applicable to adolescents (13–17 years) as well as adults, physician's attitude towards managing diabetes changed dramatically. Moreover, developments in the pumps made them a more attractive option generally. They are now smaller in size, have better infusion sets, are easier to use, are more reliable, more flexible, and have excellent safety features. They also provide information about bolus history other have other memory functions.

The question arose as to whether the use of pumps in children was feasible. Ahern *et al.* (2002) reported its use in 161 patients, aged 18 months–18 years, followed up for at least 1 year before start of CSII and 1 year thereafter. HbA1c dropped from 7.8% to 7.1% without any concomitant increase in weight or frequency of severe hypoglycaemic episodes. The latter in fact fell from 37 to 24 events per 100 patient years, particularly in the pre-school children under 7 years of age. The authors concluded that pumps were both efficacious and safe even in the very young. Various studies have now been published looking at the effect of switching from insulin injections to CSII in children, showing an improvement in HbA1c with no additional adverse events (Plotnick *et al* 2003; Doyle *et al* 2004).

Possible indications for using CSII include: unstable blood glucose levels, recurrent hypoglycaemic episodes, nocturnal hypoglycaemias, request by child/parent, high HbA1c, 'busy schedule' and, possibly, the very young! The major advantages of using pumps include improvement of control, reduced frequency and severity of hypogly-caemias, fewer injections and some normalization of life-style. However, it is labour-intensive, at least initially, and is a costly therapeutic modality.

A look to the future: prevention and cure

Prevention strategies for type 1 diabetes can be classified into three categories based on the timing of the intervention: (1) primary prevention, aimed at preventing the disease in high-risk populations any serological evidence of islet autoimmunity; (2) secondary prevention, aimed at delaying islet cell damage in subjects with evidence of autoimmunity who have not yet developed hyperglycaemia; and (3) tertiary prevention, aimed at preserving or even regenerating islet cell function in those who have been recently diagnosed.

The only primary prevention trial that is on-going is based on the possible role of cow's milk protein in inducing diabetes. The Trial to Reduce Insulin-dependent diabetes in Genetically at Risk (TRIGR) is an ongoing randomized controlled trial aimed at determining whether the absence of cow's milk proteins in the diet protects from type 1 diabetes progression in first degree relatives carrying high-risk HLA alleles.

The most important secondary prevention trials are the European Diabetes Intervention Trial (ENDIT) and the Diabetes Prevention Trial type 1 (DPT-1). The ENDIT trial was based on the observation that nicotinamide prevented or delayed the onset of diabetes in the Non-Obese Diabetic (NOD) mouse. First degree relatives of individuals with type 1 diabetes were screened for islet cell antibodies and those with a certain titre were randomized to receive nicotinamide or placebo. After 5 years of treatment, there was no decrease in the incidence of type 1 diabetes. In the DPT-1 insulin was administered to relatives at high risk of developing type diabetes within 5 years, the principle of the intervention was that insulin epitope can modify the natural history of autoimmune diabetes. Oral, subcutaneous, or intravenous insulin was administered but no effect on incidence of diabetes was observed after a median follow-up of 3.7 years.

In type 1 diabetes, approximately 15% of beta cells are still viable at the onset of the disease. Tertiary prevention aims at preserving the remaining beta cell function. Various agents have been tried, including the use of immunosuppressant agents (cyclosporin, azathioprine, or prednisolone), which resulted in temporary remission of no effect. Side-effects were a major problem with these treatment modalities. Monoclonal antibody treatment with anti-CD3 antibodies resulted in a reduced decline in the C-peptide response to mixed meal tolerance test and it lasted for more than 1 year. Other immune modulators, such as anti-CD20 and antithymocyte globulin, as well as other compounds (inhaled insulin and heat shock protein 60) are currently being studied including. The results of these trials are awaited.

The ultimate aim is clearly to find a cure for diabetes. The restoration of physiological insulin secretion can be achieved by engrafting the pancreas or the pancreatic islets into a type diabetic recipient. However, when dealing with paediatric diabetic patients one needs to consider the risks of long-term immunosuppressant therapy to prevent allograft rejection versus the potential benefits. Recent modifications in immunosuppressant regimens and the consequent improvement in post-transplant off insulin duration (Shapiro *et al.* 2000) have revived the interest in islet cell transplants. Long-term outcome data of these new protocols are still awaited.

One of the problems with islet cell transplantation, quite apart from the immunosuppression medication required, is the insufficient number of suitable donors to yield sufficient number of transplantable islets. A number of new strategies have been adopted to overcome this problem but the most promising area of future research focuses on the use of stem cell therapy.

Conclusions

Diabetes in childhood and adolescence is a difficult, lifelong and evolving disorder. The management of type 1 diabetes, the most common form of diabetes in childhood, centres around the triad of insulin, diet, and exercise. However, social, psychological, and behavioural factors play a pivotal role in the overall control and many other factors, such as puberty, can be disruptive. Although no cure has yet been found for diabetes some 80 years after the discovery of insulin, the recent advances in diabetes are starting to have a positive impact and help ease the huge burden on children with diabetes.

References

Abuzzahab J, Schneider A, Goddard A, Grigorescu F, Lautier C, Keller E, Kiess W, Klammt J, Kratzsch J, Osgood D, Pfäffle R, Raile K, Seidel B, Smith RJ, Chernausek SD, for the Intrauterine Growth Retardation (IUGR) Study Group (2003). IGF-1 receptor mutations resulting in intrauterine and postnatal growth retardation. *New England Journal of Medicine* **349**: 2211–2222.

Ahern JA, Boland EA, Doane R, Ahern JJ, Rose P, Vincent M, Tamborlane WV (2002). Insulin pump therapy in pediatrics: a therapeutic alternative to safely lower HbA1c levels across all age groups. *Paediatric Diabetes* **3**: 10–15.

Arslanian S (2002). Type 2 diabetes in children: clinical aspects and risk factors. *Hormone Research* **57** (Suppl. 1), 19–28.

Auchus RJ, Rainey WE (2004). Adrenarche—physiology, biochemistry and human disease. *Clinical Endocrinology* **60**: 288–296.

Carrel Al, Myers SE, Whitman BY, Allen DB (1999). Growth hormone improves body composition, fat utilization, physical strength and agility, and growth in Prader-Willi syndrome: a controlled study. *Journal of Pediatrics* **134**: 215–221.

Catagni MA, Lovisetti L, Guerreschi F, Combi A, Ottaviani G (2005). Cosmetic bilateral leg lengthening: experience of 54 cases. *Journal of Bone and Joint Surgery (Br)* **87**: 1402–1425.

Cutfield WS, Wilton P, Bennmarker H, Albertsson-Wikland K, Chatelain P, Ranke M, Price D (2000). Incidence of diabetes mellitus and impaired glucose tolerance in children and adolescents receiving growth-hormone treatment. *Lancet* **355**: 610–613.

Dahlgren J, Albertsson-Wikland K (2005). Final height in short children born small for gestational age treated with growth hormone. *Pediatric Research* **57**: 216–222.

Dattani M, Brook CGD (1996). Outcomes of neonatal screening for congenital hypothyroidism. *Current Opinions in Pediatrics* **8**: 389–395.

DCCT Research Group (1993). The effect of intensive treatment of diabetes on the development and progression of long-term complications in insulin-dependent diabetes mellitus. *New England Journal of Medicine* **329**: 977–986.

Devendra D, Liu E, Eisenbarth GS (2004). Type 1 diabetes: recent developments. *British Medical Journal* **328**: 750–754.

Doyle EA, Weinzimer SA, Steffen AT, Ahern JAH, Vincent M, Tamborlane WV (2004). A randomized, prospective trial comparing the efficacy of continuous subcutaneous insulin infusion with multiple daily injections using glargine. *Diabetes Care* **27**: 1554–1558.

Dubuis JM, Glorieux J, Richer F, Deal CL, Dussault JH, van Vliet G (1996). Outcome of severe congenital hypothyroidism: closing the developmental gap with early high dose levothyroxine treatment. *Journal of Clinical Endocrinology and Metabolism* **81**, 222–227.

Edge JA, Ford-Adams ME, Dunger DB (1999). Causes of death in children with insulin dependent diabetes 1990–96. *Archives of Disease in Childhood* **81**, 318–323.

FDA (2003). FDA talk paper: FDA approves humatrope for short stature. Available at: http://www.fda.gov.

Freeman JV, Cole TJ, Chinn S, Jones PRM, White EM, Preece MA (1995). Cross-sectional stature and weight reference curves for the UK. *Archives of Disease in Childhood* **73**: 17–34.

Godfrey KM, Barker DJ (2000). Fetal nutrition and adult disease. *American Journal of Clinical Nutrition* **71** (Suppl. 5): 1344S–1352S.

Grigorescu F, Lautier C, Keller E, Kiess W, Klammt J, Kratzsch J, Osgood D, Pfaffle R, Raile K, Seidel B, Smith RJ, Chemausek SD, Intrauterine Growth Retardation (IUGR) Study Group.

Heger S, Partsch C-J, Sippell WG (1999). Long-term outcome after depot gonadotrophin releasing hormone agonist treatment of central precocious puberty: final height, body proportion, body composition, bone mineral density and reproductive function. *Journal of Clinical Endocrinology and Metabolism* **84**: 4583–4590.

Hindmarsh PC, Brook CGD (1996). Final height in short normal children treated with growth hormone. *Lancet* **348**: 13–16.

Hokken-Koelega AC, De Waal WJ, Sas TC, van Pareren Y, Arends NJ (2004a). Small for gestational age (SGA): endocrine and metabolic consequences and effects of growth treatment. *Journal of Pediatric Endocrinology and Metabolism* **17** (Suppl. 3): S463–469.

Hokken-Koelega AC, van Pareren Y, Boonstra V, Arends N (2004b). Efficacy and safety of long-term continuous growth hormone treatment of children born small for gestational age. *Hormone Research* **62** (Suppl. 3): S149–154.

Hrytsiuk I, Gilbert R, Logan S, Pindoria S, Brook CGD (2002). Starting dose of levothyroxine for the treatment of congenital hypothyroidism: a systematic review. *Archives of Pediatric and Adolescent Medicine* **156**: 485–459.

Ibanez L, de Zegher F, Potau N (1999). Anovulation after precocious pubarche: early markers and time course in adolescence. *Journal of Clinical Endocrinology and Metabolism* **84**: 2691–2695.

Karlberg J, Albertsson-Wikland K (1995). Growth in full-term small-for-gestational-age infants: from birth to final height. *Pediatric Research* **38**: 733–39.

Laing SP, Swerdlow AJ, Slater SD, Botha JL, Burden AC, Waugh NR, Smith AWM, Hill RD, Bingley PJ, Patterson CC, Qiao Z, Keen H (1999). The British Diabetic Association Cohort Study, II: cause-specific mortality in patients with insulin-treated diabetes mellitus. *Diabetic Medicine* **16**: 466–471.

Lee PD, Rosenfeld RG (1987). Psychosocial correlates of short stature and delayed puberty. *Pediatric Clinics of North America* **34**(4), 851–863.

MacFarlane CE, Brown DC, Johnston LB, Patton MA, Dunger DB, Savage MO, McKenna WJ, Kelnar CJH (2001). Growth hormone therapy and growth in children with Noonan syndrome: results of 3 years' follow-up. *Journal of Clinical Endocrinology and Metabolism* **86**: 1953–1956.

McIntire DD, Bloom SL, Casey BM, Leveno KJ (1999). Birth weight in relation to morbidity and mortality among newborn infants. *New England Journal of Medicine* **340**: 1234–1238.

Milward A, Metherell L, Maamra M, Barahona MJ, Wilkinson IR, Camacho-Hübner C, Savage MO, Bidlingmaier CM, Clark AJL, Ross RJM, Webb SM (2004). Growth hormone (GH) insensitivity syndrome due to a GH receptor truncated after Box1, resulting in isolated failure of STAT 5 signal transduction. *Journal of Clinical Endocrinology and Metabolism* **89**: 1259–1266.

Owen K, Hattersley AT (2001). Maturity-onset of diabetes of the young: from clinical description to molecular genetic characterization. *Best Practice Research Clinical Endocrinology and Metabolism* **15**: 309–323.

Persico N, Postlewaite A, Silverman D (2003). *The effect of adolescent experience on labor market outcomes: the case of height.* Working paper number 03-036. Penn Institute for Economic Research, Philadelphia.

Plotnick LP, Clark LM, Brancati FL, Erlinger T (2003). Safety and effectiveness of insulin pump therapy in children and adolescents with type 1 diabetes. *Diabetes Care* **26**: 1142–1146.

Ramaswami U, Rumsby G, Spoudeas HA, Hindmarsh PC, Brook CGD (1999). Treatment of achondroplasia with growth hormone: six years of experience. *Pediatric Research* **46**: 435–439

Richman RA, Kirsch LR (1988). Testosterone treatment in adolescent boys with constitutional delay in growth and development. *New England Journal of Medicine* **319**(24): 1563–1567.

Rosenfeld RG, Attie KM, Frane J, Brasel JA, Burstein S, Cara JF, Chernausek S, Gotlin RW, Kuntze J, Lippe BM, Mahoney CP, Moore WV, Saenger P, Johanson AJ (1998). Growth hormone therapy of Turner's syndrome: beneficial effect on adult height. *Journal of Pediatrics* **132**: 319–324.

Rosenfield RL (1990). Clinical review 6: diagnosis and management of delayed puberty. *Journal of Clinical Endocrinology and Metabolism* **70**: 559–562.

Rosenfield RL, Ghai K, Ehrmann DA, Barnes RB (2000). Diagnosis of polycytic ovary syndrome in adolescence. Comparison of adolescent and adult hyperandrogenism. *Journal of Pediatric Endocrinology and Metabolism* **13**: 1285–1289.

Sas TC, de Muinck K, Stijnen T, Jansen M, Otten BJ, Hoorweg-Nijman JJG, Vulsma T, Massa GG, Rouwè CW, Maarten Reeser H, Gerver WJ, Gosen JJ, Rongen-Westerlaken C, Stenvert LS (1999). Normalization of height in girls with Turner syndrome after long term growth hormone treatment: results of a randomized dose-response trial. *Journal of Clinical Endocrinology and Metabolism* **84**: 4607–4612.

Sedlmeyer L, Palmert MR (2002). Delayed puberty: analysis of a large case series from an academic center. *Journal of Clinical Endocrinology and Metabolism* **87**: 1613–1620.

Shapiro AM, Lakey JR, Ryan EA, Korbutt GS, Toth E, Warnock GL, Kneteman NM, Rajotte RV (2000). Islet cell transplantation in seven patients with type 1 diabetes mellitus using a glucocorticoid-free immunosuppressant regimen. *New England Journal of Medicine* **343**: 230–238.

Silverstein J, Klingensmith G, Copeland K, Plotnick L, Kaufman F, Laffel L, Deeb L, Grey M, Anderson B, Holzmeister LA, Clark N (2005). Care of children and adolescents with type 1 Diabetes—A statement of the American Diabetes Association. *Diabetes Care* **28**: 186–212.

Stanhope R (2000). Premature thelarche: clinical follow-up and indication for treatment. *Journal of Pediatric Endocrinology and Metabolism* **13**(Suppl. 1): 827–830.

Sybert VP (1984). Adult height in Turner syndrome with and without androgen therapy. *Journal of Pediatrics* **104**: 365–369.

Tillotson SL, Fuggle PW, Smith I, Ades AE, Grant DB (1994). Relation between biochemical severity and intelligence in early treated CH: a threshold effect. *British Medical Journal* **309**: 440–445

Wickman S, Sipila I, Ankarberg-Lindgren C, Norjavaara E, Dunkel L (2001). A specific aromatase inhibitor and potential increase in adult height in boys with delayed puberty: a randomised controlled trial. *Lancet* **357**(9270): 1743–1748.

Wit JM and Rekers-Mombarg LT. (2002) Final height gain by GH therapy in children with idiopathic short stature is dose dependent. *Journal of Clinical Endocrinology and Metabolism* **87**: 604–611.

Woods KA, Camacho-Hubner C, Savage MO, Clark AJL (1996). Intrauterine growth retardation and postnatal growth failure associated with deletion of the insulin-like growth factor 1 gene. *New England Journal of Medicine* **335**: 1363–1367.

Chapter 21

Speech and language disorders and hearing problems

Maria Luscombe, Celia Harding, and
Michael Bannon

Speech and language disorders

Maria Luscombe and Celia Harding

Introduction

Identifying and working with children who have a range of communication needs in the early years population is a challenging and complex task. Speech language and communication difficulties may present in isolation or in conjunction with a range of other developmental difficulties. Similarly, the cause of these difficulties can be attributed to a range of factors within the individual themselves, or social, emotional, or environmental factors.

Primary care workers such as health visitors and GPs have a vital role in identifying which children may require further intervention. It is highly likely that these professionals will meet a number of these children as it is generally agreed that the percentage of children demonstrating speech and language difficulties is 6% of the population (Law *et al.* 2003). This therefore makes communication difficulties one of the most common developmental conditions in early childhood and consequently is of considerable public health interest.

Other studies highlight a similar number of children with speech, language, and communication difficulties. One view is that the percentage of children reaching school age with significant speech and language difficulties is about 5%, with the number of cases of very severe problems confined to speech and/or language, being 1 in every 500 (AFASIC/ICAN 1995; American Psychological Association (1944).

The numbers quoted for children with autistic spectrum disorders (ASD), are between 4.5 and 6.0 in 10 000 for the most severe forms of the disorder (American Psychological Association 1994); or 26 in 10 000 for autistic manifestations of the disorder (Gillberg and Gillberg 1989).

The average family GP has on his or her caseload about 17 000, 15% of this figure being below 16 years of age. Thus, 150 of this group will have pronounced speech and language delay (Enderby and Philip 1986). Within the UK, some 250 000 school-aged children have some degree of language difficulty (Enderby and Philip 1986) with likely additional literacy needs. Law *et al.* (1998) highlighted wide range of children assessed in studies, which may have impacted on the outcomes. The wide range of needs highlighted could be explained by the differences in the ages of the population sampled; the type of problems being identified and the level of the problems being identified.

The type of difficulties

There is a wide range of speech, language, and communication difficulties within a paediatric population. These can include children with the following:

- Difficulties in listening to and attending to spoken language in a range of contexts.
- Difficulties in understanding spoken language within a range of daily living situations.
- Difficulties in acquiring vocabulary and in developing syntactic structures to develop word linkage skills.
- Difficulties in learning how to use communication effectively to request, comment, question, and sustain an interaction event.
- Difficulties in learning specific speech sounds.
- Difficulties in speaking fluently.
- Difficulties in voice production.
- Difficulties in using oral–motor skills effectively to eat and drink.

Hall and Elliman (2002) write that speech and language difficulties are probably the most common cause of parental concern regarding development, with 20% of parents reporting anxieties with their child's speech and language development.

Children with speech and language difficulties are a vulnerable group. Communication skills are closely linked to learning and cognitive skills, which are essential underpinning abilities to enable children to learn effectively. Communication difficulties may impair considerably the quality of the interaction between carers and siblings within the home, thereby impacting on positive interactions and a stable environment within the early years.

Beitchman *et al.* (1996) and Dockerall and Lindsay (1998) highlight the link between language impairment and literacy, and the associated links between oral language problems and social/emotional and behavioural development. It is therefore important that speech, language, and communication difficulties are identified in the pre-school years so that schools are aware of the potential impact on literacy.

Communication is at the centre of the education process. Whether written or spoken, language is the most effective medium for a child to show his or her understanding of a topic being taught in class, and can enable a child to access the curriculum. Communication is also an important factor in the child's well-being and mental health, enabling them to interact at a personal and social level with friends and family. Such communication needs are likely to have significant impacts on literacy learning (Beitchmann *et al.* 1996; Dockerall and Lindsay 1998), socialization, behaviour and therefore the ability to access the curriculum effectively (Dockerall *et al.* 1997).

Communication difficulties can be a presenting feature of other severe disorders. A child's communication needs may already be impacted upon by a variety of sensory deficits such as hearing impairments, visual impairments, and/or motor delays. For children who have just expressive language difficulties, their problems may resolve and not necessarily lead to a poor outcome (Whitehurst and Fischel 1994). However, children with additional receptive difficulties are likely to have a poorer prognosis (Rickman *et al.* 1982; Hall *et al.* 1993) and are going to need longer-term strategy management to help them cope with learning environments as well as everyday living contexts.

If the 6% that Law *et al.* (2003) quote as being the size of the paediatric population demonstrating speech and language difficulties, then this presents a significant challenge to all pre-school provisions and schools.

Who is at risk?

There is a wide variation within the norm for language acquisition, particularly within the first 3 years of development. As already mentioned, 20% of parents register concerns with their child's communication difficulties (Hall *et al.* 2002). However, parents and sometimes early years practitioners are lacking in knowledge regarding language and communication development and tend to focus on quantity and quality of speech sound production, with a tendency to focus less on the understanding of language development or interaction skills. This continues to be a challenge for future training initiatives.

Of the identified group of children with communication difficulties, a significant number of these will resolve within the pre-school years through use of appropriate interventions, e.g. direct speech and language therapy intervention, parent training, nursery or playgroup position, and parents support groups. Although this may be the case, screening of children is still essential to ensure that those with possible long-term difficulties are identified. However, there is no one tool, which is sensitive enough to ascertain who those children are, who are likely to have long-term difficulties. It is essential that screening is available to all children where speech and language difficulties are an issue. A continual challenge for speech and language therapists is to highlight this group to colleagues in primary care.

Within primary care, professionals need to be fully aware of those groups of difficulties, which may predispose a child to being at risk of communication difficulties, or problems, which have a high association with speech, language, and communication difficulties such as:

- **Premature infants:** this group of infants is particularly high-risk (Hall 2002) with between 8 and 20% of cases of cerebral palsy being related to early and traumatic neonatal history and prematurity. There may additionally be cognitive, behavioural, and language difficulties within this population (Luorna *et al.* 1998; Wolke 1998).

- **Birth traumas:** evidence is available that suggests that early traumatic postnatal events may well impact on an infant's future development (Harwood *et al.* 1998; Wolke 1998).

◆ **Postnatal depression:** identification of post-natal depression is not always easy (Hall *et al.* 2002). Hall *et al.* writes that only about 50% of cases are identified unless formal enquiries are made by professionals. Naturally such a diagnosis will influence a child's development through inconsistent parental modelling and reduced opportunities to facilitate early areas of learning.

◆ **Parental mental health issues:** lack of social contact and isolation along with low self-esteem and confidence may impact on a parent's ability to manage.

◆ **Hearing loss:** hearing difficulties can be conductive, i.e. caused by diseases/obstructions in the outer and/or middle ear. Otitis media or glue ear is a common form of conductive loss, Transmission of sound is impeded and middle ear problems tend to be fluctuating. Sensorineural losses are caused by damage of the hair cells in the inner ear or nerves. This causes distortion of sound interpretation. A child may also have a mixed hearing loss, involving elements of conductive and sensorineural losses and a central loss, which is the result of the damage through experiencing a normal routines, interacting and learning with siblings and close family through experiencing a normal routine, interacting and learning with siblings and close family associates, and learning opportunities provided by playgroups and nurseries. A prolonged illness may involve repeated hospitalizations and treatments, which are likely to impact on a child's ability to gain a consistent routine and therefore opportunity for sustained language learning.

◆ **Major illnesses** such as childhood cancers may involve prolonged treatment packages, which could include the use of radiotherapy, chemotherapy, and direct surgery. It is recognized that such treatments are likely to cause structural and functional changes to the central nervous system leading to a number of long-term negative outcomes including neuropsychological problems, sensory and motor deficits and speech and language disorders (Bamford *et al.* 1976; Murdoch and Hudson-Tennent 1994a,b).

◆ **Emotional needs; neglect, abuse and environmental needs** Environment may play a part in impacting on a child's language and communication development. Hart and Risley (1995) comment that with different environmental opportunities, there may be different rates of vocabulary learning due to a variety of socio-economic back-grounds. In addition, low social-economic status accounted for 35% of variance in verbal IQ scores and that scores decreased in proportion with the accumulated number of environmental risks (Sameroff 1987). Escalona (1982) found that at 40 months of age, IQ scores of 'impoverished, former low birth weight infants' dropped from 99.8 at 15 months to 79.9 at 40 months.

An association between oral language difficulties and social and emotional needs impacting on behaviour development has been described by Dockerall *et al.* (1997). There is also evidence from clinical areas making the link between these areas. In a study by Lindsay and Dockerall (2000), which examined 69 children with speech and language difficulties, the found a higher prevalence of behaviour difficulties than would be expected in a typically developing group of children of the same age. Harter (1999) mentions that self-esteem is influenced by positive interactions with others' behaviour affecting the child's self-perceptions. Negative feedback or rejection from significant others is likely to help present an image of low self-esteem.

A child's emotional needs are likely to be affected by their peers, particularly those with speech, language, and communication needs. Conti-Ramsden and Adams (1995) noted that peer interaction between children with language impairment and their normally developing peers is 'impaired and mainly negative', with the children with language impairment having difficulties making their views known and communicating effectively.

A growing body of research supports evidence that maltreatment and neglect can impact negatively on a child's development and there is some suggestion that language development may be sensitive to environment (Law and Conway 1991). Child abuse and neglect may result in impaired social development and low self-esteem and therefore impact on a child's communication development (Coster and Cicchetti 1993). Taiz and King (1998) evaluated a sample of 260 children who had had a history of abuse or neglect and found that 33% of this sample had speech and language or other developmental delays.

◆ **Learning difficulties:** Children with syndromes such as Down syndrome, Fragile X syndrome, and Williams' syndrome, often have associated learning needs. In addition, they are likely to have speech, language, and communication needs, which can be effectively assisted by early strategy management such as signing, use of photograph cues, and use of symbol cues.

◆ **Physical difficulties:** Motor impairments, particularly with associated difficulties such as learning needs and visual impairment will have a major impact on the development of communication. Such children are often referred early to speech and language therapy due to difficulties with oral-motor function, which thus impacts on eating and drinking development. Owing to this, early language and communication intervention is likely to occur.

◆ **Autistic spectrum disorder:** Wing and Gould (1988) suggested that ASD consists of a triad of impairments including difficulties with social relatedness to other persons, limited communication skills and limited imagination. ASD visually occurs before 30 months and presents with an unusual pattern of language development, deviant social development, and restricted and abnormal stereotyped patterns of behaviour. Sometimes, ASD is picked up late by Early Years Practitioners due to it covering a wide range of abilities and needs. Sometimes, a child's range of difficulties may not fully manifest themselves until they enter a playgroup or other similar group setting where their needs become apparent within an interactive context.

Typically, parents may have concerns earlier and comment that they noticed a change in the child's development at about 18–24 months. They may additionally report that language development may have also stopped or even regressed at this point.

Early intervention for autism is recommended by the NIASA Guidelines (2003) as this may help reduce or minimize secondary behavioural difficulties that may arise as a consequence of entrenched behaviour developed by children.

◆ **Regressions:** Any regressions in a pre-schooler's early development can be associated with a range of difficulties such as Rett's syndrome, autism, possible tumour or emotional trauma. All areas include risk to speech, language, and communication development, and therefore warrant early intervention.

- **Craniofacial anomalies:** Infants born with a craniofacial anomaly such as a cleft-lip and/or palate are naturally identified quickly. Usually, speech and language intervention focuses around eating and drinking management. However, it is anticipated that speech work may be necessary. Additionally, it is good practice to ensure that other areas of communication development are progressing, or if specific intervention in these areas is required.

- **Convulsive disorders:** Epilepsy is common in childhood with a prevalence of about five per 1000 (Cowan *et al.* 1989). It is also recognized that there is an increasing prevalence of epilepsy in children with learning difficulties (Corbett 1985). Seizures may cause the language disorder or they may indicate abnormal brain development or damage, which may lead to language impairment (Robinson 1991).

- **Traumatic brain injury:** In many instances, communication difficulties may be an outcome of a brain injury. After trauma, functional language may return, although language processing skills may be impaired. If receptive skills are particularly affected, then the prognosis is not so positive, Ylvishaher (1986). Such trauma may have long-term implications for language difficulties.

- **Dysfluency:** Early non-fluent speech needs careful monitoring. The hesitant child may have periods of fluency interdispersed with non-fluent speech. On assessment, dysfluent children may present with mild language difficulties. However, a negative social and emotional impact of non-fluent speech during interaction events with peers is likely to be an outcome if support for the parent and child is not provided.

Meeting the challenges in supporting children speech, language, and communication needs

Identification

As mentioned earlier, there are a range of screening and surveillance techniques, e.g. Fluharty Pre-school Language Screening Test (1978) and the Sentence Repetition Screening Test (1996). However, it is acknowledged that these are not always sensitive enough to identify children's needs fully (Law *et al.* 2000). Imminent research would not necessarily recommend a universal screening test, although early speech and language delay should be a cause for concern as communication difficulties can be symptomatic of other difficulties or be symptomatic of a communication disorder in its own right.

Colleagues in primary care have a responsibility to ensure that children with these difficulties are identified and that they are a primary source for advice and support.

Advice and support

The key issues for Primary Care Professionals are supporting and educating parents and carers with an emphasis on positive parenting.

The Green Paper, 'Every Child Matters' (2003) highlight that supporting parents is central to a child's well-being. Parents can be fully supported through:

- Universal services, e.g. health services, educational provision.

◆ Targeted and specialist support where needed, e.g. referral to speech and language therapy, referral to clinical psychology for behaviour management, referral to pre-school education services, i.e. Portage.

◆ Compulsory action through parenting. Orders as a last resort were parents are condoning a child's anti social behaviour.

The Green Paper also states that the 'bond between the child and their parents is the most critical influence on a child's life and that 'parenting has a strong impact on a child's life and that 'parenting as a strong impact on a child's educational development, behaviour and mental health'. To promote this stable influence, the Green Paper supports Early Years Practitioners working in partnership to support parental support and implement specific intervention.

Partnership working

Sure Start have a 'Birth to Three Matters' programme, which provides a framework of effective intervention. This is supported by home visiting and enhanced health advice. It is important that this is considered within the context of the National Standards for Under Eights Day Care and Childminding (DfES 2001) and Curriculum Guidelines for the Foundation Stage (DfES/QCA 2000). The principles included are:

◆ 'parents and families are central to the well-being of the child'

◆ relationships with other people (both adults and children) are of crucial importance in a child's life

◆ a relationship with a key person at home and in the early years setting is essential to young children's well-being.

All these aspects are essential in helping the child to maximize their potential as a skilful communication and competent learner. Practitioners can also be effective in linking parents together as increasing confidence and self-esteem, as well as widening social networks and contacts can improve parents' health and therefore have benefits for children (Hall *et al.* 2002).

Primary healthcare team members should be aware of other interventions such as Homestart, founded in 1973, which is a voluntary organization. In this organization, volunteers offer regular support, friendship, and practical help to young families under stress in their own homes.

Approaches to support children with speech language and communication difficulties rely on inter-agency support and increased joint working. Such a holistic approach to child and family health may reduce speech, language, and communication difficulties, along with other risk features.

Working with speech and language therapists

Practitioners need to work in partnership with their local speech and language therapy departments developing literature for parents providing advice and support for mother and toddler groups and toy libraries and ensuring that the availability of materials external to the Primary Care Trust are available, e.g.

- Tesco Baby Club I-can pack for parents on speech and language development
- Afasic/I can web-site
- Royal College of Speech and Language Therapy website.

Practitioners should also be aware that Speech and Language Therapists have a role within prevention and education. This can take the form of the following:

- Providing training for Early Years Practitioners on early identification of risk factors, which may predispose a child to speech, language, and communication difficulties. This training may be done in conjunction with other professionals such as Portage workers and social workers. There may already be a local intervention package in use.
- Providing printed materials for practitioners to access; see Figure 21.1 from the author's Local Trust entitled 'Promoting Early Intervention'.
- Providing assessment and treatment for the conditions highlighted. Most Speech and Language Therapy Services will do their own local service delivery of a range of interventions to meet the needs of the local community. Specific parent–child programmes such as the 'Hanen Early Language Parent Programme (Manolsen 1992) may be provided to promote positive communication and general management of the child.

Parents will benefit from the support of primary care workers to encourage participation and to attend the range of programmes. As professionals, all involved have a responsibility to provide a rationale for parents so that they can see fully the benefits for their child's learning and language development. It is therefore important for professionals to make the links for parents between stimulation provided and the long-term impact of communication difficulties.

Who to refer to speech and language therapy

Glascoe (1997) indicates that parents are good identifiers of children's needs and therefore should be taken seriously. Early Years Practitioners need to be aware that parents can self-refer directly to speech and language therapy. Parents' concerns should be listened to as speech, language, and communication difficulties are often symptomatic or ore serious needs and it is safe to assume that if a parent has a concern, a referral should be made or a discussion with the local speech and language therapist should occur pre-referral. Such a discussion may provide a useful opportunity to explore possible language and communication difficulties.

The printed information sheet mentioned earlier (Figure 21.1), entitled 'Promoting Early Intervention' is used by health visitors and GPs in Harrow. This was developed in consultation with health visitors and primary care workers with speech and language therapists to provide a reference to assist in early identification of communication difficulties. Such a framework is recommended as reference material with the early screening provided. Any children who do not fit the profiles may benefit from intervention.

In addition, the following groups of children may benefit from referral to a speech and language therapist.

PAEDIATRIC SPEECH & LANGUAGE THERAPY SERVICES

A GUIDE FOR GPs AND HVs
FOR REFERRALS OF
CHILDREN 0 TO 5 YEARS

*promoting early
intervention*

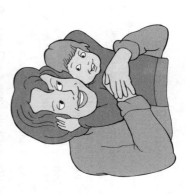

NORTH WEST LONDON HOSPITALS NHS TRUST

HOW DO YOU REFER THE CHILD?

Use referral form or write to:

Head of Speech & Language Therapy
Paediatric Therapy Services
Chaucer Unit, Level 3
Northwick Park Hospital
Watford Road
Harrow, Middx, HA1 3UJ

Tel: 020 8869 3010
Fax: 020 825 4157

Include the following in your letter:

Name, address and date of birth of the child, and telephone number.

Reason for referral

Relevant medical/ development history

Relevant social, emotional and behavioural information

Results of any hearing test

Parental concerns and consent to referral

Other professionals who are involved

COMMENT:

If you would like to comment on our service or would like to make suggestions for improvement, please contact the Head of Speech & Language Therapy.

PRE-SCHOOL CHECK:

Play:
- ✓ Starts to understand rule-based games like Snakes & Ladders
- ✓ Engages in role play / sets up pretend play situations.

Understanding:
- ✓ Understand questions with "Why?" (related to everyday experiences)
- ✓ Understand longer instructions, e.g.: "Put the cup under the cushion and give me the pencil."
- ✓ Begins to be able to reason, e.g.: "If you do X then Y will happen."

Expression:
- ✓ Links sentences using "and", "but", "so", "to"
- ✓ Pronouns "she" "we" "them" "his" used
- ✓ Child no longer repeats/ echoes words and phrases
- ✓ Child able to use a wide vocabulary without struggling to find words
- ✓ Able to talk about a wide range of events

Speech:
- ✓ Speech sounds should be generally intelligible. Clusters of sounds are still developing, but not fully established, e.g. "pade" for spade, "lue" for blue. Other <u>normal</u> errors are:
  r → w "wabbit"
  s → th "thock"

NB: Bilingual children can experience the same difficulties in communication as their English speaking peers. However, only refer if the difficulties are in both languages.

Fig. 21.1 Promoting early intervention.

WHO MAY REQUIRE SPEECH & LANGUAGE THERAPY REFERRAL?

Stammering/ Stuttering Children

Many children have a period of "bumpy speech" between 2 – 5 years. Refer to Speech & Language Therapy is:

• Stammering lasts longer than two months from onset;
• There is a family history of stammering.

Always encourage parents to praise their child's attempts to communicate and not to correct the "bumps".

Voice

Some children exhibit persistent hoarse/ croaky voice. These children should be referred directly to the ENT service who will, if necessary, reer to Speech & Language Therapy.

Eating & Drinking Skills

Therapists will assess and treat children who have severe oral and pharyngeal skills which impact on ability to swallow safely.

Speech, Language & Interaction

The following sections outline the stages in communication development. If a child has not achieved the majority of skills three months after your initial check, please refer.

9 to 12 MONTHS:
Play:
✓ Exploratory play; i.e. examines objects by shaking, mouthing and hitting them.
✓ Enjoys peek-a-boo games with parents/ carers

Fig. 21.1—cont'd

Understanding:
✓ Watches people when they are speaking;
✓ Understands "No" and "Bye"
✓ Turns to own name
✓ Understands several words in context, e.g. dinner, spoon cup
✓ Understands simple commands with gestures, e.g. "come here" and "Give it to Daddy"
✓ Begins to understand functions of objects, e.g. will brush hair

Expression:
✓ Babbles tunefully and incessantly;
✓ Begins to use consonant-vowel combinations e.g.: "baba", "mama"
✓ Imitates adults with playful vocalisations;
✓ Uses pointing with vocalisation (e.g. points at objects of interest, vocalises and looks at carer)
✓ Waves bye-bye

18 MONTHS:
Play:
✓ Demonstrates pretend play, e.g. brushing dolly's hair
✓ Plays alongside but not with other children
✓ Enjoys looking at picture books with carer
✓ Enjoys sharing play activities with carer

Understanding:
✓ Can identify a large range of familiar objects and toys, e.g. chair, table, dog
✓ Understands simple questions, e.g. "Where are your shoes?"
✓ Shows own hair, tummy etc

Expression:
✓ Continues to use unintelligible chatter to accompany play
✓ Begins to use single words (may be unclear)

✓ Draws adult's attention to objects for adult to name

Speech
✓ Emerging words are likely to be unclear.

3 YEARS:
Play:
✓ Demonstrates short sequences of pretend play, e.g. washes doll then puts it to bed
✓ Begins to play with other children
✓ Able to sit through short story book with adult

Understanding:
✓ Able to reply to questions, e.g. "Which one is for drawing?"
✓ Understands familiar action words, e.g. jump, kick, walk
✓ Understands some concepts e.g.: "Show me the big shoe", "Which cup is broken?"
✓ Understands basic prepositions, e.g. up, down, on, in.

Expression:
✓ Can hold simple conversation
✓ Will initiate a conversation with familiar adult
✓ Uses some pronouns, but not necessarily the right ones, e.g. "Me want juice!"
✓ Uses plurals, not necessarily correct, e.g. mousse, foots
✓ Asks "what?" "where?" and "who?" questions

Speech
Speech may be unclear, but should be understood by familiar adult. Examples of normal errors at this age:

Spoon	← poon	finger	← binger
Train	← tain	shoe	← do
Rabbit	← wabbit	car	← tar

- children with language delays secondary to other conditions as in the 'who is at risk?' section
- social and environmental needs in the absence of other difficulties
- children presenting with non-fluency
- children presenting with social communication disorders with an inability to interact effectively
- children who appear not to understand or who have difficulties acquiring vocabulary
- children who have difficulties with oral-motor skills.

Children who use English as an additional language naturally may display a lesser use of English until they go into an early years placement. Practitioners working with potentially bilingual or multilingual children need to consider supporting and developing language demands from all their different environments. It is safe to assume that if parents have a concern, they should have the opportunity for a speech and language therapy assessment. An interpreter will be needed as an essential part of the assessment to help assist in assessing the child in their first language (RCSLT 1996).

Speech and language therapist liaison

Once a speech and language therapist receives a request for a referral, they may have already had an in-depth conversation with the referring agent usually a health visitor or a GP. Once assessed and the child's key needs identified, it may be necessary to liase with the referring agent prior to referring on to other agencies to inform them of the actions to be taken.

The agencies referred to may include the following:

- Referral to the GP requesting that a referral be made to a consultant paediatrician for a full development assessment to ascertain if the speech, language, and communication needs are part of a more global need or to see if there are any unusual developmental patterns.
- Referral to a clinical psychologist if pervasive difficulties such as ASD are suspected or there are challenging social and behavioural issues.
- Referral to and liaison with specialist agencies at a tertiary level centre, e.g. a plastic team who repair craniofacial anomalies or an ENT team who may work with children who have voice problems.
- Referral to the education team. This may involve:
  - referral to education to notify them that a child may have long-term needs, which may impact on their ability to access the curriculum effectively.
  - referral to an Early Education Team such as Portage who can home visit and carry out early education programmes in the home.
  - referral to education to request an early years placement so that the child can benefit from peer language models and have opportunities to develop language skills through functional use with peers and with significant adults.

- referral to colleagues in social services if there are factors in a child's environment, which may impact on them achieving their full potential or where parents may benefit from some of the parent programmes already described.

Case history example

The following case history illustrates a successful early intervention through effective collaborative working between primary care workers.

Paul (not his real name), was the second child of two parents living with each other. His older sister was 2 years older than him and both parents were described as being professionals. His mother became concerned when Paul appeared to stop talking at about 21 months. They were unable to recall any significant events around this time except that he had suffered a heavy cold. She and her husband described Paul as no longer using the range of single words he had learnt to use or playing productively. Instead, he had appeared to take an interest in climbing and lining up cars and bricks. Additionally, he displayed little interest in his sister, and used his parents for needs by lifting their hands or pulling them to the desired object.

On discussion with the health visitor, Paul's mother agreed that a referral to speech and language therapy may be useful. On assessment, the therapist felt that Paul may well have difficulties within the autistic spectrum and immediately initiated a referral for a consultant paediatrician, clinical psychologist and a Portage worker having gained the parents' permission.

Speech and language therapy involved group work and individual work using a mixture of child-led and adult-led strategies to enhance Paul's communicative potential with his parents' support. In addition, transition work and training took place when Paul was old enough to go to nursery. Training took the form of highlighting Paul's communicative strengths, i.e. a mixture of some words, some symbol exchange and lifting an adult's hand and implementing these strategies into the nursery environment so that his skills could be extended further. At this time, Paul's parents also attended the Earlybird programme recently set up by the health and education departments and run by speech and language therapists and Portage workers.

Paul is now happily settled in his nursery and is making progress in all areas of his development. He had support in the classroom to enable him to access the curriculum and gain benefit from all activities on offer. Paul has a diagnosis of social and communication difficulties within the autistic spectrum.

Conclusions

Paul's case history summarizes the positive outcome of early identification and collaborative working. Early intervention made the parents feel that they were effective in developing Paul's skills through joint health and education working. They also felt supported through the support provided as well as the training opportunities available to them.

Such early intervention focused on developing and maximizing a child's communicative skills. Additionally, the parents were supported in introducing strategies into the home setting and through the input of all the professionals involved gained insight into their son's difficulties.

This successful outcome was achieved largely through parental support provided by primary care workers participating collaboratively, and such a model of identification and practice has much to recommend it.

References

AFASIC/ICAN (1995). *Principles for Educational Provision*, AFASIC, 347, Central Markets, Smithfield, London, EC1A 9NH

AFASIC Website; www.afasic.org.uk

American Psychological Association (1994). *Diagnostic and Statistical Manual of Mental Disorders* (4th edn). APA, Washington, DC.

Baker C (1993). *Key issues in Bilingualism & Bilingual Education*. Multilingual Matters. Avon.

Bamford FN, Morris-Jones P, Pearson D, Ribeiro GG, Shalet SM, Beardwell CG (1976). Residual disabilities in children treated for intracranial space-occupying lesions. *Cancer* 37: 1149–1151.

Beitchman JH, Nair R, Clegg M, Patel PG, Ferguson B, Pressman E (1986). Prevalence of speech and language disorders in 5-year old kindergarten children in the Ottawa-Carleton region. *Journal of Speech and Hearing Disorders* 51(2): 98–110.

Conti-Ramsden G, Adams C (1995). Transitions from the clinic to the school: the changing picture of specific language impaired children from pre-school to school age. *Journal of Speech and Language Studies* 5: 1–11.

Corbett J (1985). Epilepsy as part of a handicapping condition. In Ross E, Reynolds E (eds), *Paediatric Perspectives on Epilepsy*. John Wiley, Chichester.

Coster W, Cicchetti D (1993). Research on the communicative development of maltreated children: clinical implications. *Topics in language Disorders* 13(4): 25–38.

Cowan LD, Bodensteiner JB, Leviton A, Doherty L (1989). Prevalence of the epilepsies in children and adolescents. *Epilepsia* 30: 94–106.

Curriculum Guidance for the Foundation Stage (2000). QCA & DfEE.

Dale P, Simonoff E, Bishop D, Eley T, Olivier B, Price T, Purcell S, Stevenson J, Plomtin R (1998). Genetic influences on language delay in two-year old children. *Nature Neuroscience* 1(4): 324–328.

DfES (2001). National Standards for Under 5's Day Care and Childminding.

Dockerill J, Lindsay G (1998). The ways in which speech and language difficulties impact on children's access to the curriculum. *Child Language Teaching & Therapy* 14: 117–133.

Dockerill J, Messer D (1999). *Children's language and Communication Difficulties. Understanding, Identification and Intervention*. Cassell Education, London and New York, pp. 81–95.

Dockerill J, George R, Lindsay G, Roux J (1997). Problems in the identification and assessment of children with specific speech and language difficulties. *Educational Psychology in Practice* 12: 29–38.

Enderby P, Philip R (1986). Speech and language handicap; towards knowing the size of the problem. *British Journal of Disorders of Communication* 21: 151–165.

Escalona SK (1982). Babies at double hazard: early development of infants at biological and social risk. *Paediatrics* 70: 670–6.

Fluharty N (1978). *Fluharty Pre-school Speech and Language Screening Test (Fluharty)*. Teaching Resources, Boston MA.

Gillberg IC, Gillberg C (1989). Aspergers syndrome—some epidermiological considerations: a search note. *Journal of Child Psychology & Psychiatry* 30: 631–638.

Glascoe FP (1997). *Parents' evaluations of Developmental Status (PEDS)*. Radcliffe Medical Press, Oxford.

Green Paper: Every Child Matters Presented to Parliament by the Chief Secretary to the Treasury by Command of Her Majesty, September 2003 CM 5860.

Hall DMB, Elliman D (2002). *Health for all Children*, (4th edn). Oxford University Press, Oxford.

Hall NE, Yamashita TS, Aram, DS (1993). Relationship between language and fluency in children with developmental language disorders. *Journal of Speech and Hearing Research* **6**(36): 568–579.

Hart B, Risley TR (1995). *Meaningful Differences in Everyday Experiences of Young American Children*. Paul Brookes, Baltimore, MD.

Harter S (1999). *The Construction of Self: A developmental perspective*. The Guildford Press, London.

Homestart UK, 2 Salisbury Road, Leicester, LE1 7QR.

Harwood LJ, Mugridge N, Darlow BA (1998). Cognitive, behavioural and educational outcome at 7–8 years in a national very low birth-weight cohort. *Archives of Disease in Childhhod* **79**: F12–F20.

Law J, Conway J (1991). *Child Abuse and Neglect: the Effect on Communication Development—a Review of the Literature*. Available from the Association for All Speech Impaired Children, 347 Central Markets, Smithfield, London EC1A 9NH, UK.

Law J, Boyle J, Harris F, Harkness A, Nye C (1998). Screening for speech and language delay: a systematic review of the literature. *Health Technology Assessment* **2**(9): 1–184.

Law J, Garret Z, Nye C (2003). Speech and language therapy interventions for children with primary speech and language delay or disorder (Cochrane Review) In *The Cochrane Library*, Issue 3, 2003. Oxford: update software.

Lindsay G, Dockerill J (2000). The behaviour and self-esteem of children with specific speech and language difficulties. *British Journal of Educational Psychology* **70**: 583–601.

Luoma L, Herrgard A, Ahowen T (1998). Speech and language development of children born at <32 weeks gestation: a five year prospective follow-up study. *Developmental Medicine and Child Neurology* **40**: 380–387.

Manolsen HA (1992). *It takes Two to Talk*. Haven Centre Publications, Toronto.

Murdoch BE, Hudson-Tennent LJ (1994a). Differential language outcomes in children following treatment for posterior fossa tumours. *Aphasiology* **8**: 507–534.

Murdoch BE, Hudson-Tennent LJ (1994b). Speech disorders in children treated for posterior fossa tumours. *European Journal of Disorders of Communication*, **29**: 379–397.

National Autism Plan for Children (NAPC) Produced by NIASA: *National Initiative for Autism: Screening and Assessment*. Ann Le Couteue (Chair) March 2003 London. Published by National Autistic Society.

Rice M (1997). Specific language impairment: in search of diagnostic markers and genetic contributions. *Mental Retardation and Developmental Disabilities Research Reviews* **3**: 350–357.

Richman N, Stevenson J, Graham PJ (1982). *Preschool to School: a Behavioural Study*. Academic Press, London.

Robinson RJ (1991). Causes and associations of severe and persistent specific speech and language disorders in children. *Developmental Medicine and Child Neurology* **33**: 943–62.

Royal College of Speech and Language Therapists (1996). *Communicating Quality, 2. Professional Standards for Speech and Language Therapists*. RCSLT, London.

Sameroff AJ, Seifer R, Barocas R (1987). Intelligence quotient score of 4 year old children: social—environmental risk factors. *Paediatrics* **79**: 343–49.

Shields J (2001). *Parent Book*. NAS EarlyBird Programme. NAS, London.

Taitz LS, King JM (1998). A profile of abuse. *Archives of Disease in Childhood* **63**(9): 1026–1031.

Whitehurst GJ, Fischel J (1994). Practitioner review: early developmental language delay: What, if anything, should the clinician do about it? *Journal of Child Psychology and Psychiatry* **35**: 613–648.

Wing L, Gould J (1979). Severe impairment of social interaction and associated abnormalities in children: epidermiology and classification. *Journal of Autism and Developmental Disorders* **9**: 11–29.

Wolke D (1998). Psychological development of prematurely born children. *Archives of Disease in Childhood* **78**: 567–70.

Ylvishaher M (1986). Language and communication disorders following paediatric head injury. *Journal Head Trauma Rehabilitation* **1**: 48–56.

Hearing disorders in childhood

Michael Bannon

Classification of deafness in children

Type

- Conductive hearing loss is relatively common and results from abnormalities of the external and middle ear; it mainly effects the middle and lower frequency range.
- Sensorineural or nerve deafness is caused by damage or malformation of the inner ear. It is much less common than sensorineural deafness (about 1–2 babies per thousand are born with significant nerve deafness); it is permanent and has profound implicates for speech and general development.
- Mixed hearing loss refers to a mixture of sensorineural and conductive loss.

Severity

Hearing loss is measured in decibels (dB):

- normal hearing range is considered to be within 0–20 dB
- mild hearing loss is between 20 and 40 dB
- moderate loss: between 40 and 60 dB
- severe loss: between 60 and 90 dB
- profound loss: >90 dB.

Frequency

Frequency of hearing loss is measured in Hertz (Hz):

- low (<500 Hz)
- middle (500–2000 Hz)
- high (>2000 Hz).

Aetiology

Conductive hearing loss is commonly associated with otitis media with effusion and can result in middle frequency losses of the order of 40 dB. This type of hearing loss also fluctuates and usually resolves.

Sensorineural loss may result from the following causes:

- About 25% of cases are idiopathic in the sense that no demonstrable cause may be readily found despite investigation. Over 10 years ago, this proportion would be as high as 50%. Prompt diagnosis with intuitive investigation along with genetic opinion has helped to establish a likely aetiology in an increasing number of cases.

- Another 25% of cases of sensorineural deafness will be caused by variety of environmental and other causes:
  - prenatal infections especially those caused by cytomegalovirus, toxoplasmosis, glandular fever, and rubella
  - ototoxic drugs in particular aminoglycosides
  - prematurity and perinatal hypoxia are both associated with significant risk of development of sensorineural deafness
  - postnatal infections including meningitis, mumps, and measles
  - significant head injury.

- About half of all cases are now thought to have a genetic cause that may be:
  - autosomal recessive
  - autosomal dominant
  - X-linked
  - syndromic where sensorineural deafness is one feature of a larger constellation of other findings and symptoms.

Syndromes associated with deafness

There are at least several hundred known syndromes associated with deafness. Detailed knowledge of these is not required in primary care. The more commonly encountered syndromes are:

- Waardenburg's syndrome of which there are several types. Deafness is seen in association with a white forelock, wide spacing between the eyes and heterochromia iridis. Inheritance is thought to be mainly autosomal dominant.

- Usher's syndrome (autosomal recessive) represents congenital deafness in association with progressive retinitis pigmentosa.

- Pendred's syndrome is autosomal recessive and presents with goitre at about the age of 5 years. There is incomplete oxidation of trapped iodide prior to organification.

- Jervell and Lange-Nielsen syndrome is a rare but significant autosomal recessive syndrome where profound sensorineural deafness is found with prolongation of the QT interval (i.e. corrected Qc >440 ms). These children may present with syncopal attacks which if untreated may be fatal.

- Alport's syndrome (X-linked) where glomerulonephritis is associated with progressive sensorineural loss.

Many clinicians advocate a battery of screening tests when they encounter a child who is newly diagnosed with sensorineural hearing loss. This is a somewhat contentious subject due to the rarity of the syndromes in question. However, the following represent some of the investigations commonly ordered:

+ thyroid function (Pendred's)
+ ECG (Jevell and Lange-Nielses)
+ urinalysis (Alport's)
+ fundoscopy (Usher's, prenatal infection).

It must be noted, however, that unless there are clinical indicators, the rate of pick up from these tests is low.

Detection of childhood deafness

The adverse effects of delayed diagnosis of childhood deafness in terms of delayed speech and other adverse developmental outcomes are well described. Furthermore, 90% of deaf children are born to parents with normal hearing. The resulting levels of stress for families is often underestimated.

Childhood deafness is detected by the following means.

Parental concern

In general, concerns raised by parents about their child's hearing must be taken seriously and referral to a paediatric audiology clinic undertaken without delay. This is particularly appropriate in order to allay anxiety. Moreover, in very young children, apparent lack of auditory responsiveness may be a signal for other significant diagnoses than deafness, such as global developmental delay or autism.

Screening

Assessment of hearing is now part of the child health surveillance programme. It may be undertaken at different ages:

+ *Neonatal*: various methods are available including:
  - Brainstem evoked response audiometry, which is very reliable. However, it is time consuming and the child must lie still.
  - Otoacoustic emissions represent a simple form of objective audiometry that is increasingly being suggested as the most useful test for screening children. Its disadvantage is that it does not distinguish between conductive deafness and sensorineural deafness and that any children who fail the otoacoustic emission test usually have to then progress to brainstem evoked response audiometry.
+ *8 months*: The distraction test is still a reliable form of testing that requires the minimum of equipment if correctly undertaken.
+ *Pre-school*: Conditioned audiometry is feasible where a child is conditioned to perform specific tasks in response to sound inputs
+ *School age*: Pure tone audiometry remains a satisfactory method of testing when a child will allow the use of headphones and is able to reliably respond to pure tone sounds.

Management of childhood deafness

Prompt referral to a paediatric audiology clinic is required once the diagnosis is suspected. A full history (including family details) is taken and a full examination undertaken. The type and extent of the hearing loss is determined by one or more of the methods described above. If sensorineural deafness is confirmed, then referral to the genetic clinic is considered. Treatment largely consists of some form of hearing aid of which many types are available.

- The behind-the-ear hearing aid is most commonly used with children. It has the advantage being relatively easy to handle with detachable earmolds that can be remade as children grow.
- Body aids are used by people with profound hearing loss whereby the aid is attached to a belt connected to the ear by a wire.
- In-the-Ear hearing aids fit completely in the outer ear and are used for mild to severe hearing loss.

In school a radio-aid type of hearing device known as a phonic ear may be used whereby the teacher wears a microphone with transmitter while the child wears the radio receiver. This device ensures that the child can sit anywhere in the class and be in direct contact with the teacher.

Cochlear implants represent a powerful form of hearing aid where a fenestration is made surgically in the basal turn of the cochlea and electrodes on a wire are inserted into the cochlea itself. Theses implants are especially appropriate for children who have lost their hearing having previously acquired speech. A cochlear implant works in a very different manner from a conventional hearing aid. Hearing aids merely amplify sound, whereas cochlear implants compensate for damaged or non-working parts of the inner ear. A cochlear implant works by finding useful sounds electronically and sending them to the brain. The technology is expensive and should only be undertaken in specialized centres. Cochlear implantation does not suit all children, however. The device is particularly of use in children who have become deaf after having learnt speech, for example those who have had meningitis with severe acquired hearing loss.

Further reading

AFASIC/ICAN (1995) *Principles for Educational Provision*, AFASIC, London.

AFASIC Website; www.afasic.org.uk.

American Psychological Association (1994). *Diagnostic and Statistical Manual of Mental Disorders*, 4th edition, APA, Washington. DC.

Baker C (1993). *Key issues in Bilingualism and Bilingual Education* Multilingual Matters, Avon.

Bamford FN, Morris-Jones P, Pearson D, Ribeiro GG, Shalet SM, Beardwell CG (1976). Residual disabilities in children treated for intracranial space-occupying lesions. *Cancer* 37: 1149–1151.

Beitchman JH, Nair R, Clegg M, Patel PG, Ferguson B, Pressman E (1986). Prevalence of speech and language disorders in 5-year old kindergarten children in the Ottawa-Carleton region. *Journal of Speech and Hearing Disorders*, 51(2): 98–110.

Conti-Ramsden G, Adams C (1995). Transitions from the clinic to the school: the changing picture of specific language impaired children from pre-school to school age. *Journal of Speech and Language Studies* 5: 1–11.

Corbett J (1985). Epilepsy as part of a handicapping condition. In E Ross and E. Reynolds (eds) *Paediatric Perspectives on Epilepsy*. John Wiley, Chichester.

Coster W and Cicchetti D (1993). Research on the communicative development of maltreated children: clinical implications, *Topics in language Disorders* 13(4): 25–38.

Cowan LD, Bodensteiner JB, Leviton A, Doherty L (1989). Prevalence of the epilepsies in children and adolescents. *Epilepsia* 30: 94–106.

Curriculum Guidance for the Foundation Stage (2000). QCA & DfEE.

Dale P, Simonoff E, Bishop D, Eley T, Olivier B, Price T, Purcell S, Stevenson J, Plomtin R (1998). Genetic influences on language delay in two-year old children *Nature Neuroscience* 1(4): 324–8.

Dockerill J, George R, Lindsay G, Roux J (1997). Problems in the identification and assessment of children with specific speech and language difficulties. *Educational Psychology in Practice* 12: 29–38.

Dockerill J, Lindsay G (1998). The ways in which speech and language difficulties impact on children's access to the curriculum, *Child Language Teaching and Therapy* 14: 117–33.

Dockerill J & Messer D (1999). *Children's language and Communication Difficulties. Understanding, Identification and Intervention* Cassell, London 81–95.

Enderby P & Philip R (1986). Speech and Language handicap; towards knowing the size of the problem. *British Journal of Disorders of Communication* 21: 151–65.

Escalona SK (1982). Babies at double hazard: early development of infants at biological and social risk. *Paediatrics* 70: 670–6.

Fluharty N (1978). *Fluharty Pre-school Speech and Language Screening Test (Fluharty)*; Teaching Resources: Boston MA.

Gillberg IC & Gillberg C (1989). Aspergers Syndrome - some epidermiological considerations : a search note. *Journal of Child Psychology and Psychiatry* 30: 631–8.

Glascoe FP (1997). *Parents' evaluations of Developmental Status (PEDS)*, Radcliffe Medical Press, Oxford.

Green Paper: *Every Child Matters* Presented to Parliament by the Chief Secretary to the Treasury by Command of Her Majesty, September 2003 CM 5860.

Hall DMB & Elliman D (2002). *Health for all Children* (4th ed). Oxford University Press, Oxford.

Hall NE, Yamashita TS & Aram DS (1993). Relationship between language and fluency in children with developmental language disorders. *Journal of Speech and Hearing Research* 6: 36: 568–79.

Hart B & Risley TR (1995). *Meaningful Differences in Everyday Experiences of Young American Children*. Paul Brookes, Baltimore.

Harter S (1999). *The Construction of Self: A developmental perspective* The Guildford Press: London.

Harwood LJ, Mugridge N & Darlow BA (1998). Cognitive, behavioural and Educational Outcome at 7-8 years in a National Very Low Birth-weight Cohort. *Archives of Disease in Childhood* 79: F12–F20.

Law J, Boyle J, Harris F, Harkness A, Nye C (1998). Screening for Speech and Language Delay : A Systematic Review of the Literature. *Health Technology Assessment* 2(9): 1–184.

Law J, Conway J (1991). *Child abuse and Neglect: the effect on communication development - a review of the literature*. Available from the Association for All Speech Impaired Children, London.

Law J, Garret Z, Nye C (2003). Speech and Language Therapy Interventions for children with Primary speech and language delay or disorder, (Cochrane Review) In : *The Cochrane Library*, Issue 3, 2003. Oxford.

Lindsay G & Dockerill J (2000). The behaviour and self-esteem of children with specific speech and language difficulties. *British Journal of Educational Psychology* 70: 583–601.

Luoma L, Herrgard A, Ahowen T (1998). Speech and Language Development of children born at
< 32 weeks gestation: A five year prospective follow-up study. *Developmental Medicine.
Child Neuro* **40**: 380–7

Manolsen HA (1992). *It Takes Two to Talk* Haven Centre Publications, Toronto.

McCormick B. *Paediatric Audiology 0-5 years*. Whirr, 2003.

Murdoch BE, Hudson-Tennent LJ (1994a). Differential language outcomes in children following
treatment for posterior fossa tumours. *Aphasiology* **8**: 507–534.

Murdoch BE, Hudson-Tennent LJ (1994b). Speech Disorders in children treated for posterior fossa
tumours. *European Journal of Disorders of Communication* **29**: 379–397.

National Standards for Under 5's Day Care and Childminding. (DfES, 2001).

National Initiative for Autism: Screening and Assessment. June (2002). *Guidelines for Identification,
Assessment, Diagnosis, and Access to early interventions for pre-school and primary school aged children
with ASD.*

Rice M (1997). Specific language impairment: in search of diagnostic markers and genetic contributions.
Mental Retardation and Developmental Disabilities Research Reviews **3**: 350–7.

Richman N, Stevenson J, Graham PJ (1982). *Preschool to school behavioural study*. Academic Press.
London.

Robinson RJ (1991). Causes and associations of severe and persistent specific speech and language disorders in children." *Dev. Med. and Child Neurology* **33**: 943–62.

Royal College of Speech and Language Therapists (1996). *Communicating Quality, 2. Professional
Standards for Speech and Language Therapists*. Pub. RCSLT.

Sameroff AJ, Seifer R, Barocas R (1987). Intelligence quotient score of 4 year old children: social -
environmental risk factors. *Paediatrics* **79**: 343–49.

Shields J (2001). *Parent Book. NAS EarlyBird Programme*, NAS, London.

Steel P (2000). Science, medicine, and the future: New interventions in hearing impairment. *British
Medical Journal* **320**: 622–625.

Taitz LS & King JM (1998). A profile of abuse. *Archives of Disease in Childhood* **63**(9); 1026–31.

Whitehurst GJ & Fischel J (1994). Practitioner Review: Early Developmental Language Delay: What, if
anything , should the clinician do about it? *Journal Child Psychology and Psychiatry* **35**: 613–48.

Wing L & Gould J (1979). Severe impairment of Social Interaction and Associated Abnormalities in
Children : Epidermiology and Classification. *Journal of Autism and Developmental Disorders*
9: 11–29.

Wolke D (1998). Psychological development of Prematurely Born Children, *Archives Diseases Childhood*
78: 567–70.

Ylvishaher M (1986). Language and Communication Disorders following paediatric head injury.
Journal of Head Trauma Rehabilitation **1**:48–56.

Chapter 22

Child protection

Ruth Bastable and David Vickers

Introduction

This chapter aims to give you an understanding of the issues around the protection of children. It is not about all the signs and symptoms, nor about the details of the legal framework, rather it tries to help you think about the issues you may face in primary care.

What is child abuse?

Child abuse is not a diagnosis, like diabetes, but is a social construct. Abusive treatment of children is defined by society and changes with time: what was acceptable and widespread practice, such as beating children with belts and sticks (a common practice 100 years ago) is not acceptable now.

Look at the examples below in Table 22.1. Ask yourself, is this abuse?

For many, you will have answered that it depends and you would like more information.

Recognition of child abuse

The first step in recognizing abuse is acknowledging that it exists. We won't see it if we don't think of it, and we won't think of it unless and until we acknowledge its importance. Of course, it is far easier and less trouble to turn away. Child abuse is a difficult problem in the primary care context; by its very nature it tends to be hidden. The signs and symptoms may be difficult to interpret. It is also a disturbing topic and it can be tempting to ignore the signs and symptoms. Physical, emotional, sexual abuse, and neglect often coexist in varying combinations. For example, it is almost impossible to sexually abuse a child without also emotionally abusing them, so the picture can be confusing. The parents, usually the child's most powerful advocates, are also the most frequent perpetrators; they may need help, but not want to recognize that they may be actively concealing the problem from you.

Child abuse in context

Child abuse needs to be thought about in the context of vulnerable children (Figure 22.1, Department of Health, 2000). A child can suffer harm because of its circumstances but not be suffering child abuse. Here are some examples:

- A child of a mother fleeing domestic violence and living in bed and breakfast accommodation as a result. Such a child may not be dealt with in the child protection system

Table 22.1 Is this child abuse

	This is abuse	This is not abuse	Not sure/ need more information
An 18 month old is admitted to hospital with a fractured arm. He has fallen down stairs; the stair gate was left open.			
A 3 month old is noted to have facial bruising on his cheek			
A mother comes to your surgery with her 6-week-old baby. She is distraught; she has just shaken her baby because it would not stop crying. She asks for your help			
Crystal, a 6 year old from a travelling family, has had no immunizations. Her mother does not agree with them			
A 9 year old is left to look after his 4-year-old brother while his mother goes shopping			
A mother lets slip in conversation with the health visitor that she has slapped her 4-month-old baby for being 'naughty'. He draws his legs up when she changes his nappy			
A 14 year old comes to you requesting postcoital contraception. She has a 20-year old boy friend. She knows you will not tell her parents (you have posters in the waiting room saying so)			

but might still be suffering harm; the mother and the child will both be traumatized and may need help, the child may be 'in need' (see below for definition).

◆ A child may be very loved by his or her parents, and still be being abused or neglected: for example the parent with chronic mental health problems whose child is acting as carer. Within the UK, 1.4% (114 000 children) children aged 5–15 provide care; 18 000 of these children provide care for 20 hours or more a week (Donovan *et al.* 2003).

◆ Many children coming into the 'looked after' system (children in public care or otherwise accommodated) are there as a result of severe parenting problems. Such children may be offending and/or substance misusing and out of parental control; it is all too easy to lose sight of these children as victims (Mather 2003).

Some child abuse occurs 'out of the blue', with little warning and in the context of no apparent problems. However, most abuse is preventable. The challenge for primary care is to recognize children and families early in the course of their distress and offer effective and timely intervention, such that a vulnerable child does not become a child in need of child protection, (Carter and Bannon 2003).

Incidence and prevalence

Child abuse is a surprisingly common problem and an important cause of morbidity and mortality.

◆ *Incidence*. Severe abuse: 3/1000 children per year under the age of 18.

Box 22.1   Some of the reasons for not recognizing child abuse: (Bannon et al. 1999)

- *Looking for the wrong thing*: child abuse comes in different forms and is a problem that will be hidden. Looking for physical signs of physical abuse as the sole markers for child abuse misses a lot.

- *Looking in the wrong place*: parents will present their child with something other than abuse, such as an 'accident', or not present their child at all. This presents great challenges to a relationship based on trust; rather than believing the parent (which we usually do), we have to be suspicious. Primary care for children is very much 'needs led' and we rely on patients coming to us rather than seeking them out.

- *Not looking*: there is no doubt that child abuse is upsetting. It is easier to ignore the problem or seek other, more comfortable explanations for our observations. We have to think about the child, who can't ignore it.

- *The problem is hidden*: parents may be frightened or feel ashamed. They may want help, but be unwilling to accept responsibility for their actions. Rarely, they may actually induce illness (factitious induced illness, previously referred to as Munchausen's syndrome by proxy).

- *Inertia*: acknowledging that there is a problem can cause a lot of work and strife. It is less work, at least in the short term, to do nothing. The easiest way to do this is to not acknowledge the problem, and minimize or normalize it ('good enough child care for round here').

- *Not listening*: we recognize child abuse by what we see, what others tell us and what the child and parents say and do. We are also given information by other health professionals, other professionals (such as teachers) friends, relatives, and neighbours. We need to listen to all this, and to ourselves; this latter may be a small voice of discomfort or a sense of 'things not being right', but it needs to be heard.

- *Relationships*: we are often concerned for our relationship with the family; they will be angry and upset and we may fear for our safety if we raise the issue of child abuse. The family may feel betrayed by us if we express our concerns. Relationships may be fragile anyway or it may be that the family is doing their best under very difficult circumstances; we feel sorry for them, we don't want to make things even more difficult. Raising child protection concerns may also sour our relationships in the community or with professional colleagues.

- *Trust*: our relationship with our patients is founded on trust and mutual respect. Where there are suspicions of child abuse, we have to adopt a much more inquisitorial and forensic approach that cuts across this relationship of trust. We don't like to think badly of people we respect and what if we are wrong?

Box 22.1   Some of the reasons for not recognizing child abuse: (Bannon et al. 1999) *(continued)*

- *Interprofessional relationships*: working effectively in child protection demands an interprofessional approach involving at least health, education, social services, and the police. This creates problems, over confidentiality and information sharing, the different languages, cultures and expectations of the different agencies, and the practical difficulties of finding the right professional at the right time and being able to talk to them (DfES 2003).

- *Lack of confidence in the system (Haeringen et al. 1998)*: sometimes we feel that the cost of engaging the child and family in the child protection system outweighs the benefits. It can feel easier to 'go it alone'.

- *Individual freedom versus the nanny state*: child rearing practices vary; we all have a right to a private and family life without undue interference from the State. Judging someone else's child rearing practices is uncomfortable.

- *Prevalence of child abuse.* Not really known, but an NSPCC study (Cawson *et al.* 2000) of 2689 young people between 18 and 24 years found that:
  - 7% suffered serious physical abuse
  - 6% suffered serious physical neglect
  - 6% suffered serious emotional or psychological maltreatment
  - 4% of children suffered serious sexual abuse within the family (1% parent, 3% another relative, most often brother or step brother)
  - 11% of the sample had suffered sexual abuse by another non-related but known person.

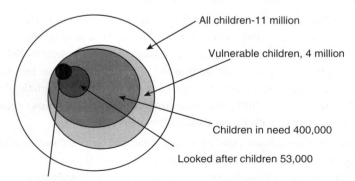

Fig. 22.1 Child abuse in context: vulnerable children, children in need, children in need of child protection and looked after children.

Box 22.2 Cause for concern? (Clever and Freeman, 1995) What are the opportunities for prevention?

583 cases from social services, police, probation, and health visitor files were studied where there was 'cause for concern' (29% of these children eventually had their name placed on the child protection register; most of the rest were referred or in some way monitored; in 16% there was no further action)

- *43% Multiproblem families*: well known families, problems include chronic ill health, poor housing, long-term unemployment, and financial and social incompetence. Petty crime and violence were common as was substance abuse or other addictions. There was a high likelihood that parents were abused themselves. Abuse tended to be multiform and included physical abuse and neglect, incest, and intergenerational sexual abuse and emotional abuse. These families tended to be stigmatized by their own communities.

- *21% Specific problem families*: these families were characterized by having 'no problems' until suspicion of sexual abuse or physical abuse arose. The problem tended to be hidden by the family. The families tended to be quite well educated and in work, but investigation opened a 'Pandora's box of guilty secrets'.

- *13% Acutely distressed families*: these families were struggling, but coping until some final overwhelming incident precipitated child abuse. Such families tended to be single or poorly supported immature parents who were physically ill or disabled. Abuse usually took the form of neglect or physical abuse.

- *The rest were 'infiltrating perpetrators' (9%) and 'outside perpetrators' (13%)*. Infiltrating perpetrators were usually male and befriended or became the new partner of a usually vulnerable (for example, learning disabled), single mother. Suspicion was aroused in cases where the male had a record of child abuse and was known to services, such as probation. There was characteristically a high degree of collusion and or denial by the mother. Outside perpetrators were usually known to, but unrelated to the family were family friends, school friends, boyfriends. Families were seldom aware of the problem until the child spoke out.

Consequences of abuse

Sadly, the morbidity from child abuse casts a very long shadow forwards on the life of the child.

There are victims and survivors. The outcome for the child depends on context, severity, and persistence of abuse and features of the child itself (some children are more resilient than others). There is no one to one relationship between abuse and outcome—cruel treatment can produce an aggressive child or a timid and crushed one. The effects can persist throughout life; for example, there is a high incidence of history of child abuse and neglect in young adult offenders, runaways, and the homeless (Cloke 2003).

Box 22.3 Effects of child abuse (Hobbs et al. 1999)

Morbidity:

- Child abuse has a profound effect on a child in terms of their physical and emotional development, their ability to form relationships and their educational attainment. There is no area of a child's life abuse does not touch.

- The effects of child abuse persist into adult life and, by affecting parenting skills, can be transgenerational.

- The effects of abuse may be transient, situational, permanent, or intermittent.

- Adults who have survived abuse have high levels of physical and psychiatric morbidity and are very frequent consulters in general and hospital practice.

- A large number of the homeless are abuse survivors.

Mortality: child death—the most severe form of child abuse:

- Child abuse is responsible for one to two deaths per week in England, 'but likely to be significantly higher' (NSPCC 2001). Somewhere between 50 and 100 child deaths occur each year in England because of child abuse and neglect (Department of Health 2002).

- Most child homicide is as a result of parental or step- parental activity with murder by a stranger is rare.

Abuse survivors are frequent general practice consulters, often presenting with symptoms for which there is not a physical explanation. They also present to hospitals and again are investigated or have surgery, but with a high incidence of no physical explanation (Smith *et al.* 1995).

> Keith is a 35-year-old homeless man with a drinking problem. He has lost count of the number of times he has attempted to take his own life. As a child, he was a victim of sexual abuse. He struggles to find any purpose in life. 'The person that did this to me got 3 years. I got life'.

The child protection register

In England, there are about 27 000 children on the child protection register. Children may be registered under one or more of four categories

- physical abuse

- sexual abuse

- emotional abuse

- neglect.

Each Social Service Department holds a central register with the names of all those children in the area who have been placed on the Child Protection Register. The decision to register the child's name takes place at an initial child protection conference. This decision is made if the child is at *continuing risk of significant harm and hence in need of a child protection plan and registration.*

The rate at which children are registered varies hugely from area to area; some social service department register almost no children, others register many. The registers are not intended to be a list of all children in the area who have suffered or are likely to suffer significant harm but are those for whom there is a need for a child protection plan.

We know that when professionals consult the child protection register they have two possible responses:

- If the child is on the register, they feel less worried and are reassured that someone else is dealing with the problem.

- They may also feel less worried and reassured if the child is not on the register!

- The important thing is, if you are worried, get help and advice, don't ignore your feelings; do something!

Knowing what you don't know: thinking holistically

One of the great strengths of primary care is the ability to think holistically about a child, his parents and family, and wider circumstances, such as their local environment. We care for children, in their own environment (home) or in the surgery (close to home) along side their families; we often know children and families for many years, sometimes across generations.

The Framework for the Assessment of Children in Need and their Families (Figure 22.2) (Department of Health 2000) is a thinking tool; it tells us what we know, but it also emphasizes what we don't know. We will often know a lot about the health and development

---

Box 22.4 Essential child protection jargon

- *Child in need*: Section 17 of the Children Act 1989: A child in need is one whose vulnerability is such that they are unlikely to reach or maintain a satisfactory level of health and development or that health and development will be significantly impaired *without the provision of services*

- *Child in need of child protection*: Section 47 of the Children Act, 1989: A child in need of child protection is one suffering from or likely to suffer from *significant harm.*

- *Significant harm*: 'has a particular meaning and establishes a threshold for concern'. Significant in the context means noteworthy, which may be through presenting seriousness or presenting implication' (Polnay 2001).

- *Looked after child* (LAC) refers to one who is accommodated by the Local Authority, whether or not a care order has been made. Children in public care may be fostered, in a children's home or otherwise accommodated by the Local Authority.

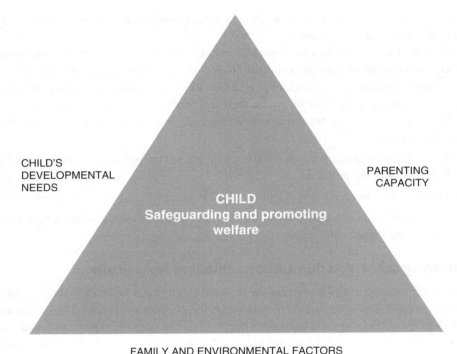

Fig. 22.2 The assessment framework.

of a child, the health of his or her sibs and parents, but we may not know much about the child's view of their problems, their schooling or wider family support.

The Assessment Framework also provides a common language; the child protection system involves at least health, education, the police, and often housing, probation, and youth justice, and sometimes others. Each of these organizations and professions has their own language and culture, but to work together effectively for a child, we must communicate effectively; the common language of the Assessment Framework encourages this.

Non-accidental or inflicted injury

Physical abuse; definition

> Physical abuse may involve hitting, shaking, throwing poisoning, burning or scalding, drowning, suffocating or otherwise causing physical harm to a child. Physical harm may also be caused when a parent or carer feigns the symptoms of or deliberately causes ill health to a child.
>
> Department of Health (2006)

An example The midwife has phoned you and asked you to see Rex aged 4 weeks. When she was on a home visit, his parents mentioned he had some bruising to his face. The explanation given by the parents for the injuries was that the father was holding Rex when he suddenly extended his head, then flexed and hit head against father's chest, causing Rex to bruise his lip. Later the same day, Rex fell off the couch onto a changing mat and banged his right cheek. You admitted him to hospital the same day, where retinal haemorrhages were found. The paediatrician thinks Rex has been shaken.

+ What made you suspect non-accidental injury in Rex?
+ Are you worried about his safety? If so, why?

Recognizing the problem

There are certain warning signs that make us concerned about inflicted, as opposed to accidental injury. There are features to do with the child's injuries and to do with the way the child is presented. Although there is not such thing as a typical abusing parent and abuse can occur in any context, some parents, like some children, are more vulnerable than others. A full history and an assessment of the child, the parents and the wider family circumstances will help but no one thing will make a 'diagnosis' of child abuse, child abuse is like a jigsaw or patch work and no one person will hold all the pieces.

Rex is particularly at risk, as he is a very young, baby with injuries for which there is an implausible explanation and we have concerns that he has been shaken. Clearly, this is a situation in which we must take urgent action to safeguard him.

Head injury caused by shaking is the major cause of fatal physical abuse; 95% of serious head injury in the first year of life is caused by abuse. In this age group, head injury due to other causes, such as household accident is rare. The injuries in shaken baby syndrome are probably caused by a mixture of acceleration/deceleration due to shaking, and impact against hard surfaces from being thrown or swung. Crucially, most babies will have prior evidence of child abuse and neglect; this is often minor injury (such as a small bruise) and may be known to professionals. Retinal haemorrhages are an important finding and are suggestive of shaking injury. The mortality varies with the severity of injury; 60% of those unconscious at presentation die or are profoundly disabled; only about 10–20% will escape unscathed.

Sexual abuse

What is child sexual abuse?

Sexual abuse involves forcing or enticing a child or young person to take part in sexual activities including prostitution, whether or not the child is aware of what is happening. The activities may involve physical contact, including penetrative (e.g. rape, buggery, or oral sex) or non-penetrative acts. They may include non-contact activities, such as involving children in looking at, or in the production of, pornographic material or in the production of online sexual images, watching sexual activities, or encouraging children to behave in sexually inappropriate ways

Department of Health (2006)

An example Marsha is 9 years old and has learning difficulties. She attends a special school. Her teachers are worried because she is exhibiting inappropriately sexualized behaviour: she was seen attempting to 'french kiss' a fellow pupil and then lay on top of another making suggestive thrusting pelvic movements. She has also been using foul language and her schoolwork has deteriorated sharply. She has problems with wetting and soiling. Her mother is also learning disabled and has health problems.

What makes you worried about Marsha?

Recognizing the problem

There are many barriers to recognizing abuse and even more to recognizing sexual abuse. It is an emotional issue, a problem that is hidden by both the perpetrator and the victim

---

Box 22.5 Features of inflicted injury (Hobbs *et al.* 1999)

The pattern of the child's injuries:

- Pre-mobile children do not get bruises or other injuries without good explanation.
- 'Babies bounce': 'Common' household accidents, such as falling from a changing mat, rarely result in significant injury (Hobbs 1994).
- Discrepant explanations: apparently minor or trivial injury, often with a discrepant explanation, may precede major catastrophic injury (NSPCC 2002).
- Injury site and type:
  - especially worrying are: bruises in or around the mouth (especially in small babies); grasp marks on the arms, legs, or chest; finger marks; symmetrical bruising; bruising behind the ears; outline bruising, e.g. hand, belt; and symmetrical bruised eyes.
  - adult bites are always inflicted.

Further reasons for concern:

- Delay in seeking help for the injury.
- Explanations for the injury that change, are implausible or accompanied by unexplained parental aggression and denial.
- Very young children are especially vulnerable to serious injury.

Parental factors:

- There is no such thing as a typical abusing parent.
  - abuse is more prevalent where parents are young and/or socially disadvantaged or socially isolated; where there is drug or alcohol misuse; or where there are parental mental health problems.
  - abuse also occurs in apparently stable, relatively affluent households where there are no apparent problems.

Remember:

- Women can and do physically abuse their children.
- There is a strong association between male perpetrated domestic violence and physical abuse of the children (BMA 1998).

and it is also intrinsically difficult to diagnose; it may go on for many years before being recognized.

You need to think about:

◆ What the child *says* (always take disclosures seriously).

◆ What the child *does* (how he or she behaves, for example, sexualized behaviour).

◆ What we *find on examination. Diagnostic* clinical findings are rare, and if you see anything which suggests to you that the child has been sexually abused you should get help from an expert.

Given Marsha's (above) very suggestive and worrying history, we probably would not examine her in the primary care setting, but ask an expert for help. However, there will be times where we will examine children; for example, vulvovaginitis presents relatively commonly in the general practice setting. A high proportion of young girls who have been sexually abused will have vulval symptoms but vulvitis is also a common and often innocent part of childhood, so we have to be alert enough to know what is normal and treat it as such, yet humble enough to know our limits. There is not an immediate physical risk to Marsha here; it's important for us to do something, but we also have time to talk to other professionals and do the right and best thing for Marsha.

The way in which sexual abuse presents will vary with age. A young child may not be able to verbalize and may exhibit symptoms such as nightmares, anxiety, or fearfulness. An older child may be too frightened or feel too guilty to talk about their problem and may express their pain through soiling or wetting, aggressive sexualized behaviour; self-mutilation, prostitution, or they may be withdrawn and socially isolated. Because of her learning disability, Marsha is more vulnerable to abuse of all kinds, and may have great difficulty in verbalizing her distress.

Both boys and girls are sexually abused and perpetrators can be male or female. Marsha's mother may be less well able to protect her because of her own learning disability. Sadly, her mother is vulnerable to being targeted by paedophiles.

Neglect

What is neglect?

Neglect is the persistent failure to meet a child's basic physical and or psychological needs, likely to result in the serious impairment of the child's health or development. Neglect may occur during pregnancy as a result of maternal substance abuse. Once a child is born, neglect may involve a parent or carer failing to provide adequate food and clothing, shelter, including excluding from home or abandonment, failing to protect a child from physical and emotional harm or danger, failure to ensure adequate supervision including the use of inadequate care-takers, or the failure to ensure access to appropriate medical care or treatment. It may also include neglect of, or unresponsiveness to, a child's basic emotional needs.

Department of Health (2006)

An example Damien is 4 years old. He has had difficult to manage asthma all his life. He was born prematurely; his twin died while being ventilated on NICU. Damien has frequent admissions to hospital with his asthma, and often has contact with the out of

Box 22.6   Features of sexual abuse (Hobbs *et al.* 1999)

Strongly associated with sexual abuse:

- disclosure by the child
- STDs
- pregnancy
- sexualized behaviour or inappropriate sexual knowledge
- bruising or signs or injury in the genital area.

Not specific, but sexual abuse should be considered in the differential diagnosis:

- symptoms of local trauma or infection such as vaginal discharge, perineal soreness, rectal bleeding, anal trauma, genital warts
- symptoms related to emotional effects such as enuresis, encopresis, loss of concentration, change in behaviour or self-harm.

The presentation depends on the age of the child. Perpetrators can be male or female— there is no such thing as a typical abuser. Children with a disability are more vulnerable.

hours services. He is small and light for age. The reception staff have noticed that requests for his inhaled steroids are very infrequent and requests for other medications are always made at the last minute. He often misses hospital outpatient appointments and, however much you ask, does not attend planned follow-ups at the surgery. He is also very behind on his immunization. His mother keeps promising to bring him and never does. You are reluctant to immunize opportunistically, as every time you see him he is unwell. Consultations are always as a result of crisis so its very hard to get a handle on his problems or have any continuity of care.

He seems unusually affectionate towards you, and wants to sit on your knee during the consultation. He is dressed in a thin sweater and no coat in spite of it being a very cold day.

You know Damien's mother is probably doing her best; she has a lot of problems with depression.

Why are you worried about Damien?

Recognizing the problem

Neglect is the persisting failure of the carers to recognize and or meet the child's need and to comply with professionals' advice. It is strongly associated with poverty and other adverse social circumstances, but may also occur in socially advantaged household, which is even more difficult to recognize. There is often poor compliance with medication schedules and immunization. A climate of neglect makes simple medical problems difficult to deal with, complex ones impossible. Households are often chaotic and often 'known to' other agencies, such as housing, police, and educational welfare. Problems may have persisted over many months or years and there may have been extensive professional involvement. Neglect may be transgenerational. As with other forms of abuse, children who are disabled are more at risk.

Neglect can be insidious and therefore very difficult to recognize. It may go unacknowledged or tolerated by professionals for years; it is easy to normalize very poor care of a child because that is what we are used to seeing or feel it is the best this parent can do. Neglect may coexist with other forms of abuse, such as emotional or sexual abuse. It is often the case that it is not recognized until some other precipitating event, such as an 'accident' or physical abuse. We may suspect it when a child is not taken to the doctor when ill or frequently has to look after his or herself because parents were away, for example at work. The parents may be suffering a chronic illness, may have their ability to parent their child impaired by drug or alcohol misuse or mental ill health. Such parents may sincerely love their children and want the best for them, but in the end, because of their own difficulties, are unable to provide good enough parenting. Neglect may also involve being abandoned or deserted, or living in a home in dangerous condition.

Our problem with Damien is that he is not being cared for anything like as well as he could be. He is very at risk of having a serious and even life-threatening attack of asthma. Some of his problems with growth and development may be due to his asthma, but treatment of this is not optimal, as his mother is not properly engaged in this. He may not be growing because he is neglected. He has no coat on and it's a cold day; in what other ways are his needs not being met? Is he being properly fed and cared for? Probably not. We need to do something for him, but probably have time to take a considered view and gather information from other professionals. We will find this case hard to deal with; we feel great sympathy for Damien's mother (she is unwell herself and doing her best), but Damien is undoubtedly suffering.

Emotional abuse

What is emotional abuse?

Emotional abuse is the persistent emotional ill treatment of a child such as to cause severe and persistent adverse effects on the child's emotional development. It may involve conveying to the children that they are worthless or unloved, inadequate, or valued only insofar as they meet the needs of another person. It may feature age or developmentally inappropriate expectations being imposed on children. These may include interactions that are beyond the child's developmental capacity, as well as overprotection and limitation of exploration and learning, or preventing the child participating in normal social interaction. It may involve seeing or hearing the ill-treatment of another, serious bullying causing children frequently to feel frightened or in danger, or the exploitation or corruption of children. Some level of emotional abuse is involved in all types of ill treatment or a child, though it may occur alone.

Department of Health (2006)

An example Morag and Cain are aged 6 and 5. They have recently registered with the practice. A neighbour reports that she has observed Cain's mother putting pepper into his mouth because he swore. She says that there is always shouting in the house, and the children are constantly criticized. She describes the house as 'a tip'.

Box 22.7 Features of neglect (Hobbs *et al.* 1999)

These will depend on the age of the child and signs may be physical, developmental. or behavioural.

- *In infants.* Failure to thrive (but then gain weight well outside the home environment). Common conditions may be untreated until they become very severe. Repeated admissions to hospital. Avoidable accidents: these may be recurrent. General developmental and social delay.

- *In pre-school children.* As above, plus failure to thrive may present as short stature. The child may be dirty and unkempt, general health may be poor. Language delay, poor attention, and immaturity. Behaviour may be aggressive or overactive or passive and withdrawn. The child may show indiscriminate friendliness and seek emotional comfort from strangers.

- *In school children.* As above plus learning difficulties and lack of confidence, poor relationships, poor school progress, destructive behaviour, physical problems such as wetting, soiling.

- *In teenagers.* Short and underweight or short and obese with poor general health. They may be unkempt, dirty, and have delayed puberty. School failure, truancy, and drug/alcohol misuse. They may run away, exhibit sexual promiscuity, steal, and be destructive (of self, others, property).

The health visitor reports that the school has been concerned over Cain. He is unable to settle to tasks, cannot hold a pencil and his behaviour in class is often aimless, loud, and disruptive. Morag is a sad and withdrawn child; she has no friends at school. At home she spends a great deal of time alone in her room because she is 'naughty'. Apparently, there has been previous social services involvement.

Cain's mother is very chaotic and has problems keeping appointments.

Why are you worried about these children?

Recognizing the problem

A certain amount of emotional abuse is present in all other kinds of abuse. Emotional abuse can be difficult to recognize or may go unacknowledged, especially when it occurs alone and in a 'well off' family. Most commonly, parents will terrorize a child, threatening them with 'bogey men', or making threats against things the child loves, such as pets, or threats of being sent away. Proxy attacks may be made by the perpetrator, harming someone or something the child loves, such as a possession or a pet. Domestic violence between carers can be a form of proxy attack. The perpetrator may attempt to psychologically control and dominate by attempts to control thinking or isolating a child from its peers, A child may be controlled and punished by being locked up, or having their mouth washed out with soap and water. The child is humiliated and degraded by attacks on his or her self-worth or self-esteem that can be verbal or non-verbal. Affection may be withdrawn or withheld. There can be marked dislike of the child and it is sometimes the case that one child in a family is singled out for this treatment, whereas the others are loved and cared for apparently quite normally.

Morag and Cain are clearly suffering because of their mother's treatment of them. They will not thrive as children, and will be likely to suffer serious and long-term effects from the harm being done to them. Socially, they are not doing well, and Cain is suffering in his schooling. Although there is little immediate threat of physical harm to them, it is important to not underestimate the distress these children are suffering. We have time to think, to consult other professionals here, but it will be important to act.

What you should do (Department of Health 2003)

- Ensure the safety of the child:
  - You must always ask first, *is this child safe?* For example, if there is physical abuse in a very young child, you should consider how to ensure the immediate safety of the child.
  - If you think a child is not safe, then you need to act quickly to ensure their safety. Refer the child to social services urgently, by phone. If the child is injured or ill, he or she may need hospital treatment or admission.
- Put the child's needs first:
  - As professionals working in primary care, we have to care for the child and their family. When there is a child protection concern, we must put the needs of the child above all others (this is the 'Paramountcy Principle' of the Children Act).
- *Respond with appropriate speed:* if the child is not in immediate jeopardy (this may be the case especially in sexual abuse, neglect and emotional abuse), you have time.

Box 22.8 Features of emotional abuse (Hobbs *et al.* 1999)

These will depend on the child's stage of development

- *Babies* may show sleeping/feeding problems, excessive irritability. They may fail to thrive. They may be apathetic towards their carers or clingy and excessively attached to them.
- *Toddlers and young children.* As above, plus indiscriminate affection, language delay, fearful and anxious behaviour, inability to play. They may be withdrawn and very quiet, or may be overactive and destructive.
- *School age.* As above, but also difficult peer relationships, difficulties at school, poor educational attainment or underattainment, and poor social skills. They may also begin to develop delinquent behaviour, bullying, truanting.
- *Teenage.* As above, but also depression, aggression, anxiety, self-harm, and substance misuse.

- The detail of what you will do depends on the presentation. For example, recent history of serious sexual assault needs a rapid response. A case of neglect that has dragged on for years needs a rapid response if the child is found to be recently physically injured.

- *Gather information from the child and family:* you can discuss your concerns with the parents and the child (as appropriate), unless doing so would put the child at risk. If you suspect sexual abuse, the parent presenting the child may be the perpetrator (but remember this will be relatively rare), if so, you will need to be circumspect in your questioning as there is a risk of the child being 'coached' in his or her story.

- *Gather information from the practice team:* ask other doctors in the practice and the health visitor/school nurse, carefully check the notes of other household members for concerns. For example, there may be other concerns about the welfare of other children in the household; there may be domestic violence, or concerns about drug or alcohol misuse or history of mental ill health in the parents.

- *Make a clear and careful note of your concerns:* good note keeping is essential. Record this and all other contacts, whether by phone or face to face and think about whether you need to record anything in other household members' notes (children, parents, etc.).

- *Know your local arrangements:* local arrangements for advice and referral will vary: it's wise to find out what these are before you need them.

- *Seek advice from your named or designated doctor or nurse or from social services*: you can do this on an anonymized basis, and therefore avoid consent issues.

- *You can ask for a medical opinion:* this will usually be from either a community paediatrician or a hospital paediatrician (depending on local arrangements and the nature of your concerns).

- *Irrespective of other actions, if think there is a child protection concern you should make a referral to social services.*
  - Before making a referral, you should usually seek consent of the parent, and/or child (if this is appropriate). You can act without consent if seeking this might lead to further harm to the child or if consent is withheld and you have reason to suspect child abuse. Dealing with adolescents is particularly challenging; generally, you should try to build trust and make a referral with consent, rather than acting in a hurry.
  - You should make a referral by phone, followed up in writing within 48 hours.
  - You should expect a response from social services within 1 working day. If you have heard nothing after 3 days, contact them again to find out what is happening.

- *Good safety netting is essential:* follow cases up, make sure what you expect to happen actually does. If it doesn't happen, ask your named or designated doctor or nurse for advice. If you think your concern has not been understood, talk to the social worker again.

- *Child protection is a multi-agency process:* the inquiry into, assessment and subsequent management of any child protection issue needs a multi-agency approach. You need to know about and follow your local interagency procedure (Bastable *et al.* 2005). If you are not sure about this, the named and designated doctors and nurses and social services are there to help you

♦ *You have a continuing role:* your responsibilities do not stop at referral. You have a role in the assessment and continuing management of the problem and need to think about how you will contribute to this (Carter and Bannon 2003, Royal College of General Practitioners 2005).

Conclusions

Child protection is a difficult area of medical practice. There is no clear diagnostic test, its management involves many other people, often with a differing perspective and it tests our relationships with parents.

Prompt action may be essential to ensure a good outcome. Early intervention in distressed families may prevent escalation into child protection issues.

It is not an area of practice in which you should work alone. Share concerns within the practice team; seek advice from others with more experience, such as named and designated doctors and nurses and keep up to date. There is a need for ongoing education and training for the whole team in relation to child protection (Carter *et al.* 2006).

Remember that the child's interests should always be your primary concern.

References

Bannon MJ, Carter YH, Ross L (1999). Perceived barriers to full participation in the child protection process: preliminary conclusions from focus group discussions in West Midlands UK. *Journal of Interprofessional Care* **13**: 239–248.

Bastable R, Brimblecombe P, Ambury T, Baker M (2005). Child protection: what does the Laming Inquiry mean for GPs? *The New Generalist* **Winter**: 60–61.

BMA (1998). *Domestic Violence: a health care issue?* British Medical Association, London.

Carter YH, Bannon M (2003). *The Role of Primary Care in the Protection of Children from Abuse and Neglect.* A Position Paper for the Royal College of General Practitioners. Royal College of General Practitioners, London.

Carter YH, Bannon MJ, Limbert C, Docherty A, Barlow J (2006). Improving child protection: a systematic review of training and procedural interventions. *Archives of Disease in Childhood* **91**(9) 740–3.

Cawson P, Wattam C, Brooker S, Kelly G (2000). *Child Maltreatment in the United Kingdom: a study of the prevalence of child abuse and neglect.* NSPCC, London.

Clever H, Freeman P (1995). *Parental Perspectives in Cases of Suspected Child Abuse.* The Stationery Office, London.

Cloke C (2003). Forgotten patients—adults abused as children. In Bannon MJ, Carter YH (eds), *Protecting children from abuse and neglect in primary care.* Oxford University Press, Oxford, 111–125.

Department of Health (2000). *Framework for the Assessment of Children in Need and Their Families.* The Stationery Office, London.

Department of Health (2002). *Learning from Past Experience—a Review of Serious Case Reviews.* The Stationery Office, London.

Department of Health (2003). *What to Do If You Are Worried a Child Is Being Abused: Summary.* Department of Health, London.

Department of Health (2006). *Working Together to Safeguard Children*. The Stationery Office, London.

DfES (Department for Education and Skills), Department of Health and The Home Office (2003). *Keeping Children Safe: the Government's Response to the Victoria Climbie Inquiry Report and Joint Chief Inspector's Report Safeguarding Children*. The Stationery Office, London.

Donovan T, Drever F, Whitehead M (2003). Health of young and elderly informal carers: analysis of UK census data. *British Medical Journal* 327: 1388.

Haeringen A, Dadds M, Armstrong K (1998). The child abuse lottery—will the doctor suspect and report? Physician attitudes towards and reporting of suspected child abuse and neglect. *Child Abuse and Neglect* 22(3): 159–169.

Hobbs C (1994). Could it have happened when he fell, doctor? *Child Abuse Review* 3: 148–150.

Hobbs C, Hanks H, Wynne J (1999). *Child Abuse and Neglect: A clinician's handbook* (2nd edn). Churchill Livingstone, London.

Mather M (2003). The health needs of looked after children and the role of the primary care team In Bannon MJ, Carter YH (eds), *Protecting Children from Abuse and Neglect in Primary Care*. Oxford University Press

NSPCC (2001). *Out of Sight: NSPCC report on child deaths from abuse 1973–2000*. NSPCC, London.

NSPCC (2002). *What Really Happened? Child Protection Case Management of Infants with Serious Injuries and Discrepant Parental Explanations, (SIDE)*. NSPCC, London.

Polnay J (2001). *Child Protection in Primary Care*. Radcliffe Medical Press, Oxford.

Royal College of General Practitioners (2005). *Keep Me Safe*. The Royal College of General Practitioners Strategy for Child Protection. London, RCGP http://www.rcgp.org.uk/pdf/corp_childprotection-strategy.pdf (accessed 14 May 2006).

Smith D, Pearce L, Pringle M, Caplan R (1995). Adults with a history of child sexual abuse: evaluation of a pilot therapy service. *British Medical Journal* 310: 1175–1178.

Chapter 23

Ophthalmology

Gill Adams and Barbara Dulley

Introduction

The eye develops early in pregnancy starting about 2 weeks after conception. Infection, drugs, X-rays, or metabolic abnormalities can damage the development process. At birth the visual system is very immature and it must then develop by forming neural connections and pathways. Maturation, which occurs over the next 7–8 years, is called the critical period of visual development and once this plastic phase is completed the system and its pathways are set and cannot be altered (Wiesel 1982). As well as vision, other aspects of visual function including colour, pattern, and binocularity with stereopsis (3-D vision) develop. The critical period is divided into early and late phases and is preceded by a short 6-week latent period, which is the time before the baby's visual system is sensitized to stimulus deprivation. For example, birth haemorrhages do not lead to amblyopia (reduced acuity in one or sometimes both eyes, caused by interruption of normal visual development during the sensitive period) because they usually clear within 4 weeks of life. This is also the reason why prompt diagnosis and treatment of neonatal cataracts gives the infant the best chance of achieving good vision, with a delay in diagnosis and treatment likely to result in a poorer outcome. If the visual cortex does not receive clearly focused aligned images from each eye the child will not develop high-quality sight with stereopsis. Hence the need for the early treatment of significant refractive errors and squints to allow for good visual development

Screening

Screening and surveillance programmes are in place in the UK to detect and treat visual impairment or ocular abnormalities at the earliest opportunity. Although there is at present some variability across the UK, in 2003 a new revised programme was set out which advised specialist ophthalmic examinations of significantly premature and low birthweight babies for the detection of retinopathy of prematurity, also an eye examination of all newborn babies to detect media opacities and eye anomalies, which should be repeated at the 6–8-week infant check (Hall and Elliman 2003). The hospital paediatrician and the general practitioner usually perform the two later checks. The new programme recommends that there should be no routine ophthalmic screening examinations until primary school age when all 4–5 year olds should have primary vision screening by an orthoptist to include assessment of distance vision, squint, ocular motility, binocular function, and stereopsis.

In secondary schools if there are screening procedures running these will continue but new programmes will not be started. A child attending a Special school will have had a full visual assessment at the time of referral or admission with follow-up care continuing through the school medical officer.

If any ophthalmological concerns are reported to health professionals during other health checks or at any other time the child should be referred for further examination.

Retinopathy of prematurity (ROP)

ROP is a major cause of blindness in premature babies, and in the UK screening is for babies born weighing 1.5 kg or less and 31 weeks or less gestation. All babies who have required treatment or have reached advanced ('stage 3') disease require ongoing ophthalmic care because of the increased incidence of strabismus and refractive error. Treatment is with either cryotherapy or diode laser (Royal College of Ophthalmologists, British Association of Perinatal Medicine 1996).

Postnatal and 6–8-week eye check

The purpose of these examinations is to detect abnormalities including congenital cataract, microphthalmos, coloboma, and buphthalmos.

Other screening programmes

As well as screening programmes for all children there are recommendations for specifically targeting children with certain diseases or on particular therapies who are at risk of developing eye problems. These include examining children with juvenile rheumatoid arthritis for uveitis, optic nerve gliomas in neurofibromatosis type I, optic neuropathy in patients on ethambutol, and retinal toxicity in those on desferoxamine treatment and vigabactin.

Examination of the eye

Postnatal and 6–8-week check

The examination should start externally with the face to check for any abnormality such as the Sturge–Weber anomaly ('port wine stain'), which is associated with infantile glaucoma, lid abnormalities, including those that may be seen in dysmorphic infants, lid retraction, capillary haemangioma, or ptosis. Normally in the awake child the lower lid will cover the inferior border of the cornea and the upper lid crosses over the cornea between the pupil and the corneoscleral limbus. The conjunctiva is firmly attached to the lids and the limbus but loosely attached to the rest of the sclera. If there is fluid under the conjunctiva it will become swollen or chemotic and may even protrude out of the closed lids. Small children are often asleep when you want to do such exams so the lids may have to be lifted gently to allow observation of the external eye. Look for major anomalies such as anophthalmos (non-existent eye) or microphthalmos (particularly small eye). In most babies the sclera should be white but it may be yellow if the infant is jaundiced and a slatey grey colour in osteogenesis imperfecta. The cornea should be bright and transparent, but can be opacified in conditions such as sclerocornea or in some chromosomal abnormalities, and through it should be seen the coloured iris with the almost central pupil. Buphthalmos is the very rare condition of congenital glaucoma, with less than 50 new cases each year in the UK. It is usually bilateral and presents with enlarged eyes and hazy corneas. In the slightly older child it may present with epiphora. Most Caucasian babies will have bluish coloured iris, which can change colour over the following months. The sphincter muscle of the iris develops more quickly than the dilator muscle so the pupils in infants and small children are usually small and dilate poorly. The pupils should be inspected to check that they are round and regular. Physiological anisocoria is not uncommon and can be found in anything up to 20% of children. It is usually only commented upon in light eyed children as it is difficult to detect in dark eyed infants. It is due to an asymmetric development of the iris muscles. Horner's syndrome is a rare cause of unilateral ptosis and small pupil. The reported colour change in the iris with congenital Horner's syndrome takes time to develop so will not be evident immediately after birth. It does not require any treatment. A coloboma can be difficult to see especially in infants with dark irises if the lids are not pulled open to allow a thorough inspection. They appear as keyhole or cats eyes pupils and are caused by failure of closure of the fetal fissure during early eye formation. Use a good bright light; preferably a halogen powered ophthalmoscope or torch. A coloboma of the iris may be associated with a posterior coloboma of the retina, which may involve the macular areas and hence affect sight.

The lens should be checked for opacities. This is best done in dim light using a fully charged ophthalmoscope. Set the ophthalmoscope dial at zero if you have no refractive error or are wearing glasses, or set to correct for any required prescription if testing without glasses. Hold the lids open, look straight at the eye from a distance of 18 inches and inspect the pupillary red reflex (reflection). This will be redder in Caucasian infants and slightly paler in dark infants. In children with dark brown irises and small pupils it may be difficult to be certain if the reflex is present. In this case dilate the pupils with cyclopentolate 0.5% and phenylephrine 2.5%, and re-examine. If there is any suggestion that the red reflex is not clear, refer immediately for an ophthalmological opinion. In the UK there are about 248 congenital infantile cataracts per year diagnosed, giving an incidence of 2.49 per 10 000 children (Rahi and Dezateux 1999). There appears to be no sex difference. About two-thirds of these are bilateral, and 55% are isolated, with 45% being associated with ipsilateral ocular disease or a systemic anomaly. Only half of these children are diagnosed by 10 weeks of age, and 30% are not diagnosed until after 1 year of life.

By 6–8 weeks most infants will have smiled at their mother and can fix and follow lights. If this is not the case, in the majority of children it will be due to a delayed response called delayed visual maturation. However, it may be a sign of a more major visual problem such as a retinal dystrophy, albinism, congenital anomalies of the optic nerve or damage of the cortical visual pathways. Cortical visual impairment is now the main cause of vision impairment in North America, and is the major cause of visual disability in ex-premature babies.

The presence of nystagmus or wobbly eyes is abnormal and requires early referral for ophthalmological evaluation. The commonest cause is congenital idiopathic motor nystagmus, with other associations being albinism, severe visual loss due to dense cataracts for example, and intracranial disease. Nystagmus is often not present immediately after birth but most types will develop in the first 6 months of life.

Ptosis or droopy lid may often be mistaken as the opposite eye being larger or the affected eye being smaller than normal. It is very rare for the globes to be of different sizes. The commonest cause of childhood ptosis is a congenital dystrophy of the levator muscle, other causes include a III cranial nerve palsy, a Horner's syndrome due to sympathetic denervation or in association with the Marcus Gunn jaw-winking syndrome, where the lid is ptotic but elevates when the jaw moves.

If there is complete ptosis this can cause severe deprivation amblyopia, and will require urgent surgery. If the ptosis is partial, close monitoring of vision is required as about 20% of these children will develop amblyopia due to an anisometropic refractive error. If the vision is affected and cannot be improved with glasses and occlusion therapy, lid surgery is required. If possible, surgery should be delayed until after the child is 4 years of age.

Capillary haemangioma (strawberry mark or naevus) is a benign vascular tumour that may affect the eyelids and orbit. If the tumour involves the lids and is large, it can obstruct the visual axis producing visual deprivation but more commonly it produces astigmatism and amblyopia.

A white pupil is a significant and serious sign in a child. There are many causes of leukocoria ('white pupil'), the most important to exclude being retinoblastoma, a malignant embryonic retinal tumour that occurs in 1 in 20 000 live births. About one-third of the tumours are bilateral, the majority of these cases presenting in children under the age of 3. Some children may have a family history, but in others the tumour may arise as a new abnormality. Other causes of a white pupil include cataract, and retinal problems.

Findings that should prompt referral

- Microphthalmos
- Coloboma of iris
- Buphthalmos
- Corneal abnormality
- Abnormal or absent red reflex
- Failure to see, not smiling at parents by 6–8 weeks of life
- Nystagmus
- Leukocoria or white pupil
- Ptosis
- Enlarging capillary haemangioma involving the lids.

Examination of a child of any age with a suspected eye problem

The history defines the area of concern and while the examination will concentrate upon this area, an assessment of vision should be attempted in every case. Vision testing should be done using an age appropriate test remembering that vision develops throughout infancy and does not achieve normal levels until about the age of 2 years (see Table 23.1).

Table 23.1 Expected visual function and appropriate testing methods

Age	Expected normal acuity			Assessment
	Snellen	LogMAR	USA	
Newborn 2/12	6/240 6/90	1.6 1.18	20/800 20/300	Turns head in response to light. Closes eyes in objection to sudden bright light. Can hold gaze. Corneal reflections symmetrical. May exhibit intermittent convergent squint
3/12	6/24	0.6	20/80	Visually directed reaching begins. Changes fixation from one stimulus to another. Will follow a target across the midline. Continues to look 'squinty' at times
3/12–6/12 12/12	6/18 6/12	0.48 0.3	20/60 20/40	Will examine hands and objects closely. Blinks to threat. Preferential looking or Cardiff cards. Fixation behaviour. Steadiness and maintenance of alignment, corneal reflections
18/12 24/12	6/9 6/9–6/7.5	0.18 0.18–0.1	20/30 20/30–20/25	As above, plus recognition cards such as Kay pictures
30/12	6/6	0.0	20/20	Kay pictures. Matching tests, such as Sheridan Gardiner singles. Crowded tests
36/12—5 years	6/6+	0.0	20/20	Sonksen-Silver. Crowded Kays, Snellen, LogMAR

When testing vision start out testing both eyes together to give the child confidence in doing the test. This will give you the vision in the better eye. Then check the eye you suspect from your initial exam may have the worse vision. The effect of putting a hand over one eye may be helpful as it will give you an idea whether the child has an amblyopic eye, and gets upset or vigorously resists the good eye being covered. Occlusive patches are useful to ensure accurate vision testing without the risk of the child peeping around a hand or tissue. In some instances you may want to put a patch over the eye with suspected lower vision first, in order to gain confidence, doing only a brief test so as not to exhaust interest before you move the patch across to the other side.

Use a bright torch to examine the external eye and pupils. If a squint is suspected examine the ocular movements and perform cover tests to look for manifest or latent deviations. Check eye movements by getting the child to follow either the torch or a moving toy, keeping the head still. Dolls head rotations can be used by rapidly rotating the head to one side, initiating deviation laterally to the opposite side. If you are unsure if abduction is full, cover up the other eye and retest. Incomitant eye movement can be seen in children who have had previous squint surgery, those with squint syndromes such as Brown's and Duane's syndromes and in cranial nerve palsies, or as an outcome of congenital asymmetry of ocular muscle balance.

Check the red reflex and the fundus. This is best undertaken in dim light. Get the child to look straight ahead and fix upon a target while you look into the eye. Set the dial for zero if you have no refractive error or set to compensate for one if you remove your glasses. The disc should be demarcated with a pink neural rim and a paler magnolia coloured cup, which is usually half or less of the disc diameter. The retina of the young child may have a moist appearance. There should be a ring reflection around the macular area.

In hospital a child is often dilated in order to get a good look at the media and the fundus. It should be remembered that although rare, development of a squint or poor vision can be caused by a retinoblastoma, or other structural anomaly.

Possible red/green colour blindness can be tested using the Ishihara test. This most common form defect of colour vision occurs in 8% of boys and 0.5% of girls.

If there is concern about a possible squint, start by examining the corneal reflexes. Sit at eye level in front of the child and shine a pen torch at the pupils. The reflections will appear symmetrical and central if the eyes are aligned. If there is a convergent deviation the reflection will be temporal in the deviating eye. In divergent strabismus the corneal reflection will be displaced nasally and similarly with vertical deviations the reflection will be above or below the pupillary centre. This will exclude a pseudosquint due to epicanthus where the wide nose bridge obscures nasal sclera and the eyes look squinty but are correctly aligned with centred light reflexes. Then perform cover/uncover and alternate cover tests.

The cover/uncover test is best performed with a round edged opaque occluder and a fixation target. With an infant use a light or interesting, brightly coloured, squeaky toys. Cover the suspected squinting eye first and observe any movement of the fellow eye. If there is no deviation and central fixation, the eye will remain still, fixating on the target. This eye is now covered and the same observation made. No movement means the eyes are straight, unless the eye has extremely poor vision and cannot take up fixation.

Eye deviations are therefore categorized as follows:

- an outward movement of the uncovered eye to take up fixation denotes a manifest esotropia or convergent squint
- an inward movement denotes a manifest exotropia or divergent squint
- a downward movement indicates a hypertropia of that eye
- an upward movement indicates a hypotropia of that eye.

The alternate cover test dissociates the eyes to look for the presence of a phoria or latent squint, which is only revealed when the fusion of the two images is disrupted. It is carried out by alternating the occluder from one eye to the other. The eye under the occluder drifts out of alignment but is seen to recover when dissociation ceases. As with manifest deviations, the direction of recovery is opposite to that of the latent misalignment.

Abnormalities that need referral

- Reduced vision in children over 5 years initially refer to optician, under 5 refer to hospital services
- Suspected papilloedema or other fundal abnormality

- Squint or abnormal ocular movements at any age
- Double vision, as a priority.

Errors of refraction

In an eye with no refractive error (emmetropia) light rays will be focused on the retina. If the light rays are focused behind the eye, because it is shorter than normal, it is hyperopic or long sighted, and if the light rays are focused in front of the eye because the eye ball is longer than normal, it is myopic or short sighted.

Most infants and very small children are hyperopic and focus light rays by accommodation (changing the shape of the crystalline lens in the eye to make it more convex) so low hyperopic refractive errors rarely require correction. The eyeball lengthens with age or emmetropises allowing the child to focus on a near object, without the need for accommodation or spectacles. Hyperopia is corrected with convex or positive lenses.

Myopia is usually caused by the eyeball being longer than normal but can be found with abnormalities of the lens. Myopes are usually able to read without difficulty but distance acuity will be reduced. Myopia is corrected with concave or negative lenses.

Astigmatism is present when the cornea is curved more in one direction than another and is corrected with cylindrical lenses. Both near and distance acuity may be reduced.

Anisometropia is present when there is a difference in refractive error between the two eyes of more than one dioptre. The eye with the less crisp image may become amblyopic.

Very small children and infants are not able to complain about poor sight and do not know what 'normal' vision should be and for this reason may present late with visual failure. School age children will complain of difficulty seeing at school or be noticed to screw up their eyes (often described as squinting) when watching television. In general the need for glasses does not cause headache.

In the older child vision can be checked on a Snellen or LogMAR chart and then retested using a pin hole (simply made by pushing a hole in a card or sheet of paper with a ball point pen). Using the Snellen chart the visual acuity is recorded as a fraction: (the distance at which the letter is read)/(distance at which the letter should normally be read). If the pinhole test improves the vision the child should be referred to an optometrist for the provision of glasses. It is more difficult to test younger children accurately and they also run the risk of developing amblyopia with an uncorrected refractive error so they should be referred either to a vision clinic or to the hospital eye service. In small children refraction requires that the pupils be dilated to relax the accommodation. This is usually with cyclopentolate but in dark eyed children atropine may be used. Older children can be tested without cycloplegia.

Glasses should be worn all the time except for sport or activities where they may get damaged. Prescription goggles can be obtained for swimming.

Squints

Squint and amblyopia are common in childhood with about 2% of children having a squint, and up to 5% an amblyopic or lazy eye. A squint or strabismus is present when the visual axes of the two eyes are not aligned and bifoveal fixation does not occur. The effects of a squint can be to produce amblyopia and subnormal or absent binocular function. The commonest causes of amblyopia are squint, and refractive error but it can also be caused by visual deprivation from a media opacity or ptosis. Treatment for amblyopia is worthwhile, because poor vision in one eye may later debar the child from certain jobs because they fail vision standards (in particular they may not be able to hold a Class II professional driving licence) (Adams and Karas 1999). Potential for stereoscopic vision may be lost. There is also the risk of future visual handicap because of damage or disease to the good eye (Rahi *et al.* 2002). Treatment of moderate levels of amblyopia with glasses and occlusion has been shown by a recent trial with children aged 3–5 years, to be positively beneficial (Clarke *et al.* 2003), but those with mild visual loss (6/12–6/9) show little benefit from therapy. Delay in starting treatment until the age of 5 years does not appear to influence final visual outcome if reduced acuity is not worse than 6/18. Glasses alone do not improve vision; occlusion is the added important influence.

Children at risk of developing strabismus are those who have been treated for ROP or who have had stage 3 ROP, those with cerebral palsy or craniofacial disease, or those who have a family history of squint, amblyopia or high hyperopia.

Many children have neonatal malalignments, where their eyes turn usually inward, and these are commonest at the age of 7 weeks of life and disappear by 15 weeks of life (Pediatric Disease Investigator Group 2002a). These episodes of apparent convergent squint represent early flexing of the relationship between focusing and converging the eyes and are thought to be beneficial in setting up appropriate links for future development (Horwood 2003). This should be distinguished from infantile esotropia, which is a large angle, usually alternating convergent squint developing within the first 6 months of life in a normal child (Pediatric Disease Investigator Group 2002b). Large exotropia in young children is uncommon and may be a sign of neurological or ophthalmic disease. If there is a constant unilateral strabismus, amblyopia is likely to develop.

Treatment

The aims of managing any child with squint are to provide the best vision in each eye, to align the eyes, to correct any abnormal head posture and if possible to obtain binocular function (Royal College of Ophthalmologists 2000). Treatment may have to be continued until the age of visual maturity and usually involves appropriate glasses and treatment for any amblyopia. Occlusion of the better eye or atropine penalization, which dilates and blurs the vision in the better eye, encourage improved sight in the weaker eye (Pediatric Eye Disease Investigator Group 2002c). Although the number of children needing squint surgery is declining, those that need it are benefiting from intervention when younger, which gives the optimal potential for the development of 3-D vision and long-term ocular alignment (Birch *et al* 2000; Birch 2003).

What should be referred

- Divergent squint in a young child
- Large convergent squint after 10 weeks of age

- Any squint after 15 weeks of age
- Double vision
- Restricted eye movements
- Reduced vision in one or both eyes with no refractive cause, or not improved with glasses after these have been worn for 2 months.

Sticky eyes

In children watery, sticky eyes are common. The cause will vary with the age of the child.

Neonatal conjunctivitis

Conjunctivitis within the first month of life is called neonatal conjunctivitis and its potential to cause blindness should not be forgotten; in the nineteenth century ophthalmia neonatorum due to gonoccocal infection was the main cause of childhood blindness. Because of the risks of neonatal infection prophylactic eye treatment with silver nitrate solution or topical tetracycline are used in some countries but not the UK. An infant may acquire an eye infection during delivery (if the mother has a vaginal infection or it is born in an unhygienic environment) or from caregivers after birth.

The commonest identifiable infectious cause is *Chlamydia trachomatis* (Preece *et al.* 1989) with other causative organisms including *Staphylococcus aureus*, *Streptococcus viridans*, enterococci, and *Neisseria gonorrhoeae*. *Gonococcal conjunctivitis* is rare but can be devastating, rapidly resulting in corneal perforation and blindness. Herpetic keratoconjunctivitis can be passed to a baby born to a mother with genital herpes infection.

The infant presents with injected conjunctivae, lid swelling and a conjunctival discharge. Although the causative organism cannot be accurately diagnosed from the clinical presentation gonoccocal conjunctivitis tends to be more severe with an earlier onset than chlamydial infection, which has a creamy white discharge and a velvety appearance to the conjunctiva. Staph infection tends to have a yellow discharge.

Appropriate swabs should be taken. The conjunctiva is friable and may bleed after swabbing so the parents should be warned about this so as not to feel that intervention has worsened the baby's condition.

In practical terms an infant with mild to moderate neonatal conjunctivitis without a history of maternal vaginal infection can be treated with lid hygiene and topical antibiotics. If chlamydia infection is suspected or there is a history of maternal vaginal discharge systemic therapy is required as topical therapy alone is insufficient to clear chlamydia infection from the eye (Heggie *et al.* 1985). Treatment with erythromycin for 14 days should be used and the mother and her partner should be investigated and appropriately treated (Sandstrom 1987).

Dacryocystitis (acute infection of the lachrimal sac) in the infant is due to a developmental obstruction in the nasolacrimal system and there is swelling of the lacrimal sac at the medial corner of the eye with a mucopurulent discharge. Treatment is with sac massage to reflux mucopus into the eye from which it can then be cleared. Topical antibiotics may be required initially if the eye is injected.

Persistent discharge after a course of treatment suggests a blocked nasolacrimal duct.

Blocked nasolacrimal duct

Congenital blockage of the nasolacrimal duct is common and is usually caused by a membranous obstruction at the lower end of the lacrimal system. It affects between 5 and 20% of newborn infants but will resolve spontaneously in 95% of cases within the first year of life. The obstruction results in a watery, sticky eye with regurgitation of mucopurulent material with pressure over the ipsilateral lacrimal sac. The eye is usually white and the cornea clear. Occasionally a mucocoele of the lacrimal sac can develop. Because of the high rate of spontaneous cure expectant treatment should be employed until after the child is 1 year of age. The treatment is with massage of the lacrimal sac before every feed to discharge the stagnant material. Vaseline applied to the skin of the lower lid will stop any matter sticking to the skin and make cleaning easier. Topical antibiotics are usually only required if the eye becomes injected, which is rare with regular nasolacrimal massage. If still symptomatic at 1 year the standard treatment is syringing and probing under general anaesthesia. More than 90% of children will be cured by one probing if they have a simple membranous lacrimal obstruction (MacEwen *et al.* 2001). Probing will fail if there is a bony obstruction of the nasolacrimal system or stenosis of the lacrimal canaliculi, in these cases dacryocystorhinostomy may be required.

If the cornea is not clear, consider buphthalmos and corneal or conjunctival disorders such as staphylococcal keratoconjunctivitis, dendritic ulcers, and foreign bodies.

Conjunctivitis in pre-school and school age children

Sticky eyes, often associated with upper respiratory infections, are very common in children, with over half of all treatments for bacterial conjunctivitis occurring in the 0–9-year-old age group (Lichtenstein *et al.* 2003). The child may have an associated upper respiratory tract or ear infection. The bulbar and palpebral conjunctiva will be erythematous, but rarely haemorrhagic with a conjunctival discharge. The infection is normally bilateral. The vision is unaffected (except by discharge filming over the cornea) and the pupils react normally. Treatment is with topical antibiotics and lid cleaning to remove any discharge matted into the eyelids. In the UK the single commonest ocular antibiotic prescribed is chloramphenicol, usually used as one drop four times a day for a week. In North America topical chloramphenicol is not as commonly used because of the fear of causing aplastic anaemia, a risk that appears to be insignificant with a reported 0.36 cases per 1 million weeks of treatment (Isenberg 2003). Alternatives are topical ofloxacin four times a day or fucidic acid ointment twice a day. If the eye is particularly sticky, it is helpful to instil one drop of topical antibiotic every 1–2 hours for the first 2 days, and then four times a day for the following 3 days, in a 5-day treatment regimen, combined with warm lid soaks to remove encrusted matter.

In very young children nasal blockage may play a significant part in recurrently watery and infected eyes and nasal Otrivine is often helpful to reduce nasal blockage and improve lacrimal drainage.

Adenovirus conjunctivitis can start as unilateral disease. There may be significant peri-orbital swelling. There may be haemorrhagic change in the conjunctiva or even membrane formation in the lower lids. Pre-auricular lymph node enlargement and systemic malaise are often present. There is no topical antiviral to combat adenovirus, but a topical antibiotic may be useful to prevent secondary bacterial infection. Very rarely topical steroids are required if the cornea becomes involved with reduction in vision. Adenovirus is highly contagious, and the parent or caregiver should be warned about the risks of cross-contamination and the need for scrupulous hygiene measures to prevent transmitting it to other members of the family, or to those in contact with the child.

Allergic eye disease

Allergic conjunctivitis presents with bilateral watery itchy eyes, and there may be oedema of the conjunctiva (chemosis) with a mucoid discharge, or strings of mucus may be seen in the lower fornix. The child may be a known atope or have been exposed to an irritant such as pollen or dust. Treatment of the acute event is with a short course of topical Otrivine and systemic antihistamine if severe. In children with recurrent or persistent disease treatment with topical Opticrom or Opantanol may be helpful. Some children with severe allergic disease, and corneal involvement may need topical steroid therapy but this should only be under ophthalmic supervision.

What should be referred

- Neonatal conjunctivitis with maternal infection or significant discharge
- Persistent or recurrent infections or epiphora
- Allergic conjunctivitis not responding to Opticrom
- Conjunctivitis with reduced vision.

The acute red eye in children

Most of the causes of a red eye are common to all age groups with a few exceptions such as acute glaucoma, which is an age-related condition and does not occur in otherwise normal children. In children the commonest cause is probably bacterial or viral conjunctivitis.

Subconjunctival haemorrhage

Subconjunctival haemorrhage produces a bright red eye, with no effect on vision. It is likely to occur in children following trauma, and may also be seen in children with leukaemia. It requires no treatment and will resolve spontaneously.

Lid margin disease

Staphylcoccal lid margin disease with conjunctival and corneal involvement can produce a red and photophobic eye. The child presents with an injected eye with crusty erythematous lids. There may be associated styes or meibomian cysts. Initially, treatment should be with lid cleaning followed with topical antibacterial ointment massaged into the lid margin.

Persistent problems will need long-term low-dose systemic antibiotic usually with erythromycin and lid cleaning.

Foreign body

Foreign bodies may get into the eye and be trapped underneath the upper lid as a sub-tarsal foreign body, adhere to the conjunctiva or cornea, or be loose in the lower fornix. The eye should be examined with a torch and the lower lid pulled down. In the older child a foreign body may be removed, after the instillation of topical anaesthetic, with a cotton wool swab or the edge of a needle. In younger children a general anaesthetic for removal of even the most simple foreign body may be required, as it is dangerous to attempt to remove a foreign body in a child who cannot remain still. If the foreign body is underneath the lid there may be linear abrasions of the cornea demonstrable after the instillation of fluorescein. A subtarsal foreign body can be removed in the cooperative child after everting the lid by sweeping a swab stick along the lid. In a very small child it may be possible to wrap the child in a blanket evert the lid and wipe off the foreign body. If in doubt a general anaesthetic will be required to examine the eye. After removal topical antibiotic is usually required and if there were corneal abrasions a pad is helpful.

Corneal abrasion

An abrasion is caused when the corneal epithelium sloughs off, resulting in an extremely painful, red, watery photophobic eye. It may be diagnosed by instilling fluorescein. It is treated with topical antibiotic ointment, topical cycloplegic to relieve iris spasm and a pad. The pad should remain in place for approximately 24 hours. After the pad is removed topical treatment with antibiotic may be needed for a number of days for comfort and to reduce the risk of infection.

Dendritic ulcer

Herpes simplex type 1 infection of the cornea causes a dendritic ulcer and is treated with Zovirax topically five times a day. Recurrences are common. In a small number of cases there is corneal scarring due to herpetic keratitis. Primary herpes infection may also cause a conjunctivitis with a vesicular skin rash around the lids.

Trauma

Blunt trauma to the eye may cause a hyphaema with blood in the anterior chamber, or even an orbital blow-out fracture. In children, orbital blow-out fractures do not always cause a red eye but there are restricted eye movements due to ocular muscle trapping or herniation. Both of these findings require specialized eye examination and treatment.

Penetrating trauma can occur in all age groups and while an older child can give a history of the eye being hit by a sharp object very small children cannot describe what happened and may simply present with a red eye. The signs to be looked for include an irregular pupil or iris prolapse. The child should be referred immediately for ophthalmological care. Do not use a pad as this can put more pressure on the eye but if you can, use a plastic shield to protect it from further damage. Penetrating trauma in children, especially if the lens is damaged, is likely to lead to significant visual problems.

Lid margins can be cut or torn and this requires ophthalmological attention.

Contact lenses

Older children, or children who are aphakic, may wear contact lenses. If a child who wears a contact lens develops a sore red eye, the contact lens should be removed and spectacles worn. They may have an abrasion or a corneal infection. Fluorescein should be instilled after removal of the lens, as soft lenses will be stained by the dye. If the eye does not settle within 24 hours or the cornea is hazy, the child should be referred promptly for an ophthalmic opinion.

Iritis

Inflammation of the iris is called iritis. It is uncommon in children, and is probably most commonly seen in juvenile rheumatoid arthritis when the eye may be white and pain-free. Usually in iritis the child will complain of a red, watery, irritable eye. Vision may be reduced with ciliary hyperaemia, and a small pupil due to spasm of the iris sphincter muscle. There will be anterior chamber activity with flare and cells, and there may be keratic precipitates on the posterior surface of the cornea. Posterior synechiae, with adhesions between the iris and the lens, is a sign of chronic, untreated uveitis, and if seen in juvenile arthritis is a poor prognostic sign for the development of cataract. Treatment is with topical steroid or Acular and mydriatic drops.

What should be referred

+ Red eye with reduced vision
+ Non-healing abrasions
+ Cases of trauma
+ Contact lens-related problem either not settling after 24 hours or with corneal involvement
+ Foreign body that is not safe/possible to remove.

Orbital cellulitis

The orbit is the bony cavity that contains the eyeball and its muscles, nerves, and blood vessels. The orbital septum is the sheet of fascial tissue that is the framework for the eyelids, and is attached to the bones of the orbit, and medially passes behind the lacrimal sac. This sheet of palpebral fascia acts as a diaphragm for the orbital cavity and divides it into two spaces, pre- and retro-orbital. Infection anterior to the septum is described as pre-septal cellulitis while infection posterior to the septum is called orbital cellulitis. Pre-septal cellulitis is much more common than orbital cellulitis.

Orbital cellulitis

Infection posterior to the orbital septum has the potential to cause blindness, meningitis, cavernous sinus thrombosis, and brain abscess. Up to 85% of cases are associated with sinusitis, particularly of the ethmoid sinus. Other routes of infection are orbital trauma and bacteraemia from dacryocystitis, ear and upper respiratory tract infections. *Haemophilus influenzae* used to be the commonest pathogen in orbital and pre-septal disease, but has reduced significantly since the introduction of the Hib vaccination in the late 1980s (Ambati *et al.* 2000).

A child with orbital cellulitis is likely to be unwell and febrile with lid oedema, chemosis and proptosis, or limitation of eye movements. In addition there may be reduced vision, an afferent pupil defect, reduced colour vision, or papilloedema. In practical terms if there is either proptosis or ophthalmoplegia orbital infection should be assumed. The child should be admitted, blood cultures and swabs of any ocular discharge taken, and intravenous antibiotics started. A computed tomography scan may be helpful, especially if the clinical situation does not improve rapidly on antibiotic therapy. The commonest pathogenic organisms, assuming the child has been Hib vaccinated are *Staph. aureus* and *Strep. pneumoniae*; appropriate intravenous antibiotic therapy should be started. An appropriate regimen based on the most likely pathogens is a third generation cephalosporin, flucloxacillin, and metronidazole (Fergusson and McNab 1999). An ENT opinion should be requested if the child is not improving, as surgical drainage of infected sinuses or orbital abscess may be required. If there is any suggestion of a retained foreign body in the orbit, surgical exploration will be required. Other reasons for a child not improving on treatment for what is thought to be orbital cellulitis include rhabdomyosarcoma or an orbital secondary from a neuroblastoma. Rhabdomyosarcoma is the commonest orbital malignancy in childhood, and usually presents before the age of 7 years with rapid proptosis.

Pre-septal cellulitis

Pre-septal cellulitis is infection anterior to the orbital septum, and confined to the lids and peri-orbital structures. It usually follows lid trauma or a lid infection but may be associated with an upper respiratory tract infection. The vision is normal, the lids are swollen with normal ocular movements, no proptosis and no chemosis. If the child is well, afebrile with a white eye, full ocular movements and no proptosis, the child has presumed pre-septal cellulites. Broad-spectrum oral antibiotics should be started and the child reviewed in 48 hours. If at that point the child is no better, or unwell, they should be admitted and treated as for orbital cellulitis.

What should be referred

- Suspected orbital cellulitis.
- Pre-septal cellulitis not settling after 24 hours oral antibiotic treatment.

References

Adams GGW, Karas MP (1999). Effects of amblyopia on employment prospects. *British Journal of Ophthalmology* 83(3): 380.

Ambati BK, Ambati J, Azar N, Strappon L, Schmidt EV (2000). Periorbital and orbital cellulitis before and after the advent of haemophilus influenzae type B vaccination. *Ophthalmology* 107: 1450–1453.

Birch EE (2003). Binocular sensory outcomes in accommodative ET. *Journal of AAPOS* 7: 369–373.

Birch EE, Fawcett S, Stager DR (2000). Why does early surgical alignment improve stereo acuity outcomes in infantile esotropia? *Journal of AAPOS* 10: 410–414.

Clarke MP, Wright CM, Hrisos S, Anderson JD, Henderson J, Richardson SR (2003). Randomised control trial of treatment of unilateral visual impairment detected at pre-school vision screening. *British Medical Journal* 327: 1251–4..

Fergusson MP, McNab AA (1999). Current treatment and outcome in orbital cellulitis. *Australian and New Zealand Journal of Ophthalmology* 27: 375–379.

Hall D, Elliman D (2003). *Health for all Children*. Oxford University Press, London. Chapter 18.

Heggie AD, Jaffe AC, Stuart LA, Thombre PS, Sorensen RU (1985). Topical sulfacetamide vs oral erythromycin for neonatal chlamydial conjunctivitis. *American Journal of Diseases of Children* 139: 564–56.

Horwood A (2003). Neonatal ocular misalignments reflect vergence development but rarely become esotropia. *British J Ophthalmology* 87(9): 1146–1150.

Isenberg SJ (2003). The fall and rise of Chloramphenicol. *Journal of AAPOS* 7: 307–308.

Lichtenstein SJ, Rinehart MD, the Levofloxacin Bacterial Conjunctivitis Study Group (2003). Efficacy and safety of 0.5% Levofloxacin ophthalmic solution for the treatment of bacterial conjunctivitis in pediatric patients. *Journal of AAPOS* 7: 317–324.

MacEwen CJ, Young JDH, Barras CW, Ram B, White PS (2001). Value of nasal endoscopy and probing in the diagnosis and management of children with congenital epiphora. *British Journal of Ophthalmology* 85: 314–318.

Pediatric Eye Disease Investigator Group (2002a). Spontaneous resolution of early-onset esotropia: experience of the Congenital Esotropia Observational Study. *American Journal of Ophthalmology* 133: 109–118.

Pediatric Eye Disease Investigator Group (2002b). The clinical spectrum of early-onset esotropia: experience of the Congenital Esotropia Observational Study. *American Journal of Ophthalmology* 133: 102–108.

Pediatric Eye Disease Investigator Group (2002c). A randomised trial of Atropine versus patching for the treatment of moderate amblyopia in children. *Archives of Ophthalmology* 120: 268–278.

Preece PM, Anderson JM, Thompson RJ (1989). Chlamydia trachomatis infection in infants; a prospect of study. *Archives of Diseases in Childhood* 64: 525–529.

Rahi JS, Dezateux C (1999). National cross sectional study of detection of congenital and infantile cataract in the United Kingdom; Role of childhood screening and surveillance. *British Medical Journal* 318: 362–365.

Rahi JS, Logan S, Timms C, Russell-Eggitt I, Taylor D (2002). Risk, causes and outcomes of visual impairment after loss of vision in the non-amblyopic eye: a population-based study. *Lancet* 360: 597–602.

Royal College of Ophthalmologists (2000). *Guidelines for the Management of Strabismus and Amblyopia in Children*. London.

Royal College of Ophthalmologists and British Association of Perinatal Medicine (1996). Report of a Joint Working Party. Retinopathy of prematurity: guidelines for screening and treatment. *Early Human Develoment* 46: 239–258.

Sandstrom I (1987). Treatment of neonatal conjunctivitis. *Archives of Ophthalmology* 105: 925–928.

Wiesel TN (1982). Postnatal development of the visual cortex and the influence of environment. *Nature* 299: 583–591.

Chapter 24

Autism for primary care

Paul Gringras

Introduction

> Children with early infantile autism were the offspring of highly organized, professional parents, cold and rational, who just happened to defrost long enough to produce a child
>
> Kanner Time, 25 July 1960

Over the last 30 years there has been an explosion of research into the aetiology, prevalence, and treatment of autism. Increasing public interest and awareness over the last 10 years brings new challenges. With very little effort anyone can access hundreds and thousands of internet sites on autism. Many sites describe anecdotal case reports or non-peer-reviewed articles and parents often look to professionals to help them separate the wheat from the chaff.

We have left behind damaging hypotheses from the fifties that suggested autism arose as a consequence of abnormal parenting, but despite recognizing a major genetic contribution, the causes of autism still remain poorly understood. Autistic spectrum disorders (ASD) affect at least 1 in 100 children (Baird *et al* 2006), and local services are struggling under the pressure of continuing new referrals. Well-established multidisciplinary secondary and tertiary assessment centres are unequally distributed throughout the UK and at present see only the tip of the iceberg and have long waiting lists. Given the benefits of early identification and early intervention, primary care services can play a vital role in recognizing children at risk, and initiating nationally agreed referral pathways to specialist services as required.

In an effort to avoid a review that simply covers the 'science of autism' this chapter enrols the help of two groups of people to help also tell the real story. The extracts/quotes are about children with autism (or from their parents) that have been seen across two national referral units over the last 7 years. Their questions are often taxing, incisive, and with a welcome ability to leave politics and formal diagnostic definitions behind. The chapter also draws on support from some of the gifted writers, who themselves have ASD, and write so eloquently about their lives, opinions and experiences. (See addendum for recommended reading.)

Diagnosis

> I knew something was wrong four years ago. Why didn't anyone tell me it was autism?

The first area where families may experience difficulty is in obtaining both a correct and timely diagnosis with about 40% of all children with autism waiting more than 3 years for a clear diagnosis (Howlin and Asgharian 1999).

Over the last 5 years DSM-IV (APA 1994) and ICD-10 (WHO 1993) have produced diagnostic criteria for autism that are almost identical (WHO 1993). To meet criteria for autism individuals must show abnormalities in each of the three categories (social reciprocity, communication, and restricted behaviours and interests) and fulfil a total of six or more criteria. This seemingly simple operational definition is difficult to apply in reality. There is no single behaviour deviant for all individuals with autism and there is variation in behaviour across individuals and over time. Furthermore we still have no 'gold standard' biological marker.

Developmental domains of impairment

people just assume that because he flaps his hands and doesn't talk much he must be stupid.

Although two children may share the same diagnostic label, they will each be unique, with the label acting as no more than a clue to understanding their range of abilities and difficulties.

A useful concept in autism is to remember there are a range of domains that all need consideration and each may be impaired to different degrees.

This has been termed the 'graphic equalizer model' and quoted by both professionals and mentioned in Luke Jackson's wonderful book *Freeks, Geeks and Asperger's Syndrome*.

The first three bars of this model come from the fundamental concept of a triad of impairments commonly seen in all individual with ASD (Waterhouse *et al* 1996).

Social abilities

There is a typical impairment in the ability to engage in reciprocal social interactions. The range is, however, wide with the most severely affected individuals seeming aloof

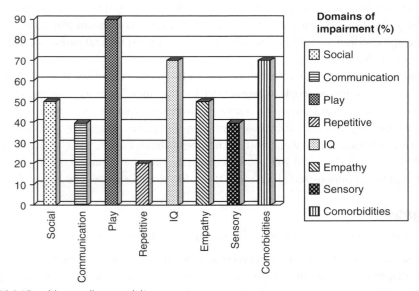

Fig. 24.1 'Graphic equalizer model'.

and uninterested in people, while others desire contact but seem unsure as to how to go about it. Social interactions may be gauche, awkward, and one-sided.

> One 9-year-old highly intelligent girl with autism keen on dancing would initiate interactions with peers by spontaneously performing a complex dance in front of them. She completely lacked any concept of personal space, often dancing within a few inches of their body, and failing to monitor their expressions or responses—usually to walk away.

Communication abilities

Here again linguistic skills range from those children who are unable to speak to those who learn language at a precocious age and use complex, grammatically correct, if often pedantic, speech. In more able children with superficially good language skills, understanding of concepts such as proverbs, or metaphors can be surprisingly literal. Nonverbal communication is also often impaired and this may be an early marker for ASD. Poor use of pointing to share interests, reduced eye contact with a paucity of gestures, and a decreased variety of facial expression are common. Joint attention behaviours are attempts to monitor or direct the attention of another person. They include gaze monitoring, pointing, and showing. These behaviours are normally present by age 9–14 months but are rare or absent in autistic children

> A child referred with a suspected expressive language delay was noted to have very poor non-verbal skills and poor social interaction. Formal language testing revealed she actually had a normal expressive and receptive language abilities. What was missing was her 'communicative intent', i.e. the desire to use language socially.

Imagination and pretend play

A history of limited or absent pretend or symbolic play is common. In its place are often extremely repetitive and seemingly non-functional play routines. The generation of new ideas can be difficult without structure. Some individuals with higher abilities develop an almost encyclopaedic knowledge of highly focused topics, that may well be of no interest to their peers.

> Some of these routines are not immediately obvious. One child appeared to enjoy playing well in the school playground on a range of activities. It was only by the end of his first term that teachers had realized that he would in fact always play of the same playground activities in the same order and in the same manner every day. Tantrums would ensue if he was interrupted in any way.
>
> Our efforts to divert one child's interest from burglar alarm circuits to computer games enjoyed by his peers were unfortunately unsuccessful.

Repetitive and stereotyped behaviours

Although people are familiar with the image of autistic children obsessively lining up toys, repeatedly spinning objects, or flapping their hands in the periphery of their vision, these behaviours do not differentiate children from autism from children with severe learning difficulties from a variety of causes.

> A wonderfully sociable child with Down syndrome was referred because of concerns about hand flapping and spinning behaviours but no 'core' features of autism.

Cognitive abilities

It is becoming more widely accepted that autism can occur at all levels of functioning with probably no more than 15% of individuals with autism having learning disability. However, in the severe learning difficulty group, as many as one in three children will have autism (Gillberg and Soderstrom 2003).

> A child with autism was referred with increasingly challenging behaviours at his school for children with severe learning difficulties. He was socially very cut off and teachers felt he was failing to make any academic progress on account of his severe learning difficulties. In fact on formal testing his verbal and non-verbal skills were in on the 90th percentile for his age. He was bored and inappropriately placed educationally—both learning and behaviours improved on moving him to a mainstream school with a base for children with autism.

Empathy

Although often conceptualized as part of a general difficulty in social understanding, lack of empathy can be a huge problem. Without an appreciation of a child's inability, or difficulty to moderate their behaviours as a result of another's response, any conventional behavioural advice may fail.

> One 7-year-child with autism was repeatedly hitting his younger sibling after returning from school. He also frequently pulled the dogs tail. Lengthy explanations about the distress it was causing his sister did not help. The suggestion that 'good behaviour would make mummy and daddy pleased' also produced no change. Neither did the statement that 'we shouldn't be cruel to animals'. The behaviours stopped when a visual timetable with the strict instruction that 'no hitting of younger sister (with photograph) or pulling the dogs tail (with photograph) was allowed in this house'. The reward identified for this particular child was more time to play with the family's old lawnmower, which he could dismantle and rebuild in a matter of minutes.

Unusual responses to sensory stimuli

Perhaps 'underrated' extreme sensitivity to noises, smells, textures, and visual stimuli are all well described. These can be seen across a wide range of children with ASD and can be particularly disabling.

> A particular child would scream, moan, and hunch under his desk—always in one or two lessons that took place in an upstairs classroom. It transpired that the content of the lessons were not the problem. He was in fact able to discern the hum of an aging fluorescent light and was incredibly sensitive to this particular noise. Changing the lighting strip solved the problem.

Comorbidities

Each one worthy of a separate domain, these are the commonly associated behavioural and neuropsychiatric conditions that can themselves cause as much or more problems than the autism itself. These are discussed in more detail later, but include attentional difficulties, depression, anxiety, tics, sleep disorders, aggressive, and self-injurious behaviours.

Early diagnosis and screening tools

> But he's now 12 years old. Couldn't you have diagnosed it earlier?

The benefits of early diagnosis have rightly been emphasized and the Checklist for Autism in Toddlers (CHAT) has served to emphasize key early aspects of social behaviour; lack of sensitivity and specificity makes this tool unlikely to be advocated widely for screening (Baron-Cohen *et al.* 1996). Despite attempts to develop 'checklist' aids to the identification of relevant behavioural profiles, there do not seem to be any shortcuts to accurate diagnosis and appropriate assessments can still take time and require experienced multidisciplinary teams (Lord and Risi 1998).

High functioning autism and Asperger syndrome

Why did one paediatrician say he's got high functioning autism but then another say it's definitely Asperger syndrome?

The cumulative hours that have been spent debating whether Asperger syndrome has a right to exist outside the autistic spectrum syndrome are enormous. According to current criteria early language and cognitive development is the principal divider. Whereas typical autistic individuals have delayed speech development (phrase speech after 36 months of age) and very unusual speech patterns, typical children with Asperger syndrome are said to have no clinically significant cognitive or language delay. Although they do demonstrate difficulties with prosody, pragmatic, and non-verbal aspects of communication they do not develop the more severe communication disorder seen in autism.

These discussions are either fascinating or pedantic depending what side of the fence you sit on. Some clinicians are 'splitters' who enjoy subgroups and increasing numbers of diagnostic categories and some are 'lumpers' who see it all as variations on a theme. Perhaps the splitters will do the best research particularly for genetic studies, but the lumpers will see more patients and do just as good a clinical job. Lorna Wing who first translated Asperger's original account beautifully puts the whole debate in context in *Past and Future of Research on Aspergers Syndrome*. She begins 'Since the publication of my paper on Asperger's work (in 1981) I have felt like Pandora after she opened the box.' (Wing 2000).

Studies of individuals with high-functioning autism and Asperger syndrome, find little evidence for a distinction between autism and Asperger syndrome. Even when cohorts are divided on criteria of early language development, follow-up studies showed found no difference in social outcomes or language abilities (Howlin 2003b). Despite IQ in the normal range (and, sometime, reaching quite high academic levels) sadly the majority of individuals in both groups had no close friends, remained highly dependent on families for support, and employment status was low.

There is little to support the view that individuals with Asperger syndrome require different education or management programmes. As the children get older, social demands and the need to deal with social situations independently increase significantly. These children need the tools to deal effectively with these situations to minimize isolation and victimization. It should be recognized that for all high-functioning individuals with an autistic spectrum disorder there is a need for much improved services throughout childhood and adulthood if the long-term outcome is to be significantly enhanced.

Epidemiology

There's definitely an epidemic of autism in our school. There needs to be a real enquiry into the food and stuff they give the kids.

Claims that autism was on the increase supported more recent robust epidemiological studies (Baird *et al* 2006). Recent apparent rises in prevalence of autism in some regions have been mirrored by decreases in the rate of children with learning disabilities. As there is no reason for this decrease, which has not been reported elsewhere it seems likely that some children that would have previously fallen into the learning disability ('mental retardation' in the USA) are now being diagnosed as having ASD. Whatever the exact numbers, autism as currently defined is more common than was previously realized and a number of possible explanations have been proposed (Fombonne 2003). Whether or not a proportion of this increase is 'real', the current prevalence data must be used to plan for the health, educational, and social needs of children with autism in the UK. Figures produced by the National Autistic Society estimated that at least 500 000 families in the UK are affected by autism.

Breaking the news

The importance of breaking the news well, to both parents if possible, and with recorded or written summaries cannot be overemphasized. In contrast to a number of lifelong disabilities, parents are constantly reminded how 'normal' their children look, and therefore how expectations of members of the public expect children to behave well with their parents. Anything less is automatically taken to be a failure of parental discipline and poor family values. In reality the excessive noise, number of strangers, and often long queues means that supermarkets, car parks, shopping malls could have been specifically designed to precipitate the most disruptive behaviour in any child with autism.

> she looked so beautiful, lovely blue eyes, such a good child—we couldn't believe anything was wrong

Siblings are affected and often forgotten. The attention, hospital visits, and special schools results in well-described combinations of jealousy, guilt, and resentment. The Early Years Service in Nottingham have produced a number of excellent publications, including one for siblings of children with autism or Asperger syndrome. As short and informative booklets they also have a useful role in helping grandparents and family members reluctant to accept the diagnosis.

Professionals are unfortunately faced with conflicting pressures when trying to reach early diagnoses of autism. On the one hand they are under constant pressure to reach a speedy accurate early diagnosis. However, accurate diagnosis is difficult before 2 years of age, with maximal accuracy being reached at about age 5. Furthermore, although early behavioural/educational intervention is a reasonable goal, lack of such provision in many areas means that parents can be left with a devastating potential diagnosis and little more. It is of little surprise that the rates of depression in parents of children with autism are so much higher than in parents of controls and children with physical disabilities.

> the doctor told me he had something called childhood autism when he was 2 and it was all a question of getting into the right school. Nothing then happened and no one gave us any information. In the end we learned everything from the internet and other parents we then met.

A number of programmes have been developed to try and fill his early and stressful gap, with the National Autistic Society Early Bird schemes being one notable example. This scheme aims to support parents in that difficult period between diagnosis and school placement. Parents also learn skills to help improve children's behaviours, hopefully at an early enough age to prevent the later development of more challenging behaviours.

In a number of cases the diagnosis of autism or Asperger syndrome is made so early that there is no discussion of breaking the news to the child him- or herself. As a 'lifelong' diagnosis this issue will, however, arise and deserves a book in itself. We have found that the news should be broken at the child's own pace, and every child is ready at a different stage.

Labelling is for jam-jars

A commonly voiced opinion is why bother with all these labels. Potential misdiagnosis, stigmatization and describing pathology in a normal spectrum are reasons given. Many who work in the field will have experienced the converse. Children are often victimized, misdiagnosed as oppositional or stupid, and fail to receive adequate support without the correct descriptive label. Luke Jackson, a gifted young man with Asperger syndrome writes on this topic:

> Doctors and professionals who can give a diagnosis, this is where not giving one causes a big problem … You may think that if the child or person you are seeing has lots of AS traits but you can't fit them neatly into your checklist of criteria, then you are doing them a favour by saying they haven't got it. In fact it doesn't make them not have AS. It just muddles them up and makes them and all around them think that they are even more 'freakish'.

Claire Sainsbury has Asperger syndrome, received a First in philosophy and politics from New College, Oxford and wrote in her book *The Martian in the Playground*:

> I think that I might be an alien who has been put on this planet by mistake; I hope that this is so because this means that there might be other people out there in the universe like me … In the next few years I would work out that the spaceship was never going to come and rescue me, but it wasn't until I was twenty that I finally found a name for my differences, when I was diagnosed with Asperger's syndrome … If the right people had only been given the right information, more than a decade ago my life might have gone very differently.

Assessment pathways

Parents often tell stories of changing professional diagnoses that remind one of the story about the four blind men describing an elephant differently based on the parts they happen to be feeling; depending on the therapist and assessment tool employed, a child with Asperger syndrome could receive a diagnosis of developmental co-ordination disorder, semantic pragmatic disorders, or non-verbal learning difficulties. Snapshot assessments conducted in unfamiliar environments, over short periods of time, often miss crucial clinical features. Hastily reached clinical impressions of intelligence and communication in this group of children are often shown to be inaccurate when checked by formal tests. However, formal tests alone can also be misleading, and informal observations in a school playground are invaluable to observe a child's real life social skills within an appropriate peer group.

> ...failure to be integrated in a social group is the most conspicuous feature...
>
> Leo Kanner (1943)

There is unfortunately still much regional, national, and international variation in assessment pathways and service availability for autism. In 2002 research commissioned by the National Autistic Society found that although 92% of GPs recognized having seen a patient with confirmed or suspected ASD in the last year, one in eight of them did not know how or where to refer such patients (http://www.nas.org.uk/content/1/c4/34/68/gps.pdf).

The National Autism Plan for Children (NAPC) was published under the banner of The National Autistic Society in collaboration with the Royal College of Paediatrics and Child Health and the Royal College of Psychiatrists. The aim to address identification, assessment, diagnosis, and access to early interventions for pre-school and primary school age children with ASD. It emphasizes the potential of existing child development surveillance programmes undertaken by primary care teams, including health visitors. Although there remains no ideal whole population screening test for autism, tools such as the CHAT will help to train all involved professionals in the 'alerting' signals of possible ASD both at pre-school and school age. Parents' concerns invariably precede professionals and concern about any developmental problems should trigger referral to a locally available child development service or equivalent. The NAPC proposes timely referrals for such assessments with delays audited. The next stage is then for a general multidisciplinary developmental assessment. Stage 2 is a multi-agency assessment, ideally with the teams' core members available locally and with feedback to the family given within 17 weeks from initial referral. Finally remains the possible need for referral to a tertiary ASD assessment. Such referrals may occur for complex cases requiring second opinions, diagnostic uncertainty, assessment of treatable comorbidities with advice and possible short-term interventions. Of particular relevance for primary care is the recommendations that in every local area there should be:

- an agreed written referral pathway for children with suspected ASD, both pre-school and school age, accessible to all professionals and parents: this may be the same as for all developmental problems
- a local ASD co-ordinating group for strategic planning of training and service needs/development in each local area with representation from all statutory and voluntary services together with users of the service.

Aetiology and medical investigations (Figures 24.2 and 24.3)

[T]hese children have come into the world with innate inability to form the usual biologically provided affective contact with people, just as other children come into the world with innate physical or intellectual handicaps

Kanner (1943)

Since the first reports describing autism there have been several attempts to find a common cause or biochemical markers among the many children that display symptoms

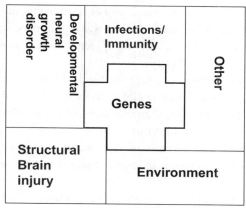

Fig. 24.2 Piecing together the autistic puzzle.

of autism. Accumulating research indicates that autism is a biological disorder that originates during brain development. The limited autopsy data show no evidence of lesions or scarring to indicate postnatal insult. Neuropathology suggests neurological immaturity and developmental failure due to abnormalities during the gestation period.

> surely you know what causes it now. We've got the whole genome after all and there are enough children with autism aren't there?

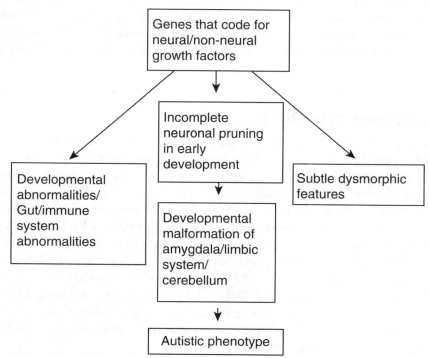

Fig. 24.3 A hypothetical pathway of causation from genotype to phenotype.

The race to find the most important genetic and environmental variables continues. The prominent role of genetic influences in autism was emphasized by twin studies where any excess of affected identical twin pairs compared with non-identical pairs is due to genetic factors, not environmental factors.

These have showed a heritability of over 90% for the liability of autism, more than for depression and schizophrenia (Bailey *et al.* 1995). Family studies that broaden the concept of autism to look for subtle language and social difficulties find that 20% of relative show similar but much milder symptoms of autism. What is without doubt is that in individual families a moderate number of genes act together to cause the phenotype. Unfortunately there is little evidence to suggest that the same group of genes act in all families.

At present chromosome and DNA anomalies are reported in approximately 5% of cases, the most common being fragile X followed by maternally inherited trisomy or tetrasomy of chromosome 15q11.2.

Recurrence risks

With this increasing awareness of the importance of genetic influences on autism, there is now a demand from families with an affected member for advice regarding their risk of having a further autistic child. The first stage must always be to exclude causes of autism due to known medical disorders, many of which have known inheritance patterns. After excluding fragile X, tuberous sclerosis, phenylketonuria, and variety of chromosomal anomalies many would use the term idiopathic autism; for this diagnosis an empirical recurrence rate in siblings of 5% has recently been quoted (Simonoff 1998).

Investigations (Table 24.1)

Knowing precisely which investigations are warranted remains unclear. The frequency with which known medical conditions are associated with autism ranges in the literature between 10 and 30% (Filipek *et al.* 1999). This question may end up needing to be answered by community-based studies that avoid the pitfalls of referral bias to specialist centres. There is dubious rationale in carrying out non-routine and invasive procedures in the absence of clinical indications and evidence of their utility. Chance associations, often seen in tertiary referral centres, do not prove causation and premature conclusions can and have impacted adversely on wider public health issues, particularly in the recent case of the MMR vaccination. Given the heterogeneity of the disorders origins a 'standard range of tests' for every child is likely to be unhelpful and may distract from the importance of a good clinical history and examination. Rationale for a few potential investigations are presented in Box 24.2. Formal recommendations are covered in a number of texts (Filipek *et al.* 1999).

Table 24.1 Sample of investigations for autism and their rationale

Investigation	Rationale
Chromosomes-karyotype	To exclude a range of aneuploides, translocations, deletions and rearrangements. Essential before genetic counselling
MRI scan	Particularly if neurocutaneous stigmata on Wood's light examination suggestive of tuberous sclerosis
EEG-Sleep deprived or 24-hour monitoring most valuable	If clinical features suggestive of seizure disorders or in cases of unusually marked regression with fluctuating course
Metabolic studies	Likely to be normal unless clinical features and specific suggestive history. Urine to exclude Sanfillippo syndrome may be helpful
Thyroid hormone	If learning difficulties
Polymerase chain reaction (PCR)/DNA tests	If clinical suspicions, e.g. Fragile X/Angelman/William's syndrome/22q11 deletion/Prader–Willi

Late onset autism and MMR

Are babies born with autism?

Clinically, some babies are 'autistic from birth', very difficult to manage, and won't even tolerate the early touch of parents. Changes in head circumference (at birth normal head circumferences have led to suggestions of abnormal regulation of early brain growth (Courchesne *et al.* 2003). By 1 year of age, experts looking at videos have been able to identify the majority children who would go on to have autism. Behaviours including not turning to name, not following pointing, and not showing objects of interest have helped to discriminate cases (Mars *et al.* 1998).

However, this is not always the picture, and it is the group of children who tragically lose language and social skills between 1½ and 2 years, that cause great concern and inevitably lead to a scrutiny of any environmental factors coincidentally occurring around the time of regression. Regression has always been described in a percentage of children presenting with autism. The actual proportion of children who present with regression has, in fact, remained astonishingly constant at about 30%. In one review on MMR, Regression and Autism, six papers dating back to 1966 are summarized and all show a rate of regression between 20% and 50% (Fombonne and Chakrabarti 2001). MMR immunization was not associated with a shift towards an earlier rate of first parental concerns, with 19 months being the average age of first concerns in a number of studies, both before and after the introduction of the MMR. While there may well be an increased rate of gastrointestinal problems in children with autism and Asperger syndrome, there is still a lack of robust or replicated evidence to support a distinct syndrome of MMR-induced autism or of MMR-induced autistic enterocolitis.

But I've already got two children with autism–where's the research for my situation

Despite the likelihood this all arose out of unfortunate timing of MMR administration, new concerns about the high total thiomersal (mercury) levels from certain vaccination programmes, has provoked additional concerns, such that the decisions for many parents remain difficult, with a potent brew of politics, psychology, and fear continually stirred by the media.

> banning the single vaccines didn't work did it? It was supposed to prevent a lack of confidence and keep vaccination rates up but it didn't

Therapeutic approaches

Educational and behavioural

Early educational approaches are still one of the few proven strategies for increasing the potential of children with ASD. Different methods are advocated with evangelical zeal that at times detracts from their usefulness. Thankfully robust studies and evidence-based approaches have begun to define a number of key factors common to many approaches. From a clinical perspective, the unsurprising observation that can be made about seemingly diametrically opposed approaches is that the good therapists all inspire families, help children, and seem to use similar skills. Approaches range form those using operant techniques and the shaping of behaviour through reinforcement, prompting, and fading procedures, and use of positive reinforcers that are functional to those that advocate joining in children's repetitious behaviours such that they actually become more engaged, more socially available, and more motivated to be with others. All interventions advocate starting early and with intensive input—often up to 40 hours per week being recommended for best results. In a quest for evidence-based interventions, and maximum cost-effectiveness where resources are scarce important questions still remain: How much is dependent of the training and skill of the individual therapist? How much time is really needed per week; how much can one deviate from the initial descriptions of a therapeutic intervention and still expect similar results (Howlin 2003a).

> They told us it would take a year to be seen by the team that will confirm the diagnosis. But he's already four and everything we read seems to say that you need to intervene early

The NAPC document proposes a co-ordinated programme of early intervention to be discussed with the family (National Initiative for Autism:Screening and Assessment Working Group 2003) With support from a key worker, within 6 weeks of the end of the multi-agency assessment. It also recommends 15 hours per week of appropriate ASD specific expertise. These may be school or home based and do not imply wither segregated ASD provision nor 1:1 working. While most areas would fail to provide even this level of care, advocates of early intervention would still insist more than 15 hours per week are necessary, and thus expensive educational tribunals are still occurring.

The situation becomes even more difficult by secondary school. The nirvana of inclusive education often fails in reality for this group of children. In her book Claire Sainsbury gives her views and the accounts of others with autism and Asperger syndrome at schools (Sainsbury 2000). Bullying seems a particular problem, as are frequent misunderstandings when instructions and rules are interpreted too literally. Low mood and anxiety arising from the pressures of unpredictable situations and large numbers of peers can result in aggressive behaviours that often seem to escalate quickly. A survey by the National Autistic Society showed children with autism and Asperger syndrome are on average 20 times more likely to be excluded from school than their peers. The situation was worse still for the more able children with autism where 29% have been excluded from school at one time or another.

Pharmacological approaches

Cures for core symptoms

> You better give him those secretin injections. They are the only thing that can cure it and you're supposed to be his doctor. I bet it's all about money?

New 'cures' for autism continue to emerge and range from those with potential to those that are merely wishful thinking. The concept that one drug could affect core symptoms in most children with autism is clearly appealing to both professionals and parents. It is, however, difficult to understand at a scientific level if the causes of autism are as multi-factorial as research has suggested. It is vital to realize that the existence of a plausible biological explanation does not mean it is right, or that it should guide treatment. It has always been easier for scientists to tell good stories, than to prove them. Naltrexone, fen-fluramine, and now secretin belong in the above category and share three important characteristics. First, each has caused excitement and hope that a cure for autism is on the way. Second each has occupied a pivotal role in elegant, although largely unproven, unifying biological hypotheses explaining the origins of autism. Third, although case reports and open trials have shown promise, randomized trials have not managed to demonstrate any impact on the core symptoms of autism. Randomized controlled trial of secretin injection have taught us more than simply that saline is more efficacious; they have reminded us that the placebo effect is present and considerable in ASD, should be exploited therapeutically, and means that no putative new therapies should be allowed to avoid the rigours of a robust randomized controlled trial.

Treating associated symptoms (Figure 24.4)

Although there is still no medication, which has been shown to 'cure' autism, the more conventional psychopharmacological approaches are valuable in treating many of the associated difficult behaviours that can affect everyday functioning in autism (Gringras 2000; Hollander et al. 2003) (Table 24.2).

Unfortunately having autism or Asperger syndrome does not protect against depression, attention deficit hyperactivity disorder, Tourette's syndrome, self-injury, sleep disorders, and challenging behaviours. All in fact are seen more commonly, and may respond to similar groups of psychotropic medications that play a valuable role in children without autism. Gradually the concept of treating comorbidities has evolved such that children with treatable neuropsychiatric disorders who also have autism, are not deprived trials of the appropriate medications. Methylphenidate for example may help hyperactive symptoms, without of course altering core social impairments (Quintana et al. 1995). Serotonin reuptake inhibitors appear efficacious in treating compulsions, stereotypies, and self-injury in some cases. Antipsychotic drugs, particularly

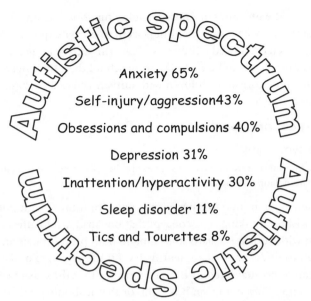

Anxiety 65%

Self-injury/aggression43%

Obsessions and compulsions 40%

Depression 31%

Inattention/hyperactivity 30%

Sleep disorder 11%

Tics and Tourettes 8%

Fig. 24.4 Important comorbidities in autism and Asperger syndrome. Modified from: Tsai LY (1996), Comorbid psychiatric disorder of autistic disorder. *Journal of Autism and Developmental Disorder* **26**: 159–163.

risperidone have a valuable role in reducing challenging behaviours whether they are aggression towards others or self-injury (McDougle *et al.* 1998; Zarcone *et al.* 2001). Sleep disorders are extremely common in children with ASD and a major source of family stress. The hormone melatonin seems likely to have has a valuable role in reducing sleep onset problems (Lord 1998).

Treatment needs to be provided in safe environments (Table 24.3). Although often initially prescribed by secondary and tertiary clinics, close liaison with schools and primary care services is essential, and careful follow-up or clearly defined systems of shared care essential (Gringras and McNicholas 1999).

Medication should not be considered in isolation, and finding the right school and optimizing behavioural management in all settings is crucial. Applied behavioural analysis and other education approaches have shown their efficacy in systematic evaluations and must always be considered early on in any proposed treatment.

Diet and vitamins

Gluten- and casein-free diets, high doses of vitamin supplements, and essential fatty acid supplementation, belong to the ever-growing range of internet publicized, potentially interesting, but non-evidence-based, therapeutic approaches. All have fervent supporters and case reports of successes abound. Clearly a lack of robust evidence does not equate to a lack of effect—it just indicates the need for larger, better designed controlled trials.

It has been suggested that megavitamin therapy may globally improve some individuals with autism, but again robust trials are lacking, although there is much enthusiasm

Table 24.2 'Tailor-made' approach to paediatric psychopharmacology in autism

Associated behaviour	Medication (in order of preference)	Specific notes (This table is intended only as summary of the associated review and not as a guide to treatment in isolation)
Hyperactivity	1. Methyphenidate	Best in high functioning/Asperger's syndrome. Increase in adverse effects if associated learning difficulties
	2. Clonidine	Useful if also tics. Watch for sedation
Ritualistic/compulsive behaviours	1. Fluoxetine	Watch for early increase in anxiety
	2. Other SSRI	Although not recommended by CSM for depression, still have a role to reduce obsessions and autistic stereotypies
Tics/Tourette's syndrome	1. Risperidone	Effective but worrying adverse effects
	2. Clonidine	Less effective but less worrying adverse effects
Self-Injury	1. Risperidone	Difficult to treat-always accompany with behavioural interventions
	2. Naltrexone	No evidence for effect
Sleep	1. Melatonin	Only after analysis of sleep pattern and attempt at behaviour modification
Aggressive behaviour	1. Risperidone	Effective but significant adverse effects, especially weight gain and matabolic concerns.
	2. SodiumValproate 3. Carbamazepine	If mood stabilization is also required, 'very little support from clinical trials'

Adapted from Gringras P (2000). Practical paediatric pharmocolgical prescribing in autism: the potential and the pitfalls. *Autism* 4(3): 229–248.

about their potential (Rimland and Edelson 1996). Pfeiffer *et al.* (1995) concluded that even though the majority of studies report a favourable response, their interpretation is hampered by methodological shortcomings (Pfeiffer *et al.* 1995). In a randomized controlled trial of high-dose magnesium and pyridoxine administration no benefit was demonstrated (Findling *et al.* 1997).

Gluten- and casein-free diets are one example of therapeutic approaches for autism that remain popular but with unproven effects (Various 2001). Trials have been small thus far and poorly controlled. Many case reports of improvement exist but there needs to be more research before such measures can either be recommended or advised against.

It is at times difficult to know what to advise when a child is taking a range of unproven and potentially harmful 'cures' from the internet or other sources. In keeping with the principle of concordance rather than compliance, clinicians play an important part in helping parents evaluate therapies. Those that are unproven need careful observation, and even those that are 'proven' will not be beneficial for every child. The previously mentioned placebo effect is valuable, and clinicians need to temper cynicism about wishful treatments, as this does not help families. As always the imperative remains to avoid harm to the child—many herbal remedies have the potential for serious interactions,

Table 24.3 Potential and pitfalls of medication in autism

No medication will treat core symptoms
Environmental manipulations, including behavioural treatment, may more effective
Idiosyncratic responses of children
Living arrangement must allow safe and consistent administration and monitoring
Long- and short-term side-effects
Lack of evidence for long-term benefits from robust clinical trials
The need for ongoing multidisciplinary work and continuing behaviour management
Licensing and informed consent issues
Unknown interactions
Decide goals in agreement with parent and child
Monitor beneficial and adverse effects
Inform parents, child, and school fully
Printed guidelines/protocols/information
Evaluate and share results with other professionals

dietary supplements in excess of physiological requirement can do harm, and restrictive diets can become a threat to adequate nutritional intake. We must never forget that 'conventional treatments' may have just as much potential to also cause harm as alternative treatments. Hopefully we will not be looking back on the current range of psychopharmacological medications with the same concern as when we look back on common practice in 1954 when 500 'autistic' children (127 under 7 years of age) were given ECT because:

> It is necessary to remove the child from the anxiety ridden home to the hospital

> > Bender (1954)

and use ECT

> to stimulate biological maturation, to pattern primitive embryonic plasticity, to mobilize anxiety in the apathetic autistic child.

> > Bender (1954)

References

Bailey AJ, Le Couter A, Gottesman I, Bolton P, Simonoff E, Rutter M (1995). Autism is a strongly genetic disorder. Evidence from a British twin study. *Psychological Medicine* 25: 6–16.

Baird G, Simonoff E, Pickles A, Chandler S, Loucas T, Meldrum D, Charman T (2006). Prevalence of disorders of the autism spectrum in a population cohort of children in South Thames: the Special Needs and Autism Project (SNAP). *Lancet* 368: 210–215.

Baron-Cohen S, Allen J, Gillberg C (1996). Can autism be detected at 18 months? The needle, the haystack and the CHAT. *British Journal of Psychiatry* 168: 839–843.

Bender L (1947). One hundred cases of childhood schizophrenia treated with electric shock. *Trans Am Neurol Soc* 72:165–169.

Courchesne E, Carper R, Akshoomoff N (2003). Evidence of brain overgrowth in the first year of life in autism. *JAMA* **290**(3): 337–344.

Diagnostic and Statistical Manual of Mental Disorders, Fourth Edition, Text Revision (2000). Washington, DC, American Psychiatric Association.

Filipek PA, Accardo PJ, Baranek GT (1999). The screening and diagnosis of autistic spectrum disorders. *Journal of Autism and Developmental Disorder* **29**: 437–482.

Findling RL, Maxwell K, Scotese-Wojtila L, Huang J, Yamashita T ,Wiznitzer M (1997). High-dose pyridoxine and magnesium administration in children with autistic disorder: an absence of salutary effects in a double-blind, placebo controlled study. *Journal of Autism and Developmental Disorder* **27**: 467–478.

Fombonne E (2003). Epidemiological surveys of autism and other pervasive developmental disorders: an update. *Journal of Autism and Developmental Disorder* **33**(4): 365–382.

Fombonne E, Chakrabarti S (2001). No evidence for a new variant of measles-mumps-rubella-induced autism. *Pediatrics* **108**(4): E58.

Gillberg C, Soderstrom H (2003). Learning disability. *Lancet* **362**: 811–821.

Gringras P (2000). Practical paediatric pharmocolgical prescribing in autism: the potential and the pitfalls. *Autism* **4**(3): 229–248.

Gringras P, McNicholas F (1999). Developing rational protocols for paediatric psychopharmacological prescribing. *Child: Care, Health and Development* **25**: 223–233.

Hollander E, Phillips AT, Yeh CC (2003). Targeted treatments for symptom domains in child and adolescent autism. *Lancet* **362**(9385): 732–734.

Howlin P (2003a). Can early interventions alter the course of autism? *Novartis Foundation Symposium* **251**: 250–259.

Howlin P (2003b). Outcome in high-functioning adults with autism with and without early language delays: implications for the differentiation between autism and Asperger syndrome. *Journal of Autism and Developmental Disorder* **33**: 3–13.

Howlin P, Asgharian A (1999). The diagnosis of autism and Asperger syndrome: findings from a survey of 770 families. *Developmental Medicine and Child Neurology* **41**(12): 834–839.

Kanner L (1960). The Child is Father *Time Magazine USA* Jul. 25: 111.

Kanner L (1943). Autistic Disturbances of Affective Contact. *Nervous Child* **2**: 17–50.

Lord C (1998). What is melatonin? Is it a useful treatment for sleep problems in autism? *Journal of Autism and Developmental Disorder* **28**(4): 346.

Lord C, Risi S (1998). Frameworks and methods in diagnosing autistic spectrum disorders. *Mental Retardation and Developmental Disabilities Research Reviews* **4**: 90–96.

Mars AE, Mauk JE, Dowrick P (1998). Symptoms of pervasive developmental disorders as observed in prediagnostic home videos of infants and toddlers. *Journal of Pediatrics* **132**: 500–504.

McDougle CJ, Holmes JP, Carlson DC, Pelton GH, Cohen DJ, Price LH (1998). A double-blind, placebo-controlled study of risperidone in adults with autistic disorder and other pervasive developmental disorders . *Archives of General Psychiatry* **55**(7): 633–641.

National Initiative for Autism: Screening and Assessment Working Group (2003). National Autism Plan for Children (NAPC)London: NAS Publications.

Pfeiffer SI, Norton J, Nelson L, Short S (1995). Efficacy of Vitamin B6 and magnesium in the treatment of autism: a methodology review and summary of outcomes, *Journal of Autism and Developmental Disorder* **25**: 480–493.

Quintana H, Birmaher B, Stedge D, Lennon S, Freed J, Bridge J, Greenhill L (1995). Use of methylphenidate in the treatment of children with autistic disorder. *Journal of Autism and Developmental Disorders* **25**: 283–294.

Rimland B, Edelson SM (1996). Brief report: alternative approaches to the development of effective treatments for autism. *Journal of Autism and Developmental Disorder* **25**: 237–241.

Sainsbury C (2000). The Martian in the Playground—Understanding the schoolchild with Asperger syndrome. The Book Factory, London.

Simonoff E (1998). Genetic counselling in autism and pervasive developmental disorders. *Journal of Autism and Developmental Disorders* **28**(5): 393–405.

Various (2001). MRC Review of Autism Research Epidemiology and Causes From: http://mrc.ac.uk/pdf-autism-report.pdf

Waterhouse W, Morris R, Allen D, Dunn M, Fein D, Feinstein C, Rapin I, Wing L (1996). Diagnosis and classification in autism. *Journal of Autism and Developmental Disorders* **26**: 59–86.

Wing L (2000). Past and future of research on Asperger syndrome. In. Klin A, Volkmar FR, Sparrow S (eds), *Asperger Syndrome*. The Guildford Press, New York, pp. 418–432.

World Health Organization (1993). The ICD-10 Classification of Mental and Behavioural Disorders: diagnostic criteria for research. 1 Mental Disorders-classification 2. Mental Disorders- diagnosis. World Health Organization, Geneva.

Zarcone JR, Hellings JA, Crandall K, Reese M, Marquis J, Fleming K, Shores R,Williams D, Schroder SR (2001). Effects of risperidone on aberrant behavior of persons with developmental disabilities: 1. A double-blind crossover study using multiple measures, *American Journal of Mental Retardation* **106**(6): 525–538.

Reading suggestions

The available literature is too extensive for any one reading list for all purposes. This is therefore a selected number of books the author of this chapter likes, has recommended to families and professionals in the past, and that usually receive positive feedback.

For everyone

Haddon M (2004). *The curious incident of the dog in the night time*. Doubleday, USA/London.

Although a work of fiction, this book shows an uncanny insight into the world of a child with Asperger syndrome. The book is superbly written (a Whitbread winner) and is both poignant with a positive message.

By individuals with autistic spectrum disorders

Books by Luke Jackson, Donna Williams and Claire Sainsbury. Both personal accounts by talented individuals with autism/Asperger syndrome. Each author has a different story to tell, every story is worth reading, and every story contains lots of lessons to learn from.

Jackson L (2002). *Freeks, Geeks and Asperger syndrome: a user guide to adolescence*. Jessica Kingsley Publishers Ltd, London.

Sainsbury C (2000). *The Martian in the Playground—Understanding the schoolchild with Asperger syndrome*. The Book Factory, London.

Williams D (1998). *Nobody Nowhere: The Remarkable Autobiography of an Autistic Girl*. London.

For parents who may also have autism

No better book than *Pretending to be Normal*.

Liane Holiday Willey, Jessica Kingsley, *Pretending to be Normal: Living with Asperger's Syndrome*. London 1999.

This excellent account tracks a mother's discovery about her own difficulties whilst trying to find help for her daughter.

For Professional/parents learning about autism

These again can now be found in abundance. I prefer a few listed below, for their clarity, clinical usefulness and where they also contain useful information for families.

Atwood T (1998). *Asperger's Syndrome: a guide for parents and professionals.* Jessica Kingsley, London.

Howlin, P. 1997, *Autism:Preparing for Adulthood* Routledge, London.

Wing L (1996). *The Autistic Spectrum: a Guide for Parents and Professionals.* The National Autistic Society, London.

Electronic media

Cambridge University Autism Research Centre (2002). *Mind Reading: the interactive guide to emotions.* Human Emotions.

This is a medium that one suspects will start to expand rapidly. *Mind Reading* is an interactive guide to emotions based on research by Cambridge University. It is slickly assembled, and serves as a fascinating tool that will hopefully prove to be a useful educational tool for individual with a range of autistic spectrum disorders Cambridge University Autism Research Centre 2002).

Web sites

The number of web sites on autistic spectrum disorders has grown exponentially. Its very difficult to keep track of the good ones that keep emerging. The National Autistic Society Website is continually updated and redesigned. It has a huge number of helpful resources on a wide range of subjects and a massive list of publications. I would recommend starting here to any family in the UK and then moving on according to their particular interests: http://www.nas.org.uk

Chapter 25

Child health promotion programme

Doug Simkiss

Introduction

In the late 1980s the British Paediatric Association set up a multidisciplinary working group chaired by David Hall to review routine health checks for young children. The report of this working party was published as a book in 1989. *Health for all Children* is now in its fourth edition and is the definitive text on these issues (Hall and Elliman 2003). Each new edition has seen a shift from a medical model of screening for disorders to an approach including health promotion, primary prevention, and active intervention for children at risk, whether for medical or social reasons. The fourth edition encompasses services to school age children, updating the *Health needs of school aged children* report (Polnay 1995).

The National Service Framework (NSF) for Children, Young People and Maternity Services (Department of Health 2004) adopted the recommendations of *Health for all children*. Standard 1 of the NSF lays out a new Child Health Promotion Programme (CHPP) designed to promote the health and well-being of children from pre-birth to adulthood. It replaces the Child Health Surveillance (CHS) Programme.

The change in terminology, although initially confusing, is important. Child Health Surveillance describes 'activities related to secondary prevention i.e. the detection of defects' (Hall and Elliman 2003). Child health surveillance is one component of CHPP. Unfortunately, much of what has been done in the past as part of child health surveillance does not meet the criteria for a screening test (Hall and Elliman 2003; UK National Screening Committee 2005). The term 'screening' should be confined to the evidence-based programmes agreed by the Child Health subgroup of the National Screening Committee.

A key aim of the CHPP is to change the relationship between parents, children, and health professionals, moving to one of partnership rather than supervision, in which parents are empowered to care for their own health and to make use of professional services and expertise according to their needs. It is clear that families will require different input to achieve this and the CHPP encourages targeted services for children and families in special circumstances.

The Child Health Promotion Programme

The CHPP is laid out in full in Table 25.1, it differs from the CHS programme it replaces in three important ways; a reduction in screening interventions, it's emphasis on health promotion activities, and interventions focused on families with more complex needs.

Table 25.1 Child Health Promotion Programme (adapted from Department of Health, 2004)

Age	Intervention
Antenatal	Antenatal screening and a preliminary assessment of child and family needs. Provide advice on breast feeding and general health and well-being, including healthy eating and smoking cessation where appropriate. Arrangements are put in place, including sharing of information, to ensure a smooth transition from the midwifery to health visiting service
Soon after birth	General physical examination with particular emphasis on eyes, heart, and hips. Administration of vitamin K (if parents choose vitamin K drops, these are administered during the first week after birth). BCG is offered to babies who are more likely to come into contact with someone who has TB. The first dose of hepatitis B vaccine is given to babies whose mothers or close family have been infected with hepatitis B
5–6 days old	Blood spot test for hypothyroidism and phenylketonuria. Screening for sickle cell disease and cystic fibrosis is also being implemented. See www.newbornscreening-bloodspot.org.uk
Within first month	Newborn hearing screening now being rolled out to all areas. If hepatitis B vaccine has been given soon after birth, the second dose is given
New birth visit (usually around 12 days)	Home visit by the midwife or health visitor to assess the child and family health needs, including identification of mental health needs. Distribution of 'Birth to Five' guide and the Personal Child Health Record if not already given out antenatally. Information / support to parents on key health issues to be available (e.g. support for breastfeeding, and advice on establishing a routine).
6–8 weeks	General physical examination with particular emphasis on eyes, heart and hips. First set of immunizations against polio, diphtheria, tetanus, whooping cough, pneumococcus Hib, and meningitis C. Review of general progress and delivery of key messages about parenting and health promotion. Identification of postnatal depression or other mental health needs. If hepatitis B vaccine has been given after birth, the third dose is given at 8 weeks
3 months	Second set of immunizations against polio, diphtheria, tetanus, whooping cough, Hib, and meningitis C. Review of general progress and delivery of key messages about parenting and health promotion, including weaning
4 months	Third set of immunizations against polio, diphtheria, tetanus, whooping cough, Hib, and meningitis C. Opportunity to give health promotion pneumococcus advice to parents and to ask about parents concerns
By the first birthday	Systematic assessment of the child's physical, emotional, and social development and family needs by the heath visiting team. This will include actions to address the needs identified and agree future contact with service
Around 13 months	Immunization against measles, mumps, and rubella (MMR) hib, pneumococcus and meningitis C is given. Review of general progress and health promotion and other advice to parents. If hepatitis B vaccine has been given soon after birth a booster dose is given and blood test arranged
2–3 years	The health visiting team is responsible for reviewing a child's progress and ensuring that health and developmental needs are being addressed. The health visitor will exercise professional judgement and agree with the parent how this review is carried out. It could be done through early year's providers or the general practice or by offering a contact in the clinic, home, by post, telephone, or email, etc. Use is made of other contacts with the primary care team (e.g. immunizations or visits to the general practitioner)

Table 25.1 (continued) Child Health Promotion Programme (adapted from Department of Health, 2004)

Age	Intervention
3–5 years	Immunization against measles, mumps, rubella (MMR) and polio and diphtheria, tetanus and whooping cough. Review of general progress and delivery of key messages about parenting and health promotion.
4–5 years	A review at school entry provides an opportunity to check that: immunizations are up to date, children have access to primary and dental care, appropriate interventions are available for any physical, developmental or emotional problems that have previously been missed or not addressed, to provide children, parents and school staff with information about specific health issues, to check the child's height and weight (from which the body mass index can be derived as a public health indicator), and to administer the sweep test of hearing. National orthoptist-led programme for pre-school vision screening to be introduced. Foundation stage profile—assessment by the teacher to include a child's • personal, social and emotional development; • communication, language and literacy; • physical development, and • creative development
Ongoing support at primary and secondary schools	Access to school nurse at open sessions/drop-in clinics and clinics by parents, teachers or through self-referral. Provision for referral to specialists for children causing concern. Children and young people with medical needs and disabilities may receive nursing care within the school environment according to their needs
Secondary school	Tetanus, diphtheria, and polio vaccines are given between 13 and 18 years. Check other immunizations are up to date. The school programme for BCG vaccination is being replaced with an improved targeted neonatal and others at risk-based programme (Department of Health 2005a)

A reduction in the whole population screening interventions

The pre-school years

In the CHS programme, all children were offered appointments to see a member of the primary care health team in the first few days of life, at 6 weeks, 9 months, 21 months, and 3 years with selective school medical assessments carried out at school entry. The uptake of these assessments after the first year of life and their diagnostic yield was low. The CHPP reduces routine contacts allowing the health visiting team to spend time in more effective ways, targeting vulnerable families.

The neonatal and 6–8-week physical examination are retained as the only whole population physical examinations now recommended. Some aspects of these can be seen as screening; examination of the eyes for congenital cataract, the heart for congenital heart disease and the hips for developmental dysplasia of the hip. In boys, undescended testes at 6 weeks require referral. Many primary care teams combine the first immunization and the physical examination at 8 weeks. *Health for all children* is clear that this is acceptable but only when 8 weeks is the latest date for examination as there is a short time frame to prevent the visual impairment associated with congenital cataract and hip deformity associated with developmental dysplasia of the hip. Rapid referral is also necessary to allow surgical correction of biliary atresia, identified initially with a prolonged conjugated hyperbilirubinaemia.

Universal neonatal hearing screening with automated otoacoustic emissions and automated auditory brainstem response audiometry is being implemented across the UK. Consequently, the distraction hearing test at 9 months will be withdrawn. It is clear that some sensorineural hearing loss is progressive and these children may pass a neonatal screen; therefore, it is, of course, always important to take a family's concern about hearing seriously and arrange testing.

A new requirement in the CHPP is for the health visiting team to 'systematically assess a child's physical, emotional, and social development and family needs by the first birthday. Actions to address the needs identified and agreed future contact with the service should be established' (Department of Health 2004a). On average, children see their general practitioner nine times in the first year. Each contact should be viewed as an opportunity to detect health issues and concerns and where relevant to provide health promotion advice. This requires a quick method for eliciting parental concerns, observational skills for identifying possible problems affecting health, growth, development and well-being in the child and sensitivity to parental physical or mental health disorders that might affect the child. Close liaison within the primary healthcare team with the health visitor in a pivotal role is essential to a complete assessment of the child and family.

A standardized approach (called the Common Assessment Framework) to conducting an assessment of the needs of a child and deciding how those needs should be met, which is based on the five outcomes in *Every Child Matters* (HM Treasury 2003) and the three dimensions of the Framework for Assessment (Figure 25.1) (Department of Health 2000), is being developed for children likely to have complex needs (Department for Education and Skills 2005). The Common Assessment Framework has a pre-assessment checklist. This is a single page document that could act as a foundation for a systematic assessment of any child at any age (Figure 25.2) (Department for Education and Skills 2005).

Between 2 and 3 years of age, the health visiting team is again responsible for reviewing a child's progress and ensuring that health and development needs are being addressed. The health visitor can exercise clinical judgement and agree with the parent how the review is carried out. Once again the Pre-assessment checklist of the Common assessment Framework could be a good place to start.

Recently, Early Years provision has expanded and most localities will include day nurseries, nursery schools, or Sure Start projects and this will continue to increase with the development of children's centres. Concerns about children may first surface in these settings and staff in these facilities will have expertise in recognizing children with health or developmental concerns. The health visiting team could involve staff within the Early Year's settings in the assessment of a child's progress. This is an effective way to ensure broad coverage of children on a health visitor case load and health visitors could provide drop in sessions to Early Years settings to see children of concern.

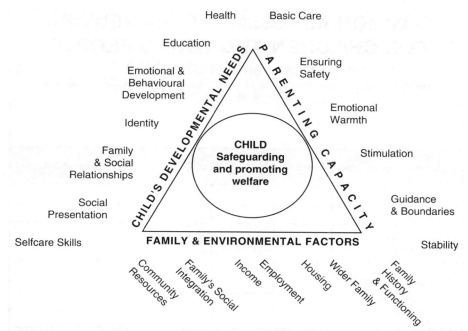

Fig. 25.1 The assessment framework (Department of Health 2000).

Early Year's staff may need training, but a developmental tool such as the Parents' Evaluations of Developmental Status (PEDS), is simple to use and has been validated in studies of more than 900 families whose socio-demographic characteristics capture the diversity of families seen in primary care (Glascoe 1997, 2000). PEDS can be administered very quickly and parents concerns used either alone, or in occasional combination with a second assessment, detect 70–80% of children with and without disabilities (Glascoe 2000) (Figure 25.3).

It is important that health visiting teams have expertise in developmental assessment beyond the 10 questions set out in PEDS. There are a variety of tools that would be suitable including the *Denver Developmental Screening Test II* (Denver Developmental Materials Inc) or *Schedule of Growing Skills* (2nd edition, nferNelsen), which are straight forward developmental tests that only take a few minutes in experienced hands and provide an objective measure of development that allows decisions on referral to be made.

School age children

At school entry, measurement of height and weight to allow body mass index calculation and a sweep hearing are recommended. Vision screening can be stopped once an orthoptic led assessment is in place between 4 and 5 years of age. The reduction in routine health screening in school within the CHPP and the changes in the BCG vaccination programme recently announced (Department of Health 2005a) allow a focus on health

COMMON ASSESSMENT FRAMEWORK FOR CHILDREN AND YOUNG PEOPLE
Pre-Assessment Checklist

Identifying details of baby, child or young person (i.e. name, date of birth) and contact with them/their family.

Does the baby, child or young person appear to be ...	Yes	No	Not Sure	Evidence/Comment
• healthy?				
• safe from harm?				
• learning and developing?				
• having a positive impact on others?				
• free from the negative impact of poverty?				

If you answered "no", what additional services are needed for the baby, child or young person or their parent(s), carer(s) or family?

Can you provide the additional services needed?

Yes	No

If you answered "no" or "not sure", or if it is not clear what support is needed, would an assessment under the Common Assessment Framework help?

Yes	No

Who will do this assessment?

I will	Another practitioner will

Name of practitioner	
Agency	
Date completed form	

Fig. 25.2 Pre-assessment checklist from the Common Assessment Framework (Department for Education and Skills 2005).

promotion and children with medical needs. School nursing plays an important part in a number of new ways (Table 25.2) and the National Healthy School Programme (Department for Education and Skills 2004) and the development of extended schools provide opportunities for school nurses to help in delivering a whole school approach to promoting health.

PEDS RESPONSE FORM

Child's Name Roger J.   Parent's Name Malinda J

Child's Birthday 8/8/03   Child's Age   2   Today's Date 8/10/05

Please list any concerns about your child's learning, development, and behavior.

I'm worried about how my child talks and relates to us. He says things that don't have anything to do with what's going on. He's oblivious to anything but what he is doing. He's not doing as well as other kids in many ways.

Do you have any concerns about how your child talks and makes speech sounds?

Circle one: No   (Yes)   A little   COMMENTS:

He repeats odd things like "Wheel of Fortune"

Do you have any concerns about how your child understands what you say?

Circle one: No   (Yes)   A little   COMMENTS:

I can't tell if he doesn't understand, doesn't hear well or just ignores us

Do you have any concerns about how your child uses his or her hands and fingers to do things?

Circle one: (No)   Yes   A little   COMMENTS:

He's good with manipulatives but does a lot of the same things over and over: spinning wheels on cars, flicking light switches, flipping pages

Do you have any concerns about how your child uses his or her arms and legs?

Circle one: (No)   Yes   A little   COMMENTS:

He's very coordinated and very fast!

Do you have any concerns about how your child behaves?

Circle one: No   Yes   (A little)   COMMENTS:

still lots of tantrums but headbanging is almost gone. Behavior therapy has been helpful and his tantrums are less severe and shorter

Do you have any concerns about how your child gets along with others?

Circle one: No   Yes   (A little)   COMMENTS:

He doesn't seem interested in watching other kids, let alone playing with them

Do you have any concerns about how your child is learning to do things for himself/herself?

Circle one: (No)   Yes   A little   COMMENTS:

He's very independent

Do you have any concerns about how your child is learning preschool or school skills?

Circle one: (No)   Yes   A little   COMMENTS:

He's too young for any of that!

Please list any other concerns.

We spend lots of time playing with Roger and talking to him. This seems to be helping him be more engaged. I still wonder about his hearing.

Fig. 25.3 Parental evaluations of developmental status (Glascoe 1997).

The National Healthy Schools Standard (NHSS) is the mainstay of the healthy schools programme and was introduced in 1999 as a vehicle to support delivery of Personal, Social and Health Education (PSHE). The NHSS and PSHE framework are designed to support each other and engage staff, pupils, governors, parents, and the wider community in a whole school approach to improving educational achievement, health and emotional

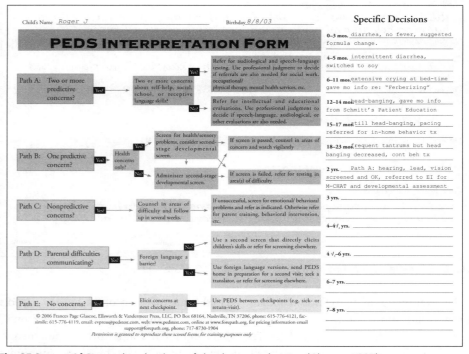

Fig. 25.3—cont'd Parental evaluations of developmental status (Glascoe 1997).

Table 25.2 The role of the school nurse (Hall and Elliman 2003)

Safeguarding the health and welfare of children
- Children with medical problems may need support in school with medication (e.g. asthma inhalers, adrenaline pens in anaphylaxis, medication in attention deficit hyperactivity disorder).
- Inclusion of children with statements of special education need may require administering nasogastric or gastrostomy feeds, the care of a tracheotomy or regular turning to prevent pressure sores.
- Special educational needs coordinators (SENCOs) and other teachers need to be fully informed about childrens health problems.
- Enabling all children to participate as fully as possible in school activities, including outings and journeys.
- Identifying emerging emotional and behavioural problems and disorders, learning difficulties and physical illnesses such as epilepsy.
- Helping to review and implement school policies on bullying and racism.
- Dealing with infectious diseases in school in collaboration with the Consultant in Communicable Disease Control

A confidante for children and young people
- To children experiencing stress, anxiety, depression, bereavement, abuse, domestic violence that want confidential support, advice, and intervention.
- Young people want a health service that offers them private and personal advice on issues such as eating disorders, obesity, menstrual problems, sexual health, skin problems (like acne), migraine and alcohol and drug issues.

Health promotion
- Children want an environment that facilitates the positive promotion of health, for example, the National Healthy Schools Standard (Department for Education and Skills, 2004) incorporates measures to support mental health (emotional literacy), good nutrition, exercise and physical activity, avoidance of harmful behaviours, sufficient sleep.
- Preparation and support for transitions—from primary to secondary school and leaving school.
- Extended child and family support
- Early interventions for conflicts between parents, child and school and for pupils at risk of dropping out of school
- Special additional support for children known to be at very high risk—looked after children, homeless children, excluded pupils and pregnant school girls are examples.

well-being, and making schools a safe, secure and healthy environment in which young people can learn and develop.

The NHSS includes eight key areas of activity:

- personal, social, and health education
- citizenship
- drug education (including tobacco and alcohol)
- emotional health and well-being
- healthy eating
- physical activity
- safety
- sex and relationship education.

Schools are able to work directly with health and social care partners to develop their own outreach services. The concept of Extended Schools was developed in the 2002 Education

Act and provides flexibility for governing bodies to enter into agreements with other partners such as a Primary Care Trust to provide services on school premises. These can be tailored to the needs of their individual school or wider local community and could include: smoking cessation clinics, dental clinics, family health centres or teenage health walk-in clinics (for issues such as bullying, drugs, eating disorders, and sexual health).

Special Schools and other schools with specialist resources such as consulting rooms may be particularly well suited to provide these types of services.

Health promotion activities

The CHPP schedule (Table 25.1) is underpinned by a health promotion programme that focuses on priority issues such as healthy eating, physical activity, safety, smoking, sexual health, and mental health as highlighted in the NHSS. This should be delivered by all members of the primary care health team who come into contact with children and young people. Establishing an evidence base for these interventions is a priority and the best available evidence is reviewed later in this chapter.

Interventions focused on families with more complex needs

Children in special circumstances are a theme running through the NSF and Box 25.1 identifies some vulnerable and socially isolated groups.

Box 25.1 Vulnerable and socially isolated groups (Hall and Elliman 2003)

- Children in transition (e.g. from one location to another, changing schools, changing from paediatric to adult healthcare)
- Children not registered with any general practitioner
- Children living away from home
- Children excluded by language barriers
- Traveller families
- Families living in temporary or bed and breakfast accommodation
- Children of troubled, violent or disabled parents
- Children who care for disabled parents
- Children who are involved with, or whose families are involved with, substance abuse, crime, or prostitution
- Runaways and street children
- Asylum seekers and refuges, particularly if unaccompanied
- Children locked up
- Children of parents in prison

The CHPP allows a flexible approach so that resources can be targeted on these children and their families. There is compelling evidence that these groups of children fare less well than their peers, whether it is children looked after by the local authority (Department of Health 2002), children in domestic violence refuges (Webb *et al.* 2001), children whose parents misuse alcohol or drugs (Tunnard 2002; Advisory Council on the Misuse of Drugs 2003) or have mental health problems (Cleaver *et al.* 1999), or young people who become parents while still teenagers (Social Exclusion Unit 1999). The research evidence for effective services to support these children was reviewed in the development of the NSF (Statham 2004).

The primary healthcare team will need to work within a multi-agency approach to these families and the Common Assessment Framework focused on the five outcomes from *Every Child Matters*; being healthy, staying safe, enjoying and achieving, making a positive contribution and achieving economic well-being, will be an important tool to facilitate effective joint working.

Looked after children are an example of a vulnerable population where the primary healthcare team can make a very significant contribution. Primary Care Trusts should have a designated doctor and nurse lead for looked after children but the role of health visitors and school nurses in completing health assessments on some of these children is invaluable (Department of Health 2002).

Organization of Child Health Promotion Programme in the primary care team

As CHPP has evolved from CHS, the involvement of different parts of the primary healthcare team has changed. The detection of physical abnormalities remains a key component of the CHPP, but the role of the doctor has lessened with only one examination of all children required at 6–8 weeks (it is likely that the neonatal examination will be done by hospital staff in most cases). Immunization remains a cornerstone of the programme.

Health visitors and school nurses are the lead professionals in the primary healthcare team for the CHPP. The programme is challenging as it requires three different ways of working brought together; promoting health and development, identifying abnormalities and disorders and taking a public health approach to prevention and community development. Individuals will bring differing experience in these three ways of working and it is important that the team has a skill mix that incorporates these different approaches. There are examples of services that have successfully worked in this way for a number of years (Swann and Brocklehurst 2004).

Quality assurance and audit

Quality assurance and audit are components of an effective clinical governance framework. Primary healthcare teams need to plan to use information to undertake these exercises. Helpful measures should be collected with an emphasis on outcomes. However, because adverse outcomes may be uncommon or may occur years after the healthcare was provided (or omitted), process measures that correlate with outcome may need to be monitored. For example, the uptake of immunization (process) is likely to be a more useful measure than the incidence of diseases such as tetanus or diphtheria (outcome) (Hall and Elliman 2003).

Children or young people failing to attend clinic appointments following referral from the primary healthcare team may trigger concern, given that they are reliant on their parent or carer to take them to the appointment. Failure to attend can be an indicator of a family's vulnerability, potentially placing the child's welfare in jeopardy. It can equally be an indicator that services are difficult for families to access or considered inappropriate, and need reviewing. A system should therefore be in place to identify children or young people who do not attend an appointment following a referral for specialist care; so that the referrer is aware they have not attended and can take any follow-up action considered appropriate to ensure that the child's needs are being met. This could include a home visit or telephone contact to find out, for example, whether the appointment is no longer necessary.

The CHPP should be made available to the whole population and skills in assessing and mapping the health needs of a population are important in matching provision to need. This could be done by health visiting case load, school population or on a Primary Care Trust basis with the input of the Director of Public Health. Mapping provision to need may mean that differing levels of resource are needed for individual groups, services, or areas, and that existing resources should be redistributed, this can be done in creative ways (Swann and Brocklehurst, 2004).

Training requirements

Box 25.2 outlines the training and development issues identified for the primary healthcare team in implementing the CHPP. This provides a syllabus for a rolling programme of training that a Primary Care Trust or Children's Trust could provide for primary healthcare staff, along side professionals from other agencies such as teachers and social workers.

Evidence-based practice

The CHPP makes health promotion a important role for the primary care team. So what is the evidence that this is effective? There is thorough and regularly updated information on key health promotion priorities in the Cochrane Library. The National Institute for Health and Clinical Excellence has taken over the role of producing regular Evidence Briefings from the Health Development Agency. All these are available via the National Electronic Library for Health website; www.nelh.nhs.uk. In the development of the NSF, a review of the evidence for promoting and protecting the health of children and young people was commissioned and published (Licence 2004; Department of Health 2005b). Implementing the NSF is a 10-year plan and the evidence underpinning its recommendations, including the CHPP, is evolving (Table 25.3).

In adolescence, there is significant evidence that health risk behaviours (such as smoking, drinking, illicit drug use, sexual intercourse, and suicidal behaviour) may form a

Box 25.2 Training requirements (Department of Health, 2004b)

All staff who come into contact with children in all agencies need to be competent in the following core areas:

- child and young person physical and psychological development
- safeguarding children/child protection, including risk and protective factors
- effective communication and engagement (listening to and involving children and working with parents, carers, and families.
- supporting transitions (maximizing children's achievements and opportunities and understanding their rights and responsibilities)
- multiagency working (working across professional and agency boundaries)
- sharing information.

Depending on their role, staff working with children may also need training to ensure they are competent in the following areas:

- assessing children and young people's developmental needs in the context of their family and environmental factors (including school and community) and parenting capacity
- understanding of the impact of disability on the child and family
- understanding the key vulnerability factors for children in special circumstances and responding to their needs, including through referral and joint working
- identifying the early warning signs of mental health problems in children and young people such as attention deficit hyperactivity disorder, depression, eating disorders, substance abuse, and self-harm
- recognizing inequalities and ethnic diversity and addressing them proactively
- promoting healthy life-styles and directing families to local services
- issues of confidentiality and consent
- record keeping

single entity related to family connectedness and mental health factors. This has led to research on resilience and protective factors in the lives of young people (Resnick *et al.* 1997; Resnick 2000) and the development of 'social development model' interventions that have been shown to be effective in improving long-term mental health and risk behaviours (Hawkins *et al.* 2005).

Conclusions

The CHPP has evolved from Child Health Surveillance. It was proposed by *Health for all Children* (Hall and Elliman 2003) and adopted by the National Service Framework for Children, Young People and Maternity Services (Department of Health 2004a). It contains

Table 25.3 Evidence for health promotion strategies

Home visiting	There is evidence that home visiting programmes are associated with: ◆ improvements in parenting ◆ reported improvements in some child behaviour problems ◆ improved cognitive development, especially among some subgroups of children such as those born prematurely or born with a low birthweight ◆ a reduction in unintentional injury among children ◆ improved detection and management of postnatal depression. There was either no evidence or inconclusive evidence for the impact of home visiting on other outcomes reviewed including child abuse, increased uptake of immunization, reduced hospital admission or maternal participation in education or in the workforce (Bull *et al.* 2004)
Breast feeding	A recent Cochrane review found five studies (including 582 women) that evaluated the effect of health education on the initiation of breastfeeding. When all studies were combined for meta-analysis, a statistically significant increase in the number of women starting to breast feed was demonstrated as a result of the health education interventions (relative risk (RR) 1.53, 95% confidence interval (CI) 1.25–1.88). These interventions were all conducted among women on low incomes in the USA (Dyson *et al.* 2005).
Unintended injury prevention	Multifactorial injury prevention interventions have been shown to reduce injuries in the home and on the road. Towner *et al.* found good evidence for cycle helmet education campaigns and child restraint loan schemes. They found reasonable evidence for education aimed at parents about pedestrian injuries, cycle training, child restraint, and seat belt education campaigns. In the home, there is good evidence for smoke detector programmes and child resistant packaging and reasonable evidence for window bars, parent education on hazard reduction and general safety measures (Towner *et al.* 2001; Millward *et al.* 2003). However, a review of common home alterations include the installation of locks on cupboards and covers on electrical sockets, improvement of lighting in halls and stairways, and the removal of rugs and other falls hazards found that there is insufficient evidence from trials to show that such changes reduce the number of injuries in the home (Lyons *et al.* 2003)
Obesity and overweight prevention	Interventions to prevent obesity in children were the subject of a Cochrane review and treatment and a Health Development Agency Evidence Briefing. There is evidence to support the use of multifaceted, school-based interventions to reduce obesity in school children, particularly girls. These interventions include nutrition education, physical activity promotion, reduction in sedentary behaviour, behavioural therapy, teacher training, curricular material and modification of school meals and tuck shops. Currently there is limited evidence to support school-based health promotion (classroom curriculum to reduce television, video tape and videogame use) and a lack of evidence of the effectiveness for school-based physical activity programmes led by specialist staff or class room teachers for the prevention of obesity and overweight in children (Mulvihill and Quigley 2003; Summerbell *et al.* 2005). The same Cochrane group reviewed treatment for child hood obesity; there was a limited amount of quality data on the components of programs to treat childhood obesity. The research team concluded that no direct conclusions can be drawn from this review with confidence (Summerbell *et al.* 2003).
Positive mental health	Most of the reviews on this topic have found that school-based mental health promotion programmes can be successful. Those that include environmental and cultural change within the school and promote positive mental health amongst

Table 25.3 (continued) Evidence for health promotion strategies

	staff as well as students, tend to be more successful than those that are purely curriculum-based (Durlak and Wells, 1997; Wells *et al.* 2003). Programmes that aim to provide children with individually focused mental health promotion and attempt to help children negotiate through stressful transitions have also been successful. It appears that implementing preventative programmes over prolonged periods of time (more than 1 year) improves the outcomes for some children
Prevention of teenage pregnancy	There are differing opinions on the effectiveness of strategies to reduce teenage pregnancy. A systematic review showed that a range of interventions, including sex education, school-based clinics, family planning clinics and community programmes, did not delay initiation of sexual intercourse for young men or women nor improve contraceptive use. There was limited evidence to suggest that multifaceted programmes have potential to reduce the number of pregnancies in young women (DiCenso *et al.* 2002). However, the Health Development Agency finds there is good evidence for school-based sex education, particularly linked to contraceptive services (measured against knowledge, attitudes, delaying sexual activity, and/or reducing pregnancy rates). School-based clinics may be effective as part of multifactor programmes (Swann *et al.* 2003)
Prevention of sexually transmitted infections	The Health Development Agency has found sufficient review-level evidence to demonstrate that school-based sex education can be effective in this regard (Ellis and Grey 2004)
Avoiding smoking	Smoking rates in adolescents are rising. An estimated 9% of children aged 11–15 were regular smokers in 2004 (Department of Health 2005c). Helping young people to avoid starting smoking is a widely endorsed goal of public health, but there is uncertainty about how to do this. Schools provide a route for communicating with a large proportion of young people, and school-based programmes for smoking prevention have been widely developed and evaluated. Sixteen good quality randomized controlled trials of school-based programmes to prevent children who had never smoked becoming smokers were identified in a Cochrane systematic review (Thomas 2002). There is little evidence that information alone is effective but there is review level evidence that supports the use of school-based 'peer' or 'social type' interventions (Naidoo *et al.* 2004). These combine a variety of curricular components including ◆ information on the short-term health consequences of smoking ◆ information on the social influences that encourage smoking ◆ correction of students' normative expectations for smoking ◆ provision of training, modelling, rehearsal, and reinforcement of techniques to resist social pressures to smoke ◆ training on resistance to smoking messages in advertisements and in the media ◆ making a public commitment not to smoke. It is possible that the impact of these programmes could be improved if ◆ they are delivered early, about age 10–11 years. ◆ same age peer leaders play a substantial part in delivering the programme ◆ they are part of a multicomponent health programm ◆ booster sessions are included in subsequent years ◆ peers are not overtrained
Drug use prevention	There is little evidence available as to what constitutes an effective intervention. The available evidence suggests that broadly based and more

Table 25.3 (continued) Evidence for health promotion strategies

	specifically focused interventions can have an effect. The provision of booster sessions and multi-component programmes may have the potential to have a positive effect on drug prevention programmes. (Canning *et al.* 2004 Faggoano *et al.* 2005)
Alcohol use prevention	Many studies that have evaluated educational and psychosocial prevention of alcohol misuse programmes were considered and appraised in a systematic review. A number of programmes showed evidence of ineffectiveness. Those that reported longer-term evaluations (over 3 years follow-up) were examined in more detail and several promising studies were re-analysed to provide a better indication of the potential impact of the prevention programme. On the basis of this re-analysis, the Strengthening Families Programme (SFP) in particular but also culturally focused skills training appear to offer promise. However, all of the studies included in the review showed some methodological weaknesses and it is therefore necessary to replicate these studies with more robust design and analysis, and across different settings (Foxcroft *et al.* 2002).
Dental and oral disease prevention	Fluoride in water as 1 part per million has been shown to be the most effective method of reducing tooth decay. However, only 10–15% of people in the UK receive fluoridated water (Hall and Elliman 2003). There is little evidence that individual health education improves oral health in the long term, although short-term improvements in knowledge may be achieved through simple information giving approaches (Department of Health 1998). Individual oral health education can be effective at reducing plaque levels in the short term

evidence-based screening activities but reduces the number of contacts recommended for the whole population. It emphasizes health promotion, primary prevention, and focused activity with the children and families in most need. The evidence to underpin health promotion is evolving.

References

Advisory Council on the Misuse of Drugs (2003). *Hidden Harm: Responding to the Needs of Children of Problem Drug Users*. Home Office, London.

Bellman M, Longam S, Aukett A. *Schedule of Growing Skills* (2nd edn) nfer Nelson, London.

Bull J, McCormick G, Swann C, Mulvihill C (2004). *Ante- and Post-Natal Home Visiting Programmes: a Review of Reviews*. *Evidence Briefing*. Health Development Agency, London.

Canning U, Millward L, Raj T, Warm D (2004). *Drug Use Prevention Among Young People: a Review of Reviews*. *Evidence Briefing*. Health Development Agency, London.

Cleaver H, Unell I, Aldgate J (1999). *Children's Needs-Parenting Capacity: the Impact of Parental Mental Illness, Problem Alcohol and Drug Use, and Domestic Violence on Children's Development*. The Stationery Office, London.

Department for Education and Skills (2004). *Healthy Living Blueprint for Schools*. Department for Education and Skills, London.

Department for Education and Skills (2005). *Common Assessment Framework*. Department for Education and Skills, London. www.everychildmatters.gov.uk/deliveringservices/caf/ Accessed 28.7.05

Department of Health (1998). *National Diet and Nutrition Survey 1997: Young People Aged 4–18 Years*. Volume 2: *Report of the Oral Health Survey*. The Stationery Office, Norwich.

Department of Health (2000) *Framework for the Assessment of Children in Need and their Families.* The Stationery Office, London.

Department of Health (2002). *Promoting the Health of Looked after Children.* Department of Health, London.

Department of Health (2004a) *National Service Framework for Children, Young People and Maternity Services.* Department of Health, London.

Department of Health (2004b). *Primary Care Version. National Service Framework for Children, Young People and Maternity Services.* Department of Health, London.

Department of Health (2005a). *Changes to the BCG Vaccination Programme.* Department of Health, London.

Department of Health (2005b). *Evidence to Inform the National Service Framework for Children, Young People and Maternity Services—Promoting health and well-being, identifying needs and intervening early.* Department of Health, London. http://www.dh.gov.uk/assetRoot/04/11/24/05/ 04112405.pdf (accessed 4.8.05)

Department of Health (2005c). *Smoking, Drinking and Drug Use Among Young People in England in 2004.* Department of Health, London.

DiCenso A, Guyatt G, Willan A, Griffin L (2002). Interventions to reduce unintended pregnancies among adolescents: systematic review of randomised controlled trials. *British Medical Journal* **324**: 1426–1435.

Durlak JA, Wells AM (1997). Primary prevention mental health programs for children and adolescents: a meta-analytic review. *American Journal of Community Psychology* **25**: 115–152.

Dyson L, McCormick F, Renfrew MJ (2005). Interventions for promoting the initiation of breastfeeding. *The Cochrane Database of Systematic Reviews*, Issue 2.

Ellis S, Grey A (2004). *Prevention of Sexually Transmitted Infections (Stis): a Review of Reviews Into the Effectiveness of Non-Clinical Interventions. Evidence Briefing.* Health Development Agency, London.

Faggiano F, Vigna-Taglianti FD, Versino E, Zambon A, Borraccino A, Lemma P (2005). School-based prevention for illicit drugs' use. *The Cochrane Database of Systematic Reviews*, Issue 2.

Foxcroft DR, Ireland D, Lowe G, Breen R (2002). Primary prevention for alcohol misuse in young people. *The Cochrane Database of Systematic Reviews*, Issue 3.

Glascoe FP (1997). *Parents' Evaluations of Developmental Status.* Ellsworth and Vandermeer Press, Nashville, TN. http://edge.net/~evpress.

Glascoe FP (2000). Evidence-based approach to developmental and behavioural surveillance using parents'concerns. *Child: Care, Health and Development* **26**(2): 137–149.

Hall DMB, Elliman D (2003) *Health for all Children.* Oxford University Press, Oxford.

Hawkins JD, Kosterman R, Catalano RF, Hill KG, Abbott RD (2005). Promoting positive adult functioning through social development intervention in childhood: longterm effects from the Seattle Social Development Project. *Archives of Pediatric Adolescent Medicine* **159**: 25–31.

Her Majesty's Treasury (2003). *Every Child Matters.* The Stationary Office, London

Licence K (2004). Promoting and protecting the health of children and young people. *Child: Care, Health and Development* **30**: 623–635.

Lyons RA, Sander LV, Weightman AL, Patterson J, Jones SA Lannon S, Rolfe B, Kemp A, Johansen A (2003). Modification of the home environment for the reduction of injuries. *The Cochrane Database of Systematic Reviews*, Issue 4.

Millward LM, Morgan A, Kelly MP (2003). *Prevention and Reduction of Accidental Injury in Children and Older People. Evidence Briefing.* Health Development Agency, London.

Mulvihill C, Quigley R (2003). *The Management of Obesity and Overweight, an Analysis of Reviews of Diet, Physical Activity and Behavioural Approaches. Evidence Briefing.* Health Development Agency, London.

Naidoo B, Warm D, Quidley R, Taylor L (2004). *Smoking and Public Health: a Review of Reviews of Interventions to Increase Smoking Cessation, Reduce Smoking Initiation and Prevent Further Uptake of Smoking. Evidence Briefing.* Health Development Agency, London.

Polnay L (1995) *Report of a Joint Working Party on Health Needs of School Age Children.* British Paediatric Association, London.

Resnick MD (2000). Resilience and protective factors in the lives of adolescents. *Journal of Adolescent Health* **27**: 1–2.

Resnick MD, Bearman PS, Blum RW, Bauman KE, Harris KM, Jones J Datter Jones J, Jabor J, Beuhring T, Sieving RE, Shew M, Ireland M, Bearinger LH, Udry JR (1997). Protecting adolescents from harm. Findings from a National Longitudinal Study on Adolescent Health. *JAMA* **278**: 823–32.

Social Exclusion Unit (1999). *Teenage Pregnancy.* SEU, London.

Statham J (2004). Effective services to support children in special circumstances. *Child: Care, Health and Development* **30**: 589–598.

Summerbell CD, Ashton V, Campbell KJ, Edmunds L, Kelly S, Waters E (2003). Interventions for treating obesity in children. *The Cochrane Database of Systematic Reviews*, Issue 3.

Summerbell CD, Waters E, Edmunds LD, Kelly S, Brown T, Campbell KJ (2005). Interventions for preventing obesity in children. *The Cochrane Database of Systematic Reviews*, Issue 3

Swann B, Brocklehurst N (2004). Three in one: the Stockport model of health visiting. *Community Practitioner* **77**: 251–256.

Swann C, Bowe K, McCormick G, Kosmin M (2003). *Teenage Pregnancy and Parenthood: a Review of Reviews. Evidence Briefing.* Health Development Agency, London.

Thomas R (2002). School-based programmes for preventing smoking. *The Cochrane Database of Systematic Reviews*, Issue 2.

Towner E, Dowswell T, MacKereth C, Jarvis S (2001). *What Works in Preventing Unintentional Injuries in Children and Young Adolescents? An Updated Systematic Review.* Health Development Agency, London.

Tunnard J (2002). *Parental Drug Misuse—A Review of Impact and Intervention Studies.* Research in Practice, Dartington, UK. www.rip.org.uk/publications/research reviews.htm.

UK National Screening Committee website; http://www.nsc.nhs.uk/whatscreening/ whatscreen_ind.htm. Accessed 04.08.2005

Webb E, Shankleman J, Evans M, Brooks R (2001). The health of children in refuges for women victims of domestic violence: cross sectional descriptive survey. *British Medical Journal* **323**: 210–213.

Wells J, Barlow J, Stewart Brown S (2003). A systematic review of universal approaches to mental health promotion in schools. *Health Education* **103**: 197–220.

Chapter 26

The transition to parenthood: the role of the health visitor

Jane Barlow and Angela Underdown

Introduction

Traditionally the safe arrival of a newborn infant is perceived as one of the happiest and most natural events in the human life cycle. However, while much energy is put into the physical preparations for a new baby, the evidence suggests that there is much less preparation for the inevitable emotional transitions facing partners who become parents. The negotiation of positive, cohesive relationships within a growing family is a major concern because of the potential impact of disruptions to the parents' relationship on the mental health of the infant. Increasing knowledge about the psychological and biologically driven processes that men and women face during the transition to parenthood, coupled with evidence about the effects of early interactions on infant development mean that this is a crucial period in terms of children's future mental health.

This chapter provides an overview of the evidence about the transition to parenthood and highlights the role of health visitors in supporting parents during this period. It will be argued that parents-to-be need accessible evidence-based information and support in relation to the emotional processes taking place during the transition to parenthood. The chapter begins with an overview of the research about the transition to parenthood alongside evidence about the importance of sensitive interactions for the infant's later development. The second part of the chapter addresses the role of health visitors in supporting parents during this time, and highlights a number of innovative ways of intervening that are being developed nationally and internationally. It will be argued, that there is need for key professionals such as health visitors to develop a 'new mindset' in terms of why and how they intervene to support the transition to parenthood.

Policy context

There has long been recognition of the need to promote the physical health of women during pregnancy and immediately following childbirth. During the past few years, however, there has been increasing recognition both professionally and politically of the importance of supporting some of the 'non-physical' aspects of parents' well-being during pregnancy and the first few years of a child's life. The need for such support was highlighted as one of the key recommendations of the Acheson Report (1998), which acknowledged that the quality of the relationship between parent and infant is affected by the nature of the transition men and women make when they become parents. This report called for policies that promote the social and emotional support of parents and children, and for the further development of the role and capacity of health visitors to provide such support to both expectant parents, and parents with young children (ibid).

Similarly, the Royal College of Paediatrics and Child Health produced a report that stated:

> Parenting starts with the unborn child and much more can and should be done to recognise potential problems and provide support to parents during the antenatal period. This requires antenatal services that provide time to talk with parents about their concerns and antenatal classes that address the emotional needs of parents and babies
>
> Royal College of Paediatrics and Child Health (2002, p. 22).

The National Framework for Children, Young People and Maternity Services also points to the need for maternity services to provide 'good clinical and psychological outcomes for the woman and baby while putting equal emphasis on helping new parents prepare for parenthood' (Department for Education and Skills 2004).

The 10-year strategy for childcare has introduced a number of significant changes in terms of parental leave, to enable parents to balance work and family life particularly during the transition to parenthood (Department for Education and Skills 2004).

When partners become parents

While childbirth has come to be defined in physical terms, the potential for emotional crisis in new parents was recognized during the middle of the last century (Le Master 1957). Since then, evidence has accumulated to show that the relationships of many couples are severely challenged and may break down after the birth of a baby (Cowan and Heatherington 1991; Belsky and Kelly 1994). Cowan and Cowan (1992, pp. 212–213) researched the transition to parenthood and argued that the 'conspiracy of silence that surrounds this period leaves the couple feeling that they are the only ones having a hard time', whereas the research shows that:

◆ new fathers as well as mothers are at risk of depression

◆ the level of stress and distress couples experience during pregnancy may predict difficulties with parenting

◆ conflict or distress in the family while the child is young is accompanied by less optimal parent–child relationships and slower progress in the child's cognitive and social development up until and beyond starting school

◆ professional intervention with couples during the first year of parenthood focusing on the partner–parent relationship can have a significant impact in reducing the separation rate of couples, improving the quality of parenting and their child's adjustment and development.

The transition to parenthood: a stressful time?

Stress during the pregnancy is common. For example, one longitudinal study of low-risk parents-to-be showed that a substantial number of couples experienced 'psychological distress' at this time. This study showed that the couple had more concerns about emotional and relationship issues than about aspects of the birth or childcare, that there was a distinctive 'fatherhood constellation', and that support from external sources was low forcing the couple to support one another, thereby increasing tensions between them. This study also showed that satisfaction with the couples' relationship declined after birth, and that lack of attention to the different needs of men and women in antenatal classes increased distress in both parent–parent and infant–parent relationships (Parr 1998).

There is also increasing recognition that depression during pregnancy is common. For example, a recent cohort study showed that depression scores were higher at 32 weeks of pregnancy than 8 weeks postpartum, with 13.5% of women scoring above the threshold for probable depression between 18 and 32 weeks gestation (Evans *et al.* 2001). An earlier study showed that such depression was associated with both marital conflict and severe doubts about having the baby (Kumar and Mordecai Robson 1984).

Stress and depression during pregnancy have also been shown to be associated with poor outcomes for the infant. For example, a recent study showed that antenatal anxiety predicted emotional and behavioural problems at 4 years of age in both boys and girls (Glover and O'Connor 2002).

A number of other processes are taking place during pregnancy that are not commonly recognized or talked about. For example, between the fourth and seventh months of gestation the mother develops internal representations about the baby-to-be (i.e. feelings about the fetus) (Stern 1986). These are shaped not only by the biological changes taking place but also by psychic and social factors such as the mother's memories of her own early relationships, her family traditions, her hopes, her fears, and her fantasies. The research also suggests that while this process discontinues around the seventh month it begins again with the birth of the baby. The significance of these representations is that they may be 'laden with excessive fears' or even with 'idealized expectations about their imagined baby', and these can interfere with the process of establishing a relationship with the 'real baby' (Raphael-Leff 2001). It has therefore been suggested that pregnant women require support that is aimed at helping to increase the mothers' awareness of 'the inevitable ambivalence that pregnancy and parenthood will bring' (ibid).

Many women also become preoccupied with the physical changes and excitement about their own creativity, which may cause the couple to become emotionally closer. Clulow (1991) refers to this state as 'the fantasy of fusion'. In contrast, some men may resent their lack of control, and the attention being given to their partner, and domestic violence may become a feature of the relationship (Hedin *et al.* 1999).

In all cultures pregnancy and childbirth are embedded in rituals and customs, that may be protective, but that can also exert powerful social and emotional pressures. American families, for example, may celebrate the impending birth by hosting a 'baby shower', when family and friends visit and literally shower the family with gifts for the new baby. This places the mother-to-be at the centre of attention but may also make her feel that she has to conform to expectations, grow the perfect baby and be the ideal mother. Expectant mothers who are not part of that affluent life-style may experience the social pressures of not being 'good enough' as a mother because poverty, reflected in the lack of expensive equipment, is a powerful symbol of inequality of life chances.

Furthermore, there are many cultural contradictions surrounding pregnancy, childbirth, and parenthood that may also make the transition to parenthood more difficult. For example, prevalent beliefs about pregnancy and motherhood being a 'natural' and happy time in a woman's life are frequently in sharp contrast to the woman's lived experience. In addition, while childbirth is viewed as 'natural', it has also been located within a pathological or illness model, which has implications for the way in which women experience and make sense of this event (Miller 2000).

Antenatal classes are one of the main sources of preparation for parenthood, and are intended to prepare men and women for childbirth itself, by building confidence and self-esteem to enable parents to be in control of the labour and birth. The reality, however, may be somewhat different. Indeed, some have questioned the purpose of such classes suggesting that they actually function to 'programme' the woman for a 'passive acceptance of medicalized childbirth' (Oakley in Taylor 1985), while others have suggested that the teaching approaches used in such classes 'often promote dependency among clients rather than nurturing the decision-making skills required by a consumer-driven maternity service' (Nolan 1997). Indeed, it has been suggested that: 'Less that half of pregnant women attend any sort of class, needs and service provision are mismatched, certain parents are missing out, men are excluded, the focus of the classes is too narrow, aims are unclear, the quality is poor and there is lack of specialized training, management and support for those providing the services' (Parr 1998).

While women of different cultures may rely on different sources of support, a survey of white, Indian, and Mixed origin women in South Africa showed that all groups irrespective of ethnicity felt that they had received a poor preparation for most aspects of their experience of becoming a parent (Chalmers and Meyer 1994).

Bronfenbrenner's ecological systems theory (1979) depicts how first-time parents need to re-negotiate new relationships and boundaries in every system, and how history and culture can be a powerful help or hindrance to their ability to create a family in which parents and children can thrive. It describes the complex interaction the child, his immediate family/community environment, and background of society. This has two implications: changes or tension in one layer will effect other layers and to study a child's development then, it is essential to not examine immediate environment, but also interactions of the larger environment.

Child birth

Childbirth, like death, might appear to be one of the few inevitable rites of passage, which rely totally on nature. Most cultural groups, however, surround these life transitions with a series of rituals which are intended to make order out of the 'chaos' caused by nature. Cultural rituals are intended to control the unpredictability of nature and may offer protection for the new mother and her child. (A ritual may be defined as a patterned, repetitive, and symbolic enactment of a cultural belief or value' (Davis Floyd 1987, p. 480) and as such communicate a range of meanings.) For example, traditionally in Jamaica the woman had a period of seclusion following the birth, which was aimed at giving the new mother a rest and possibly preventing infection (Kitzinger 1982). This contrasts with current practice in the UK in which women are frequently discharged from medical care after 24 hours and before they have rested or had a chance to establish feeding.

Less technologically advanced societies may allow a woman to deliver in a more natural way than her counterpart living in a medically advanced society, where birth is often conducted in a hospital (the domain of the diseased). Davis Floyd (1992, p. 1) argues that 'the removal of birth to the hospital has resulted in a proliferation of rituals surrounding this natural physiological event more elaborate than any heretofore known in the 'primitive' world.' A severe shortage of midwives in the UK means that the physical safety of the mother and baby have to be prioritized with medical practitioners reflecting their high degree of scientific training by concentrating on the physiological aspects of birth, and treating the woman's body as a machine that has a task to perform. This machine is often perceived as 'faulty', as is highlighted by the use of terminologies such as 'failure to progress' and 'incompetent cervix'.

The Winterton Report (1992) followed by Changing Childbirth (Expert Maternity Group 1993) both acknowledged that the woman should be the focus of care in order to maximize her control. However, pregnant women are still disempowered in terms of childbirth, with the expectant mother's 'condition' being treated in isolation from the rest of her life (Helman 2000) and with little account being taken of her new 'social' birth as a mother.

The arrival of a baby and parenting

The postnatal period involves further emotional and psychological transitions for new parents. Factors such as adapting to the needs of a new baby, tiredness, and the loss of other identities that are associated with the transition to parenthood, requires that women make complex physical and psychological changes during the postnatal period (Woollett and Parr 1997). While many of these are similar for men, a survey of new mothers and fathers showed that men's feelings and experiences during this time differed in a number of important ways from those of women. Both parents, however, viewed parenthood as having a negative impact on their sex life due in the part to the associated changes in women's bodies and their identities as parents (ibid).

The 'fantasy of fusion' that draws couples together during pregnancy is often expected to continue after the baby is born. Following childbirth, however, there is frequently a polarization of goals and expectations as men and women negotiate their new roles (Belsky and Kelly 1994). Stern (1986) explains how this experience of polarization is influenced by the 'motherhood constellation', which, he argues, is a temporary period in which the mother is preoccupied with several themes. One of these, the 'life growth theme', is biologically driven, making the mother's need to keep the baby alive her top priority (ibid).

Couples are often unprepared for these fundamental changes in sense of self and without the recognition that they may affect their relationship, there may be resentment and blame. For example, after childbirth the mother may seem more concerned with the man as a father than as a sexual partner. Although the baby may be the focus of this change, it is often the fundamental changes in the parents that cause the disunity, and couples may need to mourn the loss of their close relationship before they can celebrate their new roles. In addition, there may be deep tensions between the cultural aspirations of a contemporary woman living in the developed world and the experience of deep biological drives associated with motherhood. These tensions may be exacerbated by the transition from being a 'competent woman' in control of her life to an 'incompetent' or inexperienced mother. As support networks loosen and traditional rituals decline, the challenge to health professionals lays in ensuring the healthy birth of the social mother and father.

In addition to these 'normal' transitions, as many as 15% of women will experience postnatal depression (Wickberg and Hwang 1997) with some surveys showing a prevalence of 27.5% of women and 9.5% of men (Ballard *et al.* 1994). This level of depression is strongly associated with a reduced capacity for functioning including mother–infant relationship difficulties and in some cases, rejection of the infant (Loh and Vostanis 2004).

These changes are important because the earliest years of life are a critical period when young children are making emotional attachments and forming the crucial first relationships that lay the foundations for future mental health (Bowlby 1969, 1988; Sroufe 1996; Steele 1996; Stern 1998). It is the quality of the parent–infant relationship in particular, that will create the conditions for establishing healthy patterns of functioning (Stein *et al.* 1991; Murray *et al.* 1996). Murray has demonstrated that the more the parent is sensitive in identifying the infant's signals and cues at two months the better the outcomes for cognitive and emotional development (Murray 1992). Postnatal depression is strongly associated with poorer outcomes in both emotional (Caplan *et al.* 1989) and cognitive functioning in children (Cogill *et al.* 1986), and a healthy couple relationship has also been shown to impact on the bonding and attachment processes that are fundamental to a child's short- and long-term health and well being (see for example Heinecke and Guthrie 1992).

Recent research has added a biological basis to the argument for the importance of early interactions and the advent of new techniques for imaging the functioning of the brain has indicated that: the infant's transactions with the early socio-emotional environment indelibly influence the evolution of brain structures responsible for the individual's socio-emotional functioning for the rest of the lifespan' (Schore 1994, p. 540).

Support in pregnancy: the role of health visitors
The role of health visitors

There is an urgent need for health visitors to begin focusing on supporting parents during the transition to parenthood, and on promoting the parent–infant relationship in a way that is consistent with research about the benefits of such support for parents, and thereby for infant development. A number of recent policy documents have highlighted health visitors as being the prime group to support parents during this period (e.g. Department of Health 1999; Department for Education and Skills 2001).

What should health visitors be doing?

The prenatal phase

Health visitors currently provide very little support to pregnant women and their partners. The reason for this is that at a professional level, pregnancy is viewed as being the terrain of the midwife. There is increasing evidence to suggest, however, that midwives and health visitors should be working together during this period, not only to address the many difficulties that may arise during this time, but also to help parents without specific difficulties to address the many physical and psychological changes that occur.

During pregnancy health visitors are ideally placed to work alongside midwives to identify specific problems that parents may be experiencing at this time. This includes problems such as antenatal anxiety or depression, dysfunctional attitudes towards the pregnancy or baby, drug and alcohol abuse or other problems such as domestic violence. Health visitors may also use this period to help to prepare first-time parents for some of the emotional changes that will take place in terms of the parent–parent relationship, and for some of the changes that will be necessary following the birth of the baby.

A new method of healthcare workers such as midwives and health visitors identifying families in need of extra support during the antenatal period has recently been developed. The European Early Promotion Project (EEPP) consists of trained primary healthcare workers (most of whom are health visitors in the UK) conducting 'promotional inter-views' immediately before and after all new births. The aim of the interview is to identify women who are experiencing problems antenatally and/or postnatally with a view to addressing such problems in order to promote positive interaction between parent and child during infancy and childhood. For example, the health visitor might as ask part of the antenatal interview, 'How did you feel when you learned that you were pregnant'? This provides the opportunity for the health visitor to endorse any positive feelings or to explore and talk further about any negative feelings. The health visitor then works intensively using parent counselling techniques with those families identified using the interviews, as being in need of further support.

This method of intervening during the perinatal period is currently being evaluated in a number of European countries including the UK (Puura et al. 2002). Early evidence shows that primary healthcare workers found the training useful in increasing their understanding and skills, in addition to improving their sensitivity to families' psychoso-cial needs and their accuracy in identifying psychosocial problems. Families were also significantly more satisfied with services (ibid).

Parenting programmes are another means of intervening with parents during the peri-natal period. Parents in Partnership Parent–infant Network (PIPPIN) is a group-based parenting programme that is provided by health visitors and midwives to parents-to-be during the antenatal and immediate postnatal period. The aim of this programme is specifically to support and promote the transition to parenthood. It is provided to groups of first-time parents for a period of 2 hours during pregnancy and postnatally with one visit at home following birth—a total of 35 hours of support. The programme focuses on parent–infant communication and relationships, as opposed to the type of topics that are typically included in antenatal classes such as the 'mechanics' of labour, delivery, and infant care. It is based on a range of activities that are designed to raise the self-confidence and self-esteem of parents about their own parenting abilities and to promote the kind of nurturing parenting that research suggests is more likely to result in healthy attachment relationships between parents and their infants

The results of a controlled study showed a significant increase in psychological health of parents, increased confidence as a parent, increased satisfaction with the couple and parent–infant relationship, and more nurturing child-centred attitudes as regards infant care (Parr 1998).

Birth and the postnatal phase

Following the birth, health visitors have a central role in promoting bonding on the part of the mother and attachment in the infant. The first year of life is particularly important for the optimal development of infants who have three broad developmental requirements. Social and emotional competence requires that they are able to develop trust and to become securely attached. Intellectual competence requires that the infant is alert and curious, and behavioural competence requires that the infant gradually learns to control their impulses.

Three types of parenting have been identified as being important in meeting these developmental needs. Nurturance, particularly the quality of the parent–infant relationship (e.g. sensitivity, attunement, bonding, and continuity of care). More recent research has also highlighted the importance of maternal reflective function. This suggests that the capacity of the parents to experience the baby as a 'mentalizing' and 'intentional' being rather than simply viewing them in terms of physical characteristics or behaviour, is what helps the child to develop an understanding of mental states in other people and to regulate their own internal experiences (Fonagy et al. 2002). Verbal and cognitive stimulation are also important, including verbal responsiveness and interaction, being read to, and the provision of an appropriate physical environment (e.g. acceptance of the child, the provision of learning materials, parental involvement, and variety of experience). Finally, the parent should also offer behavioural and emotional regulation through the provision of positive experiences, in addition to positive discipline. All of these forms of parenting are of course interlinked. For example, the type of parenting or care that promotes the development of trust and attachment (e.g. nurturance) also meets the infant's needs for intellectual development and impulse control.

Health visitors are ideally placed to provide parents with the sort of support that can help them to provide infants with this sort of care, and to identify any specific problems, such as postnatal depression, which may interfere with effective caregiving. Not only are these sorts of care not always known about 'naturally' by parents, but the place where many such parenting skills were traditionally learned (e.g. the extended family) has been transformed, with many families comprising just one parent, and isolation and loneliness being a common experience (Parentline Plus 2005).

All of the methods of promoting mother–infant interaction described below are aimed at enhancing the parent–infant interaction cycle by increasing the parents' sensitivity to their infant, improving their ability to empathize and thereby think about their baby in more positive ways, and by providing concrete ways of responding to the infant productively (Davis *et al.* 2002).

The Brazelton Neonatal Behavioural Assessment Scale (NBAS) (Brazelton 1995) can be used in hospital or at home, and involves the health visitor demonstrating the infant's behavioural characteristics to the mother and highlighting the baby's capabilities. This technique is used to increase the parents' interest in and knowledge about their baby, and also helps the parent to get to know about things such as their baby's characteristic body tone, how they are soothed, areas in which the baby interacts positively and areas in which they are less strong (Rauh *et al.* 1988). Parents are sometimes taught to perform the activities themselves. The use of this technique in hospital and at home with parents of low birthweight babies has been shown to improve maternal representations and infant cognition (ibid).

Once mother and baby are home there are a number of things that the health visitor can be doing to promote sensitive caregiving and to help the new parents get to learn about their 'social baby'. Many of these interventions are quick and simple, but can reap big rewards in terms of promoting good parent–infant relations. For example, increasing the amount of physical contact between the mother and infant can improve their relationship. One study showed that increased physical contact through the use of infant carriers improved maternal sensitivity and infant attachment in black and Hispanic first-time mothers (Anisfeld *et al.* 1990). Teaching mothers how to massage their infants may also be helpful, particularly if mothers are experiencing postnatal depression. One study, for example, showed that the use of infant massage resulted in less distress behaviour in the infant, less disturbed sleep patterns in infants, improvements in mothers' moods and behaviours, and improved mother–infant interactions (Onozawa *et al.* 2001).

Other methods of promoting mother–infant interaction include the use of songs and music, and baby dance. PEEP (Peers Early Education Programme) helps mothers to learn about songs, music and books, and is based on the growing body of evidence that links the early development of language, literacy, and personal and social development with outcomes relating to higher educational attainment, improved behaviour, and crime prevention. The aim of PEEP is to promote learning and cognitive development during the first few years of a child's life. Parents are invited to weekly group sessions where they are offered mutual support and group-based interactive activities with their baby including sharing a book everyday, songs and rhymes, listening games, playing with shapes, and using the library. A longitudinal study comparing a cohort of 300 babies from a PEEP area with a sample from a matched non-peep area showed improved verbal comprehension, vocabulary, concepts about print, phonological awareness, writing, early number concepts, and self-esteem (Evangelou and Sylva 2002).

Baby dance involves mother and baby engaging in a structured series of interactions, which the baby is able eventually to anticipate. This provides mothers and infants with the opportunity for joyful exchanges (Maattenen 2001).

This is also a period during which health visitors are approached by parents who are experiencing sleeping, eating, toileting, and behaviour problems. The Solihull Approach (Douglas 2000) is spreading rapidly throughout the UK and provides health visitors with a new means of addressing these problems based on the concepts of containment, reciprocity, and behaviour management. This involves health visitors addressing infant problems by focusing on the *relationship between the parent and infant*, and by the health visitor helping to contain the parents' anxieties. Preliminary evaluation suggests that this approach can improve the consistency of approach of health visitors and increase confidence in their skills (Douglas and Ginty 2001) and that it may be effective in improving the presenting problem and reducing parental anxiety about such problems (Douglas and Brennan 2004).

The Sunderland Infant programme at Sure Start Thorney Close offers an intervention aimed at the early identification of attachment problems and the promotion of sensitive parenting. The health visitor screens all consenting new mother–infant dyads by videotaping a 3-minute period of the mother and infant interacting together. The videotape is viewed by the health visitor alongside a clinical psychologist in order to identify parents who are having problems in providing sensitive parenting, e.g. they are usually either too intrusive or too passive. Mothers who are identified as having difficulties in providing sensitive parenting are offered developmental guidance or interaction guidance by the health visitor. This involves the health visitor watching the tape with the mother and identifying areas of strength in order to encourage more sensitive caregiving. Reports from the health visitors working on this project indicate that the process of helping mothers and infants synchronize their interactions, has been paralleled by professionals developing more sensitive relationships with the families. Anecdotally, health visitors have reported having better tools to do the job thereby enabling them to be more skilled in encouraging sensitive parental responses, and a lessening of infant feeding and sleeping difficulties after the intervention.

Parents who are identified as having more significant problems are offered parent–infant psychotherapy. Family or couple therapy may also be offered if appropriate. The aim of the parent–infant psychotherapy is to help the mother to resolve issues surrounding trauma, loss, and attachment. The aim is also to help the mother reflect on her own experiences of being parented.

This intervention is currently being evaluated and early findings demonstrate a significant increase in maternal sensitivity and in infant co-operativeness (Svanberg, personal communication).

Perhaps most importantly, health visitors should remember that every interaction with the mother during the postnatal period is an opportunity to (1) assess how things are progressing in terms of bonding and attachment, and (2) to increase maternal sensitivity by helping parents to get to know their 'social baby'.

Hard-to-reach and 'vulnerable' parents

While home visiting programmes are frequently less effective with vulnerable parents than centre-based programmes, they can nevertheless be an effective way of reaching families who will not attend centre-based programmes.

Home visiting primarily consists of visits to the mother in the home, but is different from the sort of home visiting that health visitors typically undertake in that the visits are delivered over an extensive period of time (often up to 2 years), on a fairly frequent basis (sometimes weekly), to families who have been identified as being particularly vulnerable (i.e. mental health problems, domestic violence, drug abuse, etc.). They also involve the use of particular techniques such as listening skills (Wiggins *et al.* 2004) or cognitive and behavioural approaches (Barlow *et al.* 2004). Most health visitors who have undertaken this role to date have been specially trained for the work (Percy and Barker 1986; Morrell *et al.* 2000; Wiggins *et al.* 2004; Barlow *et al.* 2005).

The most recently published Health Development Agency review of the effectiveness of home visiting programmes delivered during the antenatal and postnatal period showed that they can be effective in improving a range of important outcomes for mothers and babies including cognitive development, accidental injury, and the detection and management of postnatal depression (Bull 2004). The authors also concluded, however, that there were important outcomes for which the evidence was inconclusive, including child abuse, uptake of immunization, and hospital admissions.

While recent experience of the use of home visiting programmes in the UK has not proved to be effective in achieving many of these outcomes (see for example, Morrell *et al.* 2001; MacAuley *et al.* 2004; Wiggins *et al.* 2004; Barlow *et al.* 2005), one study showed that while both home visitors and health visitors delivering routine services, were able to identify families in which child abuse was an issue, there were significantly more infants removed from the home in the home visiting group than in the routine health visiting control group (6% compared with none). This suggests that home visitors were better placed to continue monitoring the lives of these high-risk babies and to intervene to remove the infant where necessary. The results also showed better maternal sensitivity in the home-visited mothers and more co-operativeness in their infants (Barlow *et al.* 2005).

In addition, participating health visitors contrasted the 'crisis management' approach of routine health visiting with home visiting, which was depicted as allowing health visitors to work in accordance with a more preventive model of care. Specifically, in contrast with their routine work, health visitors felt that an intensive approach helped them to be more focused on facilitating change, relationship-building, and on the needs of both mother and baby including the mother–baby relationship. They felt that they were less directive, and that the time available to develop trusting relationships with families made it easier for them to challenge particular attitudes and behaviours that might be deleterious to the well-being of the infant, in addition to being able to address issues in accordance with the readiness of family members. The participating home visitors also perceived themselves to have made an important difference in terms of a number of key aspects of maternal and child functioning.

In-depth interviews with women who had received the home visiting service showed a high level of satisfaction across the board, and provided moving testimony concerning the impact of this intervention on the lives of vulnerable women and children. A number of themes were identified that showed that despite their initial concerns and negative preconceptions about health and social service professionals, participating women greatly valued the relationship with their home visitor and identified a number of ways in which they had benefited. These included increased confidence, improved mental health, improved relationship including closeness with baby, fewer child behaviour problems in the infant's siblings, and changes in their attitudes toward professionals. Although some participants clearly resented the involvement of social services, no adverse effects of the intervention were reported.

The evidence

The findings of two recent systematic reviews of the evidence about the effectiveness of interventions during pregnancy and early childhood suggest that early intervention programmes should concentrate on enhancing individual and family strengths not just focusing on risk factors (Barnes and Lagevardi 2003; Bakermans-Kranenburg et al. 2003). They recommend the use of an ecological approach that involves intervening at a structural level in addition to trying to change individual behaviour, and to match individual need with provision.

These reviews suggest that the best results are achieved with at-risk, clinically referred and first-time parents especially where they are directed at both parent and child (ibid). Many universal approaches such as baby carriers and infant massage can, however, be inexpensive, quick to deliver to large groups of parents, and highly productive in terms of outcome.

These reviews also suggest that the most effective interventions begin during pregnancy and continue into the postnatal period, although one of the reviews also showed that intervening during the postnatal period only, was sometimes the most effective approach. Both reviews show that the most effective way of intervening is with fewer high-intensity rather than more low-intensity components.

A new way of working

Many of the above innovative interventions are being delivered effectively by health visitors. In almost all cases the delivery of the intervention has involved the health visitor in undertaking additional training. This suggests that the current model of training is inadequate in providing health visitors with the sort of skills that both the research evidence and the requirements of their new role, indicate as being necessary.

For experienced health visitors, this may mean being willing to take part in brief training programmes that will provide them with additional evidence-based skills that have been shown to help them to be even more effective in supporting parents during the transition to parenthood. It may also mean structuring their workload in a way that permits them to work in this way. For example, the development of skill-mix teams may provide health visitors with the opportunity to share skills with other workers (e.g. infant massage) or to offload routine tasks that could be effectively undertaken by less skilled professionals in order to enable them to undertake for example, the delivery of more intensive home visiting to vulnerable families, or the conduct of promotional interviews with all new parents-to-be in order to identify potential problems.

There is little evidence about the effectiveness of routine health visiting, and the opportunity for health visitors to engage more effectively with families has now arrived. Perhaps most importantly, health visitors need to shift their focus away from physical issues, to the emotional needs of parents individually and as a couple, and to the parent–infant relationship. Bonding, attachment, parental sensitivity, and the social baby are key words that should guide *every* interaction with new parents, no matter how mundane or brief. One simple explanation to a new parent of what a baby's action means, could be the difference between a lack of knowledge, and a whole new way for a parent to understand and enjoy their baby, with very important consequences for the baby's future health.

References

Acheson D (1998). *Independent Inquiry into Inequalities in Health Report.* The Stationery Office, London.

Anisfeld E, Casper V, Nozyce M, Cunningham NL (1990). Does infant carrying promote attachment? An experimental study of the effects of increased physical contact on the development of attachment. *Child Development* **61**(5): 1617–1627.

Bakermans-Kranenburg MJ, Ijzendoorn MH, Juffer F (2003). Less is more: meta-analyses of sensitivity and attachment interventions in early childhood. *Psychological Bulletin* **129**(2): 195–215.

Ballard CG, Davis R, Cullen PC, Mohan RN, Dean C (1994). Prevalence of postnatal psychiatric morbidity in mothers and fathers. *British Journal of Psychiatry* **164**(6): 782–788.

Barlow J, Davis H, Stewart-Brown S (2005). *The Oxfordshire Home Visiting Study.* Internal report, University of Warwick, Coventry.

Barlow J, Jarrett P, Mockford C, Kirkpatrick S, Davis H, Stewart-Brown S (2006). The role of home visiting in improving parenting and health in families at risk of abuse and neglect: Results of a multicentre randomised controlled trial and economic evaluation. *Archives of Disease in Childhood.*

Barnes J, Lagevardi (2003). *From pregnancy to Early Childhood.* London: Mental Health Foundation.

Belsky J, Kelly J (1994). *The Transition to Parenthood: How a First Child Changes a Marriage.* Vermillion, London.

Bowlby J (1969). *Attachment and Loss*, Vol. 1. *Attachment.* Hogarth Press, London.

Bowlby J (1988). *A Secure Base.* Routledge, London.

Brazelton TB (1995). Neonatal Behavioural Assessment Scale Clinics. In *Development Medicine,* No. 50. Blackwell, London.

Bronfenbrenner U (1979). Ecological systems theory. *Annals of Child Development* **6**: 187–251.

Bull J, McCormick G, Swann C, Mulvihill C (2004). *Ante- and post-natal home-visiting programmes: a review of reviews.* Health Development Agency, London.

Caplan H, Cogill S, Alexandra H, Robson K, Katz R, Kumar R (1989). Maternal depression and the emotional development of the child. *British Journal of Psychiatry* **154**: 818–823.

Chalmers B, Meyer D (1994). Preparing women for pregnancy and parenthood: a cross-cultural study. *Community Practitioner* **6**: 27–42.

Clulow C (1991). Partners becoming parents: a question of difference. *Infant Mental Health Journal* **12**(3): 256–65.

Cogill SR, Caplan HL, Alexandra H, Robson KM, Kumar R (1986). Impact of maternal postnatal depression on cognitive development in young children. *British Medical Journal*, **292**: 1165–1167.

Cowan C, Cowan P (1992). *When Partners Become Parents.* Erlbaum, London.

Cowan P, Heatherington M (1991). *Family Transitions.* Lawrence Erlbaum Associates, Hillsdale, NJ.

Davis H, Day C, Bidmead C (2002). *Working in Partnership with Parents: The Parent Adviser Approach.* London: The Psychological Corporation.

Davis Floyd R (1992). *Birth as an American Rite of Passage.* University of California Press, Berkeley, CA.

Department of Health (1999). *Making a Difference: Strengthening the Nursing, Midwifery and Community Nursing Contribution to Health and Health Care.* The Stationery Office, London.

Department for Education and Skills (2001). *Supporting Families.* The Stationery Office, London.

Department for Education and Skills (2004). *Every Child Matters*. London: Stationery Office.

Douglas H, Brennan A (2004). Containment, reciprocity and behaviour management: preliminary evaluation of a brief early intervention for families with infants and young children. *International Journal of Infant Observation* **7**: 89–107.

Douglas H, Ginty M (2001). The Solihull Approach: evaluation of changes in the practice of health visitors. *Community Practitioner* **74**: 222–224.

Evangelou M, Sylva K (2002). *The Effects of PEEP on Children's Developmental: Progress Towards Effective Early Childhood Interventions*. DfES, London.

Evans J, Heron J, Francomb H, Oke S, Golding J (2001). Cohort study of depressed mood during pregnancy and after childbirth. *British Medical Journal* **323**: 257–260.

Expert Maternity Group (1993). *Changing Childbirth* (Parts 1 and 2). HMSO, London.

Fonagy P, Gergely G, Jurist E, Target M (2002). *Affect Regulation, Mentalisation, and the Development of the Self*. Analytic Press, New York.

Glover V, O'Connor T (2002). Effects of antenatal stress and anxiety: implications for development and psychiatry. *British Journal of Psychiatry* **180**(5): 389–395.

Hedin LW, Grimstad H, Moller A, Schei B, Janson PO (1999). Prevalence of physical and sexual abuse before and during pregnancy amoung Swedish Couples. *Acta Obstricia et Gynecologica Scandinavica* **78**(4): 310–315.

Heinecke MH, Guthrie DG (1992) Stability and change in husband-wife adaptation, and the development of the positive parent-child relationship. *Infant Behavior and Development*, **15**: 109–127.

Helman C (2000). *Culture, Health and Illness*, (4th edn). Arnold, London.

Kitzinger S (1982). The social context of birth: some comparisons between childbirth in Jamaica and Britain. In MacCormack C (ed.), *Ethnography of Fertility and Birth*. Academic Press, London, pp. 181–203.

Kumar R, Mordecai Robson K (1984). A prospective study of emotional disorders in childbearing women. *British Journal of Psychiatry* **144**: 35–47.

Le Master E (1957). Parenthood as a crisis. *Marriage and Family Living* **19**: 352–355.

Loh CC, Vostanis P (2004). Perceived mother-infant relationship difficulties in postnatal depression. *Infant and Child Development* **13**(2): 159–171.

Maattanen K (2001). *Dialogical Baby Dance—A Parent's Guide*. South-EasternHealth Centre at Herttoneime.

McAuley C, Knapp M, Beecham J, McCurry and Sleed (2004). *Evaluating the Outcomes and Costs of Home-Start Support to Young Families Experiencing Stress: A Comparative Cross Nation Study*. York: Joseph Rowntree Foundation.

Miller T (2000). Losing the plot: narrative construction and longitudinal childbirth research. *Qualitative Health Research* **10**(3): 309–323.

Morrell CJ, Siby H, Sewart P, Walters S Morgan A (2000). Costs and effectiveness of community postnatal support workers: randomised controlled trial. *British Medical Journal* **321**: 593–598.

Murray L (1992). The impact of postnatal depression on infant development. *Journal of Child Psychology and Psychiatry* **33**: 543–561.

Murray L, Fiori-Cowley A, Hooper R (1996). The impact of post-natal depression and associated adversity on early mother-infant interactions and later infant outcomes. *Child Development* **67**: 2512–2526.

Nolan ML (1997). Antenatal education—where next? *Journal of Advanced Nursing* **25**: 1198–1204.

Onozawa K, Glover V, Adams D, Modi N, Kumar RC (2001). Infant massage improves mother-infant interaction for mothers with postnatal depression. *Journal of Affective Disorders* **63**(1–3): 201–207.

Parentline Plus (2005). www. Parentlineplus.org.uk, accessed 8 March 2005.

Parr M (1998). A new approach to parent education. *British Journal of Midwifery* **6**(3): 160–165.

Percy P, Barker W (1986). The child development programme. *Midwife, Health Visitor and Community Nurse* **22**: 235–240.

PEEP (2000). *Learning Together With Babies.* PEEP, Oxford.

Puura, Kaija; Davis, Hilton; Cox, Antony; Tsiantis, John; Tamminen, Tuula; Ispanovic-Radojkovic, Veronika; Paradisiotous, Anna; Mantymaa, Mirjami; Roberts, Rosemarie; Dragonas, Thalia; Layiou-Lignos, Effie; Dusoir, Tony; Rudic, Nenad; Tenjovic, Lazar; Vizacou, Semeli (2005). The European Early Promotion Project: Description of the Service and Evaluation Study. *International Journal of Mental Health Promotion.* Vol 7(1) Feb 2005, 17–30.

Raphael-Leff J (2001). *Pregnancy: The Inside Story.* Karnac Books, London.

Rauh V, Achenbach T, Nurcombe B, Howell C, Teti D (1988). Minimizing adverse effects of low birthweight: four-year results of an early intervention program. *Child Development* **59**: 544–553.

Royal College of Paediatrics and Child Health (2002). *Helpful Parenting.* Royal College of Paediatrics and Child Health, London.

Schore A. (1994). *After Regulation and the Origin of the Self: The Neurobiology of Emotional Development.* Erlbaum, Hilsdale, NJ.

Sroufe A (1996). *Emotional Development: The organisation of emotional life in the early years.* Cambridge University Press.

Steele H, Steele M, Fonagy P (1996). Associations among attachment classifications of mothers, fathers and their infants. *Child Development* **6:** 541–555.

Stein A, Gath D, Bucher J, Bond A, Day A, Cooper P (1991). The relationship between postnatal depression and mother-child interaction. *British Journal of Psychiatry* **158**: 46–52.

Stern D (1986). *The Motherhood Constellation.* Karnac Books, London.

Stern D (1998). *The Interpersonal World of the Infant.* London: Karnac.

Svanberg PO (personal communication). *Promoting Attachment Security in Primary Prevention Using Video Feed-Back: the Sunderland Infant Programme.*

Taylor A (1985). Antenatal classes and the consumer: mothers' and fathers' views. *Health Education Journal* **44**(2): 79–82.

Wickberg B, Hwang C (1997). Screening for postnatal depression in a population-based Swedish sample. *Acta Psychiatrica Scandinavica* **95**: 62–66.

Wiggins M, Oakley A, Roberts I, Turner H, Rajan L, Austerberry H, Mujica R, Mugford M (2004). *Postnatal Support for Mothers Living in Disadvantaged Areas: a Randomised Controlled Trial and Economic Evaluation.* Health Technology Assessment. York.

Winterton (1992). House of Commons Health Committee, 2nd Report, Maternity Services, Vol 1, HMSO.

Woollett A, Parr M (1997). Psychological tasks for women and men in the post-partum. *Journal of Reproductive and Infant Psychology* **15**: 159–183.

Chapter 27

Immunization

David Elliman and Helen Bedford

Immunization is one of the most cost-effective health procedures currently available. In countries with effective vaccination programmes with high uptake of vaccines, the incidence of vaccine preventable diseases and the associated morbidity and mortality has decreased to low levels. For example, polio has been eradicated from the Western hemisphere and the prospects for global eradication look good. As a result of a two-dose programme of MMR vaccination, indigenous measles, mumps, and rubella have been eliminated from Finland (Peltola *et al*.1994).

Delivery of immunization should be relatively simple as it is offered to the whole population of children as part of a standard national programme. There are very few contraindications. Parents often find the experience of having their child immunized distressing. This may the first time they have seen their child in pain and professionals are not always sensitive to the anxiety parents' feel. This, coupled with well-publicized scares about the safety of vaccines makes it extremely important that primary healthcare professionals have sufficient knowledge and confidence to respond effectively and empathetically to parents' concerns.

Current programme

The guidance in the current publication 'Immunization Against Infectious Disease' should form the basis of immunization practice. The web based version is regularly updated (http://www.dh.gov.uk/PolicyAndGuidance/HealthAndSocialCareTopics/GreenBook/fs/en). The last hard copy was published in December 2006.

The routine schedule changes over time with the addition of new vaccines or extra doses. Recent changes to the routine schedule:

1. Although very safe, oral polio vaccine (OPV) can occasionally result in vaccine associated paralytic polio (VAPP) in recipients (at a rate of about 1 in 1 million) or in unimmunized contacts of a recently immunized individual, most commonly through failing to wash hands following nappy changing. OPV boosts immunity to polio in the community and also prevents transmission of wild virus. When polio poses a significant threat, this is a considerable advantage. However as polio has become rare and the threat of imported cases is extremely low, the risk of vaccine-associated paralytic polio (VAPP) becomes less acceptable and the pressure to substitute inactivated polio vaccine (IPV) increases. It is on this basis that the policy in the UK changed in 2004.

2. At the same time, a five-component acellular pertussis vaccine with efficacy similar to the traditional whole cell vaccine has become available. Unlike the three component vaccine, this can be mixed with the *Haemophilus influenzae* type b vaccine without any loss in efficacy.

3. Universal BCG vaccination that was previously administered to school children will be replaced by a more targeted approach where individuals at high risk will be identified and vaccinated

4. From September 2006, pneumococcal vaccination will form part of the childhood immunization programme; in addition, it will be offered to all children under the age of 2 years as part of a catch up campaign.

The currently recommended programme (Autumn 2006) for the UK is as follows (Table 27.1):

   High-risk groups:

1. In addition to the above, bacillus Calmette-Guérin (BCG) vaccine should be given to all infants who live in areas of the UK where the annual incidence of tuberculosis is 40/100 000 or greater.

2. Babies born to mothers who are chronically infected with hepatitis B virus or to mothers who have had acute hepatitis B during pregnancy. This involves a dose of hepatitis B vaccine given at birth with further doses at 1, 2, and 12 months.

Table 27.1 The currently recommended programme (Autumn 2006) for the UK

When vaccineshould be given	Vaccine	Administration
2 months	Diphtheria/tetanus/pertussis/polio/Hib (DTaP/IPV/Hib)	One injection
	Pneumoccocal (PCV)	One injection
3 months	Diphtheria/tetanus/pertussis/polio/Hib (DTaP/IPV/Hib)	One injection
	Meningococcal C (MenC)	One injection
4 months	Diphtheria/tetanus/pertussis/polio/Hib (DTaP/IPV/Hib)	One injection
	Meningococcal C (MenC)	One injection
	Pneumococcal (PCV)	One injection
12 months	Hib/MenC	One injection
13 months	Measles, mumps, rubella (MMR)	One injection
	Pneumococcal(PCV)	One injection
3 years 4 months–5 years	Diphtheria/tetanus/pertussis/polio (DTaP/IPV) or (dTaP/IPV)	One injection
	Measles, mumps, rubella (MMR)	One injection
13 years–18 years	Tetanus, diphtheria, polio (Td/IPV)	One injection

aP, acellular pertussis; Hib, *Haemophilus inflenzae* type b; IPV, inactivated polio vaccine; Td, Tetanus + low dose diptheria vaccine.

The likely adverse effects and contraindications are to some extent predictable depending on whether a vaccine is live or 'dead'. It is not uncommon for vaccines to cause mild local reactions and systemic upset. Live vaccines may also produce a mild form of the disease. It is important that parents are given information on the likely adverse events and how to manage them.

Contraindications and children with 'problem histories'
General contraindications

As immunization is an elective procedure, it is advised that except under rare circumstances, no vaccine should be given when an individual has an acute illness with fever or systemic upset. However, there is no evidence that doing so either exacerbates the acute illness, gives rise to an increased incidence of adverse reactions or renders the vaccine less effective. Minor illnesses, such as an upper respiratory tract infection, are not a contraindication. A vaccine, like any medication, should not be given to a pregnant woman unless there are very pressing reasons. None of the vaccines in current use have been shown to harm the fetus, but with some there is only limited experience (Tookey *et al.* 1991 Bar-Oz *et al.* 2004). On the other hand, tetanus vaccine is routinely given to pregnant women in many countries to prevent neonatal tetanus and 'flu vaccine is frequently given to pregnant women in USA.

A vaccine is contraindicated if a person has previously had an anaphylactic reaction to the vaccine or a constituent.

Table 27.2 Types of vaccine

	Live (attenuated)	Inactivated, component or toxoid
Vaccines given as part of the routine childhood programme	BCG Measles/Mumps/Rubella (MMR)	Diphtheriapart *Haemophilus influenzae* type b Meningococcal C conjugate Pertussis (acellular) Polio (inactivated—IPV) Tetanus
Other vaccines	Polio (oral—OPV) Smallpox Typhoid (oral) Varicella Yellow fever	Anthrax Cholera Hepatitis A Hepatitis B Influenza Japanese encephalitis Meningococcal A&C Meningococcal A, C, W135 & Y Plague Pneumococcal (plain and conjugate) Rabies Tick-borne encephalitis Typhoid (inactivated)

Live vaccines

In some immunocompromised people, administration of a live vaccine may result in severe adverse reactions such as a severe form of the disease being vaccinated against. Such patients include those with congenital and acquired immunodeficiencies; those on immunosuppressive treatment, including high doses of systemic corticosteroids; and those who have had a bone marrow transplant. However, it is not always clear-cut and whether or not a vaccine should be given depends on both the particular vaccine and the nature of the immunosuppression. For example, MMR should certainly be given to someone with asymptomatic HIV infection and possibly to someone with AIDS. This is a complex field and advice should be sought from the consultant looking after the patient. More detail can be found in *Immunization of the Immunocompromised Child* (Royal College of Paediatrics and Child Health 2002).

Pertussis

The only absolute contraindications to the vaccine are the same as for any killed vaccine. In the past a family or personal history of febrile convulsions or cerebral damage in the neonatal period were considered 'problem histories' and reasons for 'special consideration'; this has confused both parents and professionals. Children with well controlled epilepsy should have the vaccine. Those who have what is termed 'an evolving neurological disorder' should have the primary course of vaccination postponed until the condition is stable (Department of Health 1996). These children will be under the care of a specialist. Administration of the meningococcal C vaccine does not need to be delayed.

MMR vaccine

Single measles vaccine was used in UK from 1968, until 1988, when it was replaced by the combined MMR vaccine. Before the use of MMR vaccine, rubella vaccine was offered selectively to schoolgirls and susceptible adult women to provide them with individual protection against rubella infection in pregnancy. Although this policy resulted in a reduction in the number of cases of congenital rubella syndrome as well as terminations of pregnancy for proven infection or contact with a case, some women remained susceptible. As rubella is a childhood disease, it continued to circulate and cases of congenital rubella syndrome were not totally eliminated. The rationale behind the introduction of MMR vaccine at 12 months was to wipe out the disease entirely. Mumps vaccine had never been used routinely.

The contraindications to MMR are as for any live vaccine with the exception of HIV. Whether the vaccine should be given to a child with AIDS depends on the individual case.

About 5% of recipients of a first dose of MMR vaccine experience mild measles 5–11 days after the vaccine. Mild mumps may occur 21 days after vaccine and mild rubella some time later. None of these are transmissible. More rarely, convulsions occur at a rate of about 1 in every 3000 doses and idiopathic thrombocytopenic purpura at a rate of 1 in every 32 000 (Miller *et al.* 2001).

About 5–10% of individuals given a first dose of MMR vaccine do not produce protective antibodies to measles. Since 95% of the population have to be immune to prevent outbreaks of the disease, from 1996 it has been recommended that two doses of MMR vaccine are given. The rate of seroconversion after a second dose is very high, with 90% of those who did not respond the first time gaining protection. The rate of adverse reactions is much lower after the second dose than after the first (Virtanen *et al.* 2000). In countries where a two-dose programme has been in place for some time and high uptakes have been achieved, notably Finland, all three infections have been eliminated (Peltola *et al.* 1994). Even in the USA, the overwhelming majority of these infections are imported. Until 2006, there had been a significant reduction in the numbers of reported cases in the UK and only one death attributed to an acute attack of measles since 1992 (Health Protection Agency 2006a). However in 2006, there was one death and more cases of measles than there had been in a whole year for the last decade. This was a direct result of the 'MMR scare'.

Travel vaccines

Foreign travel potentially exposes children to infections that are uncommon in the UK. They may require vaccines not routinely recommended in the UK. This subject is complex and advice should not be given lightly as the risks of some diseases varies over time and it can be difficult to keep up to date. Whether a particular vaccine is indicated will depend on the age of the children, the countries being visited, the part of the country in which the child will stay, the type of accommodation (especially eating arrangements), the duration of the visit, the time of year, and any underlying medical disorders. Advice should be based on the most up to date information available and should also include topics such as the care of food and drink, and where appropriate, avoidance of malaria risks and malaria prophylaxis. Apart from advice from the Department of Health (2001), there are a number of useful internet sites (National Travel Health Network and Centre 2004).

New developments
Pneumococcal vaccine

A conjugate pneumococcal vaccine is now recommended by the Department of Health for all children. It is given to ill children under 2 years old and to at-risk children up to 5 years old. Children over 2 years old who are at-risk should be given the plain poly sac-charide vaccine. This will mean that children at-risk, aged 2 to 5 years will receive both types of vaccine. Further details are in the Green Book (Department of Health 2006).

Varicella zoster

A live vaccine to protect against varicella zoster infection is available for use in children at high risk of complications or severe disease but has not been licensed for routine use. If it were to be introduced into the routine schedule, considerable thought would need to be given to the best timing for this vaccine, as the previous scare over the safety of the combined MMR vaccine, may preclude its inclusion in a quadrivalent vaccine.

Meningococcal B

Meningococcal B infection remains the commonest cause of septicaemia and bacterial meningitis in the UK and a vaccine is highly desirable. However, it is proving challenging to develop such a vaccine and it will be some years before it becomes available. It is important to emphasize, when giving the meningococcal C vaccine, that it only protects against one form of meningitis and parents should still be alert to the possibility that an ill fully vaccinated child may still develop meningitis.

Organization of services

An effective immunization programme depends on highly organized services. At practice level, one individual should be identified as being responsible for immunization. This individual should be the key person who arranges appointments, orders supplies, and ensures they are properly stored. Recording of vaccines given is vitally important and this should include recording the information in the clinical record and on the child's personal child health record (PCHR) as well as communicating the information to the child health system.

Talking with parents, effectively, empathetically, with enough time and ensuring they have sufficient information to make an informed decision about immunization is a key component of any immunization service. When it is not clear whether or not a child should receive a vaccine, or where parents require more in depth discussion referral for a specialist opinion should be made rather than denying immunization.

Within each Primary Care Trust there should also be an immunization lead who fulfils the role of the former District Immunization Co-ordinator (Elliman and Moreton 2000).

Some questions parents ask

• **I have read about concerns over safety of the MMR vaccine. Is there any reason to be worried?**

In 1998 a paper was published in which it was suggested that autism and bowel problems were linked (Wakefield *et al.* 1998). Many parents remembered their children's difficulties beginning soon after they had had MMR vaccine. The authors were very clear in stating: 'We did not prove an association between MMR vaccine and the syndrome described'. Subsequently, three of the authors have voiced their concerns that there may be a link and advised the use of separate antigens rather than combined MMR vaccine. This view has received disproportionate publicity and understandably many parents and health professionals are now confused and concerned about the safety of the combined vaccine. Since publication of this paper a significant body of research has failed to find any evidence for a link between MMR vaccine and autism or bowel disease (Madson *et al.* 2002; Taylor *et al.* 2002; Anon 2003). Despite this the uptake of MMR has been adversely affected with outbreaks of disease. At the time of writing uptake of the vaccine is 79% overall, with lower uptake particularly in inner cities and there is evidence that measles is on the brink of becoming endemic again (Health Protection Agency 2003; Jansen *et al.* 2003).

♦ **My child is allergic to eggs. Can he still have the MMR vaccine?**

MMR vaccines in use in most countries contain small quantities of egg and so there has been concern about giving the vaccine to children who are allergic to egg for fear that they might have a serious reaction to it. However, there is considerable experience of using the vaccine in such children without any serious adverse effects. Therefore, most experts would advise that the vaccine should be given but it may appropriate to give it in a hospital setting where there has been an anaphylactic reaction to egg (Lakshman and Finn 2000). This is more to reassure the parents than of medical necessity. There is no good evidence that skin testing helps in the management of these children.

♦ **I understand there is mercury in some vaccines. Isn't this harmful?**

Some vaccines contain a mercury-containing preservative, thiomersal. This was often added because many vaccines were dispensed in multidose containers and it was important to prevent bacterial contamination. In other vaccines it was part of the manufacturing process. There are no safety limits for the injection of mercury, but there are some for its oral ingestion. However, these vary widely. In 1999, it was noted that if an infant was given all the recommended vaccines in the US programme, in the first 6 months, they would exceed one of these limits. However, the amount would still be below many other thresholds including those set by WHO and the American FDA (Ball *et al.* 2001; Offit and Jew 2003). Bearing in mind the precautionary principle and the fact that, in many countries, routine infant vaccines are rarely dispensed in multidose containers, manufacturers were asked to move towards thiomersal-free vaccines. In the UK, even if an infant had been given all the routine vaccines according to the schedule in operation until September 2004, the amount of mercury received would not even have exceeded the lowest of the recommended safety levels. All vaccines in the current routine childhood immunization schedule are free of thiomersal.

♦ **Doesn't giving all these vaccines overload the immune system?**

Some parents and complementary practitioners have suggested that giving a number of vaccines together may overload the immune system, making children susceptible to other infections, autoimmune disorders, and atopy. There is no scientific rational behind this in that the immune system is constantly being bombarded by foreign antigens and its capacity is enormous (Offit *et al.* 2002). A number of studies have shown that serious infections are no commoner in children in the period immediately after they have been immunized (Black *et al.* 1991; Miller *et al.* 2003). There are a number of studies that show no association between atopy and immunizations (Nilsson *et al.* 2003; Offit and Hackett 2003). It is more difficult to disprove a link with autoimmune disorders. However, there have been no convincing studies supporting a link (DeStafano *et al.* 2001, 2003; Offit and Hackett 2003).

♦ **Wouldn't it be better to delay giving the vaccines until the baby's immune system is stronger?**

Almost all babies produce an adequate immune response to the vaccines given at 8, 12, and 16 weeks (Ramsay *et al.* 1991). However, some very premature infants may not develop protective antibody levels to hepatitis B and polysaccharide conjugate vaccines (Freitas *et al.* 2002; Heath *et al.* 2003). Consideration should be given to checking antibody levels after they complete the course of primary immunizations. If anything, side-effects such as fever and sore injection sites are commoner when the immunizations are delayed (Ramsay *et al.* 1992). Diseases such as *Haemophilus influenzae* type b, pertussis, and meningococcal C are more prevalent in younger children. Therefore, by delaying vaccines, infants are subjected to a double whammy—they are more likely to have side-effects and protection against major infectious diseases is not there when it is most needed.

This is just a selection of the many questions that parents may ask. It may be difficult to find answers to all in a single source, but the further reading list should help.

References

Anon (2003). MMR vaccine—how effective and how safe? *Drugs and Therapeutic Bulletin* **41**(4): 25–9.

Ball LK, Ball R, Pratt RD (2001). An assessment of thimerosal use in childhood vaccines. *Pediatrics* **107**(5): 1147–1154.

Black SB, Cherry JD, Shinefield HR, Fireman B, Christenson P, Lampert D (1991). Apparent decreased risk of invasive bacterial disease after heterologous childhood immunization. *American Journal of Diseases of Children* **145**: 746–749.

Department of Health (1996). *Immunisation Against Infectious Disease*. HMSO, London. Also now on the web at http://www.dh.gov.uk/PolicyAndGuidance/HealthAndSocialCareTopics/GreenBook/fs/en. (Accessed 11 August 2006).

Department of Health (2001). *Health Information for Overseas Travellers*. The Stationary Office, London. https://www.the-stationery-office.co.uk/doh/hinfo/index.htm (Accessed 17 January 2004).

DeStefano F, Mullooly JP, Okoro CA, Chen RT, Marcy SM, Ward JI, Vadheim CM, Black SB, Shinefield HR, Davis RL, Bohlke K; Vaccine Safety Datalink Team (2001). Childhood vaccinations, vaccination timing, and risk of type 1 diabetes mellitus. *Pediatrics* **108**(6): E112.

DeStefano F, Verstraeten T, Jackson LA, Okoro CA, Benson P, Black SB, Shinefield HR, Mullooly JP, Likosky W, Chen RT. Vaccine Safety Datalink Research Group, National Immunization Program, Centers for Disease Control and Prevention (2003). Vaccinations and risk of central nervous system demyelinating diseases in adults. *Archives of Neurology* **60**(4): 504–509.

Elliman D, Moreton J (2000). The District Immunisation Co-ordinator. *Archives of Disease in Childhood* **82**(4): 280–282.

Freitas da Motta MS, Mussi-Pinhata MM, Jorge SM, Tachibana Yoshida CF, Sandoval de Souza CB (2002). Immunogenicity of hepatitis B vaccine in preterm and full term infants vaccinated within the first week of life. *Vaccine* **20**(11–12): 1557–1562.

Health Protection Agency (2003). *CDR Weekly* **39**(13). http://www.hpa.org.uk/cdr/PDFfiles/2003/cdr3903.pdf (Accessed 11.8.2006).

Health Protection Agency. *Measles. Deaths, by Age Group*, 1980–2002. http://www.hpa.org.uk/infections/topics_az/measles/data_death_age.htm Accessed 17.1.2004.

Heath PT, Booy R, McVernon J, Bowen-Morris J, Griffiths H, Slack MP, Moloney AC, Ramsay ME, Moxon ER (2003). Hib vaccination in infants born prematurely.*Archives of Disease in Childhood* **88**(3): 206–210.

Jansen VAA, Stollenwerk N, Jensen HJ, Ramsay ME, Edmunds WJ, Rhodes CJ (2003). Measles outbreaks in a population with declining vaccine uptake. *Science* **301**: 804.

Lakshman R, Finn A (2000). MMR vaccine and allergy. *Archives of Disease in Childhood* **82**(2): 93–95.

Madsen KM, Hviid A, Vestergaard M, Schendel D, Wohlfahrt J, Thorsen P, Olsen J, Melbye M (2002). A population-based study of measles, mumps, and rubella vaccination and autism. *New England Journal of Medicine* **347**: 1477, 1482.

Miller E, Waight P, Farrington CP, Andrews N, Stowe J, Taylor B (2001). Idiopathic thrombocytopenic purpura and MMR vaccine. *Archives of Disease in Childhood* **84**(3): 227–229.

Miller E, Andrews N, Waight P, Taylor B (2003). Bacterial infections, immune overload, and MMR vaccine. Measles, mumps, and rubella. *Archives of Disease in Childhood* **88**(3): 222–223.

National Travel Health Network and Centre. http://www.nathnac.org/healthprofessionals/index.html (Accessed 11.8.2004).

Nilsson L, Kjellman M, Bjorkstein B (2003). Allergic disease at the age of 7 years after pertussis vaccination in infancy. *Archives of Pediatric Adolescent Medicine* **157**: 1184–1189.

Offit PA, Hackett CJ (2003). Addressing parents' concerns: do vaccines cause allergic or autoimmune diseases? *Pediatrics* **111**(3): 653–659.

Offit PA, Jew RK (2003). Addressing parents' concerns: do vaccines contain harmful preservatives, adjuvants, additives, or residuals? *Pediatrics* **112**(6 Pt 1): 1394–1397.

Offit PA, Quarles J, Gerber MA, Hackett CJ, Marcuse EK, Kollman TR, Gellin BG, Landry S (2002). Addressing parents' concerns: do multiple vaccines overwhelm or weaken the infant's immune system? *Pediatrics* **109**: 124–129.

Peltola H, Heinonen P, Valle M, Paunio M, Virtanen M, Karanko V, Cantell K (1994). The elimination of indigenous measles, mumps and rubella from Finland by a 12-year, two-dose vaccination program. *New England Journal of Medicine* **331**: 1397–1402.

Ramsay ME, Corbel MJ, Redhead K, Ashworth LA, Begg NT (1991). Persistence of antibody after accelerated immunisation with diphtheria/tetanus/pertussis vaccine. *British Medical Journal* **302**: 1489–1491.

Ramsay ME, Rao M, Begg NT (1992). Symptoms after accelerated immunisation. *British Medical Journal* **304**(6841): 1534–1536.

Royal College of Paediatrics and Child Health (2002). *Immunisation of the Immunocompromised Child.* http://www.rcpch.ac.uk/publications/recent_publications/Immunocomp.pdf). (Accessed 11.12.2004).

Taylor B, Miller E, Lingam R, Andrews N, Simmons A, Stowe J (2002). Measles, mumps, and rubella vaccination and bowel problems or developmental regression in children with autism: a population study. *British Medical Journal* **324**: 393–396.

Tookey PA, Jones G, Miller BH, Peckham CS (1991). Rubella vaccination in pregnancy. *CDR* (Lond Engl Rev). **1**(8): R86–88.

Virtanen M, Peltola H, Paunio M, Heinonen OP (2000). Day-to-day reactogenicity and the healthy vaccinee effect of measles-mumps-rubella vaccination. *Pediatrics* **106**: e62.

Wakefield AJ, Murch SH, Anthony A, Linell J, Casson DM, Malik M, Berelowitz M, Dhillon AP, Thompson MA, Harvey P, Valentine A, Davies SE, Walker-Smith JA (1998). Ileal-lymphoid-nodular hyperplasia, non-specific colitis, and pervasive developmental disorder in children. Lancet **351**: 637–641.

Further reading

Department of Health. *Immunisation: immunisation for life.* http://www.immunisation.net. (Accessed 11.12.2006).

Department of Health. *MMR The Facts.* http://www.mmrthefacts.nhs.uk/ (Accessed 11 December 2006).

Health Protection Agency. *Vaccination of individuals with uncertain or incomplete immunisation status.* http://www.hpa.org.uk/infections/topics_az/vaccination/algorithm_2006_Septl.pdf. (Accessed 11 December 2006).

Institute of Child Health, Great Ormond Street Hospital for NHS Trust. *Immunisation.* (Accessed 11 December 2006).

Kassianos GC (2001). *Immunization: Childhood and Traveller's Health.* Blackwell Science, Oxford.

World Health Organization (2006). *International Travel and Health.* World Health Organisation, Geneva. http://www.who.int/ith/ (Accessed 11 December 2006).

Chapter 28

Accidental injuries in childhood

Denise Kendrick

The use of the term 'accident' is often criticized because it implies randomness and unpredictability suggesting that these events are inevitable and not preventable. However, epidemiological studies have shown that many accidents are in some sense predictable, as children, families, and environments that have a high risk of accidents can be identified. In addition, reviews of coroner's records following accidental deaths have found the majority of deaths were preventable (Bannon *et al.* 1992). Although 'unintentional injury' is now the preferred term, as this is not commonly used among those working in primary care in the UK, the term 'accidental injury' has been used in this chapter.

Why are accidental injuries an important problem?

Accidental injuries are responsible for more deaths among children aged 1–14 years than any other cause. They have been the major threat to the life of children in the UK for the last 50 years, and they continue to be the greatest challenge to child health today (British Medical Association 2001). They result in more childhood deaths than cancer, congenital abnormalities, or neurological diseases. Figure 28.1 shows death rates for the most common causes of death in childhood in England and Wales in 1995.

In England and Wales, 993 children aged 0–14 years died from accidental injury between 1998 and 2000. Table 28.1 shows the number of deaths by age and gender.

Although the number of deaths is smallest in children aged less than 1 year, they have the highest death rate from accidental injuries (Figure 28.2).

Where and how do fatal accidental injuries occur?

In pre-school children the death rate is highest for accidental injuries occurring at home, and for school age children it is highest for accidental injuries occurring on the roads, second highest for those occurring at home and lowest for those occurring during leisure activities (Figure 28.3).

Road traffic accidents are responsible for the greatest number of deaths (46% of all child accidental deaths). The most common road traffic accidents resulting in death are pedestrian injuries (25% of all child accidental deaths), followed by car passenger injuries (12%) and cyclist injuries (7%). For deaths not occurring on the roads, suffocation (18%) is the most common cause of death followed by drowning (9%) and fires (9%), falls(5%) and poisonings (4%) (Figure 28.4).

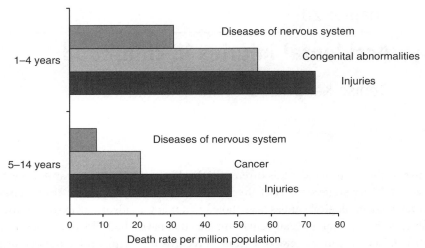

Fig. 28.1 How do accidental injuries compare with other child health problems?
Source: Mortality statistics childhood, infant and perinatal review of the Registrar General on
deaths in England and Wales, 1995. Series DH3 no 28. London. The Stationery Office (1997).

The type of accident causing death varies markedly with age. For example, suffocation
and choking on foreign bodies dominate the accidental injury deaths of children under 1
year. Among children aged 1–4 years a similar proportion of accidental deaths result
from road accidents, fire, suffocation, and drowning. Among school-aged children road
traffic accidents are responsible for the majority of accidental deaths (Figure 28.5).

Trends in fatal accidents

Death rates from accidents have been falling over the last 10 years, at approximately 6%
per year (Roberts *et al.* 1998). The UK has one of the lowest child accidental death rates
among developed countries, but if the UK had experienced the same death rate as
Sweden (the country with the lowest death rate) between 1991 and 1995, 454 child accidental deaths would have been prevented (UNICEF 2001). Although child accidental
death rates are falling, deaths in childhood from other causes are also falling, so the
proportion of all child deaths due to accidents is increasing. In developed countries the
proportion of all child deaths due to accidents rose from 25% to 37% in the last 25 years
of the twentieth century (UNICEF 2001).

Table 28.1 Numbers of deaths from accidental injury* of children aged 0–14 years in England
and Wales 1998–2000

	<1 year	1–4 years	5–14 years	0–14 years
Male	53	180	410	643
Female	43	130	177	350
All deaths	96	310	587	993

*Deaths with an external cause code E800-E949. Source: Data from ONS Mortality statistics DH4 Series 23–25.

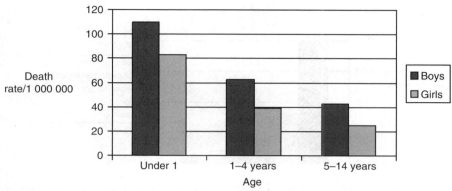

Fig. 28.2 Childhood accidental injury death rate per 1 000 000, by gender, England and Wales 1999. Source: Mortality statistics. Injury and poisoning. Review of the Registrar General on deaths attributed to injury and poisoning in England and Wales, 1999. Series DH4 no 24. London. The Stationery Office (2001).

Non-fatal accidents

Deaths represent only the tip of the iceberg of accidental injuries. Each year accidental injuries are responsible for many hospital admissions, A&E department attendances, and attendances at primary care. Many minor accidental injuries also occur that are treated at home, as do many 'near misses', where an event happens that could have resulted in an injury, but fortunately did not. A recent study found that over a 2-week period 56% of children aged between 3 and 12 months had a near miss and 44% had a minor accidental injury that did not require medical attention (Marsh and Kendrick 2000).

Hospital admissions for accidents

In England in 2001, 110 000 children were admitted to hospital following an accidental injury (Department of Health 2001/2)). A recent study in the Trent region found falls were

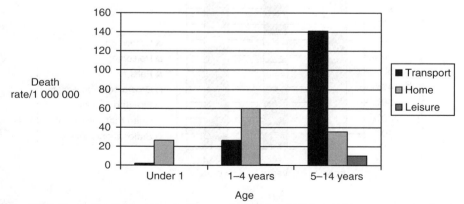

Figure 28.3 Place of accidental deaths, by age, England and Wales, 1999. Source: Mortality statistics. Injury and poisoning. Review of the Registrar General on deaths attributed to injury and poisoning in England and Wales, 1999. Series DH4 no 24. London. The Stationery Office (2001).

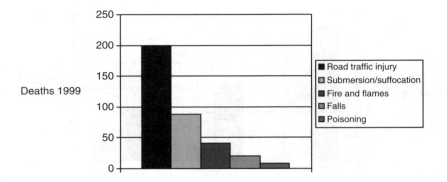

Fig. 28.4 Mechanisms of accidental death in children aged 0–14, England and Wales, 1999. Source: Mortality statistics. Injury and poisoning. Review of the Registrar General on deaths attributed to injury and poisoning in England and Wales, 1999. Series DH4 no 24. London. The Stationery Office (2001).

the most common accident leading to hospital admission in both pre-school (39% of all accidental injury admissions) and older children (49%). Poisoning (22%) and burns and scalds (7%) were the second and third most common accident leading to hospital admission in pre-school children, and pedal cycle injuries (10%) and pedestrian injuries (5%) were the second and third most common in older children (Hippisley-Cox *et al.* 2002).

Accident and emergency department attendances

In the UK in 1999, more than 2.25 million children attended A&E departments following an accidental injury. Accidents at home accounted for 580 000 attendances in children

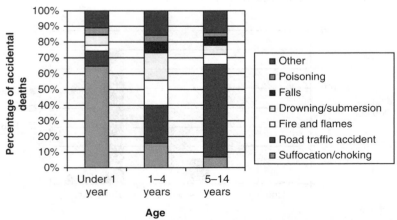

Fig. 28.5 Mechanism of accidental deaths in children of different ages: England and Wales 1998–2000. *Deaths with an external cause code E800-E949. Source: Data from ONS Mortality statistics DH4 Series 23–25.

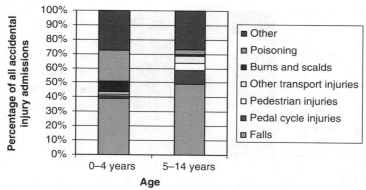

Fig. 28.6 Hospital admissions following accidental injury by age and injury mechanism, Trent Region, 1992–1997. Source: Hippisley-Cox J, Groom L, Kendrick D, Coupland C, Webber E, Savelyich B (2002). Cross sectional survey of socioeconomic variations in severity and mechanism of childhood injuries in Trent 1992–7. *British Medical Journal* **324**(7346): 1132.

aged 0–4 years and 460 000 among children aged 5–14 years. Accidents occurring during leisure activities accounted for 160 000 attendances in children aged 0–4 years and 1 080 000 among children aged 5–14 years. Five per cent of children aged 0–4 years attending A&E and 4% of those aged 5–14 years are admitted to hospital (Department of Trade and Industry 2001).

Falls are the most common accident leading to A&E department attendances for children of all ages. Poisonings, foreign bodies, and burns and scalds are more common under 5 years, while being struck by an object and cutting or piercing are more common over 5 years (Figures 28.7 and 28.8).

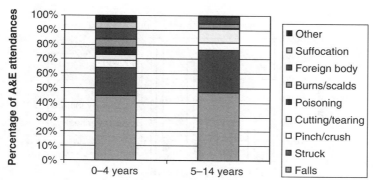

Fig. 28.7 Accident and emergency department attendances resulting from accidents at home, UK, 1999. Source: Department of Trade and Industry. 23rd annual report of the Home and Leisure Accident Surveillance System—1999 data.

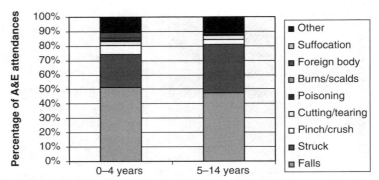

Fig. 28.8 Accident and emergency department attendances resulting from accidents during leisure activities, UK, 1999. Source: Department of Trade and Industry. 23rd annual report of the Home and Leisure Accident Surveillance System—1999 data.

Road traffic accidents

In addition to accidents at home and at leisure, large numbers of children are injured on the roads. In Great Britain in 2002, 14 231 children were killed or injured in pedestrian accidents, 4809 in cycling accidents and 13 359 as passengers in cars. The number of child pedestrian casualties, by age, is shown in Figure 28.9, child cyclist casualties in Figure 28.10, and child car passenger casualties in Figure 28.11.

Disability caused from injuries

Injury-related ill health does not end with the hospital episode. It has been estimated that accidental injury is responsible for 30% of the total burden of disability among children in the industrialized world (UNICEF 2001). One recent study found one in three children who had been admitted to hospital suffered a short-term disability immediately

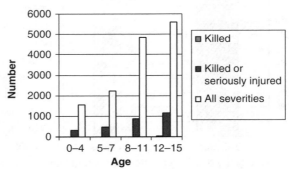

Fig. 28.9 Number of child pedestrian casualties aged 0–15 years, Great Britain, 2002. Source: Department for Transport. Road Casualties in Great Britain: The Casualty Report (2002).

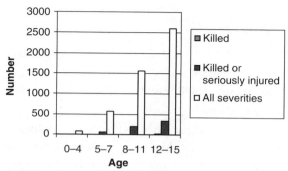

Fig. 28.10 Number of child cyclist casualties aged 0–15 years, Great Britain, 2002. Source: Department for Transport. Road Casualties in Great Britain: The Casualty Report (2002).

following the injury, most often limitations in toileting, dressing, bathing, and running. Six months following the injury, 12% of children were still experiencing limitations in running and 8% in walking (Gofin *et al.* 1999).

Which children are most likely to have accidents?

Not all children are at an equal risk of an accident. There are a number of factors which are associated with an increased risk of injury. These are:

- age—the risk of injury varies with injury type
- male gender
- socio-economic deprivation
- ethnicity
- children who have already had an injury
- hyperactive, aggressive, or impulsive behaviour

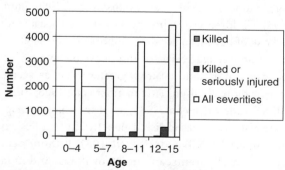

Fig. 28.11 Number of child car passenger casualties aged 0–15 years, Great Britain, 2002. Source: Department for Transport. Road Casualties in Great Britain: The Casualty Report (2002).

- ◆ children living in:
  - single parent and step families
  - families with three or more children
  - families with a teenage mother
  - families experiencing stressful life events
  - families where the mother is depressed.

As children grow, their strength, capabilities and range of activities increase. Patterns of injury can be identified that reflect a child's age and stage of development (Baker 1975; Rivara 1982). At all ages boys have higher accident rates than girls, for both fatal and non-fatal accidents (Rivara et al. 1982). The difference in death rates increases as children get older, so that by 5 years of age the death rate for boys is twice as high as that for girls.

Accidents are strongly associated with socio-economic circumstances. The social class gradient is steeper for accidents than for any other cause of death in childhood. Overall, children from social class V are five times more likely to die as a result of an accident than children from social class I. Furthermore the gap in death rates between the classes widened between 1981 and 1991 (Roberts and Power 1996). The social class gradient is steeper for some accidents than others. The death rate among children from social class five is 16 times greater for deaths from fire and flames, seven times greater for falls, 4.5 times greater for drowning or suffocation, four times greater for cycling accidents, three times greater for poisoning, and 2.5 times greater for pedestrian accidents than that for children from social class I (Roberts 1997).

The picture is similar for non-fatal accidents, with children from the most deprived wards having hospital admission rates for pedestrian injury that are four times higher than children from the most affluent wards and three times higher for burns and scalds and poisonings (Hippisley-Cox et al. 2002).

South Asian children have been found to have lower self-reported major and minor accident rates (Erens et al. 2001), and lower rates of attendance at fracture clinics, admission to hospital, and a prolonged hospital stay resulting from an accident (Tobin et al. 2002).

Children who have already had an accidental injury requiring medical attention are two to three times more likely to have another accident requiring medical attention than those who have not (Manheimer et al. 1966; Eminson et al. 1986; Bijur et al. 1988; Sellar 1991; Kendrick 1993). Children whose brothers or sisters have already had an accident are also at increased risk of having an accident (Johnston et al. 2000).

Children with hyperactive, aggressive, or impulsive behaviour are at increased risk of accidents (Lalloo et al. 2003). Children are at greater risk of an accidental injury if they are from large (three or more children) (Manheimer et al. 1966; Bijur et al. 1988a–c) or single parent families (Wadsworth et al. 1983), or if they have teenage mothers (Taylor et al. 1983). They are also at increased risk if they live in families experiencing recent stressful life events (Sibert 1975; Beautrais et al. 1981; Bithoney et al. 1985), such as moving house, separation of parents, and death or illness and in families where the mother is suffering from depression (Brown and Davidson 1978; Russell 1998; O'Connor et al. 2000).

The costs of accidents

Accidents in childhood are costly to children, families, the NHS, and to wider society. In addition to the costs of pain, grief, and suffering, parents may need to take time off work to care for injured children and children may need to take time off school to recover from accidents. Children disabled as a result of an accident may require long-term care and rehabilitation, including extra educational support and adaptations to the home and to vehicles and work places as they reach adulthood. Children and families may also require emotional and psychological support following an injury.

Childhood injuries are estimated to cost the National Health Service more than £200 million per year (Child Accident Prevention Trust 1992). The NHS costs grossly underestimate the true costs of accidents as they do not include the cost of providing long-term care for severely injured children, or the cost to the child and the family of the suffering and distress and the parental costs of caring for an injured child. Recently, published estimates of the costs of childhood accidents include:

*   the cost to the community in Great Britain of childhood injury (road and home) is over £10 000 million each year (Roberts *et al.* 1998)
*   the value to society of preventing injuries in the home to 0–14 year olds is £9460 million (Roberts *et al.* 1998). Road traffic fatalities (0–14 year olds) can be valued at £180 million (Roberts *et al.* 1998)
*   the cost of child pedestrian injuries in Great Britain in 2000 was £776 256 210 (Department of Health 2002b)
*   the cost of child cyclist injuries in Great Britain in 2000 was £202 732 330 (Department of Health 2002b).

Preventing accidental injuries in childhood

The importance of preventing accidental injuries in childhood is emphasized in the Government's Health Strategy for England *Our Healthier Nation* (Department of Health 1999), in the Government's Cross-Cutting Review on inequalities and the subsequent programme to tackle health inequalities (Department of Health 2001, 2002a), in the Department for Transports Road Safety Strategy (2000) and in the Office of the Deputy Prime Ministers White Paper on the Fire and Rescue Service.A national task force was established to advise the Government on preventing accidental injuries in 2001. It had a separate working group considering accidents in childhood. The final report of the Task Force was published in 2002 (Department of Health 2002c), which included recommendations regarding action primary care organizations and primary healthcare teams should be taking in relation to preventing accidents in childhood. In addition, a series of targets have been published, to which primary care organizations and the agencies and organizations with which they work, will need to respond. These include:

*   *Our Healthier Nation* (1999) (Department of Health 1999):
    *   to reduce the death rate from accidents by at least a fifth and to reduce the rate of serious injury from accidents by at least a tenth by 2010.

- *Tomorrow's Roads—Safer for Everyone* (Department for the Environment, Transport and Regions 2000):
  - a 50% reduction in the number of children killed or seriously injured; and
  - a 10% reduction in the slight casualty rate, by 2010.
- *Sure Start* (Department of Education and Employment 1999):
  - to reduce by 10% the number of children aged 0–4 admitted to hospital as an emergency with gastroenteritis, a lower respiratory infection or a severe injury.
- Our Fire and Rescue Service (Office of the Deputy Prime Minister 2003):
  - to reduce the number of accidental fire-related deaths in the home by 20% by 2010.

How can accidental injuries be prevented?

The prevention of accidental injuries can be considered using the same framework as for the prevention of other diseases, such as coronary heart disease. The three levels of prevention are:

- primary prevention
- secondary prevention
- tertiary prevention.

Accidents do not always result in injury. A child can fall down stairs and not be injured, but an accident has still occurred. It is therefore important that both the events leading to the (potential) injury and the injury resulting from the event are considered in terms of prevention. Primary prevention aims to prevent the events that cause injuries, secondary prevention is intended to prevent or reduce an injury occurring during the event and tertiary prevention is aimed at reducing the consequences of an injury that has already occurred. Examples of each type of injury prevention are given in Table 28.2.

Within these three levels of prevention there are three different approaches, which can be used:

- education
- engineering
- enforcement.

Table 28.2 Examples of injury prevention at the primary, secondary and tertiary levels

Primary	Secondary	Tertiary
Fire guards	Cycle helmets	First aid at site of an accident
Cupboard locks	Smoke detectors	Ambulance service
20 m.p.h. zones	Child car seats	Treatment for injuries
Child resistant containers for medicines	Seat belts	Rehabilitation services

Educational approaches

Educational approaches can be directed at a range of people and organizations. They may be targeted towards the general population, at children and families, at health or social care workers, at those working in social services, housing or environmental health departments of Local Authorities, or at managers and policy makers. Education is also important in paving the way for accident prevention initiatives using the engineering or enforcement approaches, as in the Australian educational campaigns prior to the introduction of cycle helmet legislation. Most members of the primary healthcare team and of the Primary Care Trust (PCT) will have had little, if any, training in accident prevention (Marsh P et al. 1995; Kendrick et al. 1995a,b, 2003; Morgan 1996). It is therefore important that primary care staff and those developing and implementing the accident prevention strategy for the PCT are adequately trained and supported to carry out accident prevention.

Members of primary healthcare teams will most often use educational approaches with the families and children they care for, and those working at the level of the PCT may be involved in developing and implementing educational accident prevention interventions. There are a range of health education models that can be used for educational interventions, including the preventive, empowerment, and radical models.

The preventive model

This model involves providing information and advice for parents and children. However, factors such as poverty, a lack of control over rented accommodation, insufficient support with child care, lack of safe play areas, poor quality housing, poor public transport or language barriers may all make it difficult for parents to take advantage of the advice they have been given. Providing information without attempting to address these barriers is unlikely to be effective.

The empowerment model

The empowerment model of health education attempts to increase the control that individuals have over their environment by increasing self-esteem and facilitating the development of the skills required to achieve greater control. Examples of this model would include helping parents to obtain and fit safety equipment or teaching first aid to parents.

The radical model

The third model is the radical model. This aims to change society rather than changing the individual family or child. Examples of this model would include helping parents to campaign for more safe play areas or lobbying for an improved public transport system to reduce road traffic injuries.

Engineering approaches

The engineering approach to injury prevention involves the design, manufacture, and use of products and environments to make them safer. The design and implementation of area-wide traffic-calming schemes to reduce the speed and volume of traffic in residential areas and the design and use of safety equipment such as stairgates, fire guards, child-resistant containers, or cupboard locks, are all examples of the engineering approach.

Enforcement approaches

The enforcement approach involves the use of standards, regulations, or legislation to enforce safer behaviour, safer products, and safer environments. Legislation regarding drink driving and motor cycle helmet wearing is aimed at enforcing safe behaviour, the use of the British Safety Standard on products ensures their manufacture to particular specifications and building regulations are aimed at ensuring the safety of the home environment.

Active versus passive prevention

Active prevention of accidental injuries requires some action, and often repeated action, on the part of a parent or child. For example, preventing poisoning by storing medicines in a cupboard out of a child's reach requires the parent to always put the medicine in the same place. Passive prevention does not require any action on the part of the parent or child, e.g. fitting a thermostat to the hot water supply would prevent hot water scalds without the parents having to take any action. Passive injury prevention measures are often more effective than active measures.

What interventions reduce accidental injuries in childhood?

Tables 28.3–28.5 summarize the evidence regarding the effectiveness of a range of interventions aimed at reducing accidental injuries in childhood. They are based on recent systematic reviews (DiGuiseppi and Higgins 2000; DiGuiseppi and Roberts 2000; Elkan *et al.* 2000; Klassen *et al.* 2000; Towner *et al.* 2001; Duperrex *et al.* 2002), the Health Development Agency Evidence Briefing (Health Development Agency 2003) and data from trials published subsequent to those systematic reviews (King *et al.* 2001; DiGuiseppi *et al.* 2002;

Table 28.3 Effective educational and parental support interventions

Intervention	Effect
Home injuries	
Ante and postnatal home visiting programmes to mothers of infants, by health professionals or lay workers	Reductions in home hazards and reduced accidental injury rates
Advice and safety equipment provided in clinical settings by health visitors, GPs, or paediatricians to 'childproof' the home (including for the prevention of falls, poisoning, cuts, burns, choking, house fires, suffocation and drowning)	Increased safety equipment use and other safety behaviours and reductions in home hazards, especially if free or low-cost home safety equipment provided
Community and individual education and free window guards	Reduction in window falls and mortality from window falls

Table 28.3 (continued) Effective educational and parental support interventions

Intervention	Effect
Smoke alarm give away programmes	Most unfitted alarms will not be fitted and working 12–18 months later. Fitted alarms are likely to remain functional at least in the short term (especially those with long-life batteries).
Road traffic injuries	
Pedestrian skills training, pedestrian education	Increased knowledge and safer crossing behaviour
Bicycle skills training	Increased knowledge and safer cycling behaviour
Educational campaigns and subsidised cycle helmet schemes	Increased rates of cycle helmet use
Advice by health visitors and midwives in clinical settings, to increase child car restraint use	Increased restraint use in short term
Infant car seat/restraint campaigns and loan schemes	Increased restraint use

Gielen *et al.* 2002; Nansel *et al.* 2002). Some interventions have been shown to be associated with reductions in accidental injuries, others with changes in behaviour. Although some interventions may change behaviour, a change in behaviour cannot necessarily be assumed to lead to a reduction in injuries. Most benefit is likely to be obtained from focusing, where possible, on interventions that have been shown to reduce accidental injuries, or on those behaviours that have been shown to be closely associated with the injury producing event.

Table 28.4 Effective engineering interventions

Intervention	Effect
Home injuries	
Child resistant containers for medicines	Reduction in poisoning
Leisure injuries	
Barriers for domestic swimming pools	Reduction in risk of drowning
Road traffic injuries	
Cycle helmets	Reduction in risk of head, brain and severe brain injury for all ages of bicyclists. Helmets provide equal levels of protection for crashes involving motor vehicles and crashes from all other causes. Injuries to the upper and mid facial areas are also reduced
Visibility aids for cyclists and pedestrians	Visibility aids increase detection and recognition of pedestrians and cyclists by drivers
Area wide traffic calming schemes	Possible reduction in road traffic crashes and pedestrian injuries
20 mph zones	Reduction in traffic speed and in total injuries, pedestrian and cyclist injuries

Table 28.5 Effective enforcement interventions

Intervention	Effect
Home injuries	
Smoke detector legislation	Possible reduction in fire related injuries
Leisure injuries	
Lifeguards on beaches and public pools	Reductions in drowning deaths
Road traffic injuries	
Child car seat/restraint legislation	Increased restraint use and reductions in motor vehicle occupant injuries
Seat belt legislation	Increased sear belt use and reductions in motor vehicle occupant injuries
Cycle helmet legislation	Increased cycle helmet use and reductions in cyclist head injuries

Opportunities for injury prevention

The role of the primary healthcare team

As part of their routine work, members of the primary healthcare team have many opportunities to prevent accidental injuries to the children they care for (Kendrick 1994). The programmes of antenatal care, child health surveillance, and immunization provide repeated contacts with parents and children at home, in clinics, and in surgeries. These can be used to provide age specific advice, to help parents to access items of safety equipment and to advise parents about first aid. The advice appropriate for parents-to-be, for families with children under 1 year and for families with children aged 1–4 years is shown in Boxes 28.1–28.3:

Recent changes to the child health surveillance programme with the introduction of the recommendations of the fourth Hall report (Hall and Elliman 2003), will result in

---

Box 28.1 Accident prevention advice for parents-to-be

◆ Encourage use of infant car seats and use and testing of smoke alarms

◆ Encourage families to make a plan for how to get out of the house in case of fire

◆ Discourage use of baby walkers, duvets and pillows in cots, baby bouncers on tables or work surfaces

◆ Discourage families from placing babies on beds, tables, or sofas even before the child can roll

◆ Discourage families from drinking hot drinks while holding the baby

◆ Encourage checking the suitability of toys for the child's age

Box 28.2 Age-specific advice for families with children under 1 year

- Encourage use of infant car seats and use and testing of smoke alarms
- Encourage families to start using stair gates, fire guards, cupboard locks, window locks and socket covers when the child starts to become mobile
- Discourage families from using a baby walker, drinking hot drinks while holding child, leaving child alone in the bath, using dummies or toys on strings around the babies neck
- Encourage parents to check small toys for removable parts and avoid peanuts and other small items of food, sweets, buttons or coins that could be placed in the mouth
- Teach parents first aid

Box 28.3 Age-specific advice for families with children aged 1–4 years

- Encourage use of infant car seats and use and testing of smoke alarms
- Encourage families to continue using stair gates, fire guards, cupboard locks, window locks and socket covers
- Encourage families to keep children out of the kitchen while cooking, use rear rings on the hob and curly flexed or cordless kettles
- Encourage parents to keep cleaning products, chemicals, and medicines out of reach, dispose of unwanted medicines, purchase cleaning products with child resistant caps
- Encourage parents to store sharp objects out of reach, use safety glass or film, make low-level glass visible by bright stickers, etc.
- Encourage parents to check small toys for removable parts and avoid peanuts and other small items of food, sweets, buttons, or coins that could be placed in the mouth
- Discourage parents from leaving children alone in the bath or in the care of other children, and fence off, or cover, garden ponds and pools, teach children to swim
- Encourage parents to ensure child uses a cycle helmet from the time they start riding a bike
- Encourage parents to check the safety of their garden including having an adequate fence and gate, access to garden chemicals, sharp gardening tools, ponds, and poisonous plants
- Teach parents first aid

fewer routine contacts between members of the primary healthcare team and families with pre-school children. It is therefore important that other contacts such as antenatal contacts, those for immunization, and other consultations are used opportunistically for providing age-specific advice about accident prevention. Hazards can be identified on home visits and consultations for acute injury can be used to explore how similar injuries could be prevented in the future. Following an accidental injury, parent's first aid actions can be explored with positive reinforcement of correct actions and information about action to take in case of future injury. Many parents will feel guilty following an injury to their child, so being able to discuss their feelings in a supportive and non-judgemental atmosphere is important. Paediatric liaison health visitors based in A&E departments can also notify injuries to community health visitors who can undertake post-accident support visits to provide support for the parent and child and can explore the prevention of future injuries (Laidman 1987).

Members of the primary healthcare team also have a wider public health role. They can work with organizations such as Sure Start, with local parenting programmes, programmes for teenage mothers, or community organizations. They can share their skills by teaching first aid to families and other members of the community. They can use routine contacts with families and children to provide access for other organizations and agencies such as identifying families without smoke alarms and referring these to the Fire and Rescue Service to have an alarm fitted.

The role of primary care organizations in preventing accidental injuries in childhood

A recent survey of 51 primary care organizations (PCO) in the former NHS Trent Region, UK found that most regarded the prevention of accidents as less of a priority than heart disease, cancer or mental health, the three other priority areas in *Our Healthier Nation* (Kendrick *et al.* 2003) (Figure 28.12).

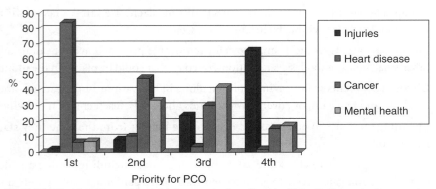

Fig. 28.12 Priority given to accidental injury and other Our Healthier Nation priority areas by members of Primary Care Organizations in Trent. Source: Kendrick D, Groom L, Hippisley-Cox J, Savelyich BS, Webber E, Coupland C (2003). Accidental injury: a neglected area within Primary Care Groups and Trusts? *Health Educ Res* **18**(3): 380–388.

Although most members of the PCO believed most accidents were preventable and accident prevention strategies can save money by reducing the number of accidents that need treatment, almost three-quarters agreed that accident prevention is predominantly the responsibility of the individual or parent and 60% that other agencies have greater responsibility for accident prevention than the PCO. One-quarter of PCO members did not believe the PCO could be effective in preventing accidents and three-quarters did not think that their PCO would increase spending on accident prevention (Kendrick *et al.* 2003).

Although PCTs are starting to develop their accident prevention work, only one-third had taken any action in relation to preventing accidents and less than one-third had a written strategy dealing with the prevention of accidents (Kendrick *et al.* 2003). Many PCTs said they would need help to develop a strategy. The Child Accident Prevention Trust has produced guidance on effective accident prevention for PCTs (Hayes 2003). This document discusses the principles of effective accident prevention, the data that are freely available to help PCTs identify priorities for action and the steps that are needed to develop a local accident prevention strategy. It gives examples of local initiatives and indicators that may be used to monitor and evaluate local initiatives. The key elements of an accident prevention strategy are:

◆ needs assessment including data on accidental injuries, which may include national, regional, or local data

◆ evidence on the effectiveness of interventions

◆ inter-agency collaboration

◆ local consultation

◆ clear aims and objectives, locally agreed targets and timetables

◆ a programme for development of skills and the identification of resources necessary to undertake accident prevention

◆ a dissemination programme including access to local policy makers, purchasing, and commissioning bodies

◆ a programme to evaluate the success of the strategy.

Evidence about the effectiveness of differing approaches to accident prevention highlights that engineering and enforcement approaches may be more effective in terms of reducing accidental injuries than education used alone. It is therefore vitally important that PCTs work with agencies and organizations that can achieve change by these means. *Saving Lives: Our Healthier Nation* emphasizes that improvements in health and reductions in inequalities will only be achieved by re-focusing local services to increase the priority given to health, and by the establishment of local partnerships where people and organizations work together to improve health (Department of Health 1999). This has been encouraged through the establishment of Local Strategic Partnerships (LSPs), which usually follow Local Authority boundaries and include PCTS. The roles of the PCT in this partnership may include the collection and dissemination of data on accidental injuries, training primary care staff in accident prevention, collaborating with other agencies and organizations, using routine contacts that primary care team members have with children and families to promote road safety or fire safety by working with road safety officers or the community fire safety team, participating in innovative schemes such as providing cycle helmets on 'prescription' or establishing or contributing towards safety equipment fitting schemes.

The recommendations of the recent policy documents regarding the roles of primary healthcare teams and the primary care organizations in reducing accidental injury in childhood are shown in Box 28.4.

Box 28.4

Tackling health inequalities (Department of Health 2001)

- PCTs have the lead in driving forward work on health inequalities and are responsible for leading and supporting partnerships in this area
- PCTs will have a key role in developing multidisciplinary family support teams
- PCTs should work with local people and agencies to set up home safety and repair schemes for vulnerable families
- PCTs should work closely with Sure Start programmes and local children's centres

The Accidental Injury Task Force Report (Department of Health 2002c)

- Local Authorities and PCTs should come together through Local Strategic Partnerships to deliver accidental injury prevention
- Health visitors should systematically identify families at risk of house fires and refer families to fire service for smoke alarms
- Health visitors should provide accident prevention advice on home visits
- Links should be made with positive parenting and grand parenting programmes to promote safety awareness about house fires

Our Healthier Nation (Department of Health 1999)

Local partnerships can:

- Conduct local campaigns on accidental injury prevention
- Provide equipment for vulnerable groups or ensure loan schemes are available
- Promote family support, accident awareness and parenting skills
- Introduce area wide road safety measures
- Develop local safe routes to school

Useful sources of information on accident prevention

Organizations

- Child Accident Prevention Trust: www.capt.org.uk
- Royal Society for the Prevention of Accidents: www.rospa.com
- International Society for Child and adolescent Injury Prevention: www.iscaip.org
- First aid: The British Red Cross: www.redcross.org.uk; St John Ambulance: www.sja.org.uk
- European Consumer Safety Association: www.ecosa.org
- European Child Safety Alliance: www.childsafetyeurope.org

Government departments

- The Department of Health: www.doh.gov.uk
- Our Healthier Nation website: www.ohn.gov.uk
- The Department for Transport: www.dft.gov.uk/roadsafety
- The Department for Trade and Industry: www.dti.gov.uk/homesafetynetwork
- The Office of the Deputy Prime Minister: www.odpm.gov.uk
- The Trading Standards Institute: www.tradingstandards.gov.uk

Journals and sources of evidence

Journals dedicated to accidental injury epidemiology and prevention

- Injury Prevention: www.injuryprevention.com
- Accident Analysis and Prevention: www.elsevier.nl/inca/publications/store/3/3/6/
- Injury Control and Safety Promotion: www.szp.swets.nl/szp/journals/ic.htm

General journals which publish articles on accidental injury prevention

- *Archives of Disease in Childhood*: http://adc.bmjjournals.com/
- *British Medical Journal*: www.bmj.com
- *Health Education Research*: http://her.oupjournals.org/
- *Health Education Journal*: http://www.hej.org.uk/
- *Health Promotion International*: http://heapro.oupjournals.org/
- *Journal of Public Health Medicine*: http://jpubhealth.oupjournals.org/
- *Journal of Epidemiology and Community Health*: http://jech.bmjjournals.com/
- *Community Practitioner*: http://www.commprac.com/
- *Journal of Advanced Nursing*: http://www.journalofadvancednursing.com/
- *Public Health*: http://intl.elsevierhealth.com//journals/pubh/

Other sources of evidence

- The National Institute for Health and Clinical Excellence: www.nice.org.uk

- Cochrane Injuries Group: www.cochrane-injuries.lshtm.ac.uk/
- Harborview Injury Prevention and Research Center: http://depts.washington.edu/hiprc/childinjury/index.htm

References

Baker SP (1975). Determinants of injury and opportunities for intervention. *American Journal of Epidemiology* **101**(2): 98–102.

Bannon MJ, Carter YH, Mason KT (1992). Causes of fatal childhood accidents in North Staffordshire, 1980–1989. *Archives of Emergency Medicine* **9**(4): 357–366.

Beautrais AL, Fergusson DM, Shannon FT (1981). Accidental poisoning in the first three years of life. *Australian Paediatric Journal* **17**(2): 104–109.

Bijur P, Golding J, Haslum M, Kurzon M (1988a). Behavioral predictors of injury in school-age children. *American Journal of Diseases of Children* **142**(12): 1307–1312.

Bijur PE, Golding J, Haslum M (1988b). Persistence of occurrence of injury: can injuries of preschool children predict injuries of school-aged children? *Pediatrics* **82**(5): 707–712.

Bijur PE, Golding J, Kurzon M (1988c). Childhood accidents, family size and birth order. *Social Science and Medicine* **26**(8): 839–843.

Bithoney WG, Snyder J, Michalek J, Newberger EH (1985). Childhood ingestions as symptoms of family distress. *American Journal of Diseases of Children* **139**(5): 456–459.

British Medical Association (2001). *Injury Prevention*. BMA, London.

Brown GW, Davidson S (1978). Social class, psychiatric disorder of mother, and accidents to children. *Lancet* **i**: 378–381.

Child Accident Prevention Trust (1992). *The NHS and Social Costs of Children's Accidents: a Pilot Study*. Child Accident Prevention Trust, London.

Department for the Environment TatR (2000). *Tomorrow's Roads: Safer for Everyone*. Department for the Environment, Transport and the Regions, London.

Department of Education and Employment (1999). *Sure Start*: DFEE Publications.

Department of Health (2001/2). *Hospital Episode Statistics 2001/2*, UK: Department of Health.

Department of Health (1999). *Saving Lives: Our Healthier Nation*. London: The Stationery Office.

Department of Health (2001). *Tackling Health Inequalities*. Department of Health, London.

Department of Health (2002a). *Tackling Health Inequalities: Cross-Cutting Review*. Department of Health, London.

Department of Health (2002b). *The Prevention of Childhood Injury: Background Paper Prepared for the Accidental Injury Task Force*. Department of Health, London.

Department of Health (2002c). *Preventing Accidental Injury—Priorities for Action. Report to the Chief Medical Officer from the Accidental Injury Task Force*. London.

Department of Trade and Industry (2001). *Working for a Safer World. 23rd Annual Report of the Home and Leisure Accident Surveillance System—1999 Data*. Department of Trade and Industry, London.

DiGuiseppi C, Higgins JP (2000). Systematic review of controlled trials of interventions to promote smoke alarms. *Archives of Disease in Childhood* **82**(5): 341–348.

DiGuiseppi C, Roberts I (2000). Individual-level injury prevention strategies in the clinical setting. *Future of Children* **10**: 53–82.

DiGuiseppi C, Roberts I, Wade A, Sculpher M, Edwards P, Godward C, et al (2002). Incidence of fires and related injuries after giving out free smoke alarms: cluster randomised controlled trial. *British Medical Journal* **325**: 995–998.

Duperrex O, Bunn F, Roberts I (2002). Safety education of pedestrians for injury prevention: a systematic review of randomised controlled trials. *British Medical Journal* **324**: 1129–1133.

Elkan R, Kendrick D, Hewitt M, Robinson JJA, Tolley K, Blair M, Dewey M, Williams D, Brummell K (2000). The effectiveness of domiciliary health visiting: A systematic review of international studies and a selective review of the British literature. *Health Technology Assessment* **4**(13).

Eminson CJ, Jones H, Goldacre M (1986). Repetition of accidents in young children. *Journal of Epidemiology and Community Health* **40**(2): 170–173.

Erens B, Primatesta P, Prior G (eds) (2001). *Health survey for England—the health of ethnic minority groups '99*. The Stationery Office, London.

Gielen AC, McDonald EM, Wilson ME, Hwang WT, Serwint JR, Andrews JS, Wang MC (2002). Effects of improved access to safety counseling, products, and home visits on parents' safety practices: results of a randomized trial. *Archives of Pediatrics and Adolescent Medicine* **156**: 33–40.

Gofin R, Adler B, Hass T (1999). Incidence and impact of childhood and adolescent injuries: a population-based study. *Journal of Trauma-Injury Infection and Critical Care* **47**: 15–21.

Hall MB, Elliman D (2003). *Health for all Children*, (4th edn). Oxford University Press, Oxford.

Hayes M (2003). *Preventing Childhood Accidents: guidance on effective action*. Child Accident Prevention Trust, London.

Health Development Agency (2003). *Prevention and Reduction of Accidental Injury in Children and Older People*. Health Development Agency, London.

Hippisley-Cox J, Groom L, Kendrick D, Coupland C, Webber E, Savelyich B (2002). Cross sectional survey of socioeconomic variations in severity and mechanism of childhood injuries in Trent 1992–7. *British Medical Journal* **324**(7346): 1132.

Johnston B, Grossman D, Connell F, Koepsell T (2000). High-risk periods for childhood injury among siblings. *Pediatrics* **105**(3 Pt 1): 562–568.

Kendrick D (1993). Accidental injury attendances as predictors of future admission. *Journal of Public Health Medicine* **15**(2): 171–4.

Kendrick D (1994). Role of the primary health care team in preventing accidents to children. *British Journal of General Practice* **44**(385): 372–375.

Kendrick D, Marsh P, Williams EI (1995a). General practitioners: Child accident prevention and 'The Health of the Nation'. *Health Education Research* **10**(3): 345–353.

Kendrick D, Marsh P, Williams EI (1995b). How do practice nurses see their role in childhood injury prevention? *Injury Prevention* **1**(3): 159–163.

Kendrick D, Groom L, Hippisley-Cox J, Savelyich BS, Webber E, Coupland C (2003). Accidental injury: a neglected area within Primary Care Groups and Trusts? *Health Education Research* **18**(3): 380–388.

King WJ, Klassen TP, LeBlanc J, Bernard-Bonnin A-C, Robitaille Y, Ba 'Pham, Coyle D, Tenenbein M, Pless IB (2001). The effectiveness of a home visit to prevent childhood injury. *Pediatrics* **108**(2): 382–388.

Klassen TP, MacKay JM, Moher D, Walker A, Jones AL (2000). Community-based injury prevention interventions. *Future of Children* **10**: 83–110.

Laidman P (1987). *Health Visiting and Preventing Accidents to Children*. Health Education Authority, London.

Lalloo R, Sheiham A, Nazroo J (2003). Behavioural characteristics and accidents: findings from the Health Survey for England, 1997. *Accident Analysis & Prevention* **35**: 661–667.

Manheimer DI, Dewey J, Mellinger GD, Corsa L (1966). 50,000 child years of accidental injuries. *Public Health Reports* **31**(6): 519–533.

Marsh P, Kendrick D (2000). Near miss and minor injury information—can it be used to plan and evaluate injury prevention programmes? *Accident Analysis and Prevention* **32**(3): 345–354.

Marsh P, Kendrick D, Williams EI (1995). Health visitors' knowledge, attitudes and practices in childhood accident prevention. *Journal of Public Health Medicine* **17**(2): 193–199.

Morgan PSAaC, YH (1996). *Accident Prevention in Primary Care. Part 4: Are the Training Needs of Community Nurses and Health Visitors Being Met?* The Royal Society for the Prevention of Accidents, London.

Nansel TR, Weaver N, Donlin M, Jacobsen H, Kreuter MW, Simons-Morton B (2002). Baby, Be Safe: the effect of tailored communications for pediatric injury prevention provided in a primary care setting. *Patient Education and Counseling* **46**(3): 175–190.

O'Connor TG, Davies L, Dunn J, Golding J (2000). Distribution of accidents, injuries, and illnesses by family type. ALSPAC Study Team. Avon Longitudinal Study of Pregnancy and Childhood. *Pediatrics* **106**(5): E68.

Office of the Deputy Prime Minister (2003). Our Fire and Rescue Service, Cm 5808: Office of the Deputy Prime Minister.

Rivara FP (1982). Epidemiology of childhood injuries. *American Journal of Diseases of Children* **136**: 399–405.

Rivara FP, Bergman AB, LoGerfo JP, Weiss NS (1982). Epidemiology of childhood injuries. II. Sex differences in injury rates. *American Journal of Diseases of Children* **136**(6): 502–506.

Roberts I (1997). Cause specific social class mortality differentials for child injury and poisoning in England and Wales. *Journal of Epidemiology and Community Health* **51**(3): 334–335.

Roberts I, Power C (1996). Does the decline in child injury mortality vary by social class? A comparison of class specific mortality in 1981 and 1991. *British Medical Journal* **313**(7060): 784–786.

Roberts I, DiGuiseppi C, Ward H (1998). Childhood injuries: extent of the problem, epidemiological trends, and costs. *Injury Prevention* **4**(4 Suppl.): S10–S16.

Russell KM (1998). Preschool children at risk for repeat injuries. *Journal of Community Health Nursing* **15**(3): 179–190.

Sellar C (1991). Occurrence and repetition of hospital admissions for accidents in pre-school children. *British Medical Journal* **302**(67): 16–19.

Sibert R (1975). Stress in families of children who have ingested poisons. *British Medical Journal* 87–89.

Taylor B, Wadsworth J, Butler NR (1983). Teenage mothering, admission to hospital, and accidents during the first 5 years. *Archives of Disease in Childhood* **58**: 6–11.

Tobin MD, Milligan J, Shukla R, Crump B, Burton PR (2002). South Asian ethnicity and risk of childhood accidents: an ecological study at enumeration district level in Leicester. *Journal of Public Health Medicine* **24**(4): 313–318.

Towner E, Dowswell T, Mackereth C, Jarvis S (2001). *What Works in Preventing Unintentional Injuries in Children and Young Adolescents? an Updated Systematic Review.* Health Development Agency, London.

UNICEF Innocenti Research Centre (2001). *A League Table of Child Injury Deaths in Rich Nations.* IRC.

Wadsworth J, Burnell I, Taylor B, Butler N (1983). Family type and accidents in preschool children. *Journal of Epidemiology and Community Health* **37**: 100–104.

Chapter 29

Eating disorders

Dee Dawson

Epidemiological studies suggest that 0.5–1% of all school children may suffer from anorexia nervosa, only 5–10% would be male. Twenty years ago, anorexia was predominantly a Western disease but recently we have been seeing more Afro-Caribbean and Asian girls and boys living in Western countries developing the illness.

In the same way, anorexia used to be an illness associated with middle and upper class children. Although still over-represented in the middle classes it is becoming more evenly distributed.

Ballet dancers, skaters, gymnasts, and athletes are particularly at risk of developing an eating disorder, probably because they believe thinness enhances their performance and is highly valued.

Whether or not the incidence of eating disorders is increasing is difficult to say. There seems to be an increase in the number of cases being treated but it could be that we are simply more aware of eating disorders now and quicker to treat them. There are few epidemiological studies involving children. Those that have been published vary enormously in their estimates of incidence, prevalence, increases in these rates and the number of boys relative to girls. Studies show that as many as 20% of female students might experience episodes of bulimia but thankfully we see very few child sufferers, 17–24 appears to be the most vulnerable time period for bulimia to develop. In the UK, there are more sufferers in private school than state schools. This is probably due to the fact that the perfectionistic children most likely to develop the illness attend these schools rather than the school themselves being at fault.

Although it is relatively rare to find a child who binges and vomits, it is not unusual to find an anorexic child who vomits because they believe that they have overeaten even though they are in fact restricting their intake. It is even more common for us to see children who turn to vomiting because we are making them eat when they would prefer to continue restricting their food intake.

Anorexia clinical signs: ICD-10 Diagnostic Criteria for Anorexia Nervosa

Weight loss or a failure to gain weight results in the child being at least 15% below a normal or expected weight for height and age.

1. weight loss is deliberate
2. a distorted body image, a perception of being fat

3. primary or secondary amenorrhoea.

Some children exhibit all the signs of anorexia but do not have or do not admit to having a distorted body image. Equally well, anorexia nervosa cannot be ruled out if a very low weight child continues to menstruate.

Bulimia Nervosa ICD-10

1. Binge eating at least twice a week on a regular basis.
2. A pre-occupation with eating.
3. A binge is often followed by
   - self-induced vomiting
   - intake of vast quantities of laxatives
   - a period of starvation
4. A fear of fatness

Bulimics can be a normal weight as they do not manage to vomit all the food they consume.

Clinical presentation: anorexia nervosa

The child will usually be convinced that she is fat and needs to lose more weight even though she may be emaciated. They have a morbid fear of fatness and are preoccupied with their body shape and very often by everyone else's too.

Typically, parents will describe a child who was a very compliant perfectionistic child who has gradually become more and more withdrawn. They will often have noticed a lowering of her self-esteem, feelings of worthlessness, and a preoccupation with food, and sometimes, exercise, which has become obsessive.

Some children continue to see their friends and behave socially while others withdraw from their peers, choosing to concentrate on schoolwork or exercise instead. As the illness progresses, friendships are usually sacrificed and even studying is neglected, they become totally preoccupied with dieting. Normally honest, outgoing, caring children become deceitful, manipulative, and increasingly isolated.

Although they do not want to eat, they love to cook and prepare food for others to eat. The control they feel when they refuse food is heightened when others are tempted into eating.

Many anorexics develop ritualistic behaviours around food. They cut up apples into tiny pieces and drop them one by one into a low calorie yoghurt. They mash their food and spread it around the plate, sometimes taking hours to consume a small meal. The presenting child is likely to be depressed. This depression is thought to be largely due to a poor diet. Low fat diets can cause depression. Their depression usually lifts once they are eating and gaining weight. Antidepressants rarely help the situation and are probably best advised at primary care level. Despite being tired, thin and cold, the child will often deny any problems, they rarely ask for help and minimize their symptoms.

Unfortunately sometimes, it is not only the child who denies a problem but the parents too. While some parents are overanxious and see faddy eating as a serious eating disorder, all too often the reverse is true. Many parents are in a state of denial and do not want to accept that there is a problem, preferring to believe their child.

To be fair to some of these families, the slow and steady decline in health and weight of their daughter is not always as noticeable to them as it is to someone who has not seen them for a while. Anorexic children are extremely deceitful and very convincing. They are experts at covering the fact that they are eating poorly. They become vegetarian, saying that they have become concerned about animal welfare when in fact it gives them an excuse to cut meat with its associated fat out of their diet. Many children give up sweets for Lent or just decide to eat more healthily. Some admit they are dieting with the intention of losing weight.

When their weight loss becomes severe, many anorexics disguise their thinness with layers of clothing, sometimes as many as three pairs of trainer bottoms and four or five tops. This could be to combat the cold they inevitably feel, it could also be that they are totally aware of how thin they have become and do not want people to notice. These garments not only weigh a significant amount but can also hide a multitude of heavy objects. It is absolutely vital to strip off the layers each time the child is weighed.

The history

When parents come to see you about their worries regarding their child, they may prefer to see you without her so that they can speak frankly without fear of her becoming angry. It is probably a good idea to see the parents together, the child alone, and then the parents and child together. Mothers' instincts about their children's eating problems are usually accurate and worthy of note. We see a lot of parents whose initial GP appointment resulted in them being told that they were neurotic and worrying unnecessarily. Once told this, the parents go home and are reluctant to ask for a second consultation. We too are contacted by obviously overanxious mothers, we know they exist but one must be sure before reassuring them that there is no real cause for their anxiety. Many of these anxious parents will recount a story that would take hours to tell, the GP needs to elicit a few concrete facts early in the consultation.

1. *Is your daughter having regular periods?* This one question immediately alerts you to a possible eating problem.

2. *Has your child lost any weight?* It may be that the child has not lost weight but has not gained weight as they should and finds themselves well below a normal weight. Any weight loss in a child should ring instant alarm bells.

3. *Does your child eat cheese, chips, and chocolate?* Most children love at least the last two of these and a recent history of 'eating healthily' or being vegetarian could be suggestive of an eating disorder.

Physical examination

It is useful to ask about a family history of eating disorders. Ask about any obsessive compulsive problems such as hand washing or overexercising.

If a thin girl tells you she is having periods when you take her menstrual history, be sure to ask about the contraceptive pill. Many parents believe that the pill reinstates the menstrual cycle and omit to mention it.

Discuss any mood or character changes the family have noticed. Finally, ask the parents to list everything their child ate yesterday, take care to elicit exact quantities. You need to know how many cornflakes constitute a bowlful! Parents will often list food they gave her but omit to mention that she left most of it.

If there has been weight loss, it will be necessary to establish a fear of fatness or deliberate dieting behaviour in order to exclude a physical cause.

It is important to weigh and measure the child and then calculate her weight–height ratio. Body mass index is not a useful measure to use in children, weight–height ratio or body mass index centiles are better predictors. Coles, the people who produce the pink and blue paediatric weight charts, market a slide rule that costs under £10 and allows the clinician to calculate the weight–height ratio and a target weight in seconds. You need an accurate height, weight, and age in years and months. An accurate height requires bare feet and for the person measuring to ensure that the child's jaw is at a right angle to the body, not with the chin thrust out and the head back as is often done. Pushing back the head can reduce the height by 1–2 cm and will make the calculation inaccurate. Likewise, children must be weighed in their underclothes and without shoes. Anorexic children put stones, coins, and kitchen weights into shoes and pockets, which will be missed if weighed in clothes and shoes. They frequently put batteries under their armpits and in their hair bands, under their hair. The practice nurse needs to be aware of all such tricks. The most common trick of all, and one that can only be overcome with the parents help, is drinking water to inflate their weight. To prevent this, the parent has to bring the child to be weighed at random times and without warning so that they do not have an opportunity to 'tank' before being weighed. Unfortunately we have heard of several mothers who have used a measuring jug to assist their child in gaining the necessary weight in order to avoid hospital admission.

One should be concerned about any child who is less than 90%, especially if the parents are worried about the child's eating. When a child's weight–height ratio drops to 80% the child has lost almost all her body fat and is beginning to use her own muscle as a source of energy. The heart muscle also becomes affected. Below 75%, the child probably needs to be admitted to hospital unless she is able to gain a steady and regular 0.5 kg a week at home. If the weight–height ratio is over 95% it is still necessary to re-weigh the child in a week to see if she is losing weight. Some anorexic children were overweight before they dieted. It is true that some parents panic, but not all and serial weights over 4 weeks are the only way to reassure yourself and parents.

Restricting the blood flow to the peripheries is one of the first compensations made by a starving body. The extremities are often cold and blue. Ankles can be oedematous.

Hypotension and a bradycardia are late but serious sign that the circulatory system is failing and the child needs urgent referral to hospital. Many anorexic children restrict their fluid intake and dehydrate. Small children can become dehydrated very quickly.

You may spot calluses on the dorsum of their fingers, a sign that the child is inducing vomiting.

During a physical examination it is necessary to look at the sacrum, which can be sore and even ulcerated from continued friction against a carpet while doing sit-ups. Muscle wasting can be demonstrated by asking the child to rise unaided from a squatting position.

The new NICE guidelines published in February 2004 suggest that the following laboratory investigations are undertaken: full blood count, erythrocyte sedimentation rate, blood biochemistry, liver functions tests, blood glucose, and urinalysis. They also suggest doing an ECG if there are signs of cardiac compromise. If a child is suspected of vomiting or abusing laxatives, it is important to check her potassium levels.

One must bear in mind, however, that even if serum potassium levels are normal, total body potassium could be seriously depleted, which could lead to arrhythmias and sudden death. Children can be extremely ill and still have near normal blood chemistry results. Pulse and BP are the best indications as to whether the child is coping or not and must be checked regularly in a child who is not gaining weight. An abnormal potassium, dehydration, or persistent vomiting are all clear indications that a child should be in hospital.

The younger the child, the greater the physical risk of starvation. As they have a lower percentage of body fat, young children can become emaciated without severe weight loss.

Parents are often concerned about bone density and want their child to take calcium supplements and to have bone density studies done. We do not use calcium supplements at Rhodes Farm as the children are all eating a normal diet and are receiving sufficient calcium.

If a child has been at a safe weight for a year and does not seem to be developing normally for her age or has not regained her periods, it might be helpful to send her for an abdominal ultrasound and to measure her luteinizing hormone and follicle-stimulating hormone. In boys gonadotrophin levels can be measured but there are no other investigations, which are useful in assessing pubertal delay. The size of the uterus and the endometrial thickness as well as the size of the ovaries and the presence or absence of follicles are useful indicators but if no development is seen, there is no useful treatment other than continuing to see that the child eats healthily.

There is no evidence that calcium absorption is increased by putting children on the contraceptive pill and is contraindicated in young adults as it leads to premature fusing of the epiphyses.

Long-term effects of eating disorders

When parents are in denial, not wanting treatment and clearly not taking their child's illness seriously, they need to be told very plainly about the long-term and short-term effects of this dreadful illness. A frank and honest discussion very often shocks the parents into agreeing to co-operate.

Children who starve lose their periods, many parents do not understand how serious this can be. If they remain at low weights, these children risk long-term infertility but their low oestrogen levels means that calcium is not taken up by the bones and they are at great risk of developing osteoporosis. Parents need to know that neither the pill nor calcium supplements will help and that the lost calcium will not be caught up later. Malnutrition also causes growth failure and anorexic girls very often remain short and even stunted by their starvation. In pre-pubertal children, puberty will often be delayed, the child will not develop breast tissue and will retain their pre-pubertal shape.

Parents need to be in no doubt that although many of the ill-effects of starvation in young adults can be reversed, this is not always the case with children. Children should not be allowed to starve themselves, it is clearly the responsibility of the adults caring for them to see that it does not continue.

A paper published in the *British Medical Journal* in January 2004 shows that starvation especially between the ages of 9 and 15 causes an increase in circulating concentrations of growth hormone and cortisol, both of which regulate blood pressure. Starvation may cause a permanent disruption of blood pressure regulation and appears to lead to raised blood pressure, excess mortality from ischaemic heart disease, and strokes. Given that the majority of children who starve will tell you that they avoid fat because it is bad for their health, they need to know the long-term risks they are running. Osteoporosis results in bones that fracture very easily and later in life causes intense pain as vertebrae collapse. Both parents and children need to be told the horrible consequences of continuing malnutrition.

Short-term effects of anorexia nervosa

Quite apart from the long-term effects of starvation noted above, there are very many serious short-term effects. Her ECG is likely to show abnormalities, in the very worse case there can be arrhythmias, which lead to sudden death. Vomiting and laxative abuse can also cause hypokalaemia and possible death. Children who restrict their food intake very often become anaemic.

Starvation, especially a lack of fat in the diet can cause depression and lack of concentration. Many parents will have recognized that their child is depressed but because they see them working so hard on their school work and achieving so well they find it difficult to admit that their child is ill. Anorexic children are determined individuals who can push themselves to the limit, both physically and mentally. They continue to exercise when they are weak and exhausted and study fanatically despite being ill.

Starving children have dry hair and skin, their hair sometimes falls out. More commonly they develop a fine, downy, dark hair covering their entire body. Many anorexics admit to sleeping very badly.

Effects of bulimia nervosa

The dangers of bulimia nervosa are very similar to those of anorexia nervosa. Bulimia has the added complication of predisposing sufferers to develop cysts on their ovaries, which can have a serious effect on fertility. Bulimics who vomit and take laxatives run the risk of hypokalaemia. Many girls who vomit do not know their salivary glands can hypertrophy giving them a hamster appearance. Their teeth are severely damaged by the gastric acid. Bulimics often have swollen hands and feet. It is common to see lesions on the back of their hands caused by their teeth when they induce vomiting. Bulimics are very often depressed.

If this catalogue of potential problems still does not mobilize the parents into seeking treatment, then the one thing that usually concentrates their mind is to explain that their daughter is not well enough to go to school. For many of these families, children and parents alike, academic achievement is highly valued. The child and the parents need to understand that it is not safe for a child who is not eating properly to remain at school.

Target weights

Target weight calculated on the Coles Growth Slide rule is a weight that cannot be negotiated. The research from Great Ormond Street Hospital has shown that most girls will menstruate at a 98% weight-for-height ratio. Of course there will be a percentage of children would menstruate at a slightly lower weight but as we have no way of knowing who they are, we have no choice but to err on the side of caution.

Do not be drawn into discussion about the fact that the family 'has small bones' or 'light bones'. The weight–height ratio calculated takes the height and age of the patient into account, nothing else needs to be considered. We are often told that the child would be more co-operative and would agree more readily to reach target if it could be set a little lower. Anyone who treats anorexic children will know that whatever target weight is agreed, the child will always endeavour to try to negotiate a few kilos less. There is not a weight at which the child feels happy about the way she looks, the proof is that she has already dieted way past the weight she is now claiming she would be happy with.

In our experience, ovarian function is very sensitive to a few kilograms and many of our patients lose their periods again when they drop even 1–2 kg below the weight we have set.

Another common complaint we hear is 'that weight is too much, she has never been that weight before'. Children can gain up to 7–8 kg in a year when growing normally so if a child has been ill for anything more than 6 months her target weight is always going to be greater than her pre-morbid weight. This is certainly not an indication that the target weight is too high. Another argument often raised is 'she had periods at several kilos below that before she was ill'. Exactly the same arguments applies, her periods have stopped because she has failed to keep up with her growth and development. It is also true that having damaged their ovaries through starvation, it is often necessary for the child to be at a slightly higher weight than before to 'kick-start' the ovaries into functioning. Beware of becoming embroiled in target weight discussions. Use the slide rule, show them how you have arrived at your figure and don't negotiate.

Nutrition

Anorexic children are often able to persuade their parents that they are eating normally unless the parents have some idea about nutrition and specifically about calories. Parents will often sit with their emaciated child denying any problem on the strength that she 'eats very well'. This comment clearly has to be taken with a pinch of salt when you are presented with a malnourished child. The parents may want you to carry out all sorts of tests and investigations that can be easily avoided if a truthful dietary history can be elicited. The restricting child can fool everyone by eating a Milky Way, a Kit-Kat, or a Crunchie everyday. These particular bars are the lowest in calories and probably consti- tute the largest part of their daily intake. A child who eats chocolate can still be extremely anorexic. It is not difficult to incorporate one of these chocolate bars into a 1000 calorie a day diet and still continue to lose weight very steadily.

Some anorexic children are fat phobic. Not only do they know that fat contains twice as many calories per gram than protein or carbohydrate, but they are also deluded about the effect of fat. I refer to their problems as delusional because no matter how much edu- cation they receive, they remain fixed in the idea that fat makes fat. Even when refeeding, these children will try to avoid fat even though the calories are being counted accurately.

I am afraid that our nation's obsession with healthy eating has led to a lot of misunder- standing among lay people about what constitutes a healthy diet. We hear constantly that we should be eating less fat, but rarely is it explained that there is a bottom line when it comes to cutting fat from our diet. Fat is a vital part of our daily food requirement, chil- dren are not healthy if they cut their fat intake below 30%, adults should not cut theirs below 20%.

Many anorexic children come from families who worry about fat and it is worth spending some time discussing the importance of fat with parents.

Why do children develop an eating disorder?

It seems as though anorexic children are born with a genetic predisposition to develop anorexia. These children tend to be obsessive, compulsive perfectionistic characters. If you are an anxious, obsessive type of person and you are surrounded by people who constantly worry about their health, weight, their food, and exercise, it is highly likely that you will take on those worries. Of course, anorexia is rarely just a diet gone wrong, in most cases there are many factors in the child's life that appear to be beyond her control and her weight is the one thing she can still control. Losing weight and being thin clearly has major advantages for these anorexic children. They are usually very reluctant to give it up even when ill and emaciated. In most cases the attention from the rest of the family increases enormously when someone begins to starve. Busy parents or warring parents often neglect their work and argue less when they have a sick child to look after. If this is the case, the child does not have a huge incentive to recover and see her family return to the way it was before she was ill. Her illness is serving a useful purpose, it may even be keeping together parents who were heading for separation.

In other cases, there can be a secret in the family, the secret can be the abuse of a child or spouse, or problems with alcohol or depression. A starving child may find herself in a setting where it is safe to reveal what is happening and again, starvation has served a use- ful function.

Sometimes at or around puberty, children begin to feel very insecure about their aca- demic abilities, their own personalities, and about their abilities to make friends. Sometimes they have high achieving siblings and they worry about whether they will be able to do as well. For them, being sick means that everyone's expectations of them are lowered. They cannot take examinations, they cannot make friends and socialize because they are ill. Again, if they are afraid of life, then life stops when anorexia takes over, to give it up and get on with life again is a daunting prospect.

Factors, which might precipitate anorexia nervosa, are many and varied. They include the traumas of body changes at puberty, the pressure of school, bereavement, social problems, and school problems. It is usually a combination of these pressures, which trigger a vulnerable youngster into an eating disorder.

Although anorexia is not usually caused by dieting alone, on occasions it does seem as though it originated either from overzealous dieting or following an illness that caused the child quite appropriately to lose their appetite. When the illness has gone, the child becomes reluctant to eat and worries about regaining the weight they have lost. There are many reported cases of prisoners, who have deliberately gone on hunger strikes developing anorexia nervosa when the reason for their starvation has long gone.

In a child who has suffered from anorexia nervosa for many months, factors, which precipitated the illness, may not be the same as the ones which are perpetuating it. By the time the illness is established, the family dynamics and the effect the illness is having may be what keeps the child anorexic. In a society that puts such enormous emphasis on weight and shape, it is not surprising that a troubled child could begin to focus her thoughts on her appearance.

While most of us survive with our feelings of inadequacy regarding our shape, there will always be a small minority for whom not being thin enough will wreck their lives if allowed to do so. We must take their problems and delusional thoughts seriously and do all we can to prepare them for the real world of imperfections.

Other eating problems

In children it is not always easy to distinguish between food avoidance emotional disorder (FAED) and anorexia nervosa. FAED resembles anorexia nervosa in that the child restricts their food and loses weight. The main difference is that they do not have a distorted body image, they know they are thin, and on the whole once their emotional problems are identified and acknowledged they eat very well with no worries about gaining weight.

Reducing the parents' level of anxiety can in some cases be an important factor in encouraging these children to eat more variety or simply to eat more. As long as they can be convinced that their child is unlikely to become physically ill, parents are usually able to relax.

Faddy eaters usually have a very small range of foods that they are prepared to eat but in most cases their diet provides for them nutritionally and they gain weight and grow normally. As they mature, these children usually bow to peer pressure and expand their repertoire of foods. Mothers become very panicked by their child repeatedly eating the same foods.

Restrictive eaters usually eat a normal range of foods but have a poor appetite and never seem to seek out and enjoy any particular food. They are usually at the lower end of normal limits of weight and height but develop and grow normally. By the time they reach puberty they are more reasonable about eating and are usually co-operative and accept dietary advice. Both faddy eaters and restrictive eaters can sometimes run into trouble when they experience a growth spurt just before puberty and it is important to see that they stay on their height and weight centiles.

Families

Most research seems to indicate that family therapy or family counselling is the most effective treatment for anorexia nervosa in young people. In the early stages of the illness and in the absence of any severe problems within the family, help advice and support in the form of family meetings could be sufficient to put the child on the road to recovery. It is probably more useful to see the family frequently for short periods of time rather than longer less frequent meetings. It is important when beginning to work with these families not to make the family feel blamed for their child's illness. The family are usually riddled with guilt and are sure that they are at fault. Whether or not they were responsible initially or whether they are responsible for the perpetuation of the illness, nothing can be gained for making the family feel inadequate.

Initially it might be better to approach the problem by explaining that it doesn't always help to go over the past (although inevitably this will happen at some stage) we need to move on. We need to find a way to help the child feel that she can eat with her family again. Anorexic families are described as being non-confrontational and over-enmeshed. Neither of these make working with the family easy. By the time the family presents with an anorexic child, they have usually totally lost control of the child and the child is firmly in the driving seat. Family counselling should be aimed at getting the parents back in charge, where they should be. Children often fight for control but in reality do not benefit from it. Children feel safer and more secure when their parents are in charge. I vividly remember a family therapy session where the child screamed 'you've never cared about me, you've always let me do exactly what I want'. A very telling statement from a child who had been fighting to do what she wanted. Children see lack of boundaries and a lack of supervision as not caring. They are not proud of parents who are weak and can be trampled upon.

In very general terms, the parents we see could be divided into three groups.

- The first group, respond very quickly to good advice and their children get better rapidly.

- The second group of parents are more difficult to manage, their children do recover but make slower progress.

- The third group of parents are the most resistive to treatment. They seem unable to take control of their child's illness. No amount of advice, counselling or therapy seems to make a difference. They carry non-confrontation to its limits and their child only recovers if they can do it on their own. Those who cannot, remain ill and move on to become chronic anorexics.

In the first group, the parents are instinctively authoritarian. They do not negotiate or back down, they expect obedience from their children. Their child, like many anorexics, has always been a perfect child. The parents have never had to exert their authority or practise their parental skills until the day she developed anorexia.

If this family is given good advice and counselling early on in the primary care setting, their child's anorexia can be brought under control before it becomes established and more difficult to treat.

We often see parents who have been told by professionals that the way to deal with a determinedly, anorexic child is to let her go her own way. When parents complain that the child only wants to eat cereals, baked beans, and vegetables, they are told that the diet is totally adequate and that they should not worry. They are told that as long as she is eating, what she eats does not matter. This would be good advice if the child was a faddy eater and not losing weight. When the parents explain that their child wants to eat alone in her room, they are told that that is what teenagers do and not to be anxious. When the parent reports that she is exercising excessively, they are told that exercise is healthy and normal. Although the parents intuitively feel that this advice is not sound, they bow to the professional and the child carries on, fully in control and her weight spirals down.

Advice in managing weight gain

Many anorexic children react very positively to being taken in hand and are desperate for help but don't feel able to ask. They do not want to be left alone with their illness. The three major treatments for eating disorders are individual therapy, family therapy and refeeding. Refeeding advice is easily dealt with in a primary setting, anorexic children do not necessarily need dieticians, they simply need to eat what normal children eat. Clearly the parents need to be aware of the different food groups and how important it is to see that the child has a varied diet. Children who are being refed need to gain 0.5 kg a week if being treated as an outpatient. One has to overeat 7000 calories in order to gain 1 kg. Therefore to gain 0.5 kg a week one has to eat 3500 calories, i.e. 500 calories a day over and above one's normal requirements. As a rule of thumb, most children need about 2000 calories a day, 2500 calories a day therefore should guarantee 0.5 kg a week increase.

One way to help children to gain weight is to use a calorie book. Initially parents need to weigh and measure their child's food to make sure she is taking the required amount. Parents need to be warned not to confuse kilocalories with kilojoules also printed on food packets.

Most cakes, bread, sweets, prepared meals, and tins have the calories clearly displayed. Warn the parents to be careful to differentiate between calories per 100 grams and calories in the entire pot or tin. Always round up and not down. Don't let the children in the kitchen. She is not to interfere with weighing, measuring, or the choice of food. Parents should be advised to be honest about the calories and not to try to pretend that foods are lower in value than they really are.

Exactly how many calories a child needs will depend on her height, weight, and the amount of exercise she is taking. Parents should weigh the child twice a week and adjust the calories up or down in order to gain 0.5 kg per week. More rapid weight gains will make the child feel out of control and the parents will lose her trust. She needs to eat at least 30% of her calories as fat, 20% as protein, and 50% as carbohydrate.

The majority of children who are admitted to our clinic claim to be vegetarian. When a good history is taken, the vegetarianism rarely pre-dates the illness. Most vegetarian children do not eat sufficient protein in their diets. While refeeding, it is probably wiser for children to eat at least chicken breast and fish rather than a completely vegetarian diet.

Butter, normal milk, and cheese are all excellent foods for a child who needs to gain weight. No harm is going to come to a child who eats a slightly higher percentage of her diet as fat for a few months while she gains weight. Cream and cheese can increase the calorific value of her meal without substantially adding to the volume and are therefore useful when refeeding. Parents who object to giving their child fat on health grounds, need to know that starving children often have exceptionally high blood cholesterol levels. It is safer to have butter than to starve. Another point to make to parents is that pizza, chips, and chocolate are standard teenage foods. If a child regains her weight but remains terrified of these sorts of food, her social life is going to be severely affected. She will refuse invitations to go out or sleep over at a friend's house because she will be worried about the sort of food she will have to eat.

Gaining the weight is only half the battle, one has to end up with a child who can eat with her friends and eat what they are eating.

School lunches can be a problem if the child is well enough to attend school. If school lunches cannot be supervised, it may be better to give the child a very small packed lunch such as a yogurt or apple and catch up the calories in a snack when she arrives home from school. A typical breakdown of the day's calories is shown in Table 29.1.

Parents do not have to eat as much as their children, they are not trying to gain 0.5 kg per week. They should, however, eat all their meals with their child and ensure the child finishes the amount served.

Table 29.1 Typical breakdown of the day's calories.

		kcal
Breakfast:	100 g crisp muesli (450 cal/per 100 g)	450
	Full cream milk	75
	Orange juice	75
	2 slices of toast or muffin with butter	200
Lunch:	(at school)	
	Yogurt	150
	Apple	50
Snacks	(at 4pm)	
	King-size Mars Bar or crisps and smaller chocolate bar	500
Supper	Main meal	500
	Dessert (pie or pudding with ice cream or custard)	500

If the parents return in a week, adamant that they have followed the plan and the child has not gained weight, there are three main reasons why this could be.

1. the child has not in fact eaten 2500 calories a day

2. she ate them but vomited

3. she exercised excessively.

If the child did not in fact eat the food, this could be because the parents calorie counting was poor, or because they failed to see the food disappearing into tissues, socks under the table or into pockets. If one suspects that a child is vomiting the family need to know how dangerous that can be. They will then need to supervise her for 3 hours following every meal and snack. Children learn to vomit silently and effortlessly, standing outside listening is not sufficient. These children will vomit into plastic bags, drawers, vases, even into their own clothes. Bags of vomit are often openly left where they can be found, a clear indication that they want to be discovered and helped.

Excessive exercising is not always easy to discover. Sometimes the parents will describe a child who never sits down, even does her homework standing up, who walks the dog several times a day, and goes to the gym. They are aware of her problem but need a firm plan in order to deal with it.

It is important to agree on a sensible exercise regime that is tailored to the child's physical condition.

Exercise can be gradually increased in line with weight gain but it is vital that it does not become a compulsion. Exercise should be fun, a social pursuit not a repetitive chore. Dancers and athletes may never be able to go back to the same level of activity they were doing before their illness.

Even at target weight, parents should be made aware that obsessive exercising could begin again if they are not vigilant.

They may need to continue restricting her exercise to relieve her of the responsibility and the guilt. If you have a child at home, eating 2750 calories a day or more and not gaining weight, she needs to be referred on, it indicates the necessary progress is not being made.

Having established the patient on a regime, which restores her weight, attention needs to be turned to why the child felt the need to starve and lose weight.

In some cases you may not identify any problem within the family and except for her dieting, the child seems well adjusted, has lots of friends and is enjoying school. If the family does not feel the need to talk and the child does not want to talk to someone individually, you do not have to worry as long as her weight gain is steady and you feel that she is behaving normally. They need to know that should they change their minds, help and support would be available.

If there are recognized problems within the family, the family counselling that you can provide might not be sufficient and they might need to see a family therapist. Children rarely ask for individual help but should be encouraged to see someone. Although recent research shows that sexual abuse among children with anorexia nervosa is probably no higher than in the general psychiatric population, it is still a significant trigger for this illness and the child needs an opportunity to be seen alone and to be asked if anyone has ever hurt them or done anything to them they have not liked.

If the family does need family therapy, it is important to refer them to an accredited family therapist, inexperienced counsellors can do more harm than good. If the child's weight does not rise steadily or you feel she is unhappy or depressed, it would be wise to refer on to the local child and adolescent psychiatrist, one who has an interest in eating disorders if that is possible. Antidepressants are seldom indicated in children with an eating disorder and could only be justified once a child was at a good weight. Most low weight children are depressed, the depression usually lifts once the child is eating a normal diet and is gaining weight.

We have talked about the group 1 parents who are easily able to be in charge of their children once they have been shown the right path. The group 2 parents are more problematic. For these parents taking control of their child does not come naturally. They are unlikely to grasp the principles of sanctions and firmness without a great deal of family work. They need constant reassurance that their child will not hate them forever if they confront her.

With help, these parents can be encouraged to stand firm against their child's illness rather than collude with it. The level of input needed to help these families is probably greater than can be provided within the primary care setting.

Case vignettes

Patient A was 13 years old when he was admitted. He had been ill for 18 months. He had a weight–height ratio of only 69% and was depressed. Following admission he ate readily in the unit, gained weight and seemed happy. He vomited spontaneously before his first weekend at home and ate very badly and lost weight during the weekend. Despite very frequent family sessions, he lost weight every time he was sent home and it soon became apparent that he did not want to be there. A year after admission we were able to persuade social services that he needed fostering. *A* agreed that this would be a good idea.

Six months after his placements with foster carers, he was eating and growing normally, thriving at school and had friends for the first time in his life.

Patient B was a long distance runner. Her father had also been a runner in his youth. *B* was admitted at a weight–height ratio of 62%. She was still training daily at her local athletics club. Her low weight meant that initially she could only do our gentle stretch and relaxation classes. Her parents came to plead on her behalf for her to be allowed to swim and do aerobic classes, even though she was still emaciated. *B* tried to exercise whenever she could and at one stage needed to eat 4000 kilocalories a day in order to gain her 1 kg per week. When put on one to one supervision we were able to reduce her calories substantially. Her exercise problem was discussed regularly in family sessions, her parents often pressing us to allow her to do more exercise.

During weekends at home, *B* was allowed to swim for an hour each day and go on several long walks. She ate huge quantities of food and kept her weight up. Despite our pleas for caution, *B* was allowed to return to her athletics club immediately after she was discharged. Initially she was able to disguise her weight loss by hiding weights and drinking water but eventually she was discovered to be 8 kg below target and needed readmission. This cycle was repeated several times before her parents agreed to control her exercise.

Patient C was a ballet dancer. Her parents argued about her target weight, despite the fact that *C* was 15 years old and showing no signs of pubertal development. Her parents explained that she was 'on the pill' so she was having regular periods and they were not worried about her bones. *C*'s mother said she had been anorexic, she remained extremely thin. Mother explained that they 'ate healthily', never used butter, never ate chocolate, hated chips, and were vegetarian.

During weekends at home *C* was given salads, pasta, and cereal with skimmed milk. She did not lose weight but her diet was severely deficient in fat. *C*'s mother had promised her that she would allow her to lose 2–3 kg once discharged as she thought her target weight was too high.

Two years after her discharge their GP sent her for an abdominal ultrasound and a bone scan. It revealed very poorly developed ovaries and an abnormal bone density. Only after these investigations did her mother restrict her to one ballet class a week. She also insisted that she restored her weight and ate a one-third of her calories as fat. *C*'s mother continued on her ultra-low fat diet and not surprisingly their relationship deteriorated. *C* left home at 16 and immediately began to eat normally and gain weight.

Conclusions

The first port of call for the parents of a child with an eating disorder is their GP. The GP first has to distinguish between faddy eating, anxious parents, and the more serious eating disorders. Having diagnosed an eating disorder, the next step is to decide if the patient can be managed in the practice, if she needs referring to the local child and adolescent mental health services team or as is sometimes the case, she needs urgent admission to hospital. Her physical condition and the ability of her parents to manage her eating with your help will be your best indicators for the advisability of referring on.

The NICE guidelines mention that many GP's lack training in eating disorders, which can lead to a delay in diagnosis. Let us hope that more training will be given in future.

They also suggest that the pathways between primary and secondary care are often too slow. In children, it is difficult to say whether this delay is due to a reluctance to refer on or to the lack of specialist services to refer to. I am sure that GP's would use the pathways if they were clearly signposted.

Chapter 30

Childhood obesity in primary care

John Reilly, Laura Stewart, and David Wilson

Introduction and aims

Obesity is now very common in children and adolescents across the world, and prevalence continues to rise. Among health professionals and patients there is widespread ignorance and confusion over issues such as the aetiology, diagnosis, complications, and management of paediatric obesity. The present chapter aims to provide a concise, evidence-based but still practical summary of these issues, with a primary care perspective.

Diagnosis and prevalence

Body mass index (BMI) for age: the basis of diagnosis

Obesity is a body fat content that is sufficiently high to be harmful. As body fat content cannot be measured accurately or practically in routine clinical practice, there is a need for a simpler alternative or proxy measure of body fat content. Simple clinical assessments such as 'eyeballing' the child, or making a judgement based on the patient's weight alone, are flawed (see Scottish Intercollegiate Guidelines Network (SIGN) in references; Reilly *et al.* 2002). The only suitable option is measurement of height and weight and calculation of the BMI (weight in kg/height^2 in m^2) (see SIGN). As BMI is lower in children and adolescents than in adults, and as BMI changes with age (Figure 30.1) and differs between boys and girls, interpreting a BMI in a child or adolescent requires that it is considered as a 'BMI-for-age', i.e. a child's BMI must be compared against a percentile chart (Must 2005; Reilly 2006). Percentile charts for BMI for age are now available for many countries, notably the USA (where they are available free from the internet, downloadable at www.cdc.gov/growthcharts) and the UK (from Harlow Printing/Child Growth Foundation; see Figure 30.1).

Diagnostic accuracy of the body mass index for age

A large body of high quality and consistent evidence has shown that the definitions BMI ≥95th percentile (obesity; referred to as 'overweight' in the USA) and BMI >85th percentile (overweight; referred to as 'at risk of overweight' in the USA) provide accurate diagnostic information (see below). In the UK the percentile charts do not give 85th and 95th percentiles, and so 91st and 98th BMI percentiles should be used to define or diagnose (see SIGN; Reilly *et al.* 2002) overweight and obesity respectively (Table 30.1).

Diagnosing or defining a patient as obese in this way has high specificity (low false positive rate) but modest sensitivity (moderate false negative rate) (see SIGN; Reilly *et al.*

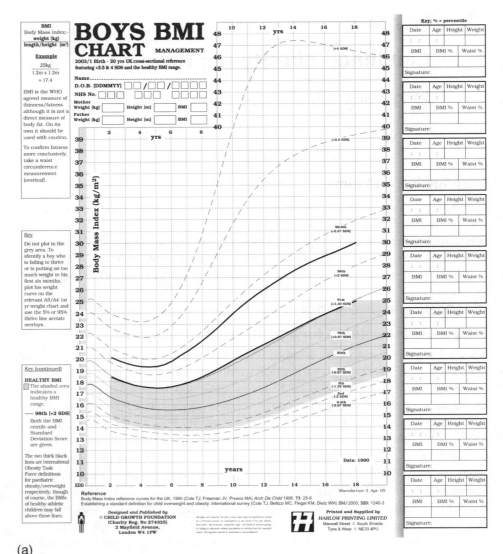

(a)

Fig. 30.1 Body mass index percentile charts for UK girls (a) and boys

2002; Reilly 2006). For the purposes of clinical diagnosis the high specificity is paramount because it provides confidence that a patient with high BMI for age really is excessively fat and therefore minimizes the risk of offering unnecessary treatment (Barlow and Dietz 1998; Must and Anderson 2005). In summary, children with high BMI for age (such as those with BMI above the 98th percentile) are highly likely to be among the fattest children in the population—they do not have high BMI as a result of a large muscle mass- and systematic reviews have also shown that they are at high risk of morbidity in childhood/adolescence *and* in later life(see SIGN; Reilly *et al.* 2002, 2003; Reilly 2006).

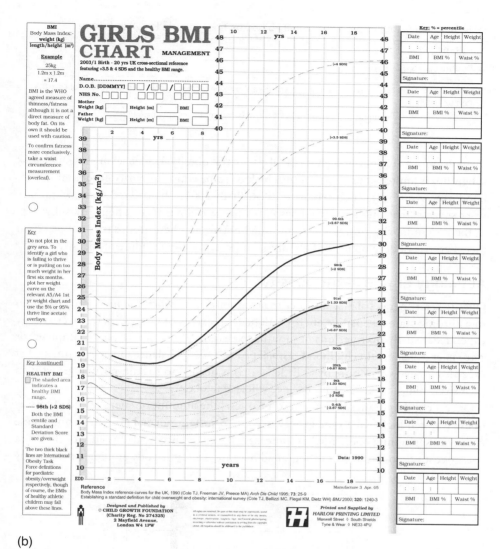

(b)

Fig. 30.1 cont'd (b). Available in the UK from the Child Growth Foundation, 2 Mayfield Avenue, London, W4 1PW; or from Harlow Printing www.harlowprinting.co.uk US BMI percentile charts available free to download from www.cdc.gov/growthcharts

Prevalence

In the UK, the paediatric obesity epidemic began in the late 1980s and prevalence continues to rise (Figure 30.2). The most recent English data confirm a continued increase and that a staggering 25% of 11–15 year olds were obese in 2004 (Health Survey for England 2004) (BMI ≥95th percentile). The UK is not unique and the epidemic of paediatric obesity is global: for evidence from other countries the reader is referred elsewhere (Ebbelling *et al.* 2002; Lobstein *et al.* 2004; Reilly 2005).

Table 30.1 Definitions of paediatric obesity based on body mass index (BMI) for age

BMI ≥85th percentile,* overweight[†]

BMI ≥95th percentile,* obese[†]

*When using UK 1990 BMI charts (Figure 30.1) overweight should be defined as BMI ≥91st percentile; obesity BMI ≥98th percentile.

[†]In the USA overweight is commonly referred to as 'at risk of overweight', and obesity referred to as 'overweight'.

Some groups are at even higher risk of paediatric obesity. Evidence on these high-risk subgroups is limited at present, but they include some ethnic minority groups and childhood cancer survivors (Lobstein *et al.* 2004; Reilly 2005). In Scotland, our preliminary work suggests that children and adolescents with special needs are a high-risk subgroup. In the USA, minority groups are at much higher risk and these groups may not just be at increased risk of development of obesity, but also of the comorbidities of obesity.

Aetiology of paediatric obesity

Obesity is an energy balance disorder that can only occur when the individual has been in a chronic state of positive energy balance (an excess of energy intake over energy expended, usually over periods of months to years). Adults should be in complete (or zero) energy balance. In childhood, a small positive energy balance (an energy intake that exceeds energy expenditure by as little as 1%) is needed to sustain normal growth; an excessively high chronic positive balance will lead to obesity.

Once a child or adolescent has become obese, the amount of energy needed to stay obese is much higher than the energy needed to sustain normal growth in non-obese children. Remaining obese further increases energy requirements because of the extra energy cost of moving an obese body, and because the larger body and higher lean body

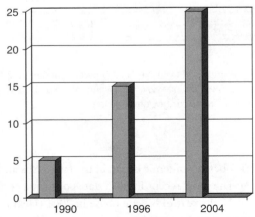

Fig. 30.2 Progress of the obesity epidemic in English children, 1990–2004. Obesity defined as BMI ≥95th percentile. Data sources: UK 1990 reference data (1990); Health Surveys for England (1996, 2004).

mass (obese children are not just fatter than non-obese children but have a higher lean body mass) requires more energy to maintain basal metabolism, even at rest.

Many parents, patients, and health professionals believe that obesity can coexist with low energy requirements, but this is a myth that is unhelpful in addressing the life-style issues in management—becoming more accurate in perceptions of life-style (the roles of eating, activity, and sedentary behaviour) is an important element of management, as described below. Treating patient/parent reports of food intake as accurate is unwise—there is good evidence that under-reporting of food intake is common. In a few very rare cases the positive energy balance required to make a non-obese child obese might have occurred secondary to some underlying pathology (such as hypothyroidism or leptin deficiency), but this is extremely rare. In the vast majority of obese patients it is their life-style over months and years that has led to their obesity, and therefore modifying their life-style over months and years is the key to treatment (see SIGN; Barlow and Dietz 1998).

Complications of paediatric obesity

Complications in the short term

Table 30.2(A) shows the principal health consequences of obesity (e.g. BMI ≥95th percentile) *in childhood and adolescence*, derived from a systematic review/critical appraisal of published evidence up to end of 2001 (Reilly *et al.* 2003). This evidence confirms that obesity *is* a health burden for children and adolescents, and the complications are many and varied. The complications or 'comorbidities' are probably more of a burden for clinical populations of obese children and adolescents, those seeking treatment, than for the obese 'general population'. Since our systematic review was published the evidence on the comorbidities of paediatric obesity has continued to accumulate with recent particular concerns over liver disease and orthopaedic complications.

Complications in the medium to long term

Table 30.2(B) shows the principal consequences of childhood obesity for the adult who was obese as a child, again based on our systematic review. The evidence (Table 30.1) is

Table 30.2 Principal health consequences of paediatric obesity

For the obese child/adolescent
Psychological ill health
Cardiovascular risk factors
Asthma
Chronic inflammation
Diabetes (type 1 and 2)
Orthopaedic abnormalities
Liver disease
Persistence of obesity
For the adult who was obese as a child/adolescent
Cardiovascular risk factors
Adverse social and economic outcomes
Premature mortality

clear that paediatric obesity matters in both the short and long term. Existing and older evidence may also underestimate the scale of complications for contemporary children and adolescent. For example, older cohort studies suggested that a majority of obese children or adolescents might 'grow out of' their obesity to become non-obese adults. In more recent cohorts the vast majority of obese children, and particularly obese adolescents, remain obese and so become obese adults (Reilly *et al.* 2003; Freedman *et al.* 2005; Reilly 2005). Growing out of obesity is particularly unlikely for the obese adolescent, for the obese child or adolescent with an obese parent, and for the more severely obese patient (Whitaker *et al.* 1997).

The evidence on the multiple comorbidities of paediatric obesity, combined with the increasing numbers of obese children and adolescents, makes a strong case not only for prevention but for the treatment of obesity in children and adolescence, and the principles of treatment are described below. It should be noted that effective treatment of obesity in childhood would also represent an obesity prevention strategy later in life, when the comorbidities become more common and more severe.

Management

Basic management principles

There are three basic questions in management: who should be treated; who should be referred from primary care; what should treatment aim for? Evidence-based answers to these questions are given in Table 30.3.

Treatment strategies: the evidence base

Evidence on specific interventions in treatment has been systematically reviewed and/or critically appraised by a number of authors in recent years (SIGN; Summerbell *et al.* 2003; Whitlock *et al.* 2005).

All of these reviews/appraisal exercises have noted a distinct lack of high-quality evidence (from randomized controlled trials, RCT) for specific interventions. Most previous

Table 30.3 Evidence-based answers to basic management questions

Who should be treated?
    Patients who are obese on basis of their BMI for age (see Table 30.1).
    Patients/families who appear motivated to seek life-style change and/or perceive their child's obesity as a problem.

Who should be referred from primary care?
    Patients who have or may have serious co-morbidity (e.g. sleep apnoea; type 2 diabetes).
    Patients where an underlying pathological cause of obesity is suspected (e.g. severe obesity in the under 2s; obesity with short stature).

What should treatment aim for?
    Weight maintenance (for most patients) not weight loss.
    Establishment of sustainable lifestyle changes.
    Resolution of comorbidity as appropriate.

treatment RCT have been relatively short term, have been underpowered, and have used interventions that are not readily generalizable to primary care. However, evidence-based 'best bets' in treatment, from recent systematic reviews and critical appraisal exercises, are given in Table 30.4, and their practical use is exemplified in case study 1.

Looking to the future of treatment

Audits of existing treatment programme for childhood obesity are frequently disappointing, characterized by high patient attrition/non-attendance and a high proportion of patients failing to maintain weight—the aim of treatment for most patients. Successful treatment may require a great many clinical consultations over a long period of time (and 'successful 'means long-term weight maintenance)—such a course is exemplified in case study 2. This creates a problem in primary care, where the reality of community care in the UK National Health Service is the expectation that this is where the majority of obese children will be treated. To compound this with poor treatment strategies and an epidemic of new cases could create despair and therapeutic nihilism.

It is clear that improvements to treatment are required, and that future treatment programmes designed for primary care are developed—that is, are potentially successful, feasible, and yet relatively inexpensive to implement. Some fairly novel treatment approaches appear to be promising: novel dietary targets such as modification of the glycaemic load of the diet (Ebbelling *et al.* 2003); combining pharmacotherapy with life-style change (Chanoine *et al.* 2005); residential treatment (Gately *et al.* 2005); surgery (Inge *et al.* 2004); and adapting the successful treatment approaches of Epstein *et al.* (1998) to make them more generalizable (Edwards *et al.* 2006). At present there is a lack of high-quality evidence for these approaches, and they may never be suitable for the treatment of large numbers of patients in primary care, so yet more carefully considered and novel approaches are likely to be necessary.

Case studies

Our first case study was a short-term intervention using simple healthy life-style messages; the second was more intensive with specific targeted life-styles. Both were successful and illustrate the necessity of the commitment and motivation of the child, parents, and the whole family.

Table 30.4 Evidence-based 'best bets' in treatment

Treat the family, not just the obese child
Modify diet, perhaps using a specific dietary scheme such as the 'traffic light diet' (Epstein et al. 1998; Stewart et al. 2005)
Encourage reduced sedentary behaviour (TV viewing and media use) to a target of <14 hours/week
Encourage increases in habitual physical activity
Encourage greater family awareness of their life-style (eating, physical activity, sedentary behaviour) by self-monitoring
Provide more time for clinic consultations, over a longer period, and more frequent consultations

Case 1

An 11-year-old boy was referred from the school health service for treatment of obesity. His weight was 83.1 kg (very much greater than the 99.6th percentile for age), height 1.54 m (on the 91st centile for age) and BMI was 35.0 kg/m^2 (very much greater than the 99.6th centile for age). Dietary review by the dietician showed that he 'grazed' all day on high energy snacks (crisps, biscuits, sweets, and ice creams). His family purchased 'take-out' meals two to three times per week and none exercised. We had a long discussion about obesity and life-style advice for the family, which emphasized:

- the need for both the child *and* the family to change their life-styles
- decreasing foods particularly high in sugar and fat (crisps, chips, sweets, etc.)
- substituting these with low energy snacks (fruit, raw vegetables, plain biscuits)
- starting a regular meal and snack pattern of eating (rather than grazing)
- giving appropriate portion sizes for different aged people
- activity: moderate exercise such as walking or cycling for at least 30–40 minutes on three to four occasions per week
- parenting skills: leading by example
- giving boundaries in terms of eating, activity, and sedentary behaviour
- installing a sensible limit on pocket money
- limiting the amount of energy-dense food purchased
- agreement on food-based weekly treats
- avoiding the use of food as a reward or for comfort.

Two issues of great importance to potential outcome were revealed during the consultation. First, the boy acknowledged that he had a problem with his weight and suggested changes that he felt he could make in terms of snacks and exercise. Secondly, the family agreed that they were all ready and willing to make necessary life-style changes. He was reviewed 6 weeks later, and all the family had made dietary and other life-style changes. His weight had decreased to 80.9 kg, and so BMI had decreased to 34.1 kg/m^2. This was shown to him on a centile chart in order to reinforce the benefits of the changes. Furthermore, his sister had lost 2.2 kg and his mother 6.1 kg over the same time period!

Case 2

A 9-year-old girl referred by community health service due to excessive weight gain. At initial consultation she weighed 60 kg (greater than the 99.6th centile for age), height was 1.52 m (on the 99.6th centile for age) and BMI was 26.0 kg/m^2 (greater than the 99.6th centile for age). Dietary review and later recording of life-style showed that she was moderately active with some weekly activities after school and that she ate a range of high energy snacks, including weekly carry outs. At first interview she gave her score for the importance of 'being slimmer' as 9/10, mum gave 8/10.

Table 30.5 Decisional balance chart

Pros of life-style change	Cons of life-style change
Wouldn't be picked on at school	Miss some favourite foods
Be lighter and be more able to walk and run faster at sports day	Not be able to watch telly very much
Be able to fit into clothes	Wouldn't be able to play some computer games I like playing
Wouldn't have to suffer watching sister eat sweets	Wouldn't be able to play board games
Wouldn't get loads of spots	
Don't want to be fat for the rest of my life	
Family more healthier	
Go as a family to the woods or something like that	

She also gave her pros and cons of changing her life-style (using a decisional balance chart) (see Table 30.5).

She was given a 'traffic light diet' scheme (Stewart *et al.* 2005) and information on increasing her physical activity levels as well as decreasing her sedentary behaviour. Emphasis was placed on the whole family undertaking any necessary life-style changes.

At her second appointment **she set her own goals** of:

♦ 1–2 chocolate biscuits per day

♦ no crisps but can have 1 packet of 'Snack a Jacks' (biscuits) per day

♦ sweets one day per week

♦ to go for a cycle during the school holiday week two to four times.

She had a total of eight dietetic appointments over 6 months. Her weight at the final appointment was 59.6 kg (greater than the 99.6th centile for age), height 1.54 m (on the 99.6th centile for age) and her BMI was 25 kg/m^2 (less than the 99.6th centile for age), i.e. her obesity grading had changed. She was very proud of herself, her mother reported an increase in her self-confidence, she was now wearing fashionable clothes and the whole family had under taken similar life-style changes. **She set her own long-term goals** as:

♦ no crisps

♦ one 'red' food per day

♦ minimum of half an hour of physical activity two to three times per week

♦ no more than 2–3 hours non-active time per day.

Six months after the completion of the dietetic intervention she had maintained her life-style changes, her weight was 60.4 kg (just below 99.6th centile for age), height was 1.58 m (just below 99.6th centile for age), her BMI was 24.3 kg/m^2 (between 98th and 99.6th centiles for age).

Conclusions

The primary care setting provides a potentially useful opportunity for both prevention and treatment of paediatric obesity (Barlow and Dietz 1998; Stettle 2004; Robinson 2006). While no specific interventions can be recommended at present, the approaches to diagnosis, management, and treatment, outlined in this chapter should be helpful for coping with the increasing numbers of obese children and adolescents presenting for treatment in primary care. Further sources of advice and information are given at the end of the references list.

References

Barlow SE, Dietz WH (1998). Obesity evaluation and treatment: expert committee recommendations. *Pediatrics* **102**: 554–570.

Chanoine JP, Hampl S, Jensen C, Boldrin M, Hauptman J (2005). Effect of Orlistat on weight and body composition in obese adolescents: a randomised controlled trial. *JAMA* **293**: 2873–2883.

Ebbelling CB, Pawlak DB, Ludwig DS (2002). Childhood obesity: public health crisis; common sense cure. *Lancet* **360**: 473–482.

Ebbelling CB, Leiding MM, Sinclair KB, Ludwig DS (2003). A reduced glycaemic load diet in the treatment of adolescent obesity. *Archives of Pediatric Adolescent Medcine* **157**: 773–779.

Edwards C, Nicholls D, Croker H, Van Zyls, Viner R, Wardle J (2006). Family based behavioural treatment of obesity. *European Journal of Clinical Nutrition* **60**: 587–592.

Epstein LH, Myers MD, Raynor HA, Saelens BE (1998). Treatment of pediatric obesity. *Pediatrics* **101**: 554–570.

Freedman DS, Khan LK, Serdula MK, Dietz WH, Srinivasan SR, Berenson GS (2005). Racial differences in the tracking of childhood BMI to adulthood. *Obesity Research* **13**: 928–935.

Gately PJ, Cooke CB, Barth JH, Bewick BM, Radley D, Hill AJ (2005). Children's residential weight loss camps can work. *Pediatrics* **116**: 73–77.

Health Survey for England (2004). Updating of trend tables to include childhood obesity data. Accessed 21 May 2006. www.ic.nhs.uk/pubs/hsechildobesityupdate

Inge TH, Drebs NF, Garcia VF (2004). Bariatric surgery for severely overweight adolescents: concerns and recommendations. *Pediatrics* **114**: 217–223.

Lobstein T, Baur L, Uauy R (2004). Obesity in children and young people: a crisis in public health. *Obesity Reviews* **5** (Suppl. 1): 4–85.

Must A, Anderson SE (2005). Childhood obesity definition, classification, and assessment. In: Kopelman PG, Caterson ID, Dietz WH (eds), *Clinical Obesity in Adults and Children*, (2nd edn). Blackwell Publishing, Oxford, pp. 215–230.

Must A, Anderson SE (2006). Body mass index in children and adolescents: considerations for population-based applications. *International Journal of Obesity* **30**: 590–594.

Reilly JJ (2005). Descriptive epidemiology and health consequences of childhood obesity. *Best Practice Research in Clinical Endocrinology and Metabolism* **19**: 327–341.

Reilly JJ (2006). Diagnostic accuracy of the BMI-for-age in paediatrics. *International Journal of Obesity* **30**: 595–597.

Reilly JJ, Wilson M, Summerbell CD, Wilson DC (2002). Obesity diagnosis, prevention, and treatment: evidence-based answers to common questions. *Archives of Disease in Childhood* **86**: 392–395.

Reilly JJ, Methven E, McDowell SC, Hacking B, Alexander D, Stewart L, Kelnar CZH (2003). Health consequences of obesity: systematic review and critical appraisal. *Archives of Disease in Childhood* **88**: 748–752.

Robinson TN (2006). Obesity prevention in primary care. *Archives of Pediatric Adolescent Medicine* **160**: 217–218.

Scottish Intercollegiate Guidelines Network (SIGN). Obesity in children and young people: a national clinical guideline. SIGN 69. www.sign.ac.uk

Stettler N (2004). The global epidemic of childhood obesity: a role for the paediatrician? *Obesity Reviews* **5** (Suppl 1): 1–3.

Stewart L, Hughes AR, Houghton J, Pearson D, Reilly JJ (2005). Dietetic management of pediatric overweight: development and description of a practical and evidence-based behavioural approach. *Journal of the American Dietetic Association* **105**: 1810–1815.

Summerbell CD, Kelly S, Waters E, Edmunds L, O'Meara S, Ashton V, Campbell K (2003). Interventions for treating obesity in children. *The Cochrane Library*.

Whitaker RC (2003). Obesity prevention in primary care: for behaviours to target. *Archives of Pediatric Adolescent Medicine* **151**: 725–727.

Whitaker RC, Wright JA, Pepe MS, Seidel KD, Dietz WH (1997). Predicting obesity in young adulthood from childhood and parental obesity. *New England Journal of Medicine* **337**: 869–873.

Whitlock EP, Williams SB, Gold R, Smith PR, Shipman SA (2005). Screening and interventions for childhood overweight: a summary of evidence for the US Preventive Services Task Force. *Pediatrics* **116**: e125–e144.

Internet-based sources of management advice

Cochrane reviews of prevention and treatment (Summerbell et al); www.nelh.nhs.uk

Evidence-based review & management guidance (Australia); www.obesityguidelines.gov.au

Evidence-based review & management guidance (Scotland); SIGN 69 www.sign.ac.uk

Expert committee report on management (USA; www.pediatrics.org/cgi/content/full/102/3/e29

Management guidance for primary care (England); www.rcpch.ac.uk/publications

Review of systematic reviews (Canada); www.caphc.org/partnerships/obesity.html

Chapter 31

Adolescence and primary care

Lionel Jacobson and Diane Owen

Introduction

> It's not that he doesn't listen ... sometimes he doesn't fully comprehend that he's talking in a way
> you can't understand ... it would help if they talked to teenagers. (Female teenager)
>   Please listen to us, we're people too you know. (Male teenager)

Adolescent patients can be forthright and give frank opinions on the care they receive
from primary care, and the above quotes may represent a distillation of some of the
issues that will become more apparent throughout this chapter. Young people can be very
sensitive to nuances of care and care provision, and this chapter will feature other teenage
voices and their comments, because we contend that communication skills may be just as
important as clinical skills when providing primary care for teenagers.

Readers with a keen eye will note that there have been three terms introduced
that technically may apply to differing age groups—namely 'adolescent', 'teenager', and
'young person'. We will not define any of these terms, partly because there is no formal
consensus as to the ages involved in each, but more importantly because the book
is devoted to practicalities not semantics. We ask that readers assume the terms to be
interchangeable throughout the rest of this chapter, and that they apply to the period
between 11 years and 19 years (Intercollegiate Working Party 2003), although there will
be elements that have relevance for older and younger patients too.

The specific age of 16 years has particular relevance because this is the age at which
patients become adults responsible for their own healthcare—technically, they are
children below this age. However, for most practical purposes the 'Gillick ruling'
(Jacobson and Wilkinson 1994) has allowed doctors and others to view patients as de
facto adult patients, provided the health provider is satisfied the patient is mature
enough to understand the consultation experience. This creates problems of how to
assess maturity, but we suggest that it takes skill and maturity to make and attend general
practice appointments without an adult presence.

We recognize that teenage patients have not been considered as patients with a voice.
A study from South Wales has demonstrated that GPs are less concerned with the
patient's presenting complaint and more concerned with dealing with the more 'public
health' issues of alcohol use, drug use, teenage pregnancy, and sexually transmitted infections (Jacobson et al. 2001). This has created a gap in how teenagers and GPs view quality
care, but it is a central tenet of this chapter that the primary care team may have little

influence on unhealthy behaviours in teenagers (Jacobson and Kinnersley 2001). None the less, we intend to show that good communication may allow more helpful health education, possibly increasing this influence.

We appreciate that there are difficulties in assessing good quality primary healthcare for teenagers (Jacobson *et al.* 1998), and that much of our considerations will be our opinions, but we will provide some evidence to back up these comments. We continue with sections on consultation patterns, communication, the role of primary care team members, teenage clinics, specific health issues, training needs, and some overall thoughts. Throughout the chapter we will emphasize what we consider to be important issues in **bold type**, separate from the main text for the ease of the reader with little time available.

- ◆ good communication skills are important
- ◆ under 16s attending alone are usually 'mature'
- ◆ primary care has little effect on 'unhealthy behaviour'.

Consultation patterns

A study of recorded care in one general practice found that the consultation rates for girls and boys below age 15 is approximately 2.5 consultations per person per year. The rates diverge above 15 years with males consulting at less than 1.5 consultations per person per year, and females consulting at the average adult pattern of four consultations per person per year (Jacobson and Owen 1993). These findings have been confirmed in other studies (Jacobson *et al.* 2000; Churchill *et al.* 2000a).

Younger teenagers are often brought to the surgery by their parents. In comparison, older teenagers may attend with their family, may attend alone, or may attend with friends for 'moral support'. The crossover from childhood patterns to consulting patterns for older patients takes place at differing ages, but in general 50% of 15 year olds consult without their parents, either on their own or with a friend.

The commonest reasons for consulting are for respiratory tract disorders, skin conditions, or minor injuries (Jacobson and Wilkinson 1994). Theoretically, this may leave time to discuss other issues, but it has been established that teenage consultations are, on average, 2 minutes shorter than consultations for any other age group (Jacobson *et al.* 1993), perhaps reflecting discomfort within the consultation from both parties.

Teenage patients may not attend for healthcare if they feel they get 'short shrift' from the GP. There have been studies demonstrating greater 'health need' than is met by GP services, and that many teenagers will not attend for healthcare because they feel the services to be 'unapproachable' (Jacobson *et al.* 1996; Kari *et al.* 1997; Donovan *et al.* 1997; Jones *et al.* 1997). A study from Nottingham showed that this may have less of an effect than previously thought, but it is significant that those teenagers who were put off attending were those who had contraception or psychological problems, both of importance to general teenage health (Churchill *et al.* 2000a).

- ◆ teenagers attend GP services infrequently
- ◆ teenagers tend to have short consultations
- ◆ teenagers may be put off consulting their GP.

Communication issues

Many studies demonstrate that a higher proportion of teenagers express dissatisfaction with GP services than proportions from other patient groups (Jacobson *et al.* 1996; Kari *et al.* 1997; Donovan *et al.* 1997; Jones *et al.* 1997). As a rough figure 20% of teenagers are dissatisfied, in comparison with the accepted figure of 10% of adults at a similar time (Rees Lewis 1994). These figures are improving, but many teenagers overtly feel that GP services can be improved (Jacobson *et al.* 2000, 2001).

Poor communication by GPs and their staff has been implicated as a source of dissatisfaction. The list of negative comments includes dismissive attitudes by bureaucratic and uncaring staff, appointment delays, unfriendly atmosphere, lack of respect for teenagers as patients, and judgemental attitudes by GPs. The following quotes illustrate some of these issues:

> Receptionists got a picture of you and what's wrong with you, don't listen to what you say.
> I'm really intimidated when I go to my doctor ... I sit there, 'Yes doctor, no doctor'.
> You got to put on such an act and you're only in there five minutes.

Confidentiality is also of great concern (Donovan *et al.* 1997, Kari *et al.* 1997). As one teenager succinctly put it: 'Teenagers know that a doctor is confidential, but individually they still worry about the doctor telling their parent.' A strategy of overtly explaining that the content of consultations is not usually divulged to other parties may be helpful (McPherson *et al.* 2001). However, teenagers from South Wales have emphasized that issues of confidentiality extend to concerns about being seen by other patients in waiting rooms, an issue that has been termed 'community confidentiality' (Jacobson *et al.* 2001)

Not all teenagers report poor communication. Studies from South Wales (Jacobson *et al.* 1996, 2001), showed that teenagers comment favourably on their care when they have a GP who treats them with respect, who listens, who is welcoming, who appears caring, and who doesn't give a judgemental opinion. Further, these 'good consulters' encourage the teenager to talk, to take their time, and to emphasize the confidential nature of consultations, either implicitly or overtly.

There are some implicit difficulties surrounding good communication: in general females tend to prefer to see younger, female GPs, and there is an associated improvement in teenage pregnancy rates (Hippisley-Cox *et al.* 2000). This clearly reflects gender and age issues, and it begs the question as to whether older, male GPs are more judgemental, or may be perceived to be so. In either instance, it appears important for all primary care team members to strive to become empathic and non-judgemental.

GPs may view good communication slightly differently: an important finding from the South Wales study was that GPs' perceptions of good communication tended to be of a respectful patient who listens to the wisdom of the GP, and will immediately act on any health education advice. This is not what teenagers report as good communication: they made it evident that health education should only be provided if asked for. To conflate these two agendas, it appears to be a required skill to learn how to respect teenagers enough to ask permission to broach helpful, individually tailored, impartial, non-judgemental advice.

- good rapport involves listening and interest
- important to emphasize confidentiality
- young people note bad communication readily
- empathy and a non-judgemental attitude are important.

Members of the primary healthcare team

An important (and frequently poorly respected) member of the team is the receptionist. Teenagers from South Wales commented about receptionists as the team member who appears the most 'challenging' to deal with (Jacobson *et al.* 2001). This may be a function of their specific role, and some receptionists are aware of their perception as 'the old dragon', but there may be possible consequences. This is illustrated by the following quote: 'She wants to know everything … is there a need to see him because he's busy … as if you're bothering them … no point going down there if you're going to get a response like that'. The receptionist should be treated as a valued member of the team, who can facilitate improved access and availability to young people, if this aspect of healthcare is considered important.

The role of the practice nurse has expanded in recent years, and most are happy to see teenagers alone at the surgery. A study in South Wales revealed that many nurses perceive themselves as more approachable and as more of a 'mother figure' than the GPs with whom they work. However, further data from the study indicated that 34% of teenagers had not visited the nurse. Furthermore, a substantial proportion was unaware of the availability of such a service (Jacobson *et al.* 2001).

There have been suggestions that the nurse can and should be more involved in providing healthcare and health advice to teenage patients (Gregg *et al.* 1998). A Hertfordshire study has confirmed that trained nurses can provide some improvements in health as measured by improvements in at least one of four behavioural areas (diet, exercise, smoking, alcohol use), although these benefits may not be maintained at 1-year follow-up (Walker *et al.* 2002).

None the less, these studies suggest that the practice nurse is an underused resource, and that greater marketing of this service should be considered, especially in light of the future changes to primary care with the advent of the new GP contract. Further, it need not be solely the practice nurse to whom young people may go, and there are suggestions to include health visitors in some initiatives (Finlay 1998).

However, it should be recognized that many teenagers have worries about the extended confidentiality of discussions between themselves and individual primary care team members. Some have reported concerns that consultation discussions may become known to other members of the primary care team, and by extension to members of their own family (Jacobson *et al.* 2001).

Furthermore, there are issues of specific training in adolescent health issues for team members who may consult with teenagers. This issue is dealt with in another section of this chapter but it is pertinent to note that some aspect of understanding of the teenage culture and agenda may be relevant for all primary care team members.

- kind receptionists can make a difference
- practice nurse is an 'underused resource'
- 'marketing' of primary care services could be better
- internal confidentiality issues may arise
- training of all team members is important.

Clinics

A survey of primary care providers indicated that 95% believed there should be dedicated services for young people, and a similar number indicated development of services should be in schools or the wider community (Intercollegiate Working Party 2003). Clearly, this may represent a 'wish list', but none the less primary care providers appear to recognize that existing services may be inappropriate and may need expansion. Therefore, teenage-specific health clinics have been set up and evaluated, although these have mostly taken place in existing GP surgery premises.

Evaluations have largely been based upon attendance rates (i.e. by the proportion of teenagers attending a service), although anecdotal reports indicate that the clinics are well received by health professionals and patients alike, and that health issues do arise which can be managed in this setting. There are reports of clinics staffed by nurses with support from GPs available if necessary (Townsend *et al.* 1991; Hibble and Elwood 1992; Walker *et al.* 2002), two utilize GPs solely (Donovan and McCarthy 1988; Cowap 1996), and one involved health visitors (Smith and Melville 1996).

Attendance rates vary from 7% in inner-city London (Cowap 1996) to 83% in Lincolnshire (Hibble and Elwood 1992), but in most instances it took some time for 'word of mouth' to spread that the service is appropriate, helpful, and congruent with teenagers' needs. However, the data from the inner city emphasized a potential drawback of clinics in the form of a new 'inverse care law for teenagers'; teenagers most 'at risk' are the least likely to seek help (Jacobson and Kinnersley 2000).

None the less, if a service is planned, the data also indicate that there must be some specific, local 'market research' to assess appropriate times and personnel, and also allowances must be made for any evaluation to take place at least 1 year after the service has been set up. Further, it should be noted that there are some inherent drawbacks to clinics too. For instance there is the problem of community confidentiality (i.e. teenagers may be recognized by others that they attended such a service and questioned by family or others as to why they went). Finally, teenagers in South Wales reported that teenage clinics can easily replicate poor communication or an inappropriate service, albeit in a different setting (Jacobson *et al.* 2001).

- specific teenage clinics may be helpful
- they may fall foul of the 'inverse care law'
- there should be 'market research' beforehand
- evaluation should be deferred for up to 1 year
- remember 'community confidentiality'.

Specific health issues

This section will cover issues related to alcohol, drug use, smoking, sexually transmitted infections, and teenage pregnancy. There will be some overlap, because many of the behaviours are interlinked. Further, many of the behaviours are linked to mental health problems; these issues are dealt with elsewhere.

The purpose of this section is to present an overview of key trends, rather than to give specific pointers, although these will be provided if any exist. The reader is still encouraged to think of each adolescent as an individual, rather than as part of the wider problem of increasing risk-taking behaviour.

Three recurring themes of relevance to the primary care team will be pertinent to all aspects of risk-taking behaviour. First, the need for support to vulnerable teenagers. Secondly, the requirement not to rush to judgements about the behaviour of individual teenagers. Finally, teenagers do want more appropriate health advice, but preferably only if sought (Jacobson *et al.* 2001).

- ◆ remember role of support
- ◆ remember non-judgemental attitude
- ◆ ask permission to broach health advice.

Alcohol

Alcohol is the most widely available drug in Britain, and girls of 13 years are reported to have little difficulty purchasing it (Willner *et al.* 2000). Further, it is socially acceptable, and as such it is the drug most open to abuse. Young people are now drinking more regularly and in larger amounts than previously reported (Hughes *et al.* 1997). In a recent study of 15 and 16 year olds, nearly 80% had reported at least one episode of intoxication (Miller and Plant 1996).

As with older age groups, the social effects of an excessive alcohol intake may become more of a concern than the physical effects of alcohol itself. There is an association with psychiatric comorbidity (Zeitlin 1999), and it is important to enquire about alcohol intake if this may be relevant to the clinical situation. None the less, there is no information on interventions that are specifically appropriate for adolescents, or on screening tests that are helpful for early detection of alcohol problems. Thus, the role of the primary care team might be limited to providing help and support as would be provided to adult patients with alcohol problems.

- ◆ alcohol use is rising among young people
- ◆ no specific interventions for adolescent drinkers.

Drug use

Illicit drug use is common, and becoming more so (Bauman and Phongsavan 1999). Over 40% of 15 and 16 year olds from a survey in 1996 had tried illicit drugs at some time, with higher levels of use associated with poor school performance (Miller and Plant 1996). The study demonstrated that reasons for drug use are similar to reasons for alcohol use, namely exploration, experimentation, a means of escape, social interaction and social acceptance among peers.

However, most drug use by adolescents does not involve dependency on drugs or formal addiction problems. Further, the use of intravenous drugs is thankfully rare (Bauman and Phongsavan 1999). The main health concerns are of injury and violence, as well as short-term adverse mental health (Bauman and Phongsavan 1999), although recently long-term mental health problems in adolescent cannabis users have been reported (Arsenault *et al.* 2002).

As with alcohol above, the role of the primary care team is to enquire sensitively about drug use if the clinical picture requires such enquiry. There are no known specific interventions for adolescent drug users, but there is clearly a role for supportive and non-judgemental care.

+ recreational drug use is increasing
+ no specific interventions for adolescent drug users.

Smoking

The proportion of adolescents who smoke regularly by the age of 16 years has continued to be in the order of 15%, and research indicates that the majority of adult smokers start smoking during their teenage years (Jacobson and Wilkinson 1994; Intercollegiate Working Party 2003). The reasons for initiation of smoking are complex, but there are associations with psychological distress in the form of low self-esteem, low confidence, increased anxiety, and a feeling of being less in control of their lives (Patton *et al.* 1996).

Nicotine dependence develops early, and data suggest that over 50% of adolescent smokers suffer withdrawal effects during attempts to stop smoking (Colby *et al.* 2000). Thus, clinicians play a part in preventing and treating tobacco use in adolescents in the same way as they do with adult patients (Vickers *et al.* 2002). However, the effects of clinicians on smoking behaviour may be limited in comparison with other, rather stronger effects such as peer pressure and advertising (Intercollegiate Working Party 2003).

None the less, there have been reports of teenagers who have at least agreed to contemplate their smoking behaviour, and have tentatively agreed to give up smoking when seen in specific teenage clinics (Townsend *et al.* 1991; Hibble and Elwood 1992; Walker *et al.* 2002), although there have been no long-term follow-up studies. It appears that teenagers are prepared to listen to advice to stop smoking if doctors and others 'make it seem really important' (Jacobson and Wilkinson 1994). Thus, teenagers can at least be encouraged to think about their smoking behaviour in a non-judgemental and non-threatening manner.

+ teenage smoking rates have not changed recently
+ health advice may have some, albeit limited, effects.

Sexually transmitted infections

Teenagers are having their first experience of sexual intercourse at increasingly younger ages. The median age of first sexual experience is now 16 years, with many having extensive sexual experience well below this age (Wellings *et al.* 2001). Sexual activity among young people is likely to be consensual, but the possibility of coercion, sexual abuse, or commercial sexual activity should be considered, although thankfully these issues are rare and will not be discussed further. There are associations between risky sexual behaviour and mental distress (Ramrakha *et al.* 2000).

There are increasing data that there is substantial sexual ill health among teenagers in the UK and that infection rates are rising. Female teenagers aged 16–19 years have the highest rates of gonorrhoea, chlamydial infection, and genital warts among all age groups (Nicoll *et al.* 1999). Almost two-thirds of 16 year olds attending GUM clinics have a sexually transmitted infection, making them three times more likely to have an infection than patients in older age groups. The increase in chlamydia infections may cause increased subfertility in future, and it has been suggested that the possibility of chlamydia should be considered if adolescents present with recurrent cystitis symptoms (Huppert *et al.* 2003).

Data from south London demonstrates that teenagers will frequently not attend for follow-up, and consequently they will not receive sufficient documented contraceptive advice (Creighton *et al.* 2002). Clearly this will include either failure to consider, or failure to act upon, suggestions for barrier methods of sexual activity, both to prevent sexually transmitted infections and to prevent unintended pregnancy.

Sexual health is an essential component of general health, and should be dealt with as such. Clearly, many teenagers may approach their primary healthcare team initially, and the professional should point the way towards the local GUM clinic where appropriate. However, the role of the primary care team includes sensitive and non-judgemental opportunistic discussion of sexual health (including discussion of barrier methods of protection against sexually transmitted infections) during other consultations, where appropriate and when the situation allows.

- sexually transmitted infection rates are rising
- chlamydia rates may create future subfertility
- many adolescents fail to attend for GUM clinic follow-up
- there is a role for sensitively provided opportunistic health advice.

Teenage pregnancy

The UK still has very high rates of pregnancy in teenagers compared with other parts of western Europe, although rates are falling, albeit very slowly (Intercollegiate Working Party 2003). The subject is contentious, partly because of the associations of prematurity, low birth weight, infant death, poor social outcomes, and isolation (Effective Healthcare Bulletin 1997; Intercollegiate Working Party 2003). However, there is also some evidence that the 'problem' of teenage pregnancy is a social construct, and is less of a problem for the young people concerned and their families (Jacobson *et al.* 1995).

There are associations between teenage pregnancy and socio-economic conditions with more teenage pregnancy in relatively deprived areas, and fewer of these resulting in terminations (Jacobson *et al.* 1995). Other factors reported by teenagers as reasons for their pregnancy include perceptions of poor information provision, confidentiality problems, and reported lack of access to services (Jacobson *et al.* 1995; Effective Healthcare Bulletin 1997).

Most teenage pregnancies are equated as being unintended, and indeed some data suggest that 80% are unplanned, although clearly some are planned and wanted (Jacobson *et al.* 1995). Recent data suggest that 71% of pregnant adolescents had discussed contraception with a GP in the year prior to becoming pregnant (Churchill *et al.* 2000b). There are further data suggesting that up to one-third of teenage pregnancies would not have been prevented, even with access to and provision of suitable services (Kives 2001). Together these studies point to the issue of teenage pregnancy being rather more complex than one where appropriate services would lead to dramatic reductions in teenage pregnancy rates.

Many teenagers feel themselves to be at low risk of teenage pregnancy, and consequently do not request emergency contraception (Free *et al.* 2002). This is a manifestation of the 'myth of immunity', whereby deleterious effects from health behaviours are perceived to occur to others but not the specific individual ('it won't happen to me') (Jacobson and Wilkinson 1994). It is certainly appropriate for primary care team members to recognize this issue, but sensitive discussion without appearing patronizing is difficult.

There are also other markers for teenage pregnancy risk, such as lapsed contraception, previous overdose, previous presentation for pregnancy tests (Houston and Jacobson 1996; Zabin *et al.* 1996; Churchill *et al.* 2002). This information may help to identify a group who may benefit from a more intense discussion of their sexual health and contraception requirements. None the less, it is important to emphasize that various primary prevention strategies have failed to result in increased contraception, or had significant effect on teenage pregnancy rates (DiCenso *et al.* 2002).

As with all other aspects of this section on specific health issues the main requirement is for a sensitive, accessible, approachable, non-judgemental service where the teenager can receive information appropriate to their requirements. This can be given on an ad-hoc opportunistic basis, as teenagers present for other services but it is crucial to re-emphasize that health advice may have only a limited effect (Effective Healthcare Bulletin 1997; Jacobson and Kinnersley 2000). Further the role of the primary care team is to provide support, whatever the outcome.

* teenage pregnancy rates remain high in the UK
* teenage pregnancy is associated with social deprivation
* not all teenage pregnancy is unwanted
* the primary care team has a role to provide sensitive support.

Training

As noted earlier, it may be appropriate for all team members who come into contact with teenage young people to at least have some understanding of adolescent culture and health concerns. Perusing some of the literature on this subject may provide this relatively easily, and we hope that this chapter will add to the existing canon.

There have been several moves to provide training for practitioners in teenage health-care, in particular in the USA and Australia (Fleming *et al.* 1994; Veit *et al.* 1996). A more recent Australian study has suggested that Australian GPs can be taught objectively improved communication skills and can feel more comfortable when they consult with teenagers (Sanci *et al.* 2000). The simulated patients involved reported no obvious improvements in communication, but this is still an important finding.

The Hertfordshire study involving practice nurses further indicates that training is feasible, and not overly time-consuming to provide (Walker *et al.* 2002). The nurses were taught communication skills, some basic elements of teenage health information, some elements of behaviour change theory, and suggestions for follow-up and/or referral if indicated. The nurses involved were happy to receive such training.

South Wales doctors did report they would like more training, with two main elements on communication, and assessment of 'risk' when consulting with teenage patients (Jacobson *et al.* 2001). It is pertinent to stress that the two are inter-twined, and that GPs do consider the 'risks' of deleterious health behaviour such as drug use or unsafe sex. However, as noted above, it is important that they impart their opinions in a respectful, helpful, non-judgemental manner, and ask permission to broach 'difficult' subjects.

We have emphasized throughout this chapter that it is important to listen to teenagers, and a quote from South Wales indicates a particularly salient final thought about training issues: 'It would be a good idea if doctors got together and had a group ... they'd know our opinion ... we'd not be telling them how to do their job'.

- training is feasible within the context of primary care
- training does not need to be time-consuming
- overt benefits in health may be difficult to ascertain.

Final thoughts

Teenagers represent 10% of the population, and are a group for whom healthcare provision at present appears to be relatively unsatisfactory. To date, the teenage voice and comments are often ignored or marginalized, although it may be that teenagers can give a more 'honest' appraisal of healthcare than many other patients. Adolescent patients need respectful, non-judgemental primary care providers, and providers need to respect today's teenagers as young people who will become tomorrow's adults and parents themselves.

However, at present, teenagers have indicated this is often not the case. They have suggested how this situation can be changed, and those who comment favourably on their care have given some pointers. In essence, teenagers would like professionals who demonstrate courtesy, respect, valuing the patient's opinions, to be given health advice in a non-judgemental manner, to allow time for the patient, and to appear to be enjoying the work.

Skills in teenage health can be taught, although sceptics will comment that improvements in communication skills will not lead to improvements in levels of teenage pregnancy, drug and alcohol use. However, perhaps better communication will facilitate a situation where individual teenagers feel more comfortable in attending an 'approachable' GP service, which will in turn lead to more appropriate and individually helpful health education messages. We recognize this principle will apply in settings outside the usual GP surgery too.

We believe the aspect that would be most helpful is for GPs and other members of Primary Care Teams to spend more time considering the health provision for their own teenage patients. Teenage health is an aspect of healthcare provision that can be improved, and perhaps making such improvements will foster opportunities to improve primary care for other groups of patients too.

References

Arsenault L, Cannon M, Poulton R, Murray R, Caspi A, Moffitt T (2002). Cannabis use in adolescence and risk for adult psychosis: longitudinal prospective study. *British Medical Journal* **325:** 1212–1213.

Bauman A, Phongsavan P (1999). Epidemiology of substance use in adolescence: prevalence, trends and policy implications. *Drug and Alcohol Dependence* **55:** 187–207.

Churchill R, Allen J, Denman S, Williams D, Fielding K, von Fragstein M (2000a). Do the attitudes and beliefs of young teenagers towards general practice influence actual consultation behaviour? *British Journal of General Practice* **50:** 953–957.

Churchill R, Allen J, Pringle M, Hippisley-Cox J, Ebdon D, Macpherson M, Bradley S (2000b). Consultation patterns and provision of contraception in general practice before teenage pregnancy: case-control study. *British Medical Journal* **321:** 486–489.

Churchill R, Allen J, Pringle M, Hippisley-Cox J (2002c). Teenagers at risk of unintended pregnancy: identification of practical risk markers for use in general practice from a retrospective analysis of case records in the United Kingdom. *International Journal of Adolescent Medical Health* **14:** 153–160.

Colby S, Tiffany S, Shiffman S, Niaura R (2000). Are adolescent smokers dependent on nicotine? A review of the evidence. *Drug and Alcohol Dependence* **59:** S 83–95.

Cowap N (1996). GPs need to be more proactive in providing health care to teenagers. *British Medical Journal* **313:** 941.

Creighton S, Edwards S, Welch J, Miller R (2002). News from the frontline: sexually transmitted infections in teenagers attending a genitourinary clinic in south-east London. *Sexually Transmitted Infections* **78:** 349–351.

DiCenso A, Guyatt G, Willan A, Griffith L (2002). Interventions to reduce unintended teenage pregnancies among adolescents: systematic review of randomised controlled trials. *British Medical Journal* **324:** 1426–1430.

Donovan C, McCarthy S (1988). Is there a place for adolescent screening in general practice? *Health Trends* **20:** 64–65.

Donovan C, Mellanby A, Jacobson L, Taylor B, Tripp J, Members of the Adolescent Working Party, RCGP (1997). Teenagers' views on the GP consultation and their provision of contraception. *British Journal of General Practice* **47:** 715–718.

Effective Health Care (1997). Preventing and reducing the adverse effects of unintended teenage pregnancies. *Effective Health Care Bulletin* **3** (1). NHS Centre for Reviews and Dissemination, University of York.

Finlay F (1998). Providing healthcare information suitable for adolescents. *Health Visitor* **71:** 16–18.

Fleming G, O'Connor K, Sanders J (1994). Paediatricians' views of access to health services for adolescents. *Journal of Adolescent Health* **15:** 473–478.

Free C, Lee R, Ogden J (2002). Young women's accounts of factors influencing their use and non-use of emergency contraception: in-depth interview study. *British Medical Journal* **325**: 1393–1397.

Gregg R, Freeth D, Blackie C (1998). Teenage health and the practice nurse: choice and opportunity for both? *British Journal of General Practice* **48**: 909–910.

Hibble A, Elwood J (1992). Health promotion for young people. *Practitioner* **236**: 1140–1143.

Hippisley-Cox J, Allen J, Pringle M, Ebdon D, McPhearson M, Churchill R, Bradley S (2000). Association between teenage pregnancy rates and the age and sex of general practitioners: cross sectional survey in Trent 1994–1997. *British Medical Journal* **320**: 842–845.

Houston H, Jacobson L (1996). Overdose and termination of pregnancy: an important association? *British Journal of General Practice* **46**: 737–738.

Hughes K, Mackintosh A, Hastings G, Wheeler C, Watson J, Inglis J (1997). Young people, alcohol, and designer drinks: quantitative and qualitative study. *British Medical Journal* **314**: 414–418.

Huppert J, Biro F, Mehrabi J, Slap G (2003). Urinary tract infection and chlamydia infection in adolescent females. *Journal of Pediatric and Adolescent Gynecology* **16**: 133–137.

The Intercollegiate Working Party on Adolescent Health (2003). *Bridging the Gaps: Health Care for Adolescents*. Royal College of Paediatrics and Child Health, London.

Jacobson L, Kinnersley P (2000). Teenagers in primary care—continuing the new direction. *British Journal of General Practice* **50**: 947–948.

Jacobson L, Owen P (1993). Study of teenage care in one general practice. *British Journal of General Practice* **43**: 349.

Jacobson L, Wilkinson C (1994). A Review of Teenage Health: Time for a new direction. *British Journal of General Practice* **44**: 420–424.

Jacobson L, Wilkinson C, Owen P (1994). Is the potential of teenage consultations being missed? A study of consultation times in primary care. *Family Practice* **11**: 296–299.

Jacobson L, Wilkinson C, Pill R (1995). Teenage pregnancy in the United Kingdom in the 1990s: the implications for primary care. *Family Practice* **12**: 232–236.

Jacobson L, Wilkinson C, Pill R, Hackett P (1996). Communication between teenagers and British General Practitioners: a preliminary study of the teenage perspective. *Ambulatory Child Health* **1**: 291–301.

Jacobson L, Matthews S, Robling M, Donovan C, Members of the Research Sub-Committee, Adolescent Working Party, RCGP (1998). Challenges in evaluating primary health care for teenagers. *Journal of Evaluation in Clinical Practice* **4**: 183–189.

Jacobson L, Mellanby A, Donovan C, Taylor B, Tripp J, Members of the Adolescent Working Party, RCGP (2000). Teenagers' views on general practice consultations and other medical advice. *Family Practice* **17**: 156–158.

Jacobson L, Richardson G, Parry-Langdon N, Donovan C (2001). How do teenagers and primary health care providers view each other? An overview of key themes. *British Journal of General Practice* **51**: 811–816.

Jones R, Finlay F, Simpson N, Kreitman T (1997). How can adolescents' health needs and concerns best be met? *British Journal of General Practice* **47**: 631–634.

Kari J, Donovan C, Li J, Taylor B (1997). Adolescents' attitudes to general practice in North London. *British Journal of General Practice* **47**: 109–110.

Kives S (2001). Desire for pregnancy among adolescents in an antenatal clinic. *Journal of Pediatric and Adolescent Gynecology* **14**: 150–154.

McPherson A, Macfarlane A, Donovan C (2001). *The Health of Adolescents in Primary Care: How to Promote Adolescent Health in Your Practice*, (2nd edn). Radcliffe Medical Press, Abingdon.

Miller P, Plant M (1996). Drinking, smoking and illicit drug use among 15 and 16 year olds in the United Kingdom. *British Medical Journal* **313**: 394–397.

Nicoll A, Catchpole M, Cliffe S, Hughes G, Simms I, Thomas D (1999). Sexual health of teenagers in England and Wales: analysis of national data. *British Medical Journal* **318**: 1321–1322.

Patton G, Hibbert M, Rosier M, Carlin J, Bowes G (1996). Is smoking associated with anxiety and depression in teenagers? American Journal of Public Health **86**: 225–230.

Ramrakha S, Caspi A, Dickson N, Moffitt T, Paul C (2000). Psychiatric disorders and risky sex in young adulthood: a cross sectional study in a birth cohort. *British Medical Journal* **321**: 263–266.

Rees Lewis J (1994). Patient views on quality in general practice: literature review. *Social Science and Medicine* **39**: 655–670.

Sanci L, Coffey C, Veit F, Carr-Gregg M, Patton G, Day N, Bowes G (2000). Evaluation of an educational intervention for general practitioners in adolescent health care: randomised controlled trial. *British Medical Journal* **320**: 224–229.

Smith A, Melville E (1996). Targeting teenagers in the primary care setting. *Health Visitor* **69**: 228–230.

Townsend J, Wilkes H, Haines A, Jarvis M (1991). Adolescent smokers in general practice: health, lifestyle, physical measurements and response to anti-smoking advice. *British Medical Journal* **303**: 947–950.

Veit F, Sanci L, Young D, Bowes G (1996). Barriers to effective health care for adolescents. *Medical Journal of Australia* **163**: 131–133.

Vickers K, Thomas J, Patten C, Mrazek D (2002). Prevention of tobacco use in adolescents: review of current findings and implications for healthcare providers. *Current Opinions in Paediatrics* **14**: 708–712.

Walker Z, Townsend J, Oakley L, Donovan C, Smith H, Hurst Z, Bell J, Marshall S (2002). Health promotion for adolescents in primary care: randomised control trial. *British Medical Journal* **325**: 524–527.

Wellings K, Nanchahal K, Macdowall W, McManus S, Erens B, Mercer C (2001). Sexual behaviour in Britain: early heterosexual experience. *Lancet* **358**: 1843–1850.

Willner P, Hart K, Binmore J, Cavendish M, Dunphy E (2000). Alcohol sales to underage adolescents: an unobtrusive observational study and evaluation of a police intervention. *Addiction* **95**: 1373–1388.

Zabin L, Emerson M, Ringers P, Sedivy V (1996). Adolescents with negative pregnancy test results: an accessible at-risk group. *Journal of the American Medical Association* **275**: 113–117.

Zeitlin H (1999). Psychiatric comorbidity with substance misuse in children and teenagers. *Drug and Alcohol Dependence* **55**: 225–234.

Chapter 32

Attention-deficit/hyperactivity disorder

Peter Hill and Jonathan Williams

Presentation

From a primary care perspective, first contact with a child with attention-deficit/ hyperactivity disorder (ADHD) will probably come in one of four ways, here ranked roughly in terms of what is most likely:

- The child's parent will bring him (it usually is him), asking for confirmation of their suspicions that he has it and asking for a referral. This may follow their reading of an article in a magazine or a discussion with a teacher. Printouts from the internet may be offered or brandished.
- A health visitor faced with a hyperactive toddler raises the question
- There is a letter from a clinic that has already made the diagnosis following a referral by a school, bypassing primary care gatekeeping, and there is a request for help with treatment.
- The GP is primarily active in making a new diagnosis, previously unsuspected.

Each pathway is associated with somewhat different demands on the GP or the primary care team. The first and third pathways may elicit some irritation.

In the case of the boy presented by a parent or health visitor already raising the question of diagnosis, or in the instance of new diagnosis, the GP will need to consider

- Whether the boy's behaviour does indeed fit diagnostic criteria
- If some other condition could cause the behaviour; the differential diagnosis
- What else is going on; the comorbidity
- What is known scientifically about the condition and its treatment as opposed to various myths and half-truths.

Diagnostic criteria

For diagnostic purposes ADHD is a pattern of behaviour with various contributing factors and no single cause for all cases; it is a behavioural syndrome. In all probability it is the final common pathway for a variety of neuropsychological processes.

To make the diagnosis of the full 'combined' form, six of nine elements from each of the two lists in Box 32.1 must be present. In addition the subsidary criteria below the list must be met. Not all parents (and not all clinicians) do this but it is absolutely necessary.

Box 32.1 Diagnostic criteria for ADHD

Inattention

- Careless with detail
- Fails to sustain attention
- Appears not to listen
- Does not finish instructed tasks
- Poor self-organization
- Avoids tasks requiring sustained mental effort
- Loses things
- Easily distracted
- Seems forgetful

Hyperactivity/impulsivity

- Fidgets
- Leaves seat when should be seated
- Runs/climbs excessively and inappropriately
- Noisy in play
- Persistent motor overactivity unmodified by social context
- Blurts out answers before question completed
- Fails to wait turn or queue
- Interrupts others' conversation or games
- Talks excessively for social context

Six of nine from each list for combined type ADHD and, for all ADHD diagnoses:

- Onset before age 7
- Evident in more than one type of situation (i.e. pervasive across situations)
- Associated with impaired functioning
- Not better explained by another disorder

ADHD is a long-standing condition evident in most areas of the child's life and associated with substantially impaired functioning. It isn't simply a matter of ticking boxes on a rating scale or checklist.

A quick glance at the elements in each list reveals that the behaviours listed are present in some degree in the general population and are particularly frequent among young boys. Cases of ADHD possess a combination of *extreme* variants of inattentive, impulsive, restless traits that are widely distributed. Substantial impairment of functioning provides a distinction from normal variation. To be included as contributing to the ADHD pattern the diagnostic elements must be outside the norm for age and situation, and this includes mental age in the case of children with general learning disability. They are also particularly common in otherwise normal pre-school children and it is wise for a non-specialist to avoid suggesting the diagnosis in this age group.

In other words, there is a short series of decisions to be made.

1. Are the elements in Box 32.1 present in sufficient number, duration and severity?
2. Do they affect most areas of the child's life?
3. Are they preventing adequate functioning (e.g. academic progress, satisfactory relationships with peers and family)?
4. Could anything else be causing this pattern?
5. What else is going on?

Confusingly, many children with ADHD can suppress their hyperactivity for half an hour or so and be quite quiet in a visit to the doctor. Testing for inattentiveness is not a straightforward process as it is most likely to be evident in a group situation that is structured and in which cognitive demands are placed on the child. Effectively that means a classroom or perhaps helping the youngster with his homework.

Answering questions 1–3 means finding out about behaviour and achievement at school and good practice is to for a clinician to do this by directly asking the teacher by phone or letter. Routine end-of-term school reports for parents tend to be bland and lack the detail required to make a clinical judgement.

If only because of these two issues, the full diagnosis of ADHD is best avoided in primary care. If the diagnosis seems likely, refer to a specialist. The exception is pre-school children. A high level of activity is a common problem in this age group and usually subsides with maturation. It is best handled on its own merits with behavioural advice and it is unlikely that medication will be used. By and large the opinion of a clinical child psychologist rather than referral to an ADHD clinic is the best option for hyperactive 2–5 year olds.

It is technically possible, though not common UK practice, to recognize subtypes of ADHD in which six of nine elements on either list are present, together with the other subsidiary criteria of pervasiveness across situations, functional impairment, onset in early life, and an absence of other disorders that could produce the picture. If this is done then it is possible to recognize ADHD-predominantly inattentive subtype, and ADHD-predominantly hyperactive-impulsive subtype. Both of these are rarer than the ADHD-combined type, which requires six of nine on both lists.

Differential diagnosis

The commonest conditions which mimic ADHD at first glance are

- normal variation of traits such as activity level
- hearing loss
- antisocial behaviour disorders

- general developmental disability (mental handicap)
- anxiety
- mild autistic spectrum conditions
- developmental language disorder.

Confusingly, any of these can also coexist with ADHD.

Comorbid conditions

ADHD is characteristically something that coexists with other developmental and psychiatric disorders. Many cases, especially below the age of about 11 years, will have associated specific developmental problems (Box 32.2). The common parental question 'is this ADHD, dyslexia or dyspraxia?' may well need to answered by 'all of the above' if the child is old enough and intelligent enough to read but can't do so at age level and is evidently clumsy with running, shoelaces, knife and fork, or bike-riding.

Rather similarly, most children with ADHD will also eventually show antisocial behaviour that may be severe enough to fulfil criteria for

- oppositional-defiant disorder (exceptional disobedience and defiance of authority)
- conduct disorder (extreme behaviour which infringes the rights or safety of others).

To make things more complicated, adolescents with ADHD are at risk for

- substance misuse (nothing to do with treatment)
- anxiety
- depression.

This is a further reason for not making a definitive diagnosis of ADHD in primary care and referring to a specialist.

Referral

Children with ADHD may be seen by paediatricians—especially community paediatricians or developmental paediatricians—or child and adolescent mental health services (CAMHS). Mature children's services will offer special clinics. Otherwise, local referral protocols may exist; they vary. If nothing formal exists, refer

- straightforward ADHD with not much apparent comorbidity to a paediatrician
- ADHD with developmental problems such as dyspraxia to a developmental paediatrician
- ADHD with antisocial behaviours, psychiatric symptoms or dysfunctional family to a child mental health service *insisting on an opinion specifically from the psychiatrist* (who will be the team member who should physically examine the child and prescribe any medication).

It follows that in a referral letter it is wise to prompt the specialist (service) to specify answer the questions

- Is this really ADHD?
- Are there are comorbid developmental or psychiatric conditions?

Box 32.2   Likely comorbid conditions

Developmental

- Dyslexia
- Dyspraxia (developmental co-ordinations disorder)
- Developmental language delay/disorder
- Tic disorder
- Autistic spectrum disorder

Antisocial behaviour

- Oppositional defiant disorder
- Conduct disorder
- Rage outbursts

Emotional

- Generalized anxiety disorder
- Depression (in adolescence)
- Low self-esteem

Substance misuse

- Illicit drugs, especially cannabis
- Alcohol
- Nicotine

Other problems

- Sleep difficulties
- Relationship problems

There is a substantial problem with the teenager who has ADHD and requires continuing treatment beyond the age of 18. There are hardly any specialist services for adults with ADHD (at the time of writing there are only four NHS services in the UK specifically for patients with ADHD who are aged over 18) and the average adult psychiatrist is not likely to know what to do. This isn't clever but is the status quo. Appropriate PCT pressure on mental health providers, particularly on arrangements for transition to adulthood, might eventually resolve the problem though. If you are faced with the problem of an adolescent who has recently turned 18 or an adult patient who seems to have ADHD (which would have been a lifelong problem for him or her) the best course of action is often to ask them to contact a support group such as Attention Deficit Disorder Information and Support Service (ADDISS) for advice and come back to you.

The internet and so forth

Although there are reputable information services such as ADDISS, there is a host of unreliable information about ADHD and its treatment on the net and in the printed media. Some of this seems to be placed maliciously. It is best not to be drawn into protracted argument but as many parents will bring their child to the practice having read quite a bit about the condition it is wise to be prepared to address some of the more common questions or objections:

It's just a posh term for naughty children

Although many children with ADHD do behave antisocially, not all do. There are also many other causes of naughtiness. Nor is it simply an alternative label for boisterousness: high and inappropriate levels of activity must coexist with inattention and impulsiveness as well as being extreme, pervasive across situation and handicapping the child's functioning.

It doesn't exist

This usually means that it is not so much a separate disease entity but an extreme variation of ordinary behaviour. Impairment of the child's functioning—academically or socially—provides a cut-off, separating cases from normal variation. There are parallels in the rest of medicine for this: hypertension, hearing impairment, or osteoarthritis in the elderly for instance.

There isn't anything in the brain you can treat and you can't prove its existence by physical investigations

This is partly true as ADHD is essentially identified as a behavioural syndrome. But there are abnormal neurological correlates (see Box 32.2) in research studies, even if physical investigations have no part to play in routine management.

Can't you diagnose it with psychological tests?

No, though certain neuropsychological patterns have been shown in research studies (Box 32.3) to be associated with ADHD. These don't help in clinical diagnosis. Each one

---

Box 32.3   Neurological findings more common in children with ADHD in research studies

- Smaller brain overall
- Absence of normal asymmetry of basal ganglia

Underfunctioning of:

- frontal lobes
- anterior cingulate gyrus
- posterior alerting circuits
- striatum when impulse control required

> **Box 32.4   Neuropsychological abnormalities, more common in children with ADHD in research studies**
>
> ◆ Deficits in working memory
> ◆ Aversion to delay
> ◆ Poor orientation to relevant stimuli
> ◆ Inefficient allocation of mental effort

does not exist in all children with ADHD; various neuropsychological abnormalities (Box 32.4) are associated with the same overall behavioural pattern. Nor is any abnormal pattern known to be only found in ADHD.

It's a genetic disorder. Is there a test?

Most cases of ADHD are largely determined genetically, probably through polygenic mechanisms. A few single genes have been discovered but these account for only a tiny contribution to the variance and are actually more common among children without ADHD. Nor do they offer any guidance as to management. Genetic testing is only feasible at a research level. There are environmental factors such as maternal alcohol intake and smoking during pregnancy, which are known to interact with genetic factors and this is possibly true for low birthweight, too. It is better to think of the genetic influences as risk factors rather than determinants.

Is it ADD, ADHD, or hyperkinetic disorder?

ADD is a term derived from the now redundant DSM-III classification system and refers to attention-deficit disorder, without hyperactivity or impulsiveness. Nowadays it would be termed ADHD-predominantly inattentive subtype. Hyperkinetic disorder is the term used in the International Classification of Diseases, tenth revision (ICD-10). At least in the diagnostic criteria for research edition of ICD-10 it is essentially the same as severe ADHD, setting more stringent criteria but using the same diagnostic elements, though combining them to a different rule.

The unexpected letter from a clinic

It is not uncommon for CAMHS to be expected to provide easy-access services, including self-referral. Education and social services can refer children in without a medical gatekeeper. In such instances CAMHS is a primary care service. The same goes for community paediatrics and a few private specialists in paediatrics or child and adolescent psychiatry. This means that sometimes the first time a conventional primary healthcare team or GP hears about a case of ADHD is a letter from a specialist service announcing the diagnosis, quite often with a request for prescription of medication.

Although this is not always welcome, be wary of shooting the messenger. The author of the letter may labour under some constraints. Some mental health trusts instruct their clinicians not to prescribe certain drugs or always to pass the task to the GP. Private health insurance companies in the UK do not reimburse for outpatient prescriptions (though American ones do, usually at about 80% of cost).

Even if you have made the referral to a clinic, you are quite likely to be asked to prescribe interim medication with the specialist clinic undertaking periodic reviews and adjustments. There may or may not be a local shared-care protocol for this. Typically such protocols require the GP to monitor growth, allow small adjustments in medication dose, and renew prescriptions.

Some children with ADHD will need off-licence prescription of clonidine, risperidone, melatonin, and the like. Feelings often run high as to who should undertake this kind of prescription. General guidance has been that so long as a consultant maintains overview, a GP would not be held negligent if any legal action were brought should adverse effects occur. This is logical as a 'licence' is a marketing authorization granted by a national regulatory body (e.g. the MHRA in England) at the request of a pharmaceutical company. Companies frequently do not carry out safety and efficacy studies on children so a licence cannot be granted for that age group. That means the company has to put a phrase such as 'not recommended for children' in the patient information leaflet. Depending upon the age group, between 30% and 90% of medications prescribed for children by paediatricians are 'off-licence', meaning that although the drug has been given a licence for a particular indication, age group of formulation, it is now being used outside these limits. It is perfectly legal to do so. The situation is nevertheless unsatisfactory as medicines used for children are not being adequately tested for safety and efficacy and there are moves to correct this.

In the UK, the Royal College of Paediatrics and Child Health issues a book *Medicines for Children*, which documents mainstream paediatric opinion as to what medicines are responsibly used for children and adolescents. There is very shortly to be a children's BNF, which will fulfil the same function.

Yet financial or perceived legal considerations sometimes come into play and some PCTs are defensive, requiring GPs not to prescribe off-licence or to prescribe from a limited list of cheaper drugs. Similarly some GPs misunderstand the concept of licensing and believe they are simply unable to prescribe off-licence or that if they do litigation is highly likely (it certainly isn't). All this can cause inconvenience or distress to families, either because recommended medication is not made available in primary care or because the GP justifies a refusal to prescribe off-licence on safety grounds, something that can give rise to unnecessary fears.

Clinic procedure

If you make a referral to a specialist clinic, what might the family expect? Practice varies according to whether it is a specialist ADHD clinic or the child is seen in routine paediatric services or CAMHS and the following are broad generalizations. In any setting, the parent(s) will be asked quite a few questions and probably asked to complete rating scales;

they should not feel criticized by this. In CAMHS and specialist clinics, reports and rating scales will be requested from the school. Paediatricians examine their cases physically and developmentally, CAMHS are less likely to. CAMHS are likely to interview the child, a practice uncommon in paediatrics. Physical and psychological investigations are not likely at a first assessment in routine services though some psychological testing may be done in specialist ADHD clinics. Assessment in a specialist ADHD clinic and in CAMHS will probably take a couple of hours. In paediatric services it will be considerably briefer.

Components of treatment

The current convention is for optimal treatment to be multimodal. There are four main components to this:

◆ educational—what do child and family need to know about ADHD?

◆ liaison between services, especially health and education—does the child's school know what to do for him and how can health services assist?

◆ behavioural management—what do the family need to do in terms of handling the child on a day-to-day basis?

◆ medication.

The first three are always required. In addition there are usually questions about diet. From the primary healthcare perspective, most of these can follow a secondary care lead. No GP should feel obliged to carry out all the above.

Education of family and child is important but fraught with pitfalls as there is misinformation and commercial interests in the field. The simplest advice is for the family to contact ADDISS, the foremost support group in the UK and have a look at the website of Children and Adults with Attention Deficit/Hyperactivity Disorder (CHADD), its American counterpart (addresses at the end of this chapter).

Liaison between services is not a primary care responsibility but should involve primary care.

Behavioural management can be complex but the principles are simple:

◆ appropriate expectations as to what the child can reasonable be expected to do

◆ clear, brief communications to the child as to what he is expected to do, often couched in terms of household rules

◆ positive parental attending to the child, using praise and encouragement with a caring, affectionate, involved feel to things

◆ the use of clear, prompt consequences for good and bad behaviour.

Medication deserves a separate section, which follows, but is intended to manage symptoms that are impairing the child's functioning and promote competencies such as academic achievement, not simply to control unacceptable behaviour.

Diet is an uncertain area, which again merits explanation at length. It should be supervised by a paediatric nutritionist/dietician, which tends therefore to take it out of the primary care arena.

Because ADHD is so commonly associated with other problems and conditions, interventions for these, such as family therapy for family relationship problems physiotherapy or occupational therapy for dyspraxia, cognitive-behavioural therapy for anger management and so forth need to be available. Conventionally it would be for the secondary care service to engage these.

Medication

Stimulants

The bedrock of pharmacological treatment for ADHD is stimulant medication—methylphenidate or dexamfetamine. There is no doubt about the efficacy of these drugs in the treatment of core features of ADHD: hyperactivity, impulsiveness, and inattention. Indeed their power, as judged by effect size (0.8–1.2) is greater than most treatments in medicine. Yet there are considerable misunderstandings about them.

Methylphenidate is used as the initial step as there is more information about it in the scientific literature. Not all cases of ADHD will respond and it will not always be acceptable or safe yet it is still by far the most widely used of all ADHD medications. It should be initiated by a specialist so the GP role is predominantly one of maintenance prescription and surveillance of possible adverse effects. Parents will quite often use the opportunity of contact with the GP to ask questions about methylphenidate, a typical range being as follows.

- *Is it an amphetamine?* Not technically but it is rather like amphetamines in its structure.
- *Is it a controlled drug?* Yes it is a class B controlled drug. Children must not take their own doses to school.
- *Is it addictive?* Not in the treatment of ADHD in childhood (the usual problem is getting them to take it). It doesn't cause euphoria though some children say they feel calmer on it because it can stop the sensation of racing thoughts. It probably reduces the risk of illicit substance misuse in adult life.
- *Isn't it the same as cocaine?* It affects the same nerve receptors as cocaine but at a much slower rate so it doesn't cause a 'rush' or euphoria when taken by mouth.
- *How does it work?* It is a competitive blocker of the dopamine transporter so that dopamine is not re-absorbed from the synaptic cleft so quickly, making more dopamine available.
- *What are the common side-effects?* Appetite suppression and difficulty getting off to sleep. Less commonly headache, epigastric pain, or rarely, worsening of tics.
- *What about long-term effects?* Not much. The effect does not wear off with time. There may be slowing of weight gain with growth but whether there is slowing or stunting of height growth is controversial. In UK practice, limitation of height growth is very rare though the follow-up of the Multimodal Treatment Study of ADHD (MTA) study in the USA did show dose-related height growth reduction, admittedly with the rather high doses used in this study.

- *Can it be prescribed as a liquid?* No.

- *Are regular blood tests necessary?* The manufacturers recommend them but the leading centres in the UK don't do them any longer because leucopenia, when it occurred, was mild and did not recur when the methylphenidate was reintroduced after stopping it.

- *Aren't children selling it in the playground?* Occasionally, yes, though this isn't at all common (in spite of what some newspapers say). It is sometimes said that crushing methylphenidate tablets and snorting these causes euphoria but this is a rare practice. In our experience, some adolescents try this but only once. The sustained release preparations can't be abused in such a way. Adults may abuse methylphenidate in order to lose weight (watch out for the sister with anorexia nervosa) or stay up all night; very rarely by using huge doses, preferably by injection, for stimulation.

- *Isn't it just a chemical cosh?* If the dose is too high, the child becomes less mobile, may stare vacantly and be rather unresponsive. This is the 'zombie' state and wears off a few hours after each dose. It shouldn't happen if the dose is carefully monitored, especially using information from the school.

- *Can't it cause psychosis and depression?* A very few children experience auditory hallucinations, usually voices, at ordinary dose levels but a paranoid psychosis is associated with enormous doses, characteristic of abuse, not treatment. A small number of children, perhaps particularly those with brain injury or who have an autistic spectrum disorder can become miserable, sometimes after several months of treatment.

For practical purposes what is said above also applies to dexamfetamine though this is more prone to abuse as it can cause euphoria. From time to time there are stories in the press that highlight possible adverse affects or scare stories and there are organizations that have a commercial or ideological opposition to the use of stimulant drugs. More complex questions should be redirected to specialists though the CHADD website is particularly good at picking up recent press stories.

Methylphenidate is available as an immediate-release form (Ritalin 10mg, Equasym 5, 10, 20 mg) as tablets. Each dose lasts about 3–4 hours so that optimal dosing means two to three doses per day. The effect on sleep lasts longer and it is generally unwise for a child to take a dose after 4pm unless there is a way of helping sleep onset with melatonin, a sedative antihistamine, or clonidine. By and large this is best left for a specialist to advise.

Sustained release preparations of methylphenidate have been developed. Concerta XL (18, 36 mg) uses a complex osmotic pump mechanism that delivers methylphenidate in three phases providing up to 12 hours from a single morning dose. Equasym XL (10, 20, 30 mg) uses a simpler system of wax-coated beads to provide a rather shorter duration of 5–8 hours, useful for children whose difficulties are mainly associated with school. This means that the child's school does not have to administer doses of methylphenidate during the day, leading to less stigmatization of the child who then does not have to join a medicine queue and be identified by other children. There still some schools that refuse to dispense medicines and many, particularly secondary schools, that require the child to remember to turn up for a dose, something that nearly always goes wrong. In such circumstances, sustained release preparations are a real advance though their restricted range of doses means less flexibility in optimal dose titration. There are other sustained-release preparations of methylphenidate available in the USA but are only occasionally seen, usually in American families passing through. They can, theoretically be obtained in the UK but a special import licence from the Home Office/Home and Health Department is required and takes several weeks. Specialist wholesalers sometimes carry limited stocks but this is a matter for specialist clinics to organize.

It is occasionally a good idea to mix immediate-release and sustained-release preparations to obtain smooth blood levels or optimal effects across the day.

Dexamfetamine only exists in an immediate release form (Dexedrine 5 mg) in the UK though sustained release preparations exist in the USA. Some children who do not respond to methylphenidate do respond to dexamfetamine though this is uncommon.

Because of their short duration of action for each dose, a number of children only take such medication on schooldays.

The primary care contribution to shared care of children with ADHD is likely to include renewing prescriptions. Stimulants are controlled drugs so that prescriptions are to be written in the prescriber's own handwriting, specifying the form of the drug (tablets) and the total amount to be dispensed in both figures and words. It is good practice to rule off the bottom of the prescription. It is commonly thought that only a month can be prescribed at a time but there is no actual limit.

A GP may also be asked to check cardiovascular signs and growth. Stimulants will increase blood pressure by about 3 mm of mercury and increase pulse rate by about 10 beats per minute. They usually suppress appetite during the day though many children eat voraciously in the evening. With this in mind, height and weight should be measured regularly—at least every 6 months—and preferably entered onto a growth chart. Although it is rare for height growth to be compromised in UK practice, slowing of weight gain is not uncommon. Simple measures such as encouraging food intake at breakfast and the evening or the use of full cream milk will often correct this.

Atomoxetine

Atomoxetine (Strattera, 10, 18, 25, 40, 60 mg) is a new agent, not a controlled drug, which can usually be given once a day. It is a noradrenaline reuptake inhibitor at the synapse by virtue of being a selective inhibitor of the pre-synaptic noradrenaline transporter. Generally speaking it is comparable with the stimulants though is not always effective and may ultimately not be as powerful. Its big advantage is that it does not affect sleep adversely so can cover evenings and early mornings. This makes it popular among parents, either because it helps with behaviour at such times or assists with homework. It also has a small beneficial effect on mood and anxiety.

Because it can induce vomiting and other gastrointestinal symptoms in the first week of administration in a minority of children it is usual to start with a low dose (0.5–0.8 mg/kg per day) for a week before instituting a full dose of 1.2–1.8 mg/kg per day.

Whether it is given in the morning or evening is a matter of choice and because drowsiness is an occasional problem, evening dosing is quite popular in the UK, even though the manufacturer suggests morning dose, in line with American practice. Some children need twice daily dosing. The full effect of treatment may not be seen for 8 weeks.

Side-effects, once full dosing is established, are not usually a problem though moderate appetite reduction is common. Occasionally irritability is an issue. Some children need the dose increasing further after a few weeks.

There was publicity given to adverse liver function tests in a very few treated children (1/50 000) but it is not thought appropriate to carry out routine liver function tests during treatment. Whether this rate of abnormal liver function results is actually greater than would be caused by stimulant medication is unclear but parents are routinely advised to consult a doctor if the child is jaundiced!

Unlike stimulants, atomoxetine needs to be taken continually and doses should not be omitted over weekends. This makes it less popular with teenagers.

Its status as a recently introduced drug means that its supervision is more likely to be the concern of the specialist service, though a GP may be asked to renew prescriptions.

Other agents

Difficulty with sleep onset is a common problem when stimulants are prescribed. Ensuring adequate sleep is always important when treating ADHD because the condition is sometimes associated with poor sleep, even in the absence of medication. It is also the case that correcting sleep abnormalities and promoting sleep quality will alleviate ADHD features in some children. Straightforward advice about the timing of medication, a bedtime routine, avoidance of stimulating computer games or television in the hour before bed and a warm milky drink at that time is the first move to make. It is unlikely that children can easily be persuaded to drink herbal teas (camomile, vervain) that might assist sleep. Otherwise a sedative antihistamine (e.g. *diphenhydramine*) or *melatonin* given an hour before bed can be useful. Melatonin is unlicensed in the UK but a number of hospital pharmacies now stock it and some retail chemists will issue it on a private prescription. Alternatively it can be purchased readily on the internet (it is classified as a food supplement in America). It seems relatively free of adverse effects but there is only limited information on its safety and dosing because of he absence of the trials ordinarily required for licensing. Usually a dose of between 1 mg and 6 mg suffices.

Clonidine is sometimes used to provide evening control of hyperactivity and its sedative effects can assist sleep onset. It is occasionally used to moderate hyperactive behaviour in pre-school children, or to control aggressive outbursts or tics in older ones. This would presumably be on the recommendation of a specialist but the primary care team might well be asked to check a child's blood pressure when new maintenance prescriptions are issued as large doses of clonidine can lower blood pressure.

Rather similarly, specialist clinics may recommend *risperidone* in order to moderate angry outbursts, control tics, and perhaps assist sleep onset though the latter would be unlikely to be a sole reason for its deployment. A marked increase in appetite is a common side-effect, though the appetite suppression of stimulant medication often masks this.

Third-line drugs for the control of core symptoms of ADHD include *imipramine* or *nortriptyline, bupropion, venlafaxine, reboxetine*, and *modafinil*. None are licensed for the treatment of ADHD. The tricyclic antidepressants are less popular now as ADHD drugs because they can have unwelcome effects on cardiac electrical activity. Even imipramine, used for years in the past as a suppressor of enuresis is to be treated with some care because of the risk of cardiac rhythm abnormalities and examining the child's cardiovascular system would be wise before using it. The others are very much the province of specialist clinics, as is the use of some of the acetylcholinesterase inhibitor dementia drugs in the treatment of predominantly inattentive ADHD.

Diet

It is popularly believed that diet and ADHD are closely linked. Finding hard evidence to support this is difficult. It is plausible that a poor quality diet is sometimes associated with problems concentrating and irritability and it may be such children who appear on television documentaries, their abilities and behaviour transformed by dietary supplements such as fish oils, which act to correct dietary inadequacies. Whether they were sufficiently inattentive and hyperactive to merit a diagnosis of ADHD is not clear. Nor is it evident that children on an adequate diet will benefit cognitively and behaviourally from supplementation with omega III essential fatty acids, though numerous commercial companies make the claim. As things stand, there are no replicated data from which to derive practice, though there is a little preliminary evidence that scores on ADHD rating scales may be improved by fish oils though it is again unclear that the children who were rated had ADHD. Whether commercially promoted fish oils are superior to cheaper cod liver oil is also unknown.

There is no value in diets that simply exclude 'E numbers' or other additives and preservatives unless it is the case that the parents have noticed a worsening of symptoms when a particular food is given. Such foods are not necessarily artificial additives and may include citrus fruits or dairy products for example. Nor is there obvious value in 'stone age' or gluten-free diets. There is no evidence to link excessive sugar intake to ADHD.

What is supported by trial data is a carefully constructed exclusion diet, starting with reduction of diet to one meat, one vegetable, and one fruit. If there is a beneficial response to this, then individual foods are introduced, one-by-one, and an adverse response noted. Foods producing an adverse behavioural response are then excluded from the eventual diet. This is time-consuming and difficult. It will not work for many children with ADHD and is only realistic for children whose food intake can be supervised—mainly pre-schoolers. It needs the assistance of a paediatric dietician. Not many ADHD clinics bother with it. Nevertheless it is an alternative approach for young patients whose families are opposed to the use of medication.

Other approaches

There are no hard data to support family or individual psychotherapy in the treatment of core features of ADHD, though each may have its place in helping with associated features such as family relationship tensions or emotional upset. Cognitive therapy can be shown to have an effect on impulsiveness in laboratory studies or selected children on summer camp placements but the gains do not translate to the real world.

EEG biofeedback has shown some promising early signs but is not generally available. Homeopathy and cranial osteopathy have their advocates but an absence of evidential support. Relaxation training is of no value.

There have been a couple of trials of L-carnitine essentially a nutritional supplement and available from health food shops, showing a beneficial effect on core symptoms at a dose of about 1 g/day, but in our experience it is hard to replicate this in practice. It can be a reasonable first step for families who are anxious about orthodox medication.

Outlook

Most children who respond to medication will remain on it for at last 2 years. Its role is to support normal development and allow ordinary developmental, social, and educational influences to operate—the 'window of opportunity' model. Medication is a symptomatic treatment, not a cure, and should be discontinued every year or two to test whether it is still required. A blind discontinuation using placebos is not normally required.

The general course is that of improvement of core features, not least because frontos-triatal pathways myelinate during adolescence. Only a small percentage of cases of ADHD still fulfil full diagnostic criteria in adulthood, though traits of impulsiveness and inattention may persist and be responsive to medication. The main problem in adult life is the persistence of associated problems and conditions: educational underachievement, low self-esteem, relationship difficulties, substance abuse, and occupational difficulties.

Other issues

Having a child or adolescent with ADHD in the family is exhausting and expensive and there may be a toll on other family relationships, especially those between siblings and the marriage. Sometimes respite through grandparents, summer camps, or social services is necessary. Specialist clinics often have details of these but may need prompting to activate them, especially when the parents present preferentially to primary care with emotional disorders or high alcohol consumption.

Rather similarly, an application for benefits such as Disability Living Allowance may require support from primary care.

Generally speaking, most children with ADHD will have special educational needs that need assessment though it is relatively unlikely that the primary care team would be involved.

Conclusions

The role of the primary health care team in the management of ADHD is usually assisting the specialist clinic as far as the treatment of core ADHD symptoms is concerned. However, there are important contributions to be made in dealing with issues of information or complications that may arise during such treatment. This can include supporting the family as well as the individual patient and alerting the specialist clinic to issues they may be unaware of.

Useful sources for families

- www.addiss.co.uk—UK self-help and advocacy group
- www.chadd.org—US self-help and advocacy
- www.adders.org.uk—useful source for parents.

Helpful source of references

Sandberg, S. (Ed) *Hyperactivity and Attention Disorders of Childhood*. Second Edition. Cambridge University Press, 2002.

Chapter 33

Encopresis and enuresis: their management in primary care

Frank Oberklaid and Daryl Efron

Encopresis

Encopresis is a devastating condition in children. It is often associated with other problems, including recurrent abdominal pain, enuresis, and an inevitable effect on self-esteem and daily functioning. Children often exhibit social withdrawal and may have behavioural and emotional problems as a consequence of the soiling. Furthermore, the issues associated with soiling—the unpredictability, the smell, the social isolation, and the additional workload in cleaning up the child and washing soiled garments—are often reflected in significantly increased family stress and tension in the relationship between the child and his/her parents.

Definition

Encopresis can be defined as 'the deposition of formed or semi-formed stools in a child's clothing on a regular basis after four years of age'. This definition implies that below the age of 4 soiling can be considered as part of delayed or unsuccessful toilet training, while the other components of the definition—'formed or semi-formed' and 'regular basis' allow for the fact the occasionally a child may have an accident, especially during an episode of diarrhoea.

Prevalence

There are no good prevalence data available, although it has been suggested that somewhere between 1 in 50 and 1 in a 100 8-year-old children may have encopresis. It is significantly more common in males, for reasons that are uncertain.

Aetiology

The aetiology of encopresis is almost always physiological, and a consequence of chronic constipation and faecal retention. This in itself is multifactorial (see later), but the faecal retention leads to a distension of the lower colon and rectum, with subsequent disturbance to the mechanics of defecation.

While a number of children have associated emotional and behavioural problems (Gabel *et al.* 1986), these are almost always the consequence of the encopresis and not the cause, and improve with successful treatment of the encopresis (Nolan *et al.* 1991).

There may be a number of predisposing factors to the child's constipation and subsequent faecal retention. The most common is simple constipation, a consequence of poor diet. This may stem from the early years of life, as many young children become constipated during weaning and the introduction of solids. The stool becomes harder and less frequent, evacuation may be incomplete, so that the amount of retention builds up over a number of years. Sometimes defecation becomes painful, leading to the child holding back, which makes the problem worse. In a small number of cases there may be an anal fissure that complicates the problem further.

In some children one of the contributing factors may date back from toddler struggles over toilet training, or a fear of the toilet. Older children may avoid going to the toilet at school, thus holding on and contributing to the faecal retention. Some children may be 'too busy' to go to the toilet, or those with attentional problems may be too impatient to sit on the toilet long enough so as to completely evacuate their bowel.

In a significant number of children there is no history of constipation as we understand it. Parents report that the stools passed by these children are of normal consistency. In many cases no clear predisposing factors can be identified.

Two very uncommon but important conditions that do need to be excluded as contributing to the faecal retention are Hirschsprung disease and neurointestinal dysplasia. Hirschsprung disease can usually be excluded by history. Children with Hirschsprung disease have a delayed passage of meconium in the newborn period, and then a history of passing ribbon-like stools infrequently, with never having passed normal bowel movements. Children with encopresis on the other hand often have a history of normal bowel movements.

Neurointestinal dysplasia is a recently described condition that causes severe constipation. It is believed to be due to the absence of a neurotransmitter in the bowel wall so that colonic contraction is affected. These children exhibit severe constipation from an early age, together with abdominal distension and pain, and frequently soiling.

Clinical features

Children with encopresis exhibit diverse clinical presentations (Levine 1975). Some will have been successfully toilet trained for both bladder and bowel, and only begin soiling many years later. Other children will never have been continent, with the longest period between accidents being days or weeks.

Some children will soil once every few days, whereas others will soil many times in a day. Sometimes children pass only small amounts into their underpants, whereas at other times there is a full bowel movement. Mostly the faeces are of normal consistency, though in some children it may be small hard pellets.

Many children seem to soil particularly in the afternoon and early evening, such that they are dirty when they come home from school, or will have an accident in the time period between coming home from school and going to bed. Sometimes there is soiling at school, and very occasionally children will soil while having a bath or in their sleep.

What all of these children have in common is an insensitivity to the desire to defecate; i.e. virtually all say that they cannot feel a bowel movement coming. A small number may become aware of defecating when the bowel movement is already at the anal verge, and often it is too late to prevent an accident. However, the majority will only become aware of having passed faeces when it has made contact with the skin of the buttock, or when they or others become aware of the smell.

The use of the toilet is also variable. Some children have occasional or even frequent bowel movements in the toilet, whereas others will defecate almost exclusively in their underwear.

As previously mentioned, recurrent abdominal pain and enuresis are frequently associated with encopresis (Levine 1975). These children almost invariably suffer loss of self-esteem and body image (Landman *et al.* 1986). Many become socially withdrawn and report that they are teased or bullied at school, and their lack of confidence affects social relationships, such that many are reluctant to spend time at other children's houses or to stay over.

Parents respond to their children's soiling in various ways. Some children, especially when they are older, are expected to clean themselves up and change their clothes, whereas in other instances, especially in younger children, parents attend to this task. Parents react to their children's soiling with anger, frustration, disbelief, exasperation, and any other combinations of emotions. Many find it difficult to believe that their child has no sensation, and sometimes children are punished for what appears to the parents to be wilful behaviour.

Evaluation

History

A careful history is obtained from the parents both to record relevant information and also to begin to establish the all important relationship with the parents and with the child. The clinician elicits any of the predisposing factors mentioned above, and documents the current pattern of toilet use. It is also important to document the pattern of soiling, in terms of frequency, timing, and severity. Does the child have any sensation or awareness, and if so is this reliable or intermittent? Other important items to note in the questioning of the parents include how the child is coping; whether there are any significant emotional or behavioural problems; what the parents do in response to the soiling, their understanding of the problem, and the level of stress that it causes in the family; what is happening at the school level, and whether the child is teased or bullied; the teacher's reaction to soiling; and any previous treatment the child may have received.

Examination

A thorough physical examination is undertaken. Any abdominal distension is noted— careful palpation of the abdomen sometimes reveals palpable stool in the left iliac fossa. Neurological conditions are excluded by inspection of the lumbosacral spine and anus, and examination of the lower limbs.

Rectal examination is not necessary as part of the assessment of children with encopresis, as it provides limited and unreliable information about the extent and severity of the faecal retention, and is uncomfortable and sometimes distressing for the child.

The diagnosis of faecal retention is made with a plain abdominal radiograph, which gives an indication of the amount of faeces throughout the colon, and especially in the rectum (Rockney *et al.* 1995). Often the rectum will be dense with faeces, such that the normal rectal shape is distorted and the lumen clearly distended. Most often the stool consistency is normal, but sometimes hard pellets are visible in the rectum.

Management

The key to management is adopt a multimodal approach, which recognizes that encopresis is a chronic condition that needs to be taken seriously. Sympathetic explanation of the condition to the child and the parents is crucial, and follow-up needs to be regular and sustained (Levine 1982).

1. *Explanation and demystification.* It is important that the child and the parents understand the reason for encopresis, and that the clinician is sympathetic to the fact that the child has no sensation. The abdominal X-ray is explained to the child and parents, and the faecal retention and the encopresis explained by the use of drawings. It is important to emphasize that the child is not to blame and is not simply lazy, but at the same time the child is told that he/she needs to take responsibility for self-management. The strength of the relationship that the clinician establishes with the child and the parents would seem to be an important contributor to the success of the treatment plan.

2. *Diet.* A high-fibre diet with adequate fluid intake is important. The child should be eating sufficient fruit, vegetables, and complex carbohydrates to increase the bulk of stools, and the amount of fat in the diet should be reduced as fatty substances decrease bowel transit time. The whole family should be encouraged to adopt good dietary habits.

3. *Regular sitting on the toilet.* This is an important part of the treatment regimen. The rationale is to increase the chance of spontaneous stooling in toilet, so reducing the risk of soiling and re-establishing normal toileting habits. The child is asked to sit on the toilet three times a day for about 5 minutes, preferably after each meal to take advantage of the gastrocolic reflex. The sits should be timed, and the child rewarded for both sitting and defecation (see below). Providing reading material for the child can help with adherence. Sometimes the clinician will need to assist in making arrangements with the teachers so that a structured toileting regimen can be implemented at school. Additionally, especially if the child tends to soil in the afternoon, sitting on the toilet as soon as he/she comes home from school is suggested. The frequency and timing of toilet use can be modified depending on the specific pattern of soiling, but a structured toileting regimen is a crucial component of management of encopresis.

4. *Behaviour modification.* A diary or star chart is often very useful to document the pattern of bowel movements and soiling, and to monitor adherence with the structured toileting regimen. It can also be very useful for behaviour modification, especially in younger children. The child receives a gold star every time he/she

defecates successfully into the toilet. The child is also urged to go to the toilet immediately when he/she feels the urge to stool, and additional stars can be awarded for the child taking responsibility. Secondary rewards, such as the child receiving a small gift when a certain number of stars are accumulated, can provide an additional incentive.

5. *Medications*. Stool softeners or bowel stimulants are used in most children with encopresis, especially in the early stages (Nolan *et al.* 1991). It does not seem to matter a great deal what type of medications are used—stool softeners, lubricants, or stimulants. They can be used either singly or in combination, and are used in doses high enough and in sufficient frequency to assist in the evacuation of the bowel in the early weeks of treatment. Parents should be warned of side-effects, such as abdominal cramps, diarrhoea, or the leakage of oil, and also that the soiling may worsen in the short term as the bowel is being cleared.

   While sometimes enemas and suppositories are advocated, most would argue that they do not offer any significant advantage over oral medications. Furthermore, they are uncomfortable for both children and for the parents who administer them.

6. *Regular follow-up*. It is important to establish a follow-up regimen that is frequent enough to provide encouragement and guidance for the child and the parents, and that is long enough to make sure that improvement or cure is sustained. As previously mentioned, encopresis should be considered a chronic condition and follow-up should be for a minimum of 6 months, and often substantially longer.

   At each visit, the child is praised and congratulated even for small gains. In most children the frequency of encopresis will slowly reduce; the child will have periods where he/she is accident-free and these will be of gradually longer duration, and slowly sensation will begin to return so the child feels the need to go to the toilet. Medications are slowly weaned, but still making sure that the child maintains a bowel frequency of at least once every 2 days.

Prognosis

Most children will respond well to this multimodal regimen. For some, the response will be rapid and sustained so that within a few months the child is essentially cured. For others there may be an initial improvement that then plateaus, or the child may even then relapse. In some instances, treatment needs to be continued for a couple of years before the child can finally be judged to be cured. Sometimes this is frustrating for the clinician as well as for the parents.

Where treatment is not successful or is prolonged, it is almost always due to poor adherence, especially with the structured toileting regimen or relates to the child not going to the toilet when he/she feels the urge to stool. Sometimes there is poor supervision of the toileting regime because the family is disorganized or otherwise stressed, and in many instances it is not until the child has achieved a certain level of maturity and takes responsibility for his/her soiling that things finally seem to get better.

Enuresis

Enuresis in children is a common presentation in general practice. It is a condition that is embarrassing for the child, often limits his social activities, and is inconvenient for the family.

Definitions

Primary nocturnal enuresis refers to children over 5 years of age who have never achieved reliable urinary continence overnight. Children who recommence wetting following a period of greater than 6 months of dryness are said to have *secondary enuresis*.

Most enuretic children have *isolated nocturnal enuresis*. However, up to 20% also have problems with daytime bladder control, with symptoms such as urinary frequency and urgency, and often dampness of underpants or frank incontinence. This is called *diurnal enuresis*. These children may suffer recurrent urinary tract infections as the constant wetness supports bacterial growth. Encopresis is sometimes an associated problem.

Prevalence and natural history

At 5 years of age 15% of children still wet the bed. Each year approximately 15% achieve dryness spontaneously, such that the prevalences at ages 7 and 10 are 10% and 5% respectively (Howe and Walker 1992). Approximately 1–2% of adolescents over age 15 still have enuresis, with some having problems into adulthood.

As with most developmental problems enuresis is much more common in boys than girls, with a ratio of about 2:1.

Aetiology

Urinary continence involves the complex neurological regulation of bladder function. Integrity of spinal cord, brainstem, and cerebral cortex is required to enable filling at low pressure, and co-ordinated voiding only when initiated voluntarily. The frequency of voiding decreases progressively from the newborn period in the early years of life as bladder capacity increases. By about age 3–4 years, most children develop the ability to suppress detrusor contractions and co-ordinate these with sphincter function. Daytime continence is usually achieved some months to years before nocturnal continence.

In most cases enuresis represents a normal developmental variant in the maturation of bladder control. Delayed nocturnal continence commonly runs in families. The strong genetic basis of nocturnal enuresis is evidenced by the much higher concordance rate among monozygotic twins than among dizygotic twins. It appears to be inherited in an autosomal dominant fashion with high penetrance. At least two gene loci have been implicated so far.

Studies have shown that children with enuresis have smaller bladder capacity than controls, However, differences observed in the awake state are not present under anaesthesia, suggesting the differences are functional rather than anatomical. Decreased antidiuretic hormone secretion, resulting in higher then average nocturnal urine production, may play a part in some patients with nocturnal enuresis. This may be secondary to small bladder volume, as bladder distension appears to promote antidiuretic hormone secretion.

It is common for parents of children with nocturnal enuresis to report that their child is a deep sleeper and hard to wake. There is some experimental evidence to support this assertion. Most enuretic episodes occur during non-rapid eye movement sleep, but at random through the night. Some characteristic EEG changes have been described in association with enuretic episodes. Obstructive sleep hypoventilation can contribute significantly to nocturnal enuresis, and in some cases adenotonsillectomy is curative.

Children with *diurnal enuresis* may have an underlying urological problems (e.g. detrusor instability, ectopic ureter) or neurological abnormality (e.g. neurogenic bladder, occult spinal dysraphism). Dysfunctional voiding can manifest as an inconsistent urinary stream and variable volumes of urine, related to incomplete bladder emptying.

Secondary enuresis may be due to urinary tract infection, diabetes mellitus, diabetes insipidus or seizures, or an emotional stress such as parental separation, death in the family, etc. However in many cases no specific cause is able to be identified.

Psychological causes are probable not a significant factor in most cases of enuresis, though there may be secondary emotional effects. The possibility of child abuse should be kept in mind if there are other indicators.

Evaluation

History

A detailed history covers frequency of wetting (whether there has ever been night-time continence, how many dry nights per week, how many times per night), timing of wetting, longest period of dryness, presence and nature of daytime bladder problems, history of urinary tract infections, bowel function, psychological effects, impact on family, family history, and interventions tried in the past.

Examination

Physical examination should include palpation for renal masses and faecal retention, palpation and percussion for a distended bladder, genitalia, inspection of lower spine for tufts of hair or dimples (raising the possibility of spina bifida occulta), neurological examination of lower limbs, and blood pressure. Wetness of underpants should be noted. A urinalysis should be undertaken to check for specific gravity, glucose, ketones, nitrites, and leucocytes. Imaging of the urinary tract is not indicated unless there have been urinary tract infections.

Management

The management of a child with enuresis is individualized according to the age and developmental stage of the child, the level of family concern, the child's level of motivation and strategies tried previously. It is important to explain to children and their parents that it is not the child's fault, and that children vary in the age at which they develop bladder control. It is often helpful for the child to hear the family history and learn that his father also wet the bed when he was a child.

Fluid management is important. Patients should be instructed to drink abundantly during the day so that they get used to having a full bladder. Parents have usually already been sensibly restricting fluids in the evenings. Caffeine such as in cola drinks should be avoided.

Parents often try waking routines, such as taking the child to the toilet when the parents go to bed. This can be successful for some children but is not reliable and sometimes parents find that the child has already wet, or wets later in the night.

Bladder training exercises have been demonstrated to be helpful in reducing enuresis. These can take the form of fun games. The child drinks two to three glasses of water, and then when he feels the need to void holds on as long as he can. This can be timed and set up as a competition, either against his own best time—aiming to 'beat my record'—or with a sibling (or parent!). Another exercise is to stop voiding mid-stream, and hold on as long as possible before emptying the bladder. The purpose of these exercises is to aid training of sensory pathways from bladder to brain, to assist in control over bladder function.

Conditioning (enuresis alarm)

The most effective therapy is the conditioning alarm (Evans 2000; Glazener et al. 2004). A sensor is placed either under the sheet (pad) or clipped to the child's underpants, and connected to the alarm by a wire. These systems vary in reliability, with cheaper versions being prone to false alarms. The alarm is activated when the sensor becomes wet, completing a circuit. It is important that the child turns the alarm off, even if the parents have to wake the child first. This is the key conditioning step. Then the child should go to the toilet to empty his bladder, and then return to help his parents change the bedsheets, before resetting the alarm and going back to sleep. Conditioning is most effective if complemented by a reward system, for example stickers in a diary. Parents (or the child) should keep a daily diary recording the size of the wetness—small, medium, or large—as well as the dry nights. When successful the wet patches becomes progressively smaller and the proportion of dry nights increases until dryness is achieved, as the child learns to tolerate a full bladder in his sleep. Parents should be instructed to praise the child abundantly for even small gains, such as a less wet bed or one or two dry nights.

Bladder conditioning is demanding and disruptive for families, many of whom have developed practical systems for dealing with the enuresis such that family life is essentially unaffected, e.g. pull-up nappies, mattress protectors. Therefore, the child needs to be motivated and the parents supportive, with no impending changes in family routines such as a holiday or house move. For the alarm to work the child needs to sleep in pyjamas or underwear, so the short-term costs are more laundry and interrupted nights as the alarm goes off.

Systematic reviews have shown that children are 13 times more likely to become dry at night with the alarm than without. Approximately 70% of children with primary nocturnal enuresis will achieve dryness with the alarm. The duration of treatment required varies from less than a week to 2–3 months, depending on a range of factors including how near the child is developmentally to achieving dryness when therapy is instituted. A significant proportion of responders relapse (between 30% and 70% in different studies); however, most of these patients then respond rapidly to a second course of conditioning, often within days.

If there is no response to the alarm within about 4 weeks then the child is probably not ready—often there is family history of bedwetting with duration beyond the child's current age. The alarm can be tried again in 6 months.

Medications

Desmopressin (DDAVP) is a very effective short-term therapy for nocturnal enuresis (Glazener and Evans 2002). It appears to work by reducing overnight urine production. It can be administered either intranasally or orally. The starting dose is 20 μg intranasally (one spray into each nostril) or 200 mg (one tablet) orally, taken at bedtime. Some patients need two to three times this dose. Desmopressin is expensive, but relatively safe. The most serious potential side-effect is water intoxication with hyponatraemia. This can present with headache, nausea, or vomiting, and in more severe cases depressed conscious state and seizures. Patients taking DDAVP should be instructed to limit fluids in the evenings. The intranasal preparation can cause mucosal irritation and epistaxis. The response rate is about up to 50%; however, most patients relapse upon discontinuation—there are no differences compared with placebo after stopping treatment. It can be used in patients in whom the alarm is not effective. Long-term therapy with DDAVP is not usually recommended. Patients should be tried off the DDAVP every few months to determine whether there has been spontaneous remission. It is very useful to cover sleepovers or camps when it is important for the child that he/she is dry.

There is some evidence that combination therapy with DDAVP and the enuresis alarm has a higher success rate than the alarm alone, particularly in families who are less supportive and children with behavioural problems (Leebeek-Groenewegen et al. 2001).

Tricyclic antidepressants are effective and were used extensively in the past. They promote antidiuretic hormone secretion, and also cause detrusor muscle relaxation. However, these drugs are not recommended now and should not be used because of the potential for side-effects (such as lethargy, sleep disturbance, and gastrointestinal) and also the risk of cardiac conduction defects if taken in overdose by the patient or a sibling.

Cases of secondary enuresis related to a clear destabilizing event often resolve spontaneously once the precipitating emotional trauma has passed or reduced in intensity, or else respond to psychological interventions. In the absence of an easily identifiable trigger the management of secondary enuresis is the same as for primary enuresis.

Diurnal enuresis is a more challenging problem. It often requires a multimodal approach, including increasing fluid intake, a structured toileting regime with the child going to the toilet at regular specific times, bladder training, and a behavioural programme. The anticholinergic drug oxybutinin is usually effective. The starting dose is 2.5 mg twice a day, although some patients need double this dose. Oxybutinin can cause constipation, so if it is to be started bowel function should be addressed pre-emptively with attention to fluids, diet, and reminders to the child to respond immediately to the call to stool.

Conclusions

Enuresis is a common paediatric problem. The conditioning alarm is the most effective treatment, and offers the best chance of long-term dryness. DDAVP has a role particularly for short-term use to cover special events such as camps or sleepovers.

References

Encopresis

Gabel S, Hegedus AM, Wald A, Chandra R, Chiponis D (1986). Prevalence of behaviour problems and mental health utilization among encopretic children: implications for behavioural pediatrics. *Journal of Developmental and Behavioral Pediatrics* **7**: 293–297

Landman GB, Rappaport L, Fenton T, Levine MD (1986). Locus of control and self esteem in children with encopresis. *Journal of Developmental and Behavioral Pediatrics* **7**: 111–113.

Levine MD (1975). Children with encopresis: a descriptive analysis. *Pediatrics* **56**: 412–416.

Levine MD (1982). Encopresis: its potentiation, evaluation and alleviation. *Pediatric Clinics of North America* **29**: 315–330.

Nolan T, Debelle G, Oberklaid F, Coffey C. (1991). Randomised trial of laxatives in treatment of childhood encopresis. *Lancet* **338**: 523–527.

Rockney RM, McQuade WH, Days AD (1995). The plain abdominal roentgenogram in the management of encopresis. *Archives of Pediatric and Adolescent Medicine* **149**: 623–627.

Enuresis

Evans JHC (2000). Nocturnal enuresis. In Moyer VA (ed.), *Evidence Based Pediatrics and Child Health*. BMJ Books, London.

Glazener CMA, Evans JHC (2002). Desmopressin for nocturnal enuresis in children (Cochrane Review). *Cochrane Library*, 3.

Glazener CMA, Evans JHC, Peto RE (2004). Alarm interventions for nocturnal enuresis in children (Cochrane Review). *The Cochrane Library*, Issue 1.

Howe AC, Walker CE (1992). Behavioral management of toilet training, enuresis, and encopresis. *Pediatric Clinics of North America* 1992; **39**: 413.

Leebeek-Groenewegen A, Blom J, Sukhai R, Van Der Heijden B (2001). Efficacy of desmopressin combined with alarm therapy for monosymptomatic nocturnal enuresis. *Journal of Urology* **166**(6):2456–2458.

Chapter 34

Common psychosocial disorders in children and adolescents: diagnosis and treatment

David Foreman

Introduction

This chapter reviews the diagnosis and treatment of common psychosocial disorders, other than behaviour disorders or abuse, in primary care. After explaining the limits of the concept of 'psychosocial disorders' an assessment programme is set out, addressing the specific needs of the primary care practitioner, in terms of disturbance, disorder, disability, and handicap. Following this, the common presentations of anxiety and depression, unexplained physical symptoms, school refusal and deliberate self-harm are presented as useful segmentations of psychosocial disorders, which can guide assessment and treatment. Cognitive-behaviour therapy (CBT) delivered by specialist workers, and serotonin-specific reuptake inhibitors (SSRIs) are identified as modes of treatment especially useful in addition to ordinary primary care across all these major segments, with other therapies having more specific applications. It is concluded that primary care has a useful role to play in the management of these problems, and can materially improve children's lives by engaging effectively with them.

General principles of assessment

The term 'Psychosocial' is an ill-defined catch-all term, which breaks all the rules of good psychiatric classification, but none the less survives because it says something useful about practitioners' experience in dealing with disturbed children. It denotes ('defines' is far too strong a word) a loose grouping of children who seem unable to cope with the circumstances of their lives. The practitioner's task is to make sense of this presentation in a useful way.

Inability to cope and child psychiatric disorder

Not all child psychiatric disorders are psychosocial, and not all psychosocial presentations have a psychiatric diagnosis. For example, autism is a neuropsychiatric disorder that is not a product of the child's social circumstances (Trevarthen *et al.* 1996), and not all juvenile presentations of deliberate self-harm indicate depression (Harrington 2001). Sometimes, one may look in vain for any problems in the child, as the presenting complaint can simply be the carer not coping with a normal child–maternal depression can present in this way. So, in dealing with psychosocial problems, the practitioner needs to distinguish between four components of a child's presentation (c.f. World Health Organization 1976). These are

1. *Disturbance.* This is the trouble the child presents to others, which leads to the presentation.

2. *Disability.* This is what the child cannot do, which a normal child in the same circumstances could. Typically, the impairment that results from disability is compounded by handicap.

3. *Handicap.* This is the component of the child's impairment that results from the child's environment. For example, in school refusal, impairment in social and educational engagement resulting from the *disability* of a separation anxiety disorder may be compounded by the *handicap* of the parents preferring that the child be at home with them rather than at school.

4. *Disorder.* This is one (or more) of a list of syndromes, i.e. groups of symptoms and signs. Currently, for child psychiatric disorders the two most authoritative lists are those of the International Classification of Diseases (version 10) (ICD-10) (World Health Organization 1992) and the Diagnostic and Statistical Manual of Psychiatric Disorders (version IV) (DSM IV) (American Psychiatric Association 1994). Either may be used, though American psychiatry is standardized on DSM IV, for which it was written, while the UK uses ICD-10.

Our examples illustrate how these components can interact. The autistic child's presentation is dominated by the disorder, and its associated disability, though handicap may also be important as the most easily reversible component of the child's overall impairment. In these circumstances, the absence of disturbance would be a disadvantage for the child, as it might prevent detection of the problem and consequential assistance. The child of the depressed mother, on the other hand, has no disability or disorder but a considerable handicap, where even normal behaviour results in intolerable disturbance. Finally, a child who attempt suicide clearly has a disability, and probably a handicap, that could be life-threatening, but may have no disorder and, if the child does not report the attempt, no disturbance.

In general, we tend to overestimate the importance of psychiatric disorder, and underestimate that of disability or handicap. At any one time, up to twenty percent of the child population present with a syndrome pattern consistent with a diagnosable psychiatric disorder, but only 3% are significantly disabled by their problems (Williams and Richardson 1995). Conversely, children who do not meet criteria for a psychiatric diagnosis but still reach general 'caseness' criteria that include impairment are as disabled as those with specific diagnoses (Angold *et al.*, 1999). So, in deciding how to manage psychosocial impairment when it presents to us, we need to consider the symptoms and signs, together with their psychosocial setting. Taylor (1982) has usefully formulated this approach in terms of 'illness' (the child's presentation) being made up of the 'disease' (the constitutional difficulties in the child) and the 'predicament' (the network of social difficulties the child is trying to manage). In the psychosocial disorders, even though primacy is presumed to lie with the predicament, we must still be aware of the 'disease', or constitutional component, as limiting the child's resilience in coping with the stressor: life is stressful, and it may not be possible to eliminate the stressor by environmental manipulation. In those cases, we need to consider ways of increasing and supporting the child's resilience.

Assessing psychosocial disorders: what should we be looking for?

From the argument just set out, it follows that our assessment should have three goals. First, we should seek to describe the problem, from the point of view of the child's symptoms and signs (remember, it may be important to establish there may be none). Next, we need to consider how the child is being impaired, both by any disabilities he or she suffers, and handicaps resulting from the child's environment. Finally, we should understand how the child's predicament contributes to the presentation, and those factors that undermine, or promote, the child's resilience.

A child psychiatry assessment in secondary care typically takes an hour and a half or more, which is simply not practical in primary care. However, the primary care practitioner has many assessment advantages that the secondary care practitioner does not: the child in question may—and often is—being seen repeatedly for a range of reasons, issues affecting other members of the child's family may be well-understood, and the child's general predicament may be accessed by the primary care practitioner in many ways. For psychosocial disorders at least, the primary care practitioner can still undertake an assessment that, while not as detailed as that offered by secondary care, none the less captures sufficient information to plan appropriate interventions.

Assessing signs and symptoms

Simplified versions of both ICD-10 (ICD-10 PC) (World Health Organization 1996) and DSM IV (DSM IVPC) (American Psychiatric Association 1995) exist for primary care practitioners. ICD-10 PC, designed as it is for worldwide use, is possibly too limited for use in primary care in the UK, e.g. it omits autism and children's emotional disorders, while the more inclusive DSM IVPC may be too cumbersome to use routinely (deGruy and Pincus 1996). A possibly more useful alternative is the National Electronic Library for Health, which provides extensive guidance on common problems the primary care practitioner might suspect, including lists of symptoms, signs and suggested treatments for common disorders, related to ICD-10 PC where possible, but not limited to it (WHO Collaborating Centre for Research and Training in Mental Health 2004). However, for psychosocial problems, matters can be simplified considerably by remembering that repeated epidemiological studies have found that children's symptomatology reliably groups into conduct, emotional, a mixture of both (mixed disorders of conduct and emotion) and other disorders (Rutter *et al.*, 1970). Conduct, or 'externalizing' disorders are characterized by antisocial and aggressive behaviour, such as defiance, lying, stealing, anger (including temper tantrums), and violence. Emotional, or 'internalizing' disorders involve mood disturbances, most typically anxiety and depression (Achenbach 1992).

Most psychosocial disorders present with either behavioural, emotional, or mixed syndromes, and the advantage for the primary care practitioner is that these can be reliably estimated by questionnaire. A full discussion of these is beyond the scope of this chapter. For primary care practitioners, the Strengths and Difficulties Questionnaire is a brief, reliable and valid (Goodman *et al.* 2000) questionnaire appropriate for common child psychopathology, which has the advantage of being freely available in electronic form, with automated electronic scoring and interpretation for both practitioner and patient, at www.sdq.com.

Assessing impairment

Impairment is the combination of disability and handicap. Though the questionnaires just mentioned do give some guidance to impairment, they are inadequate alone, as they are optimized to provide a cut-off between the normal and pathological range in terms of the symptoms they measure. So, they will not detect that part of a child's impairment that cannot be described in terms of symptoms, and a one-point difference close to the cut-off may have a quite different meaning from a similar difference at either extreme of the scale. Goodman and Scott (1997) offer a simple classification of impairment, which can guide clinical assessment. They suggest considering

1. social impairment as it impacts on
   (a) family life
   (b) the classroom and
   (c) peer relationships
2. the distress it causes the child, and
3. the disruption it causes others.

An alternative is to attempt an overall estimate of the degree of impairment resulting from all sources. This is the basis of the Children's General Adaptation Scale (CGAS), which is a 100-point scale of impairment, 70 and above being the normal range. Both it and practice examples are available online (The Washington Institute and Washington State Mental Health Division 2004). Despite its apparent crudity, it is surprisingly reliable (Dyrborg *et al.* 2000).

Though handicap and disability are the constituents of impairment, they are best evaluated as part of the next—and last—phase of the assessment.

Assessing the child's predicament and resilience

The practitioner in primary care is extremely well situated to assess both these areas. The practitioner's close and continuing relationship with both child and family will provide insight into what difficulties currently encompass the family, and how each member, including the child, has coped with stressors in the past. So, for the primary care practitioner, the issue is how this knowledge should best be organized to help guide appropriate intervention. It is both simple and effective to think in terms of risk factors, i.e. what contributes to make the problem worse, and protective factors, i.e. what seems to be preventing the problem getting worse, or is making it better. Disability and handicap contribute by making clear whether the source of the risk factor is child, environment, or both. A risk factor arising from the child is a disability, while that from the environment is a handicap. One implication of this formulation is that the presentation, itself, is defined as a risk factor. We shall see below that this apparent circularity is quite true, and is one justification for a focus on symptom relief in these conditions.

An overview of common psychosocial presentations

From what has already been said, it is unsurprising to find that there is much variation in how psychosocial problems are codified, the largest source of discrepancy being whether the problem is described in psychological or social terms, which in turn reflects the professional background of the author. The approach adopted here follows a 'presenting problem' model, i.e. discusses them as typical problems a primary care practitioner might face in daily practice, in terms of the model of assessment just set out. This has the advantage of being able to discuss them in a way that directly relates to the experience of the primary care practitioner from when the case presents. Child protection, behaviour problems and grief have deservedly received their own chapters so will not be discussed here.

The anxious/depressed child

This slightly ungainly title reflects the epidemiological fact that anxiety and depression cannot be separated in epidemiological studies (Achenbach 1993), while behaviour problems can also indicate unhappiness, e.g. bereavement (Dowdney 2000). However, the variability within this group of children means that subsets do meet diagnostic criteria for anxiety, depression, and various subtypes, including some specific to childhood, that have become the focus for elaborate codification in both ICD-10 and DSM-IV. Furthermore, not all of these syndromes are necessarily psychosocial disorders as described here. Notwithstanding all this, we shall see below that the primary care practitioner can do very well with this group of children.

Presenting signs and symptoms

The first task for practitioners is to decide what we are dealing with. As implied above, duration, pervasiveness, and intensity of symptoms is most important in judging their importance. Depressed mood needs to be continuously present for at least 2 weeks, in association with fatigue and anhedonia (loss of the sense of pleasure) before it may indicate a depressive disorder; generally anxious mood present more days than not for at least 6 months with at least one somatic symptom of anxiety before it can imply a general anxiety disorder. Social anxiety (fear of social situations) or separation anxiety (fear of separation from the child's parents or equivalent) needs to be present for at least 4 weeks before the suffix 'disorder' can be applied. The symptoms should also be disabling to at least some extent, using the criteria described above. Questionnaires focus on the intensity and number of symptoms, so they can assist, but not substitute for a conventional history and examination. The good news for primary care practitioners is that 'what you see is what you get'; a depressed or anxious child will have depressive or anxious symptomatology, though the parent or child may not mention these symptoms till specifically asked for. A very common presentation of anxiety or depression is with physical symptoms without an identifiable cause: in such cases assessing for depression or anxiety, and treating accordingly, can save many unnecessary investigations and referrals to secondary care. School refusal is a more obviously 'psychological' presentation, though of course physical symptoms may also be given as the reason for the refusal. The old idea that behavioural symptoms could mean that the child is 'really' depressed or anxious is a mistake, probably resulting from a failure to understand that many children are comorbid for both behavioural and emotional disorders (Lilienfeld 2003).

Treatment

It is worth making a stab at a conventional diagnosis in this area, as the evidence supporting most treatments is obtained from diagnostic groups. Specific phobias may be effectively treated by the behavioural techniques of flooding or desensitization. For depressive disorder, the best evidence is now for CBT, which has been applied successfully in primary care (Bushfield-Kahan 1997). Clinical experience and research evidence continues to support the value of antidepressants, and in practice primary care practitioners may find the latter more available than the former. However, drug companies' withholding of important negative and adverse clinical trial data may have led the effectiveness of such medication to have been overestimated, and currently only fluoxetine has incontrovertible evidence of its efficacy (Whittington *et al.* 2004). For depressive symptomatology that does not meet diagnostic criteria, recent adult-based outcome data suggest that outcome only relates poorly to treatment provision: watchful waiting may be sufficient, or perhaps individualized treatments negotiated with the patient as necessary (Barrett *et al.* 2001, Oxman *et al.* 2001). It seems likely that similar approaches will be appropriate for children (Asarnow *et al.* 2002). Of the anxiety disorders, separation anxiety, and simple phobias are those most likely to present to the primary care practitioner. For separation anxiety (or generalized anxiety), fluoxetine may have some benefit (Birmaher *et al.* 2003), and CBT, provided either individually, in groups or with family support also helps (Barrett 1998; Shortt and Barrett 2001). Separation anxiety typically presents to the practitioner through school refusal or somatization (Masi *et al.* 2001), so its subclinical manifestations will be considered under those headings. However, it is more likely to be undetected in those conditions than to be present, but fail to meet its diagnostic guidelines. So, while it may be important to decide whether the presentation meets diagnostic criteria for having either depression or anxiety, it is probably less important to distinguish between them in primary care, as the first-line treatments for both (aside from specific phobias) are so similar. As we have seen above, the criteria specifically include impairment and duration, so for the miserable and anxious child presenting to the primary care practitioner it is most important to use the level of impairment and its duration as a threshold for treatment.

The child with unexplained physical symptoms

This presentation follows on naturally from the last; we have seen that unexplained physical symptoms are often how depression or anxiety presents in children. However, there are also specific diagnostic categories for these problems. As usual, ICD-10 and DSM IV do things slightly differently, but it is generally accepted that both of their approaches to these disorders is unsatisfactory, even in adults (Mayou 2000). The commonest of these presentations, physical symptoms as an expression of anxiety or depressive disorders, has been discussed above. In primary care, the three other common presentations are for headache, recurrent abdominal pain (typically in younger children), and chronic fatigue (in older children). They may, of course, occur together.

Presenting signs and symptoms

It is important to note that the pain (both headache and abdominal) can be associated with nausea, pallor, vomiting dizziness, headache, and faintness, so both parental and practitioner concern is unsurprising. Simple questions can readily distinguish between tension headache and migraine; tension headache being characterized by greater duration and less intensity (Ozge *et al.* 2002; Zwart *et al.* 2003). Caffeine (from cola-based or 'energizing' drinks as well as tea, coffee, or chocolate) is worth considering (Hering-Hanit and Gadoth 2003). Symptoms that predict the presence of a space-occupying lesion include: (1) headache of less than 1-month duration; (2) absence of family history of migraine; (3) abnormal neurological findings on examination; (4) gait abnormalities; and (5) occurrence of seizures (Lewis *et al.* 2002). Psychosocial abdominal pain is variable and ill-defined, appearing anywhere from the epigastrium to the perineum. About three-quarters of recurrent abdominal pain is associated with anxiety, while the commonest non-psychological cause is distension secondary to constipation (Goldberg and Gabriel 1996). Irritable bowel disease can frequently be identified in these children (Kohli and Li 2004), but it is important to realize that much recurrent abdominal pain will not meet formal diagnostic criteria, and the presentation may vary developmentally over time (Besedovsky and Li 2004; Hyams 2004).

There are now agreed criteria for what has become known as chronic fatigue syndrome

- ◆ Inclusion criteria
  - clinically evaluated, medically unexplained fatigue of at least six months' duration that is
    - of new onset (not lifelong)
    - not the result of ongoing exertion
    - not substantially altered by rest
    - associated with a substantial reduction in previous level of activities
  - includes four of
    - subjective memory impairment
    - sore throat
    - tender lymph nodes
    - muscle pain
    - joint pain

- headache
- unrefreshing sleep
- post-exertional malaise lasting more than 24 hours

◆ Exclusion criteria
  - active, unresolved or suspected disease
  - psychosis (including psychotic depression and bipolar disorder)
  - dementia
  - anorexia or bulimia nervosa
  - alcohol or substance abuse disorders
  - severe obesity.

However, even using this definition most, though not all, cases can also be characterized by one of several other diagnoses, most typically depression, anxiety, or one of the 'somatizing disorders' coded in ICD-10 or DSM IV and mentioned above, though many will be 'atypical' and not meet the disorder's full diagnostic criteria (Sharpe and Wessely 2000).

For both of these syndromes, therefore, diagnosis is often a matter of identifying physical and psychological causes that have specific treatments, and addressing them. Following this, treatment is often better guided by the assessment of predicament and impairment. The manner of investigation and diagnosis is also an important part of the treatment, as we shall now see.

Treatment

First, there are principles relating to investigation and engagement that, correctly applied, maximize the chances of a good outcome. Complete all relevant physical investigations as soon as possible after presentation as it seems that symptomatology will not improve while investigations are ongoing. If anxiety or depression is found, treat it actively, but be prepared to combine such treatment with ones that directly address the pain or fatigue. It is usually counterproductive to enter into the debate about whether the symptoms are 'physical' or 'psychological', 'real' or 'imaginary', as this can lead to conflict and a refusal to accept psychological advice and treatment. Instead, it is better (once investigations have been completed) to honestly admit that the cause of the pain or fatigue is not understood, but the approaches the practitioner recommends may well alleviate it, even if they are also used for purely psychological problems. For chronic fatigue, two therapies, CBT and graded exercise, have been found to be effective, while antidepressant medication seems ineffective on the fatigue or depressive symptoms associated with it; in fact there was less evidence for their effectiveness than there was for food supplementation (magnesium and essential fatty acids), hydrocortisone or alternative therapies (massage, homeopathy, or osteopathy) (Bagnall *et al.* 2002). The findings regarding graded exercise mean that rest cannot be regarded as a treatment for chronic fatigue. There is currently good evidence that either relaxation therapy or CBT are effective for headache, but not other kinds of pain (Eccleston *et al.* 2003). There appears to be no useful drug for the general syndrome of recurrent abdominal pain in children

(Huertas-Ceballos *et al.* 2003), and despite the importance of constipation, diet also seems to have little overall effect (Huertas-Ceballos *et al.* 2002). If the level of impairment warrants it, such cases may benefit from the availability of a specialist worker in primary care (Bower *et al.* 2001), and for the subgroup of children who meet the criteria for irritable bowel syndrome smooth muscle relaxants may be of benefit when pain is the dominant syndrome, though there is less evidence for bulking agents (Jailwala *et al.* 2000). Evidence for other treatments is at best equivocal. Positive attention and restriction of activity can maintain symptomatology, particularly in children with low perceived self-worth and academic competence (Walker *et al.* 2002), so the primary care practitioner has a valuable contribution to make in preventing and addressing these, both directly and through support and advice to the family. Long ago, Dubowitz and Hersov (1976) recommended a programme of increasing mobilization, advice, and encouragement for all these children, while supporting their parents to help them relinquish the sick role, and it is striking how the evidence above supports, in general, this principle.

The child who avoids school

Traditionally, this presentation has been divided into truancy, defined as children who apparently acquiesce to go to school, but then do not go, and school refusal, where children overtly insist that they will not go to school, and may become distressed if they are forced. The former have been considered to be associated with behavioural disorders, while the latter were traditionally associated with emotional disorders. While this is true to some extent, more recent research suggests that many children who do not go to school display both of these behaviours (Elliott 1999).

Presenting signs and symptoms

Possibly the most important difference between school refusal and truancy is how they present to the practitioner. The former is likely to be the reason for presentation, while the latter is more likely to be just one of a long list of behavioural symptoms suggesting a conduct disorder. Children typically refuse school on first starting, when they transfer to secondary school and in the year or so before leaving. It is common to have difficulties at all three points. Unsurprisingly, separation anxiety is the most common psychological difficulty associated with school refusal, though depression—which can also occur, along with conduct disorder, in truancy—is an important alternative or addition during adolescence. Specific 'school phobia', i.e. being irrationally frightened of school is considerably rarer, certainly rarer than being rationally frightened of bullies, poor scholastic performance that may be secondary to unidentified learning disabilities, or punitive teachers. It is important not to overlook the presence of behaviour disorders. The 'distress' a child shows on being required to go to school may well be a temper tantrum, not a panic attack. Bullied children may also be bullies themselves, and this group may be more psychiatrically disabled than simple victims of bullying. Behaviour disorders may also be a marker for the poor family management that is frequently associated with this disorder (Egger *et al.* 2003). Substance abuse—both drug and alcohol—can present with school refusal: both impaired academic performance and hangovers can discourage school attendance.

Treatment

The mainstay of treatment of school refusal is CBT (King *et al.* 2000), though its effectiveness is variable; for example, children with separation anxiety disorder, social avoidance, or poor attendance at treatment sessions do less well, while antidepressants may be a useful adjuvant (Layne 2003). Additional work with families may not add significantly to work with the children (Heyne *et al.* 2002), though of course parents are important as supervisors and supporters of their children in CBT. For truancy, the most effective intervention is still probably the threat of legal action, though this remains controversial, and the Local Education Authority case workers may be reluctant to use it (Waddington 1997; Farrington 2003).

Deliberate self-harm

There are many different types of deliberate self-harm: attempted (or even completed) suicide; overdose of medication or recreational drugs (including alcohol) where death is not the intent; cutting, punching, or injuring oneself either on a single occasion, or more commonly, repeatedly. However, even experts find it difficult to reliably classify individual episodes (Wagner *et al.* 2002) so it is usually better to focus on risk assessment, i.e. the likelihood that the self-harm represents a serious threat to life or health.

Presenting signs and symptoms

Though self-harm is common (about 7% of the population) only 12% of cases come to the attention of hospitals (Hawton *et al.* 2002), so this is very much a primary care issue. The mnemonic 'SAD ADOLESCENT' (Kerr 2001) covers what is important, and is a useful frame for assessment.

- ◆ **S**ex: boys are more likely to have suicidal intent, though more girls attempt self-harm (Hawton *et al.* 2003a).

- ◆ **A**ge: in general, older children are at greater risk, and during the last decade there has been a large age-specific increase in deliberate self-harm has been among 15–24 year olds (Hawton *et al.* 2003b).

- ◆ **D**epression: it is important to realize that, even if any particular episode seems harmless or trivial, depression (as either symptoms or disorder) is a common associated finding, and the more severe the depression, the greater the risk of future self-harm, or even suicide. The assessment of depression is discussed above.

- ◆ **A**vailability of methods: this is a very important determinant of safety. Hanging, for example, has high lethality irrespective of likely intent, which may reflect no more than a transient loss or the impact of alcohol ingestion (Kosky and Dundas 2000). It is not uncommon to find young boys attempting to strangle themselves with their dressing-gown cords or belt, and the risks of this should be taken seriously—knots can be difficult to undo, and belt buckles are designed not to slip open. Fortunately, the drug of choice for overdose (the commonest hospital presentation of deliberate self-harm) has become SSRI antidepressants such as fluoxetine, which are relatively safe, while the use of more dangerous compounds such as paracetamol has declined (Hawton *et al.* 2003b).

◆ **Discordancy at home:** while arguments at home are common precipitants, more chronic family discord, including divorce and separation, is a significant general risk factor for self-harm (Fergusson *et al.* 1984).

◆ **Organization of the attempt:** this may well be the best clue to the significance of suicidal intent. Planning of the attempt over several days or weeks, e.g. by hoarding prescribed tablets; a suicide note that makes practical arrangements regarding belongings, pets, and informing people rather than announcing 'goodbye, cruel world'; taking care to hide the attempt—it is surprising how many overdoses are taken in front of someone; are all ominous. Not disclosing it or making deliberate attempts to disguise it afterwards needs to be interpreted in the light of other suggestions of intent: people who cut to relieve tension, or people who are ashamed of an episode where there was no intent, may also disguise the episode to avoid being shamed.

◆ **Lack of social support:** living in a deprived neighbourhood is a risk factor even after all other sources of risk have been allowed for (Ayton *et al.* 2003), while the termly variation in rates suggest that inability to cope with school-based stress is an important precipitant of many attempts (Hawton *et al.* 2003a).

◆ **Ever having done it before:** as ever, in mental health past performance is indeed a guide to future behaviour.

◆ **Substance abuse:** intoxication with drugs or alcohol is a very common precipitant of self-harm, and an increase in substance abuse (including alcohol abuse) problems among young people, especially boys, presenting with deliberate self-harm has been one of the biggest changes in the last decade (Hawton *et al.* 2003a).

◆ **Cognitions:** suicidal ideation, in particular, is a cognition that is particularly closely associated with deliberate suicide, and needs to be asked for, at its worst as well as currently (Beck *et al.* 1999). Hopelessness is also a risk factor, requiring direct questions to determine.

◆ **Ever known anyone else who has self-harmed:** aside from the obvious examples of family and friends, risk of self-harm also increases when a well-known public personality, either real or fictional, is presented in the media as dying or self-harming (Stack 2003).

◆ **Not agreeing to a no-suicide contract:** no-suicide contracts are discussed below.

◆ **Temper tantrums:** both these and other conduct problems are important additional risk factors in self-harming behaviour (Kennedy et al. 1999; Fergusson et al. 2000).

Treatment

The general decline in completed suicide has been ascribed to the improvements in detection and treatment of depression in primary care (Gould *et al.* 2003) and the detection and treatment of depression, described above, is the mainstay of treatment of deliberate self-harm (Cavanagh *et al.* 2003). In children who are not depressed, family interventions that improve communication have proved to be of value, though these are ineffective in preventing recurrences in children who are depressed (Harrington *et al.* 2000). Group therapy also appears to have value when the deliberate self-harm is repeated (Wood *et al.* 2001).

The 'no-suicide' contract is a useful way of establishing an informal protective network around the child. It is not, however, a complete treatment, and other conditions found in the course of assessment should receive appropriate, prompt treatment. The components are these

1. The child establishes with the practitioner likely triggers for suicidal ideation and intent. Often these involve being alone and unoccupied, particularly after stress. Strategies are jointly developed to help the child avoid these situations. Records may be kept, both as a means of monitoring progress, and as a vehicle for encouraging the child to persist in the strategies, by praising the times when the child succeeds, but do not criticize the child for those occasions the child does not succeed!

2. Working together, the child and practitioner establish a range of alternative actions that the child could take, when experiencing suicidal ideation or intent. Typically, these might include seeking out the child's caretakers, or at school going to spend time with a friend or nominated teacher.

3. The practitioner may educate and negotiate with teachers or caretakers so that the child can discuss suicidal thoughts or feelings without inducing inappropriately fearful, dismissive, or angry responses.

4. The child and caretakers have ready access to the practitioner should any feel that the suicidal thoughts or impulses are not being adequately managed. In these circumstances, the practitioner should seriously consider engaging secondary care services.

Once the contract is made, the next appointment with the practitioner should be quite soon (perhaps a week), to check if it is being adhered to. Concerns should lead to early referral to secondary care.

Conclusions

With only two specific treatments, CBT and SSRI antidepressant drug therapy used separately or in combination, the primary care practitioner is able to intervene with at least some prospect of success in most of the psychosocial problems likely to present in ordinary daily practice. It is probably better to ensure that a member of the primary care team has specific training and a remit to deliver CBT, as there is little evidence that non-specialist primary care workers delivering such treatments improve outcomes (Bower *et al.* 2001). However, this also implies that good primary care practice does itself play an important part in restoring these youngsters to good mental health. With appropriate training, experience, and confidence, there is no good reason to think that either the assessment or treatment of most of these problems cannot be appropriately managed by primary care.

References

Achenbach TM (1992). Developmental psychopathology, In Bornstein MH, Lamb ME (eds), *Developmental Psychology, an Advanced Textbook*. Lawrence Erlbaum Associates, Hillsdale, pp. 629–676.

Achenbach TM (1993). *Empirically Based Taxonomy: How to use syndromes and profile types derived from the CBCL/4–18, TRF, and YSL*. University of Vermont Department of Psychiatry, Burlington, VT.

American Psychiatric Association (1994). *Diagnostic and Statistical Manual of Mental Disorders (IV)*, American Psychiatric Association, Washington.

American Psychiatric Association (1995). *Diagnostic and Statistical Manual of Mental Disorders. 4th ed., primary care*. American Psychiatric Association, Washington, DC.

Angold A, Costello E, Farmer E, Burns B, Erkanli A (1999). Impaired but undiagnosed, *Journal of the American Academy of Child and Adolescent Psychiatry* 38(2): 129–137.

Asarnow J, Jaycox L, Anderson M (2002). Depression among youth in primary care models for delivering mental health services. *Child and Adolescent Psychiatric Clinics of North America* 11(3): 477–497.

Ayton A, Rasool H, Cottrell D (2003). Deliberate self-harm in children and adolescents: association with social deprivation. *European Child and Adolescent Psychiatry* 12(6): 303–307.

Bagnall A, Whiting P, Wright K, Sowden, A (2002). *The Effectiveness of Interventions Used in the Treatment/Management of Chronic Fatigue Syndrome and/or Myalgic Encephalomyelitis in Adults and Children*. NHS Centre for Reviews and Dissemination, University of York, 118.

Barrett J, Williams JW, Oxman T, Frank E, Katon W, Sullivan M, Hegel M, Cornell J, Sengupta A (2001). Treatment of dysthymia and minor depression in primary care: a randomized trial in patients aged 18 to 59 years. *Journal of Family Practice* 50 (5): 405–412.

Barrett P (1998). Evaluation of cognitive-behavioral group treatments for childhood anxiety disorders. *Journal of Clinical Child Psychology* 27: 459–468.

Beck A, Brown G, Steer R, Dahlsgaard K, Grisham J (1999). Suicide ideation at its worst point: a predictor of eventual suicide in psychiatric outpatients. *Suicide and Life-Threatening Behavior* 29: 1–9.

Besedovsky A, Li BU (2004). Across the developmental continuum of irritable bowel syndrome: clinical and pathophysiologic considerations. [Review]. *Current Gastroenterology Reports* 6(3): 247–253.

Birmaher B, Axelson D, Monk K, Kalas C, Clark D, Ehmann M, Bridge J, Heo J, Brent D (2003). Fluoxetine for the treatment of childhood anxiety disorders. *Journal of the American Academy of Child and Adolescent Psychiatry* 42: 415–423.

Bower P, Garralda E, Kramer T, Harrington RBS (2001). The treatment of child and adolescent mental health problems in primary care: a systematic review. *Family Practice* 18: 373–382.

Bushfield-Kahan M (1997). Managing adolescent depression in a primary care setting. [Review]. *Journal of the American Academy of Nurse Practitioners* 9(5): 235–40; quiz 242–4.

Cavanagh J, Carson A, Sharpe M, Lawrie SM (2003). Psychological autopsy studies of suicide: a systematic review. [Review]. *Psychological Medicine* 33 (3): 395–405. [erratum appears in *Psychological Medicine* 2003; 33(5): 947.]

deGruy F, Pincus H (1996). The DSM-IV-PC: a manual for diagnosing mental disorders in the primary care setting. *Journal of the American Board of Family Practitioners* 9: 274–281.

Dowdney L (2000). Childhood bereavement following parental death. [Review]. *Journal of Child Psychology and Psychiatry and Allied Disciplines* 41(7): 819–830.

Dubowitz V, Hersov L (1976). Management of children with non-organic (hysterical) disorders of motor function. *Developmental Medicine and Child Neurology* 25: 67–80.

Dyrborg J, Larsen F, Nielsen S, Byman J, Nielsen B, Gautre-Delay F (2000). The Children's Global Assessment Scale (CGAS) and Global Assessment of Psychosocial Disability (GAPD) in clinical practice—substance and reliability as judged by intraclass correlations. *European Child and Adolescent Psychiatry* 9(3): 195–201.

Eccleston C, Yorke L, Morley S, Williams AC, Mastroyannopoulou K (2003). Psychological therapies for the management of chronic and recurrent pain in children and adolescents. *The Cochrane Database of Systematic Reviews* 14651858.CD003968.

Egger H, Costello E, Angold A (2003). School refusal and psychiatric disorders: a community study. *Journal of the American Academy of Child and Adolescent Psychiatry* 42(7): 797–807.

Elliott JG (1999). School refusal: issues of conceptualisation, assessment, and treatment. [Review]. *Journal of Child Psychology and Psychiatry and Allied Disciplines* 40 (7): 1001–1012.

Farrington DP (2003). British randomized experiments on crime and justice. *Annalls of the American Academy of Political and Social Science* 589: 150–167.

Fergusson DM, Horwood LJ, Shannon FT (1984). Relationship of family life events, maternal depression, and child-rearing problems. *Pediatrics* 73: 773–779.

Fergusson D, Woodward L, Horwood L (2000). Risk factors and life processes associated with the onset of suicidal behaviour during adolescence and early adulthood. *Psychological Medicine* 30: 23–39.

Goldberg I, Gabriel H (1996). Recurrent nonorganic abdominal pain: current concepts. In Lewis, M (ed.). *Child and Adolescent Psychiatry: A Comprehensive Textbook*, Williams and Williams, Baltimore, pp. 1054–1058.

Goodman R, Scott S (1997). *Child Psychiatry*. Blackwell, Oxford, p. 8.

Goodman R, Ford T, Simmons H, Gatward R, Meltzer H (2000). Using the Strengths and Difficulties Questionnaire (SDQ) to screen for child psychiatric disorders in a community sample. *British Journal of Psychiatry* 177: 534–539.

Gould M, Greenberg T, Velting D, Shaffer D (2003). Youth suicide risk and preventive interventions: a review of the past 10 years. [Review]. *Journal of the American Academy of Child and Adolescent Psychiatry* 42(4): 386–405.

Harrington R (2001). Depression, suicide and deliberate self-harm in adolescence. [Review]. *British Medical Bulletin* 57: 47–60.

Harrington R, Kerfoot M, Dyer E, Mcniven F, Gill J, Harrington V, Woodham A (2000). Deliberate self-poisoning in adolescence: why does a brief family intervention work in some cases and not others? *Journal of Adolescence* 23: 13–20.

Hawton K, Rodham K, Evans E, Weatherall R (2002). Deliberate self harm in adolescents: self report survey in schools in England. *British Medical Journal* 325 (7374): 1207–1211.

Hawton K, Hall S, Simkin S, Bale L, Bond A, Codd S, Stewart A (2003a). Deliberate self-harm in adolescents: a study of characteristics and trends in Oxford, 1990–2000. *Journal of Child Psychology and Psychiatry and Allied Disciplines* 44(8): 1191–1198.

Hawton K, Harriss L, Hall S, Simkin S, Bale E, Bond A (2003b). Deliberate self-harm in Oxford, 1990–2000: a time of change in patient characteristics. *Psychological Medicine* 33(6): 987–995.

Hering-Hanit R, Gadoth N (2003). Caffeine-induced headache in children and adolescents. *Cephalalgia* 23(5): 332–335.

Heyne D, King N, Tonge B, Rollings S, Young D, Pritchard M, Ollendick T (2002). Evaluation of child therapy and caregiver training in the treatment of school refusal. *Journal of the American Academy of Child and Adolescent Psychiatry* 41(6): 687–695.

Huertas-Ceballos A, Macarthur C, Logan S (2002). Dietary interventions for recurrent abdominal pain (RAP) in childhood. *The Cochrane Database of Systematic Reviews* 14651858.CD003019.

Huertas-Ceballos A, Macarthur C, Logan S (2003). Pharmacological interventions for recurrent abdominal pain (RAP) in childhood. *The Cochrane Database of Systematic Reviews* 14651858.CD003017.

Hyams JS (2004). Irritable bowel syndrome, functional dyspepsia, and functional abdominal pain syndrome. [Review]. *Adolescent Medicine Clinics* 15: 1–15.

Jailwala J, Imperiale T, Kroenke K (2000). Pharmacologic treatment of the irritable bowel syndrome: a systematic review of randomized controlled trials. *Annals of Internal Medicine* 133: 136.

Kennedy HG, Iveson R, Hill O (1999). Violence, homicide and suicide: strong correlation and wide variation across districts. *British Journal of Psychiatry* **175**: 462–466.

Kerr M (2001). High school consultation. *Child and Adolescent Psychiatric Clinics of North America* **10**: 105–115.

King N, Tonge B, Heyne D, Ollendick TH (2000). Research on the cognitive-behavioral treatment of school refusal: a review and recommendations. [Review]. *Clinical Psychology Review* **20**(4): 495–507.

Kohli R, Li BU (2004). Differential diagnosis of recurrent abdominal pain: new considerations. [Review]. *Pediatric Annals* **33**(2): 113–122.

Kosky R, Dundas P (2000). Death by hanging: implications for prevention of an important method of youth suicide. *Australian and New Zealand Journal of Psychiatry* **34**(5): 836–841.

Layne AE, Bernstein GA, Egan EA, Kushner MG (2003). Predictors of treatment response in anxious-depressed adolescents with school refusal. *Journal of the American Academy of child and Adolescent Psychiarty*, **42**(3): 319–326.

Lewis D, Ashwal S, Dahl G, Dorbad D, Hirtz D, Prensky A, Jarjour, I (2002). Practice parameter: evaluation of children and adolescents with recurrent headaches: report of the Quality Standards Subcommittee of the American Academy of Neurology and the Practice Committee of the Child Neurology Society. *Neurology* **59**(4): 490–498.

Lilienfeld SO (2003). Comorbidity between and within childhood externalizing and internalizing disorders: reflections and directions. [Review]. *Journal of Abnormal Child Psychology* **31**(3): 285–291.

Masi G, Mucci M, Millepiedi S (2001). Separation anxiety disorder in children and adolescents: epidemiology, diagnosis and management. [Review]. *CNS Drugs* **15**(2): 93–104.

Mayou R (2000). Somatoform disorders and medically unexplained syndromes. In Gelder M, Lopez-Ibor J. et al (eds), *New Oxford Textbook of Psychiatry*, Oxford: Oxford University Press pp. 1074–1076.

Oxman T, Barrett J, Sengupta A, Katon W, Williams JW, Frank E, Hegel M (2001). Status of minor depression or dysthymia in primary care following a randomized controlled treatment. *General Hospital Psychiatry* **23**(6): 301–310.

Ozge A, Bugdayci R, Sasmaz T, Kaleagasi H, Kurt O, Karakelle A, Tezcan H, Siva A (2002). The sensitivity and specificity of the case definition criteria in diagnosis of headache: a school-based epidemiological study of 5562 children in Mersin. *Cephalalgia* **22**(10): 791–798.

Rutter M, Tizard J, Whitmore K (eds) (1970). *Education, Health and Behaviour*. London: Longman.

Sharpe M, Wessely S (2000). Chronic fatigue syndrome. In Gelder M, Lopez-Ibor J. et al (ed.), *New Oxford Textbook of Psychiatry*, Oxford: Oxford University Press pp. 1112–1121.

Shortt A, Barrett PM, Fox TC (2001). Evaluating the FRIENDS program: a cognitive-behavioral group treatment for anxious children and their parents. *Journal of Clinical Child Psychology* **30**: 525–535.

Stack S (2003). Media coverage as a risk factor in suicide. [Review]. *Journal of Epidemiology and Community Health* **57**(4): 238–240.

Taylor D (1982). The components of sickness: diseases, illnesses and predicatments. In Apley J, Ounstead C (eds), *Clinics in Developmental Medicine* **80**: 1–13.

The Washington Institute and Washington State Mental Health Division (2004). *CGAS SCALE* http://depts.washington.edu/wimirt/CGAS%20Scale.htm

Trevarthen C, Aitken K, Papoudi D, Robarts J (1996). *Children with Autism: Diagnosis and Inteventions to Meet their Needs*. Jessica Kingsley, London.

Waddington C (1997). The use of legal proceedings in cases of non-attendance at school: perceptions of Education Welfare Officers. *Education Research* **39**(3): 333–341.

Wagner B, Wong S, Jobes DA (2002). Mental health professionals' determinations of adolescent suicide attempts. *Suicide and Life-Threatening Behavior* **32**(3): 284–300.

Walker L, Claar R, Garber J (2002). Social consequences of children's pain: when do they encourage symptom maintenance? *Journal of Pediatric Psychology* **27**(8): 689–698.

Whittington C, Kendall T, Fonagy P, Cottrell D, Cotgrove A, Boddington E (2004). Selective serotonin reuptake inhibitors in childhood depression: systematic review of published versus unpublished data. *Lancet* **363** (9418): 1341–1345.

WHO Collaborating Centre for Research and Training in Mental Health (2004). *NeLMH: Child and adolescent disorders http://www.nelmh.org/sub_topic_list.asp?c=16andfc=011andfid=1168*

Williams R, Richardson G (eds). (1995). *Together We Stand. the Commissioning, Role and Management of Child and Adolescent Mental Health Services.* The NHS Health Advisory Service, HMSO, London.

Wood A, Trainor G, Rothwell J, Moore A, Harrington R (2001). Randomized trial of group therapy for repeated deliberate self-harm in adolescents. *Journal of the American Academy of Child and Adolescent Psychiatry* **40** (11): 1246–1253.

World Health Organization (1976). *Document A29/INFDOCI/1.* World Health Organization, Geneva.

World Health Organization (1992). *The ICD-10 Classification of Mental and Behavioral Disorders.* World Health Organization, Geneva.

World Health Organization (1996). *Diagnostic and Management Guidelines for Mental Disorders in Primary Care.* Hogrefe and Huber, Geneva.

Zwart J, Dyb G, Stovner L, Sand T, Holmen TL (2003). The validity of 'recognition-based' headache diagnoses in adolescents. Data from the Nord-Trondelag Health Study 1995–97, Head-HUNT-Youth. *Cephalalgia* **23**(3): 223–229.

Chapter 35

Multicultural paediatrics

Abdul Rashid Gatrad and Aziz Sheikh

They come to the clinic not only with the burden of their illness but also with the cultural fabric of their lives

Brown and Segal (1996)

Introduction

The 2001 census revealed that 4.6 million of the UK population class themselves as belonging to a minority ethnic group (Table 35.1). This census, for the first time, also included a question on religious affiliation, revealing that approximately three million people belong to a minority religious group (Figure 35.1). Ethnicity and religion are two key factors that shape cultural identity. Understanding the potential impact of these cultural markers on access to and provision of healthcare is important if we are to make progress in reducing the major health inequalities experienced by black and minority groups in Britain (Acheson Report 1998). Crucial to redressing these inequities is the need to improve the health outcomes of children—for health in the very earliest stages of life represents a key determinant of health status in future life (Barker 1994). In this chapter, we focus on providing the understanding needed to work with minority families and suggest practical approaches that may improve access and quality of primary health-care services for black and minority ethnic children. Although focusing on Britain, many of the issues discussed are in principal likely to be of considerable relevance to many other western European countries.

Migration and demography

Although ethnic minority groups comprise just under 8% of the general population, approximately 1 in 10 children in Britain can now be classed as belonging to a black and minority ethnic group. This discrepancy in figures is explained by two factors: the relatively younger age profile of migrant communities when compared with the indigenous population (Table 35.2) and higher fertility ratios.

It was mainly working class men that migrated from the New Commonwealth (the Indian subcontinent and the Caribbean) in the wake of rapid industrialization in Britain after the Second World War, only calling their young families over once they had realized a semblance of security. Migration from Bangladesh has been a more recent phenomenon—taking place mainly during the 1980–1990s. This too was a migration primarily for economic reasons. Such migration has now all but ceased and the most recent waves of

Table 35.1 The UK population: by ethnic group, Census 2001

	Total population		Minority ethnic population
	Count	%	%
White	54153898	92.1	n/a
Mixed	677117	1.2	14.6
Asian or Asian British			
Indian	1053411	1.8	22.7
Pakistani	747285	1.3	16.1
Bangladeshi	283063	0.5	6.1
Other Asian	247664	0.4	5.3
Black or Black British			
Black Caribbean	565876	1.0	12.2
Black African	485277	0.8	10.5
Black Other	97585	0.2	2.1
Chinese	247403	0.4	5.3
Other	230615	0.4	5.0
All minority ethnic population	4635296	7.9	100
All population	58789194	100	n/a

migration—from the Balkans, North and Central Africa, and Afghanistan—have been in the main for political reasons.

Although the majority of minority ethnic groups continue to reside in inner-city areas (London, Birmingham, Leicester, and Manchester, for example), these communities are gradually becoming increasingly geographically dispersed emphasising the importance of all health professionals having a basic appreciation of the interaction between ethnicity and health.

While retaining an inclusivist perspective, we focus in this chapter on the care of children of South Asian origin as this is the dominant broad ethnic grouping (representing over 50% of minority ethnic population) in the UK at the present time (National Census 2003).

Concept of culture and health beliefs

Culture is defined as a set of beliefs, values, and behavioural norms with institutions and customs derived from them. Anthropologists and sociologists have over the years demonstrated the many ways in which one's culture shapes outlook towards disease, health, and healing. This is particularly so with religion-based cultures where practices

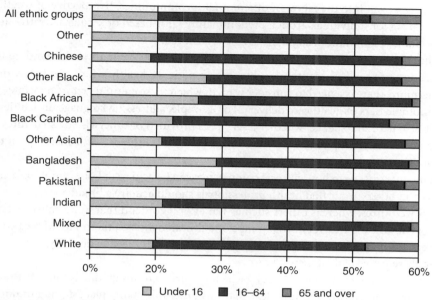

Fig. 35.1 The UK population: by ethnic group, Census 2001.

Table 35.2 Religion in Britain

	Thousands	**%**
Christian	42076	71.6
Buddhist	152	0.3
Hindu	559	1.0
Jewish	267	0.5
Muslim	1591	2.7
Sikh	336	0.6
Other religion	179	0.3
All religions	45163	76.8
No religion	9104	15.5
Not stated	4289	7.3
All no religion/not stated	13626	23.2
Base	58789	100

stem from a shared set of beliefs that are nurtured over generations and are therefore intricately woven into the fabric of different faith communities. Irrespective of whether one is caring for individuals from a predominantly faith-based or secular narrative, it is important that a minimum standard of care is achieved.

Cultural competence, according to Betancourt *et al.* (2003) entails understanding the importance of social and cultural influences on patients' health beliefs and behaviour. Furthermore, there is a need to consider ways in which these cultural factors may interact with multiple tiers of healthcare delivery. For example, addressing language difficulties is clearly a structural issue, i.e. whether a service is provided or otherwise by structures in place; access to high-quality care is a clinical issue and influence of leadership on the workforce is an organizational issue.

Arguments exist as to how cultural competency can be achieved. For example, Qureshi (1994) and others argue that health professionals should acquire a broad appreciation of minority cultures, whereas others such as Kai (1999) contend that in pluralist Britain, which is now home to a very broad range of cultural identities, there should be a commitment to equip practitioners with the attitudes and skills to value diversity and deliver culturally sensitive patient-centred care.

Acculturation refers to the process by which minority groups gradually take on aspects of the dominant culture and it is clear that this process is taking place among minority communities in Britain. This process may have advantages and disadvantages—the former include removal of language and other barriers to accessing healthcare, whereas the latter includes the erosion of traditional family and social values, such as increasing numbers of broken marriages and teenage pregnancies. A more subtle manifestation of acculturation is the breaking down of extended family bonds, which hitherto may have provided a young parent with help, advice, and support in times of need. For example a young mum who may conveniently have obtained 'in house' advice on breast-feeding techniques from her mother-in-law is likely in future to turn to the services of a health visitor. Thus the sense of friendly communities connected socially is rapidly disappearing in the face of an onslaught of social upheaval resulting from more and more nuclear families.

Perception of disease

There is now an increasing body of evidence that demonstrates cultural variations in health beliefs, values, treatment preferences, and health seeking behaviour (Coleman-Miller 2000; Gornick 2000; Willimas and Rucker 2000). These include variations in patient recognition of symptoms, threshold for seeking advice and the ability effectively to communicate experienced symptoms. Expectations of care (including preference for or against diagnostic and therapeutic interventions) and concordance with prescribed treatments are further issues to consider in understanding perception of disease by the minorities (Einbinder and Schulman 2000).

Over the years, many a government has paid lip service to the plight of minority community health needs and as a consequence many families have become dissatisfied with the health service and look elsewhere, such as to a *Hakims* (traditional herbalists), for care.

For example, research suggests that up to a third of Afro-Caribbean patients with diabetes use herbal medications (Mathias and While 2003). Increasingly, in the more affluent subsections of minority communities, private opinions from herbalists are being sought in the countries of origin.

A parent's religious beliefs may influence understanding of the nature of illness, and in turn impact on concordance with prescribed treatments (Nadar *et al.* 2003). For example, disorders such as epilepsy are sometimes believed to result from 'evil forces'. While it is important to explore health beliefs in all patients, this issue assumes even greater importance when dealing with children from ethnic and religious groups with which one is relatively unfamiliar.

Concept of time and impact on scheduled appointments

It is sometimes said that 'We in the West are ruled by the clock'. As travellers to South Asian countries will know, this is certainly not the case among these communities. It is therefore perhaps unsurprising that many first-generation migrant South Asian parents fail to appreciate the importance of punctuality when attending for scheduled appointments. Furthermore, parents whose children have recovered may fail to understand the importance of follow-up and either cancel or fail to attend; needless to say that the model of care that many poorer families are accustomed to in the third world is private and hence care is only sought when absolutely necessary. Gatrad (2000) has, however, shown that it is possible to work with communities to improve attendance rates. A special multi-cultural calendar (available from SHAP working party c/o NSREC, 36 Causton Street London SW1 4AU) costing under £5 can be purchased for clinic use and should help reception staff to quickly and easily avoid key religious festivals when booking appointments.

Communication

Difficulty in communication remains an important barrier to accessing health services particularly among recent female migrants who may otherwise live rather sheltered lives. With increasing availability of interpreters, link workers, and advocates the picture is beginning to improve although in practice many clinicians are still forced to revert to the dubious practice of using children as interpreters. Potential disadvantages of using friends and relatives as interpreters has recently been highlighted by Phelan and Parkman (1995).

Interpreters need to be appropriately trained with periodic evaluation of the quality of service they provide. However, even when available, there is evidence that they are under-used by health professionals—this in part being explained by budgetary constraints and time pressures (Levinson and Gillam 1998).

Link workers facilitate in-depth communication between patients and healthcare professionals, enhancing understanding in relation to health needs, taking into account their cultural and social environment. They were introduced in 1982 during the Mother and Baby Campaign. Evidence suggests that they have made a positive impact on delivery of care to minority ethnic women receiving maternity care, e.g. this campaign highlighted that longer maternity gowns would improve attendance for antenatal examinations (Rocheran and Dickinson 1990). Furthermore, data suggest that this service resulted in an increase in the mean birthweights of Pakistani babies (Dance 1987). More serious communication problems may arise when trying to deliver obstetric and gynaecological care, as most South Asian cultures have comprehensive codes on modesty—this explains why a large majority of women still prefer to be seen by same-sex clinicians.

Patient advocates represent patient interests to health professionals. Their service should be patient led, independent of health service providers, and accountable only to the users of this facility.

When any of these services are provided, provision for extra time for consultation should be made. Baylav and Fuller (2003) have recently reviewed the subtle differences between these three services.

Marriage, contraception, and procreation

Marriage and procreation are strongly encouraged within the indigenous cultures of many migrants (Dhami and Sheikh 2000). The fertility ratio of such families is on aver-age higher than for Caucasian families; acculturation is, however, taking place with evi-dence suggesting that there is now a trend towards diminishing family size, and in turn more nuclear families, in most ethnic communities (Modood *et al.* 1997).

Among Sikhs and Hindus there is no religious prohibition against contraception. However, traditionally, among South Asians, it is important for families to bear sons who will continue the family name and also initiate the cremation pyre (Hindus and Sikhs). Sons are also preferred for keeping inheritance within the immediate family.

Some Muslims consider contraception to be unethical because the practice is consid-ered to interfere with God's overall plan in which offspring are regarded as a divine gift. Barrier methods are in general more acceptable than the combined oral contraceptive pill (Schott and Henley 1996), which is believed by some women to 'interfere with nature' and also adversely affect fertility (Gatrad 1994).

There is an increased incidence of perinatal and neonatal deaths among ethnic minori-ties. The reasons are multifactorial, poorly understood and partly as a result of problems of accessibility and acceptability of services. However, consanguinity in Muslim commu-nities, particularly Pakistani, Arabs, and Turks (Gatrad and Sheikh 2003) contributes not insignificantly to illness and deaths in this group (Bundey and Alam 1993). The Hindu and Sikh religions do not allow consanguineous marriages, although this prohibition does not extend to the Christian and Jewish religious traditions.

With the introduction of national screening for haemoglobinopathies in 2004 it remains to be seen what impact this will have on the incidence of thalassaemia and sickle cell disease among ethnic communities.

Termination of pregnancy

In our experience, Hindus and Sikhs have a more liberal attitude to abortions for fetal abnormalities than many Muslim women. Muslims will in general consent if the mother's life is deemed to be in imminent danger (a rather unusual scenario) or if the baby dies *in utero*. Some Muslims may, however, be more likely to agree to termination for fetal abnormality before the ensoulment period of 120 days gestation. Among Hindus and Sikhs although individual attitudes vary, termination for social reasons is generally disapproved.

Naming conventions

Most babies are not named immediately after birth and some consider the choosing of a name antenatally a bad omen. Relatives, such as the sister of the baby's father, chooses a name although this practice is now changing, with the name often being agreed through consensus.

Those with South Asian backgrounds can usually deduce which religion a child has been born into simply from the name. Muslim names usually have a meaning, which it is hoped the child will aspire to. For example, Abdullah means the 'bondsman of God', whereas the female name Sakina means 'tranquil' or 'peaceful'. A religious title such as Abdul or Muhammad may precede the actual name. This, and other Muslim naming customs are discussed in detail elsewhere (Gatrad and Sheikh 2000).

A Hindu baby is often named after the sixth day—a day when Hindus believe that a child's fate is traditionally charted by the goddess of learning (Schott and Henley 1996). The choice of name depends on the cycle of the moon. The exact time of birth is important to work out the horoscope from a special book, which will give the first letter of the name. For example, if the relevant section states that the name should start with a 'G', then for a girl, Gita may be chosen. Inclusion of 'ben' after a name is customary, e.g. Gitaben. Kumari, Gouri, and Devi are also used as middle names for girls just as Kumar, Lal, and Dev are often used for boys.

Sikhs use the title Kaur (Princess) for girls and Singh (Lion) for boys. These names are often followed by the family surname, for example Dhinsa or Khera. The naming system is again based on religion. The Holy book for Sikhs called 'Guru Granth Sahib' is opened randomly and the name chosen from the opened page. There is, however, now among many Sikhs and Hindus an increasing tendency to use Western Christian names such as Tony or Simone.

From the above, it is obvious that care should be taken to accurately record names that are reproducible, as the system for all the three cultures does not necessarily follow that used in the West.

Other common customs

Birth customs vary a great deal within each religious group. We here discuss briefly some of those that that we commonly encounter.

Muslims babies after birth have religious words whispered into their ears (Adhan) and a soft piece of date (or honey if dates are unavailable) is rubbed against the soft palate. It is only Muslim and Jewish males that are routinely circumcized—this typically taking place within the first month of life. It is important to be aware that circumcision should be delayed in the event of prolonged jaundice or hypospadias as there is an increased risk of bleeding in the former group and the foreskin is used for surgical repair in the latter.

All Muslim babies have their scalp hair shaved on or around the seventh day of life (Gatrad and Sheikh 2001). Another common custom is the tying of a black string called a 'Tawiz', which may be applied around the wrist or neck. This should be treated with respect as it has a religious significance.

Hindu babies may have a white frail cotton string tied around ankles or wrists, on the sixth day. This often falls off soon after. In some communities, the family writes 'OM'—a mystical word representing the 'ultimate spirit'—on the tongue of the fledgling infant with honey or ghee (purified butter). Such a ceremony is carried out by an elder (akin to a godparent). Some parents may leave a pen and a blank piece of paper in the cot, as Hindus believe that on the sixth day after birth a child's future is charted.

A bangle called 'Kara' is an important symbol for Sikhs and is often applied to the wrists. Their babies are blessed on the 13th day of life with Amrit (holy water), during a religious ceremony. They are, however, named in their place of worship (Gurthwara) on the 40th day after birth—hence the delay in giving the baby a name. A nickname such as 'shorty' may be given in the mean time.

Most South Asian menstruating or postpartum women are considered 'unclean' and therefore may not undertake household chores such as cooking. Traditionally most mothers return to *their* parents for recuperation—this is, however, often not practical in Western countries. Some mothers may not venture out with or without their babies as is the tradition, and may therefore miss their 6-week check.

Food

Young mothers are often fed high calorie foods rich in ghee as it is often believed that this helps breast-milk production and flow. In all South Asian cultures there is also a belief in 'hot' and 'cold foods'. This has nothing to do with the actual temperature of food or how spicy it is but rather reflects the impact of the food on the personality and internal balance. Hot foods are thought to predispose to rashes, sweating, and fatigue. Cold foods have a calming effect on the body. Examples of hot foods include lentils, carrots, aubergines, grapes, brown sugar, and eggs. Cold foods include cereals, vegetables, potato, milk, yoghurt, and fruits. This becomes relevant, for example, during bleeding of pregnancy when a patient may avoid 'hot' foods, which may be thought by health professionals to be good for mother and baby.

Regional and national data show that breast-feeding is more common among South Asian mothers than whites. It is likely that with acculturation the incidence of traditional practices such as this will decline. Prolonged breast-feeding, as occurs in the Bangladeshi community can predispose children to iron deficiency anaemia—a condition that is also common in Hindus and Rastafarians. The Qur'an extols the virtue of breast feeding for a maximum of 2 years, although in practice few Muslim women will breast-feed for this length of time.

Pork and alcohol are absolutely forbidden for Muslims who only eat halal meat (special religious words are said when the animal is slaughtered). For Hindus, the cow is a sacred animal and therefore beef is forbidden. Hindus who are Gujarati are more likely to be vegetarian and indeed may bring up their children as such. Sikhs—particularly women— also tend to avoid eating beef and pork. The relevance of this is that parents may question the ingredients in medications or indeed not administer them, for example a Hindu vegetarian parent may avoid antibiotic capsules for their children in the belief that these contain animal products.

Ghee, a purified form of butter has very high cholesterol content. Pakistanis and Sikh Punjabis have a high consumption of this very fatty food. It is therefore important that health professionals opportunistically discourage its use in the early stage of a child's life, as there is a much higher incidence of coronary artery disease (Bhopal 2002) and diabetes in South Asian families (Simmons *et al.* 1991).

Smoking among South Asian men (particularly Pakistanis and Bengalis) is very high but is still thankfully relatively uncommon among females. Therefore presently smoking is an unlikely cause of a 'small for dates' baby.

Differential growth in children

Afro-Caribbean children tend to be taller than white children. Among South Asians, Gatrad has shown that Sikh children are the heaviest and the tallest of the Asians at birth, and at the age of 5 years are the heaviest and the tallest of all children, including whites (Gatrad *et al.* 1994). The Hindu and Bangladeshi babies are the smallest at birth but the latter have a much better growth during the first 5 years. The Gujarati Muslim and Gujarati Hindu babies have a similar growth pattern. Theses factors need considering when using growth charts.

Injuries to children

According to the Department of Environment, Transport and the Regions, South Asians are twice as prone to pedestrian accidents than the rest in the UK, This can largely be explained by socio-economic disadvantage and the high concentration of these communities residing in urban areas.

Non-accidental injuries are perceived to be less common among South Asians, this being particularly so with sexual abuse (Moghal *et al.* 1995). Be that as it may, data also suggests that health professionals are less likely to intervene in suspected abuse involving South Asian children. This we believe is as a result of professional insecurity that can partly be redressed by structured training programmes. The unwary may misdiagnose a blue discoloration of various sizes and shapes that not uncommonly occurs on the back and buttock area of Asians as a bruise, when in fact it is a birth mark called the Mongolian blue spot.

Travel

Asian families travel frequently to the Indian subcontinent. Many doctors are, however, still not sufficiently vigilant about imported diseases such as typhoid or malaria. Any temperature, diarrhoea, jaundice, or vomiting should raise suspicion of an imported disease in a returning traveller. Muslims travel for Hajj, which has its own health implications, particularly that of the increased incidence of meningococcaemia. Doctors in primary care should ensure that vaccination is undertaken with fully informed parental consent (Gatrad and Sheikh 2003).

Not infrequently parents take their children to the Indian subcontinent when a 'cure' cannot be found in Western countries. Such condition includes cerebral palsy, epilepsy, nephrotic syndrome, and vitilligo. It is not unusual for the Western treatment prescribed to be stopped with occasionally devastating effects; for example, a special diet for a metabolic disease. Heavy metals may be used in some of the herbal treatments from 'Hakims'.

Religious festivals

Important religious festival for Muslims are Ramadan and the two Eids. One Eid celebrates the end of the fasting season and the other the end of pilgrimage. Children over the age of 10 often fast from dawn to dusk, which could be many hours if the month happens to fall during the summer. (Muslims follow the lunar calendar and therefore the fasting month is brought forward by 10 days each year.) Apart from symptoms of a headache and weakness most children are fine. Problems arise with medications. Therefore, if possible, medications should be chosen in a way that ensures that their administration coincides with the times the patient is allowed to eat.

In spite of religious exemption for pregnant mothers from fasting, many still do during the first trimester. Mothers often report that their babies are more active at night than in the day. Interestingly, fasting during Ramadan has been shown not to affect the mean birthweight of babies at any stage of pregnancy. However, there was a non-significant increase in the prevalence of low birthweight among babies born at term when Ramadan had occurred in the second trimester (Cross and Eminson 1990).

Hindus celebrate three important festivals. Diwali (Hindu New Year eve) in October/November, Navratri, a festival of nine nights (September/October), and Holi in February/March. Although Hindus fast, most of their fasts are abstention from cooked food. Foods that are considered pure such as fruits will be eaten as the only meal in the day. These 'days' may be observed by some on certain days of the week or month but not for a period as long as Muslims.

Sikhs have two main festivals. They celebrate Diwali, like the Hindus and also have Baishki, a Spring festival in April. South Asian parents may request an early discharge for their children from the wards to celebrate these occasions or may cancel their appointments or fail to turn up.

End of life issues

Muslims are always buried. Hindu and Sikh children are buried, but the adults cremated. Muslim jurists, generally speaking, discourage post-mortems unless the law of the country demands this. Although Hindus and Sikhs do not have such a strong view, this subject needs to be approached sensitively in view of the belief in Karma. The philosophy behind this is that a person is born and reborn until perfection is achieved. With this belief in

Divine reincarnation families will undoubtedly be anxious about the return of all organs before disposal.

Burials and cremations are arranged soon after death in the Indian subcontinent in view of the high temperatures. Furthermore, culturally many hundreds of relatives come to respect the dead. Therefore it is prudent to arrange for a death certificate promptly as these visitors often stay at the 'bereaved home' till the disposal of the body.

Future strategies

It is generally accepted that black and minority patients face organizational, structural, and clinical barriers, as described by Betancourt *et al.* (2003), that preclude them from fully benefiting from the advances in health promotion and disease prevention that the host community enjoy.

When religion and culture impact on health beliefs, this inevitably creates the greatest difficulty for the health professionals particularly during pregnancy, delivery, the new-born period and 'end of life'. Our experiences suggest that nurses are more willing than doctors to engage in learning about other cultures (Gatrad 1997). But the picture is not all negative and we have shown, through work with the Acorns Children's Hospice in Birmingham that when cultural diversity is accepted and the staff adequately trained this service is widely used by all members of minority ethnic groups (Gatrad and Sheikh 2002).

More effort should be made to positively engage with minority communities in programmes for delivering health. For example, we have successfully set up a blood donor centre to encourage Asians and Afro-Caribbean's to attend. We ensure that such days do not coincide with religious days such as the fasting month or days when different groups attend their places of worship (Sheikh and Gatrad 2003). For more global change it is, however, important that those in senior management, including medical consultants, appreciate the importance of understanding diverse cultures so that those whom they lead will follow and the health of the nation will in turn improve.

In addition the Department of Health needs to work proactively with different groups in promoting health awareness and disease prevention. Such a partnership has been successful in, for example the decrease in the use of Surma (contains lead) as an eye cosmetic, the better healthcare of Muslim pilgrims returning from Hajj (Saudi Arabia) (Gatrad *et al.* 2002), and the decreased incidence of rickets after the Mother and Baby Campaign in the 1980s.

References

Acheson Report (1998). *Independent Enquiry Into Inequalities in Health. Report of the Scientific Advisory Group*. The Stationary Office, London.

Barker D (1994). *Mother Babies and Disease in Later Life. British Medical Journal* Books, London.

Baylav A, Fuller J (2003). Working with link workers and advocates. In Kai J (ed.), *Ethnicity Health and Primary Care*. Oxford: Oxford University Press pp. 75–82.

Betancourt JR, Green AR, Carillo JE, Ananeh-Firempong O (2003). *Defining Cultural Competence: a Practical Framework for Addressing Racial/Ethnic Disparities in Health and Health Care. Public Health Response*. Oxford: Oxford University Press. July–August, Vol. 118, pp. 293–301.

Bhopal R (2002). Epidemic of cardio-vascular disease in South Asians. *British Medical Journal* **324**: 625–626.

Brown CM, Segal R (1996). Ethnic differences in temporal orientation and its implications for hypertension management. *Journal of Health and Social Behaviour* **37**(4): 350–361.

Bundey S, Alam H (1993). A five year prospective study of health of children in different ethnic groups with particular reference to the effect of inbreeding. *European Journal of Human Genetics* **1**: 206–219.

Coleman-Miller B (2000). A physician's perspective on minority health care. *Finance Review* 21–45.

Cross JH, Eminson J, Wharton BA (1990). Ramadan and birthweight at full term in Asian Muslim pregnant women in Birmingham. *Archives of Disease in Childhood* **65**: 1053–1056.

Dance J (1987). *A Social Intervention by Link Workers to Pakistani Women and Pregnancy Outcome.* East Birmingham Health Authority.

Dhami S, Sheikh A (2000). The Muslim family: predicament and promise. *Western Journal of Medicine* **173**: 352–356.

Einbinder LC, Schulman KA (2000). The effects of race on the referral process for invasive cardiac procedures. *Medical Care Research and Review* **1**: 162–177.

Gatrad AR (1994). *Muslims in hospital, school and the community.* PhD thesis Wolverhampton University, p. 70.

Gatrad AR (1997). Cultural awareness audit amongst midwives. *Paediatrics Today* **5**: 82–83.

Gatrad AR (2000). A completed audit to reduce hospital outpatient non-attendance rates. *Archives of Disease in Childhood* **82**: 59–61.

Gatrad AR, Sheikh A (eds) (2000). Birth customs: meaning and significance. In *Caring for Muslim Patients*. Radcliffe Medical, Oxford, pp. 57–71.

Gatrad AR, Sheikh A (2001). Muslim birth customs. *Archives of Disease in Childhood* **84**: F6–F8.

Gatrad AR, Sheikh A (2002). Palliative care for Muslims and issues after death. *International Journal of Palliative Nursing* **8**(12): 594–597.

Gatrad AR, Sheikh A (2003). Understanding Muslim customs: A practical guide for health professionals. In David T (ed.) *Recent Advances in Paediatrics*. Royal Society of Medicine, London, pp. 151–166.

Gatrad AR, Birch N, Hughes M (1994). Preschool weights of Europeans and five subgroups of Asians in Britain, *Archives of Disease in Childhood* **71**: 207–210.

Gatrad AR, Sheikh A, Khan AR (2002). Reducing health risks to British Muslim pilgrims. *British Medical Journal* **324**: 301.

Gornick ME (2000). Disparities in medicare services: potential causes, plausible explanations and recommendations. *Health Care Financing Review* **21**: 23–43.

Kai J (1999). *Valuing Diversity*. RCGP, London.

Levinson R, Gillam S (1998). *Link Workers in Primary Care*. King's Fund, London.

Mathias M, While A (2003). *Diabetes and ethnicity*. A collaborative project between Lambeth Health care trust, Kings college and general practitioners.

Modood T, Berthould R, Lakey J, Nazroo J, Smith P, Virdee S, Beishon S (1997). *Ethnic Minorities in Britain: Diversity and Disadvantage*. Policy Studies Institute, London.

Moghal NE, Nota IK, Hobbs CJ (1995). A study of sexual abuse in an Asian community. *Archives of Disease in Childhood* **72**: 346–347.

Nadar S, Begum N, Kaur B, Sandhu S, Lip GYH (2003). Patient's understanding of anticoagulant therapy in a multi ethnic population. *Journal of the Royal Society of Medicine* **96**: 175–179.

National Census. Available from: http: //www.statistics.gov.uk/default.asp (accessed September 2003).

Phelan M, Parkman S (1995). How to do it: Work with an interpreter. *British Medical Journal* **311**: 555–557.

Qureshi B (1994). *Transcultural Medicine*. Kulwer, London, pp. 214–215.

Rocheran Y, Dickinson R (1990). The Asian mother and baby campaign. *Health Education Journal* **49**: 128–133.

Schott J, Henley A (1996). *Culture Religion and Child Bearing in a Multi-cultural Society.* Butterworth-Heinemann, Boston pp. 312–324.

Schott J, Henley A (1996). *Culture Religion and Child Bearing in a Multi-cultural Society.* Butterworth-Heinemann, pp. 304–311.

Sheikh A, Gatrad AR (2003). Promoting blood donation among British Muslims. *British Medical Journal* **326**: 1152.

Simmons D, Williams DRR, Powell MJ (1991). The Coventry diabetes study. Prevalence of diabetes and impaired glucose tolerance in Europids and Asians. *Quarterly Journal of Medicine* **81**: 1021–1030.

Williams DR, Rucker TD. Understanding and addressing racial disparities in health care. *Health Care Financing Review* **21**: 75–90.

Chapter 36

Ethical and legal issues in paediatric primary care

David Foreman

Summary

Ethical and legal issues determine how practitioners should behave at every step in the processes of assessment, diagnosis, and treatment. A model for routine ethical practice in primary care is proposed, based on three sets of assumptions: (1) that ethical practice is consistent with the four principles of beneficence, non-maleficence, justice, and respect for autonomy; (2) ethical concerns lead to legal processes, whose task is to ensure ethical practice; and (3) that we are working in the interests of our patients. Current relevant literature was organized in terms of this model, and recommendations for practice derived from it. Though there is no general ethical problem in providing routine primary care to children, ethical difficulties surround some special cases, especially when working in conjunction with other agencies or coping with non-medical frameworks. Particular care needs to be taken with confidentiality and consent, the limits of which are currently confused. The model worked well with everyday ethical problems, though more difficult cases require careful individual scrutiny.

Introduction

The provision of medical care is more than science or art. When we provide care, our patients expect us to behave ethically towards them, and the state in which we live requires us to practise our skills according to its laws. Medical law and ethics are therefore integral parts of medical practice, with their fair share of problems and pitfalls for the unwary. Children present special legal and ethical problems: they rarely present themselves for care; their ability to make decisions on their own behalf is limited; and we shall see below that the various legal frameworks that involve them are confused and contradictory. Decisions made on behalf of children can also have more profound consequences than those made at any other time in their lives, as their whole life lies before them. However, it is also true that the vast bulk of primary care offered to children does not lead to ethical or legal concern. Theoretically contentious issues, such as capacity for informed consent, are usually efficiently managed by the informal processes of ordinary consultation and examination. This chapter therefore seeks to offer a model for law and ethics that does not routinely require intense ethico-legal cogitation or elaborate procedures that would undermine the comfortable relationships essential to good primary care provision for children. Its goal is instead to alert the practitioner to when something might be amiss, give a simple approach to solving common problems, and indicate when the practitioner should seek more specialist help in resolving the dilemma.

Law and ethics: framework or toolkit?

The dominant metaphor used when thinking about ethics or the law is that of a framework. This metaphor suggests that their purpose is to keep our practice behind legally sanctioned bounds, and our professional duty is to understand where those boundaries lie. While this is all very well, both ethics and law may also be tools for making things happen. We therefore need to consider the various components of the process our patients go through as they are seen and treated by us, and examine the contribution ethics and law make at each stage, if we are to apply them to directly benefit patients, as well as set limits to our own practice.

Building the model

The first assumption: a principled approach

There is much to be said for defining ethical practice in terms of a few, easily digestible principles. Principles simplify coping with multifarious circumstances by abstracting common components from them, allowing one to generalize ethical practice consistently across many different situations. Beauchamp and Childress (1994) have developed four such principles that have proved useful in medical ethics: respect for autonomy; beneficence; non-maleficence; and justice. Respect for autonomy informs debates over issues of consent, competence, and disclosure of professional information. Respect for autonomy is more than an attitude. To show such respect, we must act in such a way that the autonomy of the patient is enabled, and limits to that autonomy are acknowledged: failure to achieve this, even when beneficence is intended, leads to unwarranted paternalism. Beneficence is what we hope to do when we treat someone. It can refer both to actions that do good, or those that prevent harm. Non-maleficence is better known as the maxim 'primum non nocere' (first do no harm). What non-maleficence is really about is distinguishing between effects and side-effects of treatment. It reminds us that the balance of benefit of intended and unintended effects of an intervention should always be positive. Justice is concerned with how people are treated by each other: in particular, justice embodies the idea that equals should be treated equally, and unequals treated unequally. While there are many definitions of justice, Rawls' explication of it as fairness (Rawls 1985) carries a close correspondence to current British health practice and policy (Daniels 1985).

Knowing the principles does not tell one how to use them. Beauchamp and Childress recommend three interrelated techniques, which they call *specification*, *dialectic*, and *balancing*. Specification describes how the principles are related to norms and practical judgements, leading to guidance towards action. Without this, principles become empty formalism, which allows one to justify any action by appeal to a judicious combination of circumstances. Dialectic involves comparing our 'considered judgement' on particular situations with the predictions of ethical theories, seeking to maximize the coherence between them. Balancing refers to the process of assigning different weights to various norms that may conflict with each other, helping one choose an appropriate course of action.

The second assumption: law is applied ethics

In the simplified model I propose here, the role of 'ethical theories' and 'norms' is taken by our current legal framework and guidance, as well as the four principles, while 'practical' and 'considered' judgements are, of course, our professional opinions.

This of course does presume that the ethics and law under consideration share their underlying values, and this may not be so. However, in England it is claimed that (Coleridge 1893), 'It would not be correct to say that every moral obligation involves a legal duty, but every legal duty is founded on a moral obligation.'

So this assumption should be broadly correct for English law, though we shall see below that the assumption occasionally breaks down even here. However, finding that the model has easily recognizable limits provides exactly the kind of warning system the practitioner needs to signal that more careful consideration is required: in particular, practice in a regime where law and medical ethics are in fundamental conflict can have dire ethical consequences (Cocks 1985).

Our legal norms

The medical management of children in primary care lies at the intersection of medical law; children's law; educational law; and criminal law. Whole libraries have been written about each of these. However, organizing their key issues in terms of the four ethical principles just discussed can provide a useful abstraction of the law the practitioner needs in order to apply our ethical principles within our current legal framework. What follows demonstrates this, using English law: an equivalent process can be adopted for other jurisdictions, but the precise cases and statutes considered will vary accordingly.

Medical law

Lord Scarman's famous 'Gillick' judgment (Gillick v West Norfolk and Wisbech Area Health Authority and Another 1986), which confirmed that children had the right to consent for treatment as soon as they were able to comprehend the treatment, its consequences, and come to a balanced decision, seems a direct specification of respect for autonomy. However, it also had a paternalistic function, as a 'flak jacket' for doctors giving treatment to children against the wishes of their parents. Paternalism also underpins the so-called 'retreat from Gillick' (Douglas 1992), which refers to a redefinition of 'Gillick competence' to set impossibly high standards for a child attempting to refuse treatment, so that competence to consent to treatment does not confer competence to refuse it (Re W 1992). Subsequent rulings have confirmed that a child below 18 years has no right to refuse a treatment if a doctor has recommended it, and someone with parental responsibility agrees (re K, W and H 1993). This paternalistic bias is very typical of the law's approach to children in medicine. It is much more apparent in the approach to confidentiality, where the law guarantees confidentiality for children's medical information only if there is no good reason for a professional to override it (Harbour 2001), and there is no clear mechanism by which children may legally access their notes: even though they have a right to do so, an application can only be made by those with parental responsibility (Kennedy and Grubb 2000a). In fact, the legal duty of a doctor to care for a child is owed to the child's parents (or others with parental responsibility) not the child if the child lacks capacity for consent (Kennedy and Grubb 2000b). Consistent with this approach, we find that the concept of a child's 'best interests', usually implicit in medical law, may be used explicitly to bar children's access to their own records (Re L 1997). We can see that medical law balances and specifies the conflict between respect for autonomy and paternalistic beneficence to favour the latter when it comes to children. The degree of this favour has meant that current mental health legislation, which applies to both adults and children, reduces, rather than increases, the doctor's rights to make treatment decisions without consultation or oversight (Paul 2004). There is the possibility that the new Mental Health Act will contain a right for children to refuse treatment, effectively creating a distinction between consenting for treatments directed at physical or mental symptoms that will, curiously, operate in the opposite way to that for adults (Department of Health 2004).

As respect for autonomy can be mapped to 'Gillick competence' and beneficence to medico-legal paternalism, so non-maleficence is addressed by negligence. This is a failure in fulfilling one's duty of care, which leads to harm (Brazier 1992). The traditional criterion, that negligent care falls below that offered by a typical practitioner of equivalent skill (the so-called 'Bolam' test) has now been extended by the requirement that the care offered must also be reasonable (Bolitho v City and Hackney Health Authority 1997). The practical effect of this is to increase the legal force of evidence-based practice and professional guidelines, as it now becomes negligent to ignore these without good reason, even if significant numbers of colleagues are doing likewise.

The medical law relating to the principle of justice focuses largely on the distribution of resources, though it is worth noting that undertaking a medical examination without consent is a potentially criminal offence (battery) (Judge LJ 1998). The NHS has an obligation to provide primary care through the child's general practitioner (National Health Service Act 1977b) that includes child health surveillance (subject to parental request) up to the age of 5 (National Health Service Act 1977b): registration with a GP is on parental request up to 16 years (National Health Service (Choice of Medical Practitioner) Regulations 1998). The only other specific duty the NHS has to children is to provide medical inspection in State and grant-maintained schools (National Health Service Act 1977a). So, community paediatric services are only offered as part of the NHS' general duty of care to all citizens and, however desirable, have no legal guarantee beyond this. NHS 'contracts' to deliver services are no such thing (Allen 1995) and, in particular (Bingham MR 1995), 'Difficult and agonizing judgements have to be made as to how a limited budget is best allocated to the maximum advantage of the maximum number of patients. That is not a judgment which the court can make.'

However, there are circumstances in which the law can intervene to compel provision of a treatment, as we shall see below.

Children's law

Unsurprisingly, beneficence takes pride of place in children's law. This is most apparent in child protection procedures, where ordinary rules of confidentiality may be set aside to allow agencies to work together to protect children (Department of Health *et al.*, 1999). The so-called 'paramountcy' of children's welfare (Children Act 1989d) is more ambiguous than it seems: it only applies to the Courts, when they are making decisions under the Children Act, and does not override other statutory requirements. The paramountcy principle is really about ensuring that children's interests take precedence over their parents', when the two conflict (Brayne *et al.* 2001), and so is more to do with (distributive) justice. The Children Act also pays considerable attention to non-maleficence, the most important example of which is the 'presumption of no order': a Court may only make an Order under the Children Act if it has satisfied itself that it is necessary for the child's welfare—'useful' or 'helpful' is not good enough (Children Act 1989f). Non-maleficence is also shown in the restriction given to the definition of 'welfare' by the 'welfare checklist', which must be met *in addition to* the general requirement that an Order be necessary, before any Order can be made (Children Act 1989b). It can be seen that respect for the child's autonomy is specifically included as the first item on the checklist.

The welfare checklist

1. The ascertainable wishes and feelings of the child, considered in the light of the child's age and understanding.

2. The child's physical, emotional and educational needs.

3. The likely effect on the child of any change in circumstances.

4. The child's age, sex, background and any characteristics of his which the Court considers relevant.

5. Any harm suffered, or risk of harm.

6. The capacity of the relevant adults to meet the child's needs.

7. The range of powers available to the Court under the Act.

For example, a Court may refuse to place a child in the care of a local authority if it does not think the authority will be able to act to improve the child's life.

Justice does not feature greatly in children's law: in some areas, for example in progress in implementing children's rights, we have been failing to meet our international obligations (United Nations 1995). Consistent with this view, children's rights of autonomy are less well protected than in medical law, e.g. children of any age have no right to refuse local authority interventions, nor can their views prevail over their parents' in Children Act matters below the age of 16 (Bainham 2000b). As social workers do not touch their child clients in assessment, the medical 'battery' defence to unwanted assessment does not hold, and more generally, negligence actions against local authorities in relation to children usually fail (Bainham 2000c).

Educational law

In educational law, the principle of beneficence is dominant, with responsibility for delivering an 'efficient' education being shared between state and parent (Bainham 2000d). For most children, respect for their autonomy in education is minimal: not only is it compulsory till 16, but 'efficient' is now defined in terms of the national curriculum (Education Act 1996), which entirely ignores the child's individuality. In contrast, children with special needs should have their choices respected, if not followed (Special Educational Needs and Disability Act 2001b), and have individualized programmes negotiated with them and their parents. However, this individuality is to be interpreted within the context of 'inclusive schooling': the programmes should, as far as possible, be provided within the ordinary school (Department for Education and Skills 2002a), and the exclusion of children from school on grounds of disability is now an illegal discrimination (Special Educational Needs and Disability Act 2001a). So, there is an increasing interest in rights-based justice in educating children, which can also be seen in the incorporation of Articles 12 and 13 of the United Nations Convention of the Rights of the Child into the statutory guidance (Department for Education and Skills 2002b) for children with special needs—the strongest incorporation yet of any part of this Convention into English law. Non-maleficence appears alien to education law. Possibly the only area where it has been effectively applied is in the abolition of corporal punishment, and even here the process took from 1950 to 1999 (Ruff 2002b).

Criminal law

It is unsurprising to discover that the criminal law relating to children is primarily concerned with retributive justice. It is perhaps more surprising to find that children *and their parents* are subject to both punishment and rehabilitation following a child's crime: parents have to attend court if their children are under 16, may be bound over (Criminal Justice Act 1991a), have to attend parenting classes (Crime and Disorder Act 1998b), in addition to making some financial contribution to any state care offered (Criminal Justice Act 1991b). Despite the joint blame applied to the parents, the age of criminal responsibility is set comparatively low, at 10 years (Crime and Disorder Act 1998a). Confidentiality is compromised, with disclosure of information being required if it is either necessary or expedient for the prevention of crime by children (Crime and Disorder Act 1998), though consent for information sharing should be sought if possible, and breaches should be made within a consistent local policy (Youth Justice Board 2004).

However, beneficence remains important and the criminal law also represents a resource for delinquent children. As well as the parenting order referred to above, the Youth Justice Board (Home—Youth Justice Board 2004) has been created specifically to address the problems these youngsters have, as part of the programme to reduce offending. Intervention can begin from when the youngster is no more than 'at risk' of offending, right through the criminal process.

The third assumption: we all work in the best interests of the child

Three things are apparent from this overview. First, that each area of law balances our four principles very differently. There is nothing inherently unethical about this, as each serves different purposes, and addresses different ethical issues. However, life is not lived in legal compartments, so—our second point—ethical difficulties are most likely to arise when more than one area of law, or by extension, relevant agency, becomes involved. Finally, our duty as practitioners requires us to ensure, if we become involved, that what we do may be justified by *our own* ethical and legal principles. This brings us to the final assumption of our model, that all the agencies we engage with, as well as ourselves, are working in the best interests of the child. This assumption sets the standard we must follow when we balance our own law and ethics with those of other professionals, if we are to achieve a good resolution.

Applying the model

Consider what happens when a child attends in primary medical care. Most typically, the child attends with a parent, worried about there being something wrong with the child. The practitioner takes a history, reassures the child as necessary then examines the child, makes some kind of diagnosis or differential, and decides either to offer treatment, further investigations or a referral to secondary care or above. Consent from the parent is implicit in their attendance and that from the child in the process of reassurance regarding the examination. We will of course, follow appropriate guidelines if any are available, and inform both parents and children, to the best of our ability and their understanding, about the reasons behind our advice or actions. Any discomfort is kept to the minimum necessary. In terms of our model, we lie entirely within medical law, and we have seen already that ordinary, reasonable medical practice is all that is needed to meet its criteria. As we would hope, the model suggests that there is nothing ethically or legally wrong with what we routinely try to do.

Defending our principles

Possibly the commonest ethical dilemma practitioners face is when parents, teachers, or others—for convenience, let us call them carers—come demanding that we confirm a diagnosis they have already made about a child, or put pressure on us to support or provide interventions they have decided the child needs. In terms of our model, we are in difficulties because we find ourselves at the intersection of our ethical domain with, at least, one other, whose principles are weighted differently. We must limit our responses to those that we can justify in terms of our own domain; if we do not, we risk ethical or even legal censure. The implication of such a limit can perhaps be best understood in terms of an example. A parent and the Local Education Authority are in disagreement about whether a child needs special schooling. The parent tells you that the education authority has got it wrong, and the child depends on your advice to ensure that the right educational provision is made. Sat comfortably at a desk, there seems to be no problem: 'state our view honestly, from our own professional perspective' seems obvious advice. However, we may know that the Local Education Authority has a poor record in recognizing such cases; or a particular school manages particularly well with that kind of problem, while the Local Educational Authority uses a school that manages the problem less well. In cases like this we feel that 'doing our professional duty' may not be doing the best for our patients. Despite the clear temptation, exaggerating or distorting our opinion 'in the patient's interests' is wrong and professionally dangerous. Being dishonest (which is what this is) may be Serious Professional Misconduct (General Medical Council 2001) and undermines the value of any future opinion we may give. However, the processes of specification, balancing and dialectic give us an alternative approach. We have seen above that education's ethical domain is insensitive to the principle of non-maleficence, i.e. the balance of benefit and harm an intervention might produce, and approaches issues of justice (fairness) very much from a 'rights' perspective. Within our own domain, our concern to achieve the best placement is ethically one of non-maleficence rather than beneficence: we are choosing the 'treatment' (placement) that has the best balance of benefits and risks for the child. We must re-specify our concerns in terms of rights, e.g. by indicating the likely prognosis, and detail the interventions that will be needed to achieve best outcome, implying the child's right to receive such intervention.

Consistent with our model, we find that this approach, though derived from purely ethical principles, is supported by law. The effect of a formal Statement of Special Educational Needs is to spell out each and every special educational need a child has, and how they will be met (Bainham 2000e), which is precisely what our intervention will address. Although Local Education Authorities have considerable latitude in deciding whether a Statement is necessary, their approach must both be reasonable and explicit (Grigson 2000).

Ethical limits to intervention and rationing

Coping with inadequate resources is the other common ethical problem practitioners face. All too often, we know what needs to be done, but the facilities are not available. In many cases, resource constraints underpin the demands we discussed above: what is sought is rationed in some way, and it is believed that we can deliver it. From our model, it follows that practitioners should understand the law governing the limits to intervention, including rationing, in outline, so that we may best represent our patients' interests.

Limiting medical provision

We have already seen above that medical rationing is acceptable in law. However, NHS Trusts do have to allocate their resources with consistency, coherence, and rationality. These questions can be subjected to judicial review. Previous reviews have held that Health Circulars (such as NICE guidelines) are legally binding on managers unless there is good reason to disregard them (R v North Derbyshire HA ex parte Fisher 1997). Secondly, if a treatment is offered the offer must be fulfilled, as it creates a 'legitimate expectation' (R v North and East Devon HA ex parte Coughlan 1999). Thirdly, if a treatment is not resourced, the reasons must both be given and be rational; in particular, the decision needs to be informed by relevant evidence (North West Lancashire HA v A D & G 1999).

Limits to intervention in children's welfare

The ancient principle of 'parens patriae' (Seymour 1994), enacted through what is called the 'inherent jurisdiction' of the High Court to children, allows the state to intervene, ultimately, in any aspect of a child's life (Department of Health 1991). The Children Act 1989 also gives extensive powers. However, duties are vague, so while the Local Authority *may* choose to act, the Children Act gives no guarantee that it will. An important distinction is made between children at risk of significant harm (Children Act 1989e) and those merely in need, defined as being at risk of not maintaining, or be impaired in attaining a reasonable standard of health or development, or be disabled (Children Act 1989c). The former group of children are managed via child protection procedures are discussed elsewhere. However, the standard of proof required, as well as the definition, limits its application. Being civil law, standards of proof under the Children Act are on the 'strong balance of probabilities', i.e. it should be considerably more likely than not that the evidence is true. This is more restrictive than is generally understood, particularly if one is seeking to remedy significant harm by the application of Care or Supervision Orders, to enforce care or supervision by Social Services (Children Act 1989a). The determination of 'significant harm' is a matter of factual proof, so it is not sufficient to claim merely that a child will do better, or even much better, under a care order (Humberside CC v B, 1993). Because harm to children is a rare event, proving that a rare event has a greater than 50% chance of happening in a particular case is demanding (Bainham 2000a). For example, the test case that established this rule held that the siblings of a child who was probably abused by the mother's cohabitee, but where a prosecution for rape had failed, could not be made subject to care orders as the standard of proof had not been met (H and R 1996). For children who are merely 'in need', specific (and so specifiable) duties are hard to find. However, Section 2 of the Chronically Sick and Disabled Persons act 1970 entitles a disabled child to help in six areas if an assessment confirms such help is needed: (a) practical assistance in the home; (b) the provision of recreational equipment, e.g. TV, radio, or personal computer; (c) provisional of recreational facilities, e.g. day centres; (d) provision of educational facilities even if they are outside local provision; (e) travel and other assistance; (f) home adaptations and disabled facilities. These are duties, not powers of provision, so may be insisted on if the child meets the Act's criteria.

Limits to educational provision

The duties of the Local Education Authority in relation to a Statement of Special Educational Needs have already been dealt with above. The definition of Special Educational Needs is very wide, including behavioural or physical problems if they impinge on the child's ability to receive education, as well as the more obvious learning difficulties (Ruff 2002a). However, the identification of Special Educational Needs and even the issuing of a proposed Statement confers no right for a Statement to be confirmed (R v Isle of Wight CC ex parte RS and ex parte AS 1993) though there are considerable rights of appeal for parents, if not the children themselves (Bainham 2000e). The Local Authority is explicitly required to consider efficient use of resources when it makes its provision, balancing resource issues against the other requirements identified. However, resource limitations cannot be used as a reason for failing to meet an educational need, though they can be part of the reason for choosing between different resources (Collins 1997).

Applying the limits

In using this information, the practitioner should not try to be a lawyer, deploying the legislation, case law and judgments just quoted as a means of obtaining resources. That requires a wholly different training! Instead, I would recommend specifying principles in relation to the problem as just described in the example, and seeing which specifications fit which limits. Choosing the specification that best fits our purposes is an example of *balancing*. Often, as our example shows, the difference between effective and ineffective action to obtain resources for our patients depends on how we specify the requirement, and to whom. It must fit the duties, not merely the powers, of the agency that owns and rations the resource we seek. Negotiating this with the relevant agency is of course the last element of the process of applying our principles: *dialectic*.

At the model's limits

The model struggles to address two areas: confidentiality and the limits of child's or family's rights of consent.

Confidentiality presents problems because GMC guidance may in some cases be at variance with case law, making balancing ultimately impossible (W v Edgell 1990). In general terms disclosure of information without consent may take place if there are concerns about child protection, lawbreaking, or harm to others, and there is also 'catch-all' guidance that covers most situations where professionals need to communicate for the good of the child. However, doubts about disclosure should encourage practitioners to seek advice from a specialist, e.g. a defence organization.

As we have seen above, setting the limits for children's consent for treatment, especially mental health treatment, is in chaos. While the decision to overrule a child's views is always difficult, overruling a family is more so, and can lead to heartbreaking results (Alderson and Montgomery 1996). Once the practitioner faces more then grumbling acquiescence, the decision to force treatment upon a competent child should be taken by practitioners trained in the Mental Health Act, and opposing a family's wishes should be discussed with other agencies, especially Social Services, as a matter to be set before the Courts. Though the model may still be helpful in framing the ethical dilemmas involved, it will probably be unable to distinguish between several, mutually incompatible solutions, without additional reflection on the case's specifics. As different solutions will be preferred by different agencies, depending on their remit, practitioners will need to ensure that whatever is decided is consistent with their own professional ethics and practice.

Conclusions

Ethical difficulties are not routine in the management of children in primary care. In cases that involve several services, civil or criminal law, demands might be placed on practitioners that conflict with good medical practice, so being clear about one's ethical principles and legal guidance is essential. The model for ethical practice set out above can help with more common dilemmas, but practitioners should seek advice in the most difficult cases.

References

Alderson P, Montgomery J (1996). *Health Care Choices: Making decisions about children*, Institute for Public Policy Research, London.

Allen P (1995). *Medical Law Review* **51**: 321.

Bainham A (2000a). *Children: The Modern Law*, Family Law, Bristol, pp. 378–379.

Bainham A (2000b). *Children: The Modern Law*, Family Law, Bristol, pp. 341–342.

Bainham A (2000c). *Children: The Modern Law*, Family Law, Bristol, pp. 355–359.

Bainham A (2000d). *Children: The Modern Law*, Family Law, Bristol, pp. 538–541.

Bainham A (2000e). *Children: The Modern Law*, Family Law, Bristol p. 567.

Beauchamp TL, Childress JF (1994). Priniciples of Biomedical Ethics. Oxford University Press, Oxford.

Bingham MR R v Cambridge Health Authority ex parte B (1995). BMLR 23 1 CA.

Bolitho v City and Hackney Health Authority (1997). *All ER(HL)*, (4) p771.

Brayne H, Martin G, Carr H (2001). Oxford University Press, Oxford, pp. 67, 85.

Brazier M (1992). *Medicine, Patients and the Law*, London: Penguin Law p. 112.

Children Act (1989a). 31(2).

Children Act (1989b). s 1(3).

Children Act (1989c). s17.

Children Act (1989d). s1.

Children Act (1989e). s47.

Children Act (1989f).

Cocks G (1985). *Psychotherapy in the Third Reich*. Oxford University Press, New York.

Coleridge L. *Regina v Instam* (1893). QB 1 453.

Collins, J. R v Hillingdon London Borough ex parte Governing Body of Queensmead School, (1997). ELR 331.

Crime and Disorder Act (1998). s 115.

Crime and Disorder Act (1998a). s 34.

Crime and Disorder Act (1998b). ss 8–10.

Criminal Justice Act (1991a). s 56.

Criminal Justice Act (1991b). s 58(2) & (3).

Daniels N (1985). *Just Health Care*. Cambridge University Press, New York.

Department for Education and Skills (2002a). Special Educational Department for Education and Skills, London Needs Code of Practice.

Department for Education and Skills (2002b). *Special Educational Needs Code of Practice*. Department for Education and Skills, London, p. 27.

Department of Health (1991). *The Children Act 1989 Guidance and Regulations*, pp. 42–43.

Department of Health (2004). *Improving Mental Health Law: Towards a new Mental Health Act*. Department of Health.

Department of Health, Home Office and Department for Education and Employment (1999). *Working Together to Safeguard Children*, HMSO, London.

Douglas G (1992). The retreat from Gillick. *Medical Law Review* **55**: 569–576.

Education Act (1996). s 357.

General Medical Council (2001). GMC, London.

Gillick v West Norfolk and Wisbech Area Health Authority and Another (1986). *FLR(HL)*, 1 p224.

Grigson, J. H v Kent County Council and SENT, (2000). ELR 660.

H and R (1996). FLR 1 80.

Harbour A (2001). The limits of confidentiality: a legal view Cordess, C (ed.). *Confidentiality and Mental Health*. Jessica Kingsley, London, pp. 151–157.

Home—Youth Justice Board (2004). http://www.youth-justice-board.gov.uk/YouthJusticeBoard/

Humberside CC v B, (1993). FLR 1 257.

Judge LJ, St George's Healthcare NHS Trust v S (1998). All ER 3 673 CA.

Kennedy I, Grubb A (2000a). *Medical Law*. Butterworths, London, pp. 1028–1031.

Kennedy I, Grubb A (2000b). *Medical Law*. Butterworths, London, p. 281.

National Health Service (Choice of Medical Practitioner) Regulations (1998). Regulation 2(3)(a).

National Health Service Act (1977a). 5(1)(a).

National Health Service Act (1977b). Part II 29–34.

North West Lancashire HA v A D & G (1999). *Lloyd's Rep Med(CA)*, p399.

Paul M (2004). Decision-making about children's mental health care: ethical challenges. *Advances in Psychiatric Treatment* **10**: 310–311.

R v Isle of Wight CC ex parte RS and ex parte AS (1993). *FLR(CA)*, 1 p634.

R v North and East Devon HA ex parte Coughlan (1999). *Lloyd's Rep Med(CA)*, p306.

R v North Derbyshire HA ex parte Fisher (1997). *Med LR(QBD)*, 8 p327.

Rawls J (1985). *A Theory of Justice*. Oxford University Press, Oxford.

re K, W and H (1993). FLR 1 854.

Re L (1997). *AC(HL)*, p16.

Re W (1992). *WLR*, 3 p358.

Ruff A (2002a). *Education Law: text, cases and materials*. Butterworths, London pp. 318–325.

Ruff A (2002b). *Education Law: text, cases and materials*. Butterworths, London pp. 277–284.

Seymour J (1994). Parens Patrice and Wardship Powers: their nature and origins. *Oxford Journal of Legal Studies* **14**: 159–188.

Special Educational Needs and Disability Act (2001a). Part 2.

Special Educational Needs and Disability Act (2001b).

United Nations (1995). United Nations, Geneva.

W v Edgell (1990). *All ER*, 1 p835.

Youth Justice Board (2004). *Guidance for Youth Offending Teams on Information Sharing*. Youth Justice Board. London. Document Number B47.

Chapter 37

The impact of bereavement on children and young people's welfare and development

Daniel Kelly

Give sorrow words: the grief that does not speak
Whispers the o'er fraught heart and bids it break.

Shakespeare, Macbeth (VII, ii)

Introduction

Helping children and families to cope with the impact of loss and bereavement is the focus of this chapter. There are particular issues for professionals to consider when seeking to support a child or family who are experiencing the threat or actuality of grief. Grief is usually taken to mean the feelings and behaviours that are evoked in response to death. These may include sadness, numbness, anger, sleep disturbances, inability to concentrate, and fatigue (Hanus 1995). In children specific behaviours may be expected depending on age, personality, and life circumstances—as well as the nature of the relationship they had developed with the dead person. The chapter will examine some of these issues by presenting childhood and young adulthood as dynamic (rather than fixed) stages in the human life course. Viewing the situation in this way allows us to provide support in a way that is most appropriate and meaningful to the child, and the family, involved. As childhood is shaped by social, cultural, psychological, and physical factors it is also important to emphasize the individual impact of loss and grief. No two families are the same, and blanket advice should be treated with caution. However, it is possible to draw on experience, as well as some empirical findings, to suggest some ways of supporting children who find themselves having to cope with the loss of a parent, sibling, friend or relative.

The nature of childhood

An ancient Chinese proverb suggests: 'A child's life is like a piece of paper on which every passerby leaves a mark.' This can be seen as a cautionary, if somewhat daunting, reminder for professionals who may feel personally unprepared when confronted with a situation where a child or family is facing bereavement or loss. It is easy to feel overwhelmed by the emotions that such a situation may evoke. Saying the wrong thing is easy and it may feel safer to say as little as possible. This is not a situation restricted to situations involving children, however. Isabel Menzies Lyth, who carried out research in hospitals in the early 1960s described ways that nurses caring for seriously ill patients would focus on routines and organizational procedures to protect them from engaging with patient's emotions directly (Menzies Lyth 1988). However, researchers who have worked with children with cancer have shown that even from a very young age they may learn how to read non-verbal cues about their situation very effectively. Bluebond-Langner (1978), for example, carried out a longitudinal ethnographic study on a children's cancer unit and described the way that children gradually learned to associate particular procedures (such as lumber punctures) with advancing disease, treatment failure, and an increased likelihood of dying from their disease.

What this suggests is that children (especially those living with a chronic illness themselves or who have experienced a sibling or parent undergoing treatment) can become very tuned in to the way that those around them react and talk, or avoid talking, about certain topics. Clearly this will depend on the age of the child and their level of cognitive or emotional maturity. However, it is important to emphasize that children and young people can develop wisdom beyond their years when exposed to situations involving serious illness or death (Kelly and Edwards 2005). What we say in such situations then, may be less important, than simply acknowledging the difficult feelings of those involved.

This introduction is intended to balance the somewhat rigid nature of developmental theories that normally underpin discussions about children's understanding of death, loss, or bereavement. The inherent value of the developmental approach to child psychology lies in its application to practice—especially when professionals need help to understand the world of the child or young person in their care.

One of the most influential theorists of childhood psychology was Piaget who suggested that children gradually understand the world around them by assimilating information as a result of enhanced cognitive skills. This theory rests on the belief that all children can be expected to pass through similar developmental stages at about the same age. The developmental approach to cognition proposed by Piaget involves the following:

- *The sensory-motor stage*, 0–2 years, is characterized by a gradual awareness that the self is separate from the world. Learning occurs mainly via the senses and explains the importance of touch, taste, and smell for infants. Babies of about 1 year will begin to explore for hidden objects and accept their existence even though they are out of sight.

- *The pre-operational stage*, 2–7 years, is focused on learning about the social and physical world. Learning can be both experiential as well as directed by others such as teachers and parents. Imaginative play is common, as well as language development and symbolic thinking. Associations may be made between actions and consequences—importantly, these associations may be incorrect, such as 'My mum is ill because I was naughty'. Usually there is limited ability to attend to multiple aspects of the same situation.

- *The concrete operational stage*, 7–12 years, demonstrates increasing evidence of logical thinking. Unlike the previous stage attention may be directed to multiple aspects of situations. The egocentrism of earlier stages also diminishes and other people's perspectives may assume more importance. There is a tendency for greater understanding of situations and objects in the world rather than appreciation of unknown experiences or possibilities.

◆ *The formal operational stage*, 12 years and over, emphasizes an emerging ability for more abstract or hypothetical thinking. Objects need not be present to be understood. Multiple sources of information may be accessed and personal opinions formed. Peer group belonging assumes greater importance.

Piaget's theories have been criticized for failing to take account of a child's individual life experiences. While acknowledging the limitations of such theoretical constructions of child development it is also important to acknowledge that they have helped to increase understanding and respect for children. Other theorists who have contributed to this debate include influential names such as Freud, Erikson, and Kohlberg (Thompson 2001). What each has contributed, in different ways, are ways of understanding the ever-changing essence of childhood and the numerous pressures that families experience—even in 'normal' situations. When considering the additional burden of bereavement, therefore, it is important to match supportive interventions with the child's stage of life and anticipated level of cognitive and emotional development.

Children's understanding of death and loss

Most studies suggest that it is difficult for children less than 2 years to understand fully the meaning of death and dying. Their reaction may be similar to those provoked by separation anxiety—including tearfulness, irritability, and searching for familiar objects or people (Thompson 2001). Between the ages of 2 and 6 years children are thought to have little knowledge or experience of death and may view it as reversible—normally being associated with separation, sleep, and loss of movement. This level of understanding may arise from witnessing the death of plants or animals. However, such children may not be able to separate fantasy from fact, e.g. 'I shot you dead, now get up and play.' After the age of 7 it is thought that children may have a more complete understanding of the finality of death. However, this may also be a time when dangerous or risk taking behaviours dominate—'It will never happen to me!' This group often may switch between denial and depression in situations where anticipated grief (for themselves or others) may be involved.

Empirical studies also confirm that younger children's perceptions of death are closely associated with cognitive development. Reilly *et al.* (1983) found that increasing age was associated with a greater level of insight about the nature of death when children were questioned. All the children taking part were between 5 and 10 years and the majority was able to express some awareness of personal mortality.

Weakness within 'broad stroke' theories of child development, such as Piaget's, become particularly apparent when considering the work of researchers such as Bluebond-Langer (1978). This suggests that children's perception of illness and death is shaped as much by the circumstances around them as their chronological age or expected level of cognitive maturity. This finding may surprise professionals who prefer to believe that children can never understand fully when negative things are happening to, or around, them. Whatever level of understanding children may have about death and dying there is a need to provide a caring and supportive response to the emotional impact of the loss involved.

The nature of loss in childhood

It is tempting to assume that physical development alone provides a measure of the level of emotional maturity achieved by a child. However, this is not always the case as has been emphasized previously (Bluebond-Langer 1978). Developmental theories may provide professionals with a useful benchmark against which the impact of disruptive emotionally challenging events (such as death of a sibling, parent, or grandparent) can be assessed; however, allowances should always be made for individual circumstances. Children who have to cope with situations involving bereavement may require psycho-logical support tailored specifically to their age group—help that can then be refined in response to their unique life circumstances (see useful contacts at the end of this chapter).

Thompson (2001) provides an example from practice of a 5-year-old child with cancer who one day lined his toys up in two groups on the bed. One group was to be taken back to the hospital and the other to 'go with him when he died.' She discusses how this child had also developed insight into the way that his parents avoided discussing the topic of death, and how the child had learned to avoid asking questions about his own situation. This may not be so far removed from the way that some adults also learn to cope with serious illnesses such as cancer. Emerging from this consideration of cognitive and emotional development is awareness that children are social beings who are constantly developing and reaffirming strong emotional attachments and relationships with the world that exists around them. When this world is changed by the death of a key figure the consequences are far reaching indeed.

Freud is among those who have emphasized the importance of these early relation-ships in shaping the adult personality. Key attachment figures in the child's world—especially the mother and father—exert a powerful influence on the way they learn to relate to other authority figures in adulthood. Other human attributes such as trust, intimacy, and responsibility may also be shaped by these early human relationships. Disruptions to formative emotional relationships, as a result of the death of a parent for instance, may have a profound effect on the way a child will view the world around them in adulthood. By feeling abandoned as a result of sudden death, for example, a child less than 10 may blame themselves for this event and gradually internalize their intense feelings of guilt: 'Perhaps of I had been better at school my dad wouldn't have died ...'.

Bereavement may also impact powerfully on the relationships between surviving members of the family. The death of a parent in childhood can mean that one of the surviving children may gradually assume the role or responsibilities of the lost parent. This may demand responsibilities beyond their years—such as caring for younger siblings while the other parent returns to work. When seen in this light the welfare of children can be effected in multiple ways long after the death itself has passed.

The impact of bereavement and loss on young people

A recent report by Ribbens-McCarthy and Jessop (2005) for the Joseph Rowntree Foundation has suggested that bereavement is a common and sometime life-defining experience for many young people. As many as 92% of young people in the UK will experience what they define as a 'significant' bereavement before the age of 16. Between 4 and 7% will lose a parent. However, there is actually very little empirical research evidence about the impact of bereavement at such a vulnerable time.

Research studies that do exist, such as Pfeffer *et al.* (2000), have compared the psychological morbidity in children whose parents died of cancer (an anticipated death) versus children whose parents died as a result of suicide (an unexpected death). Children in both groups reported normative levels of depressive symptoms; however, those children whose parents had died as a result of suicide demonstrated significantly more depressive symptoms including negative mood, interpersonal problems, general feelings of ineffectiveness, and lack of self-gratifying behaviours.

The Rowntree study (Ribbens McCarthy and Jessop 2005) found that UK mortality rates vary strongly by geography and social class—those children and young people living in disadvantaged circumstances are more likely to experience serious and multiple bereavements. This has obvious importance for public health professionals working in areas where multiple demands are already placed on the services available. Importantly, the Rowntree report also emphasizes that most research has concentrated on the impact of parental and sibling deaths—largely ignoring the loss of peers. For older children or young adults such deaths may be highly significant as they reflect the emphasis on strong peer group attachments associated with this particular stage of cognitive development.

Empirical understandings of the impact of bereavement on children and young people need to be gathered on a longitudinal basis if they are to be meaningful. The above report found that many bereaved young people had never spoken with anybody about their feelings. Counselling provision appears to be patchy at present across the UK and multiple demands are already being put on those services that are available. The Rowntree report calls for a range of bereavement services ranging from those providing basic information to in-depth individual therapy. Children and young people most at risk of enduring adverse effects of bereavement (particularly those who have experienced significant bereavement early in life or those living in disadvantaged circumstances) should be the focus of particular attention by service providers. As one of the young people in the Rowntree study said: 'I just cant get over my mother's death at times ... when it's really hard it's like losing part of yourself ... it's like learning to walk again ... Maybe the rest of them are just coping with it or looking as if they're coping with it but I'm not. There's times when I really don't cope at all.'

Specific management strategies for responding to bereavement and loss in childhood

Specific guidelines have recently been produced for use by primary care professionals on the management of bereavement in children and adolescents (National Library for Health 2005). The advice is divided into a number of sections including the presentation and assessment of grief reactions, advice for carers, and families on coping with bereavement and the possible role of medication (Black 2002).

The guidelines suggest that children may be expected, and should be allowed, to express their feelings of grief indirectly through play and social interaction. Behaviours may include believing that the dead parent will return—as well as seeming angry or appearing indifferent to others around them. Children can be expected to take part in mourning rituals (although no age-specific guidance is offered about this suggestion) but may need encouragement to do so. If the death was traumatic, post-traumatic stress symptoms may interfere with the normal grieving process.

It is also suggested that children less than 4 years will be unlikely to understand their parents' disappearance and, as suggested above, may associate this with their own 'bad behaviour.' Children experiencing bereavement will almost always display somatic symptoms; such as sleeping or eating problems, headache, abdominal pain, or oppositional or withdrawn behaviour. More generally separation anxiety as the result of a lost parent may lead to school refusal. Signs of neglect in children should also be noted as this may suggest symptoms of an enduring grief response in the surviving parent.

Specific advice for carers or families who experience bereavement include the need for awareness about the increased risk of depressive or anxiety-related disorders as bereaved children grow up. Multiple losses, such as moving home or changing carers frequently should be avoided in children who have recently been bereaved, as well as encouraging contact with previous attachment figures whenever possible. It is suggested that children over 5 may benefit from seeing the dead parent to 'appreciate the non-functionality of death.' However, it is not recommended that they view mutilated or unrecognizable bodies. Resources for children or families may be accessed from agencies such as Cruse Bereavement Care. For those who are in particular difficulty it is suggested that family therapy may assist in improving a child's psychosocial functioning following bereavement. The local Child and Adolescent Mental Health Service or other agencies may be able to arrange suitable referral (see other suggested agencies at the end of this chapter).

General management principles include the need for open reassurance that the child will be taken care of when they experience the death of a parent. Explanations should be offered as openly and honestly as possible. Younger children's 'distorted thinking' (such as blaming themselves for the death) should also be anticipated and gently challenged. Encouraging children and families to share memories of the dead person, or to start some kind of 'memory box', as well as attending the funeral, are also suggested as helpful strategies. Normal routines, such as nursery or school, should be maintained as far as possible (ensuring that the teachers are made aware of what has happened).

Reactions at the anniversary of a death should be anticipated as this is a particularly difficult time. Everyone involved is likely to have an emotional response and the child's reactions and needs should be observed closely at this time. Formal counselling or therapy may be required for those children or families who do not seem to be coping (Wiener and Sher 2002). Charitable agencies (such as the UK Charity Winston's Wish) can offer practical support in the form of groups or holiday camps for bereaved children.

Post-traumatic stress disorder should be anticipated if the death was violent, with cognitive behavioural therapy suggested as particularly helpful for dealing with ongoing and disruptive symptoms of grief. Worden and Silverman (1996) have suggested that many of the behavioural problems associated with bereavement can be expected to develop 2 years after the event. Professionals seeking to support children or young people should be aware of the long-term nature of support that may be needed.

Conclusions

This chapter has focused on the impact of bereavement on children and young people. By reviewing the needs of children at different ages it has been suggested that supportive interventions need to take account of their cognitive and emotional maturity—as well as the unique circumstances facing the child or family. While providing effective and timely support for the bereaved (whether adult or child) may seem to be a low priority in the demanding culture of primary or secondary healthcare, failure to address the issue may simply lead to significant problems at a later date. Bereavement support for children and young people undoubtedly is a complex and challenging issue for healthcare providers. This may explain why it has not received more attention to date.

Those bereavement support services that are available within the statutory and voluntary sectors need to be used wisely for those children and young people most at risk. There is also a need for increased the training available to professionals to help them assess and support children who have encountered the death of a significant figure in their life. This is important for professionals who encounter bereaved children and young people in both the education and health sectors (Thomas 1997).

The final message in this chapter concerns the outcomes of bereavement and the potential benefit for the adult that the child will become. Bereavement forces children to confront emotions that are normally only experienced later in life. However, with support it is still possible for the bereaved child to grow towards emotional maturity. In Freud's words maturity is merely the capacity to 'love and work.' Briggs (2002) adds to this the capacity to weigh up risks in life and to bear the consequent anxieties. Through a process of effective care the bereaved child can develop an enhanced ability to confront life's experiences and to make sense and cope with them. In this sense, adulthood, with its own uncertainties and losses, is merely a mirror of what bereaved young people have already endured. If so, their experience has relevance for us all.

Useful contacts and addresses

- BACP (British Association for Counselling and Psychotherapy) 0870 443 5252. www.counselling.co.uk (Advises on sources of individual and family therapy in the UK.)

- Child Bereavement Trust 01494 446 648. www.childbereavement.org.uk (Offers training for counselling bereaved children and where to obtain advice and help in the UK. The website has advice sheets for parents and young people.)

- Child Bereavement Network 0115 911 8070. www.ncb.org.uk/cbn/index.htm (Online directory of specialist bereavement support services in the UK.)

- Cruse Bereavement Care 0208 939 9530. Youthline 0808 808 1677. www.crusebereavmentcare.org.uk (Offers support, training, and direct telephone help to children and young people (12–18 years).)

- SAMM (Support after Murder and Manslaughter) 0207 735 3838. www.samm.org.uk (Offers a helpline and publications.)

- SOBS (Survivors of Bereavement by Suicide) 0870 241 3337. www.uk-sobs.org.uk (Offers emotional and practical support to those affected by suicide.)

- Winston's Wish 0845 203 0405. www.winstonswish.org.uk (Organization supporting bereaved children and young people, and anyone concerned about a child following bereavement.)

References

Black D (2002). Bereavement. In Rutter M, Taylor E (eds), *Child and Adolescent Psychiatry*. Blackwell Science, Oxford. 229–308.

Bluebond-Langner M (1978). *The Private Worlds of Dying Children*. Princetown University Press, Princetown, New Jersey.

Briggs S (2002). *Working with Adolescents*. Palgrave, Basingstoke.

Hanus M (1995). Grief in children. *European Journal of Palliative Care* 2: 73.

Kelly D, Edwards J (2005). Palliative care for adolescents and young adults. In Faull C, Carter Y, Daniels L (eds), *Handbook of Palliative Care*. Blackwell Publishing, Oxford. 317–331

Menzies Lyth I (1988). The functioning of social systems as a defence against anxiety. In Menzies Lyth I (ed.), *Containing Anxiety in Institutions: Selected Essays*. Free Association Books, London. 43–85.

National Library for Health (2005). *Primary Care Guidelines on Bereavement and Loss in Childhood* (z63.4, Grief reaction). Mental Health Specialist Library. Accessed via www.iop.kcl.ac.uk/who

Pfeffer C, Karus D, Siegel K, Jiang H (2000). Child survivors of parental death from cancer or suicide: depressive and behavioural outcomes. *Psycho-Oncology* 9: 1–10.

Reilly T, Hasazi J, Bond L (1983). Children's conceptions of death and personal mortality. *Journal of Paediatric Psychology* 8: 21–31.

Ribbens McCarthy J, Jessop J (2005). *Young People, Bereavement and Loss: Disruptive Transitions?* The National Children's Bureau, London.

Thomas J (1997). The Child Bereavement Trust: caring for bereaved families. *British Journal of Midwifery* **5**: 474–477.

Thompson J (2001). The Needs of children and adolescents. In Corner J, Bailey C (eds), *Cancer Nursing. Care in Context*. Blackwell, Oxford.

Wiener J, Sher M (2002). *Counselling and Psychotherapy in Primary Health Care*. Palgrave, Basingstoke.

Worden W, Silverman P (1996). Parental death and the adjustment of school-age children. *Omega: Journal of Death and Dying*. **32**: 91–102.

Index